Physical Fitness and Wellness

THIRD EDITION

Changing the Way You Look, Feel, and Perform

Jerrold S. Greenberg, EdD
University of Maryland

George B. Dintiman, EdD
Virginia Commonwealth University

Barbee Myers Oakes, PhD
Wake Forest University

Human Kinetics

Library of Congress Cataloging-in-Publication Data

Greenberg, Jerrold S.
    Physical fitness and wellness: changing the way you look, feel, and
perform / Jerrold S. Greenberg, George B. Dintiman, Barbee Myers
Oakes.-- 3rd ed.
            p. cm.
Includes bibliographical references and index.
    ISBN 0-7360-4696-8 (Soft Cover)
  1.Physical fitness. 2. Health. 3. Exercise. I. Dintiman, George B.
II. Myers Oakes, Barbee. III. Title.
    RA781.G799 2004
    613.7--dc22

                                        2003020642

ISBN: 0-7360-4696-8

This book was previously published in 1998 and 1995 by Pearson Education, Inc.

The Web addresses cited in this text were current as of June 10, 2003, unless otherwise noted.

Acquisitions Editor: Bonnie Pettifor; **Developmental Editor:** Myles Schrag; **Assistant Editor:** Ragen E. Sanner; **Copyeditor:** Bob Replinger; **Proofreader:** Erin Cler; **Indexer:** Pamela Homiak; **Permission Manager:** Dalene Reeder; **Graphic Designer:** Robert Reuther; **Graphic Artist:** Dawn Sills; **Photo Managers:** Kelly Huff, Kareema McClendon; **Cover Designer:** Andrea Souflée; **Photographer (cover):** PhotoDisc Royalty-Free CD; **Photographer (interior):** ©Human Kinetics, unless otherwise noted; **Art Manager:** Kelly Hendren; **Illustrator:** Mic Greenberg; **Printer:** Custom Color Graphics

We thank Parkland College Department of Athletics in Champaign, Illinois, for assistance in providing the location for the photo shoot for this book.

Printed in the United States of America

10 9 8 7 6 5 4 3 2 1

Human Kinetics
Web site: www.HumanKinetics.com

United States: Human Kinetics
P.O. Box 5076
Champaign, IL 61825-5076
800-747-4457
e-mail: humank@hkusa.com

Canada: Human Kinetics
475 Devonshire Road Unit 100
Windsor, ON N8Y 2L5
800-465-7301 (in Canada only)
e-mail: orders@hkcanada.com

Europe: Human Kinetics
107 Bradford Road
Stanningley
Leeds LS28 6AT, United Kingdom
+44 (0) 113 255 5665
e-mail: hk@hkeurope.com

Australia: Human Kinetics
57A Price Avenue
Lower Mitcham, South Australia 5062
08 8277 1555
e-mail: liaw@hkaustralia.com

New Zealand: Human Kinetics
Division of Sports Distributors NZ Ltd.
P.O. Box 300 226 Albany
North Shore City
Auckland
0064 9 448 1207
e-mail: blairc@hknewz.com

This book is dedicated to a trio of amazing women, a trio who maintained physically active lifestyles well into their 80s. The first of these women is the mother of one of the authors, the second is the mother-in-law of another of the authors, and the third is a grandmother of still another of the authors. Bess Greenberg, at age 85, walks, participates in aqua exercises, and does yoga on a regular basis. Carolyn Batson, 87, walks and swims four to five times a week. And Lady Byrd Anderson Phillips walked nearly a mile every day of her life until she died at age 83. What more appropriate dedication for this book than to these three marvelous specimens of fitness and wellness. We are indeed blessed to have known and been influenced by these remarkable women.

Contents

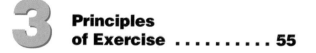

15 Designing a Program of Lifetime Fitness ... 399

16 Beyond Fitness: Becoming an Elite Performer 433

Preface

The usual bunch of guys gathered on a beautiful sunny morning for the regular Sunday pickup basketball games. About 20 men usually attended, ranging in age from 25 to 57. But this Sunday was different. You see, on this Sunday, Larry died.

Larry was physically active only on Sundays with the "boys." He played this particular day with a great deal of hustle and resolve, panting and sweating profusely. The vigorous competition was too much for his heart and, at the end of one of the games, Larry felt a pain in his chest and collapsed. Although one of the players was a physician, he could do nothing to revive Larry. In the aftermath of that Sunday morning, one of your authors resolved to write a book to help others—students, family, other readers—learn to exercise regularly and healthfully. This is that book.

Why This Book?

Given the numerous books on physical fitness, one might reasonably ask, "Why another?" The answer to this question lies within this book's unique features. We were frustrated in our attempts to find a fitness textbook that responded to the diversity of readers one might expect to be interested in reading such a book. Given the concern, we made sure to incorporate all the usual fitness content, but we did it in a way that was sensitive and appreciative of the diversity of readers.

Certainly, we discuss topics that one might expect a book on physical fitness to discuss. The book includes chapters on principles of exercise, cardiovascular fitness, weight training and body shaping, flexibility training, and the like. In other words, we present an array of valid information about physical fitness in this book, sufficient for you to become physically fit or maintain your state of fitness if it is now adequate.

Approach

We have recognized, however, that physical fitness is but one component of wellness, and not an isolated one. Therefore, we discuss physical fitness in a larger complex we describe as wellness, which views physical fitness as related to health and well-being. For that reason we also discuss topics such as nutrition, body-fat loss and weight control, stress management, chemicals and physical fitness, heart disease and cancer and other diseases (such as sexually transmitted infections, diabetes, obesity, hypertension, and kidney disease), and the prevention and care of exercise injuries. To be fit without being healthy and well is not to have finished the journey toward a full life.

Unique Features

In addition to these traditional approaches toward the topic of physical fitness, we added information unique to this book. For example, recognizing that researchers have found knowledge of physical fitness insufficient by itself to motivate people to become fit and to maintain adequate lifelong levels of physical fitness, we included a whole chapter called "Behavioral Change and Motivational Techniques." We further describe these well-researched strategies throughout the text in examples of how they might be used to overcome barriers to fitness. Most chapters have a Behavioral Change and Motivational Strategies box that describes obstacles specific to that chapter's content, which can interfere with achieving fitness, and offers behavioral change strategies that people can employ to overcome these obstacles.

We were also exasperated by the misconceptions about fitness that we encountered. Given the popularity of this topic and the legion of fitness gurus who are neither adequately trained nor qualified to teach about physical fitness, misconceptions and inaccurate information are often passed along as valid. For this reason we included a Myth and Fact Sheet box in each chapter. These boxes present general misconceptions related to the content of the chapter and correct these myths with accurate information.

Perhaps the most important unique feature of this book is the weaving of issues of diversity throughout. Many books present diversity as an aside, as we did in the previous edition of this book. This book is so committed to incorporating consideration of ethnicity, race, culture, gender, age, and physical capability as serious components of each chapter's content that every chapter has been studied, critiqued, and edited to ensure sensitivity to a diverse readership. Doing this was possible because one of the authors, although having earned graduate degrees in health and sport science, currently serves as director of multicultural affairs at a major university. This feature directs attention throughout the book to the existence and value of our differences and our similarities. We refrain from grouping everyone into the majority cultural norm, and we recognize our diversity as a strength rather than an interference.

Changes in the Third Edition

Aside from incorporating diversity into the text rather than peripheral information, we have made several other important changes in the third edition. Having the opportunity to revise *Physical Fitness and Wellness: Changing the Way You Look, Feel, and Perform,* we were able to keep the most effective features and rework the others to make this book even better than it previously was. We responded to reviewers' and readers' requests for additional content and revision of existing content. The results include these features:

- Each chapter begins with an Awareness Inventory so that readers can determine up front how much they know about the chapter's content and prepare for it.
- Each chapter also begins with an Analyze Yourself feature so that readers can determine their behavior relative to the chapter's content.
- Gender issues are considered throughout the book rather than isolated in a separate chapter, as we did with women's issues in our previous edition. Throughout each chapter, issues uniquely related to women, as well as those

uniquely related to men, are discussed as they relate to content being presented.

- New and reworked chapters from the previous edition are included in this book. Among these are chapter 7: "Weight Training and Body Shaping"; chapter 8: "Body-Fat Loss and Weight Control"; chapter 9: "Body Image"; and chapter 16: "Beyond Fitness: Becoming an Elite Performer," for readers who wish to go beyond mere physical fitness.
- Besides including end-of-chapter activities in this book, as we did in the previous edition, we have included a service-learning activity relevant to each chapter's content. Service-learning is a pedagogical tool that provides students with an opportunity to use the knowledge and skills they learned in their academic programs to provide service to others. These activities recognize readers' responsibilities to their communities' fitness and wellness.
- Researching of each content area has resulted in extensive additions and expanded currency of references in each chapter. We added approximately 200 new references. The result is a state-of-the-art text that the reader can rely on for the most current and valid information about physical fitness, wellness, and related areas.

Ancillaries

Accompanying this textbook are several electronic ancillaries that will help instructors get the most out of the book's content. An instructor's guide includes a sample class syllabus, evaluation criteria list, and a test bank of 20 test questions per chapter. A presentation package of more than 300 PowerPoint slides is included to help instructors organize book content into class sessions.

Our Goal

We have presented the information needed to engage in a physical fitness program, we have provided techniques that can motivate and encourage continued participation in this program, and we have done so in a manner that recognizes the diversity of our readers. The use of this book to achieve physical fitness, health, and high-level wellness is now up to each reader. We will feel no greater satisfaction than if we succeed in improving the lives of our readers throughout this country by having written this book. Make our day—become physically fit!

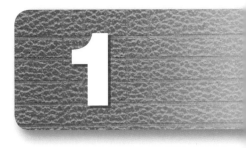

Physical Fitness, Health, and Wellness

Chapter Objectives

By the end of this chapter, you should be able to

1. define and differentiate physical fitness, health, and wellness;
2. describe the benefits of being physically fit; and
3. discuss the relationship between physical fitness and self-esteem.

Inez was an athlete when she was in college. Her basketball team always had a winning record, and she was a major reason they were so good. Still, that was long ago. Today, Inez is in her 50s, and an automobile accident has left her without the use of her legs. But she still participates in sports. She plays wheelchair basketball in her leisure time and coaches a community center soccer team on the weekends. She may not be able to run a mile, but she certainly can shoot foul shots. She may not be able to demonstrate a soccer kick, but she sure can motivate the girls she coaches.

Several years had passed—5 to be exact—since Rodney and I last saw each other. I was look-ing forward to catching up on old times. When I asked the standard, "How have you been?" Rodney replied that he had never felt better. He had taken up jogging and was now running 50 miles a week. He had given up cigarette smoking, become a vegetarian, and had more confidence than ever.

In spite of his reply, I needed further assurance. He looked like death warmed over. His face was gaunt, his body emaciated. His clothes were baggy, creating a sloppy appearance. He had an aura of tiredness about him.

"How's Cynthia?" I asked.

"Fine," Rodney replied. "But we are no longer together. She just couldn't accept the time I devoted to running, and her disregard for her own health was getting on my nerves. She is still somewhat overweight, you know, and I started viewing her differently when I became healthier myself."

You may know an Inez, a Rodney, or someone like them. Are they healthy? This is a complicated question, one that this chapter explores, first by defining physical fitness, health, and wellness and then by differentiating among them.

Physical fitness is defined differently by different people. In this text, we define it as the ability to meet life's demands and still have enough energy to respond to unplanned events. Physical fitness includes five basic components: cardiorespiratory endurance, muscular strength, muscular endurance, flexibility, and body composition. Participation in sports activities that can improve these fitness components often requires certain motor skills. Consequently, motor skills (such as agility, balance, coordination, power, speed, and

> **physical fitness**—The ability to meet life's demands and still have enough energy to respond to unplanned events.

reaction time) are often included in physical fitness programs. One can develop the five basic components of physical fitness without achieving proficiency in the various motor skills. For that reason, someone who is not a natural athlete can still be extremely fit.

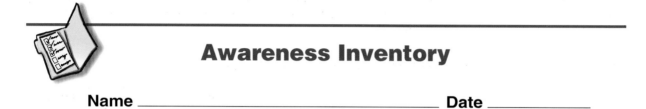

Awareness Inventory

Name _____ **Date** _____

Check the space by the letter T for the statements that you think are true and the space by the letter F for the statements that you think are false. The answers appear following the list of statements. This chapter will present information to clarify these statements for you. As you read the chapter, look for explanations for the reasons why the statements are true or false.

T ___ **F** ___ 1. Physical fitness is composed of four components: cardiorespiratory endurance, muscular strength, muscular endurance, and body composition.

T ___ **F** ___ 2. Cardiorespiratory endurance involves the provision of necessary oxygen to various parts of the body by the lungs and heart.

T ___ **F** ___ 3. The ability of the muscle to contract repeatedly is called muscular strength.

T ___ **F** ___ 4. Lean body mass is the nonfatty component of the body when added to the percent body fat.

T ___ **F** ___ 5. A person who is physically fit is considered healthy.

T ___ **F** ___ 6. Wellness is synonymous with health.

T ___ **F** ___ 7. It is estimated that 50% of the risk for heart disease, stroke, and cancer is a function of unhealthy lifestyles.

T ___ **F** ___ 8. Each decade, the federal government develops national health objectives.

T ___ **F** ___ 9. People who are physically fit may not live longer than those who are not physically fit, but they live with a better quality of life.

T ___ **F** ___ 10. The surgeon general of the United States reported that among the many benefits of physical activity are reductions in feelings of depression and anxiety, and psychological well-being.

Answers: 1-F, 2-T, 3-F, 4-F, 5-F, 6-F, 7-T, 8-T, 9-F, 10-T

From *Physical fitness and wellness, third edition,* by Jerrold S. Greenberg, George B. Dintiman, and Barbee Myers Oakes, 2004, Champaign, IL: Human Kinetics.

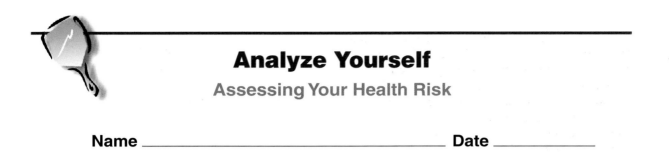

Analyze Yourself

Assessing Your Health Risk

Name _____ **Date** _____

The U.S. government developed this questionnaire to help people assess their health behavior and risk of ill health. Notice that this questionnaire has six sections. Complete one section at a time by circling the number corresponding to the answer that describes your behavior. Then add the numbers you have circled to determine your score for that section. Write your score in the line provided at the end of each section.

Health Assessment Questionnaire

Cigarette Smoking	Almost always	Sometimes	Almost never
1. I avoid smoking cigarettes.	9	4	0
2. I smoke only low-tar and low-nicotine cigarettes, or I smoke a pipe or cigars only.	1	1	0

Your Cigarette Smoking Score: 10

Alcohol and Drugs	Almost always	Sometimes	Almost never
1. I avoid drinking alcoholic beverages, or I drink no more than one or two a day.	4	1	0
2. I avoid using alcohol or other drugs (especially illegal drugs) as a way of handling stressful situations or my problems.	2	1	0
3. I am careful not to drink alcohol when I am taking certain medicines (for example, medicine for sleeping, pain, colds, and allergies).	2	1	0
4. I read and follow the label directions when I use prescribed and over-the-counter drugs.	2	1	0

Your Alcohol and Drugs Score: 10

Eating Habits	Almost always	Sometimes	Almost never
1. I eat a variety of foods each day, such as fruits and vegetables, whole grain breads and cereals, lean meats, dairy products, dry peas and beans, and nuts and seeds.	4	1	0
2. I limit the amount of fat, especially saturated fat, and cholesterol I eat (including fats in meats, eggs, butter, cream, shortenings, and organ meats such as liver).	2	1	0
3. I limit the amount of salt I eat by not adding salt at the table, avoiding salty snacks, and making certain my meals are cooked with only small amounts of salt.	2	1	0
4. I avoid eating too much sugar (especially frequent snacks of sticky candy or soft drinks).	2	1	0

Your Eating Habits Score: 8

(continued)

Analyze Yourself (continued)

Exercise and Fitness	Almost always	Sometimes	Almost never
1. I maintain a desired weight, avoiding overweight and underweight.	3	1	0
2. I do vigorous exercise for 15-30 minutes at least three times a week (examples include running, swimming, and brisk walking).	3	1	0
3. I do exercises that enhance my muscle tone for 15 to 30 minutes at least three times a week (examples include yoga and calisthenics).	2	1	0
4. I use part of my leisure time participating in individual, family, or team activities that increase my level of fitness (such as gardening, bowling, golf, or baseball).	2	1	0
Your Exercise and Fitness Score: _____			

Stress Control	Almost always	Sometimes	Almost never
1. I enjoy the schoolwork or other work I do.	2	1	0
2. I find it easy to relax and express my feelings freely.	2	1	0
3. I recognize early and prepare for events or situations likely to be stressful for me.	2	1	0
4. I have close friends, relatives, or others with whom I can talk about personal matters and call on for help when it is needed.	2	1	0
5. I participate in group activities (such as church/synagogue or community organizations) or hobbies that I enjoy.	2	1	0
Your Stress Control Score: _____			

Safety	Almost always	Sometimes	Almost never
1. I wear a seat belt while I am riding in a car.	2	1	0
2. I avoid driving while I am under the influence of alcohol and other drugs. I also avoid getting in a vehicle with a driver who is under the influence of alcohol or other drugs.	2	1	0
3. I obey the traffic rules and the speed limit when I am driving and ask others to do so when I am a passenger in a vehicle with them.	2	1	0
4. I am careful when I am using potentially harmful products or substances (such as household cleaners, poisons, and electrical devices).	2	1	0
5. I avoid smoking in bed.	2	1	0
Your Safety Score: _____			

(continued)

Analyze Yourself *(continued)*

After you have totaled your score for each of the six sections, circle the number in each column that matches your score for that section of the test.

Health Assessment Scoring Chart

Cigarette smoking	Alcohol and drugs	Eating habits	Exercise and fitness	Stress control	Safety
10	10	10	10	10	10
9	9	9	9	9	9
8	8	8	8	8	8
7	7	7	7	7	7
6	6	6	6	6	6
5	5	5	5	5	5
4	4	4	4	4	4
3	3	3	3	3	3
2	2	2	2	2	2
1	1	1	1	1	1
0	0	0	0	0	0

Source: Roger J. Allen and David Hyde, *Investigations in Stress Control* (Minneapolis: Burgess, 1980), pp. 101-105.

Interpreting Your Score

Scores of 9 or 10 are excellent! Your answers show that you are aware of the importance of this area to your health. More important, you are putting your knowledge to work by practicing good health habits. Even so, you may want to consider areas in which you can improve your health habits.

Scores of 6 to 8 indicate that your health practices in this area are good but that you have room for improvement. Look again at the items you answered with "sometimes" or "almost never." What changes can you make to improve your score?

Scores of 3 to 5 mean that your health risks are showing. You should ask your instructor for more information about the health risks you are facing. Your instructor will probably be able to help you decrease those risks.

Scores of 0 to 2 for all sections mean that you may be taking serious, unnecessary risks with your health. Maybe you are not aware of the risks and what to do about them. Consult with a health expert or your instructor to improve your health.

From U.S. Department of Health and Human Services, 1981, *Health Style: A self test* (Washington D.C.: U.S. Department of Health and Human Services).

From *Physical fitness and wellness, third edition*, by Jerrold S. Greenberg, George B. Dintiman, and Barbee Myers Oakes, 2004, Champaign, IL: Human Kinetics.

Components of Physical Fitness

Elsewhere in this book we will discuss developing the five basic components of physical fitness. First, however, we will define these components.

Cardiorespiratory Endurance

Engaging in physical activity, even breathing, requires oxygen. Without oxygen, you would not be able to burn the food you need for energy. To supply oxygen to the various parts of the body, you must have a transport system. The body's transport system consists of lungs, heart, and blood vessels. When you breathe, you inhale air that contains oxygen into the lungs. The lungs absorb oxygen into their blood vessels and transport it to the heart, where it is pumped out through other blood vessels to all parts of the body. The more efficiently and effectively you transport oxygen, the greater your cardiorespiratory endurance (*cardio* for heart and *respiratory* for lungs and breathing)—the ability to supply and use oxygen, over a period of time and in sufficient amounts, to perform normal and unusual activities.

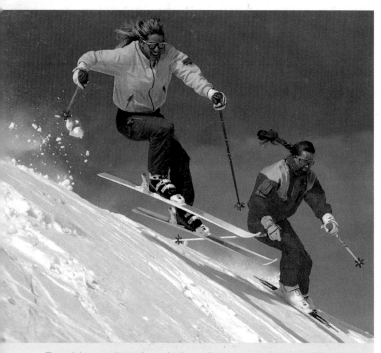

Exercising outdoors is an invigorating way to enhance spiritual health while at the same time improving physical health.

Jump/K. Vey

Muscular Strength and Endurance

The maximal pulling force of a muscle or a muscle group is called **muscular strength.** The ability of a muscle to contract repeatedly or to sustain a contraction is called **muscular endurance.** Lifting a load or moving an object depends on muscular strength. Doing that repeatedly over time requires muscular endurance. In spite of tremendous cardiovascular endurance, without sufficient muscular strength or endurance you may not be able to do the things you wish to do.

Flexibility

The range of motion around a joint, or more simply the degree to which you can move your limbs with grace and efficiency, is **flexibility.** Flexibility is important in performing exercise efficiently, safely, and enjoyably. Without adequate flexibility, you might not be able to stretch sufficiently, might overstress a muscle or ligament, and might even feel uncomfortable moving. Flexibility is probably the component of physical fitness that is most overlooked, yet the consequences of ignoring flexibility can be pain and discomfort, injury, and poor health.

Body Composition

Your body contains some parts that are made up of fats and others that are not. The fat component is usually referred to as **fat weight,** and fat in relation to the body as a whole is referred to as **percent body fat.** The nonfatty component is called **lean body mass. Body composition** is the relationship between these two components. In the past, people relied on height-weight charts to evaluate body composition. We now realize that someone can weigh many more pounds than what a chart based on height indicates is appropriate but still have good body composition. This condition can occur in a person who is muscular and has a good deal of lean body mass. Conversely, someone at just the right weight according to a height chart could be overweight because of too much fatty tissue and not enough lean body mass.

Health and Wellness

What do you mean when you think of **health?** If someone told you that Aaron was really healthy, what picture of Aaron would you have in your mind? If someone asked you to elaborate on your health, what would you say? We will help you answer that question, but first try listing five ways in which you could improve your health.

We are willing to bet that you listed ways to improve your physical health. You probably listed ways to prevent contracting heart disease, such as eating less fatty foods or exercising more, or ways to prevent cancer by not smoking cigarettes and getting regular checkups. Yet physical health is not the total picture; other components of health are just as important, including the following:

- **Social health**—the ability to interact well with people and the environment, to have satisfying interpersonal relationships.
- **Mental health**—the ability to learn and grow intellectually. Life's experiences as well as more formal structures (for example, schools) enhance mental health.
- **Emotional health**—the ability to control emotions so that you feel comfortable expressing them and can express them appropriately. Conversely, emotional health is the ability to avoid expressing emotions when it is inappropriate to do so.
- **Spiritual health**—a belief in some unifying force, which will vary from person to person but will have the concept of faith at its core. Faith is a feeling of connection to other humans, of a purpose to life, and of a quest for meaning in life.

So health is not simply caring for your body. It concerns your social interactions, mind, feelings, and spirit. Often, we decide to give up health in one area to gain greater health in another. For example, when you decide you're just not up to exercising today, you may choose to improve

muscular strength—The amount of force a muscle can exert for one repetition.

muscular endurance—A muscle's ability to continue submaximal contractions against resistance.

flexibility—The range of motion around a joint or the ability to move limbs gracefully and efficiently.

fat weight—The weight of body fat.

percent body fat—The percentage of body weight made up of fat.

lean body mass—The nonfatty component of the body.

body composition—The relationship between fat weight and lean body mass.

health—The total of your physical, social, emotional, mental, and spiritual status.

your emotional health (to seek relaxation) at some expense to your physical health. When you decide to study instead of spending time with your friends, you may be choosing mental over social health. We make decisions like these about our health all the time although we do not express them in those terms.

Now you can appreciate that physical fitness is just one component of health. In fact, it is just one component of physical health, which, in turn, is a component of overall health. Health, then, is an individual's total physical, social, emotional, mental, and spiritual status, and health is separate and distinct from illness, as shown in the continuum in figure 1.1.

Note that the continuum is a dotted line, rather than a solid line. Each dot is made up of the five health components shown in figure 1.2, and therefore everyone has some degree of health no matter where they are located on the continuum.

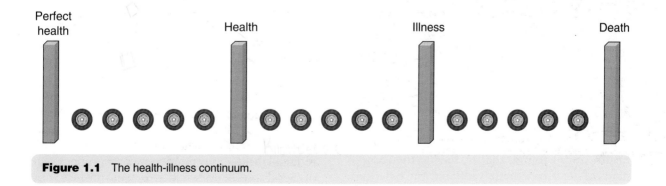

Figure 1.1　The health-illness continuum.

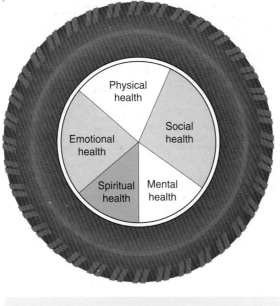

Figure 1.2   A single health-illness continuum dot.

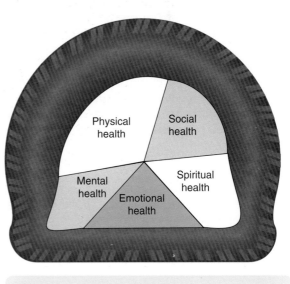

Figure 1.3   An asymmetrical dot.

Imagine that the health dot depicted in figure 1.2 is a tire on the vehicle in which you travel through life. If the tire is properly inflated, you will have a smooth ride; if it is not, the ride will be bumpy. The same is true for your health tire. If you do not pay enough attention to your health and all its components, improving (inflating) them when you can, you will experience conditions that make life more difficult and dissatisfying. For example, if you do not exercise frequently enough or properly, you may become fatigued easily or susceptible to various illnesses.

If you overdo any one component of health at the expense of the others, you may wind up with a tire like the one in figure 1.3. That tire is out of round and will not provide a smooth ride. That health tire has expanded physical health to the detriment of the other aspects of health. Rodney, introduced at the beginning of this chapter, comes to mind here. He expanded his physical health but was no longer married and looked terrible. He had no time for interacting with friends (social health), reading (mental health), or enjoying nature or participating in religious traditions (spiritual health). Even though he was more physically fit, he was probably not healthier. Further, he did not posses a high level of wellness. We refer to **wellness** as having the health tire in round, that is, having the components of health adequately inflated and balanced, paying attention to and improving all aspects of

wellness—Having the components of health balanced and at sufficient levels.

health without exaggerating any one. Inez, the other person we introduced at the beginning of this chapter, did not have the use of her legs, but she participated in physical activity at the level at which she was capable. She even learned about soccer so that she could coach a local team. Inez probably had a higher level of wellness than did the physically advantaged Rodney. That paradox is why you need to focus on your social, mental, emotional, and spiritual health as you read about physical fitness in this book. We will help you do that by regularly presenting the health and wellness implications of the content discussed.

Health Objectives for the Nation

Figure 1.4 compares the major causes of death in 1900 and today. Heading the 1900 list are diseases that are passed from one person to another or that result from unsanitary practices (tuberculosis, pneumonia, influenza). The incidence of these diseases has, for the most part, been drastically reduced through the development of proper waste disposal and sewage systems, quarantines, and other community and legislative actions.

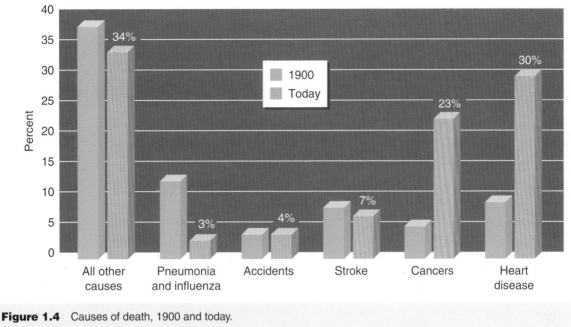

Figure 1.4 Causes of death, 1900 and today.

From U.S. Census Bureau, 2002, *Statistical abstracts of the United States* (Washington, DC: U.S. Census Bureau), 82.

The killers of today do not lend themselves to such remedies. These conditions (heart disease, cancer, stroke) are more the result of lifestyle than of a microorganism. In a democratic society we cannot legislate lifestyle. For significant decreases to occur in these diseases, people must voluntarily change unhealthy behaviors (cigarette smoking, lack of regular physical activity, lack of proper amounts of sleep, abuse of alcohol and other drugs, consumption of foods high in saturated fats, and so forth). Medical researchers estimate that 20% of the risk for heart disease, cancer, and stroke can be attributed to heredity, another 20% to environmental factors, 10% to inadequate health care, and an alarming 50% to unhealthy lifestyles (Behavior Kills, 1994).

Recognizing the need to encourage the adoption of healthy lifestyles, the surgeon general of the United States developed health goals for the nation. The first national health goals were established in 1979 and 1980. More recently, goals for the year 2010 have been announced. Although many of the national health objectives are related to physical fitness and wellness, we list only those directly related to physical fitness in table 1.1. The objectives, the baseline condition (the status of the behavior or condition when the objective was written), and the target to be achieved by the year 2010 are presented.

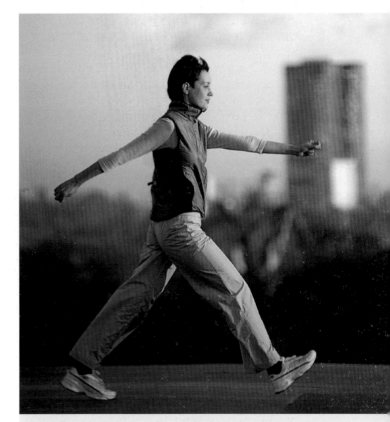

Exercise is something you should, and can, fit into your schedule to help reach an acceptable state of health.

Digital Vision

TABLE 1.1—2010 National Health Objectives Specific for Physical Fitness

Objective	Baseline	Target
1. Reduce the proportion of adults who engage in no leisure-time physical activity.	40%	20%
2. Increase the proportion of adults who engage in regularly, preferably daily, moderate physical activity for at least 30 minutes per day.	15%	30%
3. Increase the proportion of adults who engage in vigorous physical activity that promotes the development and maintenance of cardiorespiratory fitness 3 or more days per week for 20 or more minutes per occasion.	23%	30%
4. Increase the proportion of adults who perform physical activities that enhance and maintain muscular strength and endurance.	18%	30%
5. Increase the proportion of adults who perform physical activities that enhance and maintain flexibility.	30%	43%
6. Increase the proportion of adolescents who engage in moderate physical activity for at least 30 minutes on 5 or more of the previous 7 days.	27%	35%
7. Increase the proportion of adolescents who engage in vigorous physical activity that promotes cardiorespiratory fitness 3 or more days per week for 20 or more minutes per occasion.	65%	85%
8. Increase the proportion of the nation's public and private middle and junior high schools that require daily physical education for all students.	17%	25%
9. Increase the proportion of the nation's public and private senior high schools that require daily physical education for all students.	2%	5%
10. Increase the proportion of adolescents who participate in daily school physical education.	29%	50%
11. Increase the proportion of adolescents who spend at least 50% of school physical education class time being physically active.	38%	50%
12. Increase the proportion of adolescents who view television 2 or fewer hours on a school day.	57%	75%
13. Increase the proportion of worksites offering employer-sponsored physical activity and fitness programs.	46%	75%
14. Increase the proportion of trips made by adults by walking.	17%	25%
15. Increase the proportion of trips made by children and adolescents by walking.	31%	50%
16. Increase the proportion of trips made by adults by bicycling.	0.6%	2%
17. Increase the proportion of trips made by children and adolescents by bicycling.	2.4%	5%

From U.S. Department of Health and Human Services, November 2000, *Healthy People 2010: Understanding and improving health,* 2nd ed. (Washington, DC: U.S. Government Printing Office).

What Physical Fitness Can Do for You

As we have discussed, physical fitness can make you healthier and help you achieve high-level wellness. And, as you will soon see, it can even help you feel better about yourself and be more self-assured.

Benefits of Physical Activity

A friend of ours likes to kid that he gets his exercise serving as a pallbearer at the funerals of his jogger friends. Aside from simply being contentious, he is expressing an important point. Exercise itself will not guarantee a long life. Heredity sets limits on how long you will live, but within those limits is a range. Regular physical activity of sufficient duration and intensity can help you reach your upper limit. This truth is demonstrated in the studies of Harvard alumni by Paffenbarger and colleagues (1986). Paffenbarger found that mortality rates were lower for physically active alumni. By age 80 the amount of additional life attributed to adequate exercise, compared with being sedentary, was between 1 and more than 2 years. The multiple risk factor intervention trial (MRFIT) study, which involved more than 12,000 men, found that most physically active men lived longer than the least physically active did (Leon and Connett, 1991). Further, the MRFIT study indicated that any activity (not just vigorous activity) of 30 minutes five times a week decreased the risk of coronary heart disease, although more strenuous physical activity was more protective. Blair and associates (1989) found that the death rate increased as fitness level decreased. Two of the major reasons for lower death rates of exercisers can be explained by our knowledge that exercise can help prevent coronary heart disease (Donahue et al., 1988) and cancer (Krucoff, 1992), the first and second leading causes of death in the United States. Researchers have found an increase in natural killer (NK) cell activity among people who exercise as seldom as once per week (Kusaka, Kondou, and Morimoto, 1992). NK cells help prevent cancer.

Physical activity can both prevent illness and disease and help rehabilitation. In this way, it enhances physical health. Because we will discuss the relationship between physical activity and health in more detail elsewhere in this book, suffice it to say here that among the illnesses and diseases that physical activity can help prevent are the nation's leading killers: heart disease, cancer, and stroke. And this sort of activity can help prevent, and serve as a treatment for, hypertension (high blood pressure), itself a major cause of heart disease and stroke.

One reason that physical activity is so helpful in preventing and treating various conditions is that it helps people control their weight. Overweight, obesity, and malnutrition are implicated in numerous states of ill health. These conditions are also related to the amount of cholesterol in the blood (serum cholesterol), which can clog arteries leading to the heart or brain, thereby resulting in a heart attack or stroke. Some cholesterol, however, is helpful because it picks up blood fats and deposits them outside the body. This good cholesterol is called high-density lipoprotein (HDL). Exercise increases the amount of HDL in the blood (Shepard, 1989) and decreases the amount of bad cholesterol (low-density lipoprotein [LDL]) that accumulates on the blood vessel walls and can eventually block the flow of blood to the heart and other body parts.

Physical activity has also been found to be related to reduced risk of diabetes (Can Exercise Reduce Diabetes, 2001), lowered risk of breast cancer (Verloop et al., 2000), and greater bone density (Mussolino, Looker, and Orwoll, 2001). Physical activity can also result in a decreased need for hospital care (Kujala et al., 1999). Some evidence indicates that physically active women need fewer cesarean sections during childbirth (Bungum et al., 2000). Physical activity has even been associated with better sexual functioning (Krucoff, 2000).

In addition, regular exercise can be an extremely effective means of managing stress. In this way, it improves emotional health. As we will discuss in chapter 12, stress changes the body so that it is prepared to respond to a threat. The body gears up for some physical reaction. Exercise uses the built-up stress by-products and the body's preparedness to do something physical. The result is a sense of stress relief. Exercise also enhances the production of brain neurotransmitters (endorphins) that make you feel better and less stressed.

The rehabilitative benefits of exercise are almost notorious. It wasn't too long ago that people needing surgery or women giving birth were restricted to a hospital bed for days and sometimes weeks. Those restrictions are no longer observed. The benefits of physical activity in recuperating from many conditions are now well recognized. Take the case of a man we know who had a triple bypass operation in which three of the blood vessels supplying his heart were found to be obstructed. The obstructed sections were bypassed with blood vessels grafted from his legs. Shortly after the operation, he was expected to get out of bed and walk around. Although nervous at first, he soon learned that physical movement helped him get back to his regular routine. His muscular strength returned sooner than he expected, his blood circulation was enhanced by muscular contractions forcing pressure on the blood vessel walls, and his mood improved dramatically.

Physical activity can help elderly people live longer (Rakowski and Mor, 1992) and postpone the effects of aging. As people age, they become susceptible to conditions that can restrict their activities, even to the extent that they become dependent on others to tie their shoes, transport them, and shop for them. A life of regular physical activity can postpone this dependency by providing elders with the necessary muscular strength and endurance, cardiorespiratory endurance, and flexibility to manage their own affairs. Several national health objectives speak to the needs of the elderly. Table 1.2 shows the 2010 national health objectives specific to the elderly. The baseline figures refer to the state of affairs that existed at the time the objectives were written.

Physical activity has additional benefits that are often overlooked. For example, several researchers have found that workers who are physically fit are absent from work less frequently (Steinhardt, Greenhow, and Stewart, 1991; Tucker, Aldana, and Friedman, 1990). In addition, people who are physically fit are less apt to experience depression and are more likely to feel in control of their lives (Brandon and Lofton, 1991).

Physical activity can also improve spiritual health. For example, when you are exercising outdoors, you have the opportunity to experience nature and all its wonders—to feel the rush of air on your face and the heat of the sun on your skin, to hear the sound of the birds and the wind rustling through the leaves, and to sense the exhilaration of your body performing physical movement. In this way, you can feel connected—body, mind, and spirit—to a unifying force. And if you engage in physical activity with other people, you improve your social health besides all the other components of health.

Among Hispanic and African American women, a growing body of research associates spirituality with a variety of positive health outcomes (Carter, 2002). Musgrave et al. (2002) reported that for most Hispanic women, mind, body, and spirit are inseparable. This belief that man is a triune being is expressed in the practice of curanderismo among many Mexican Americans (Rojas, 1996). This religious practice integrates music, dance, and massage with herbs and ritual prayer. Many older African Americans indicate that religion provides comfort during stress (Spector, 2000). Moreover, studies indicate that spirituality builds self-esteem and a sense of belonging, lowers blood pressure, and decreases depression. These changes in turn sustain positive health behavior by providing a cardio-protective effect against stress-related disorders. Hence, the implications for health-promoting behaviors are evident among individuals who maintain a high degree of spiritual health.

Surgeon General's Report on Physical Activity and Health

In 1996 Physical Activity and Health: A Report of the Surgeon General was published. This report

TABLE 1.2—2010 Objectives Specific to the Elderly

Objective	Baseline	Target
1. Reduce the proportion of 65- to 74-year-olds who engage in no leisure-time physical activity.	51%	20%
2. Reduce the proportion of those 75 years of age and older who engage in no leisure-time physical activity.	65%	20%
3. Increase the proportion of 65- to 75-year-olds who engage in regularly, preferably daily, moderate physical activity for at least 30 minutes per day.	16%	30%
4. Increase the proportion of those 75 years of age or older who engage in regularly, preferably daily, moderate physical activity for at least 30 minutes per day.	12%	30%
5. Increase the proportion of 65- to 74-year-olds who engage in vigorous physical activity that promotes the development and maintenance of cardiorespiratory fitness 3 or more days per week for 20 or more minutes per occasion.	13%	30%
6. Increase the proportion of those 75 years of age and older who engage in vigorous physical activity that promotes the development and maintenance of cardiorespiratory fitness 3 or more days per week for 20 or more minutes per occasion.	6%	30%

From U.S. Department of Health and Human Services, November 2000, *Healthy People 2010: Understanding and improving health*, 2nd ed. (Washington, DC: U.S. Government Printing Office).

aimed to publicize the benefits of physical activity and to emphasize that people could obtain these benefits without strenuous exercise—that moderate exercise was sufficient. Among the many

benefits of physical activity touted by the surgeon general are the following:

- Reduces the risk of dying prematurely
- Reduces the risk of dying from heart disease
- Reduces the risk of developing diabetes
- Reduces the risk of developing high blood pressure
- Helps reduce blood pressure in people who already have high blood pressure
- Reduces the risk of developing colon cancer
- Reduces feelings of depression and anxiety
- Helps control weight
- Helps build and maintain healthy bones, muscles, and joints
- Helps older adults become stronger and better able to move about without falling
- Promotes psychological well-being

The surgeon general's report states that people can obtain these benefits through moderate physical activity, defined as requiring approximately 150 calories per day, or 1,000 calories per week. Figure 1.5 lists activities that meet the definition of moderate physical activity. People who are now inactive can gain the benefits just listed from participation in these moderate physical activities. People can derive even greater benefits, however, from activities requiring greater intensity, duration, or frequency.

A summary of the report's findings and recommendations specific to women, persons with disabilities, older adults, adults, and adolescents and young adults can be found in appendix C.

Washing and waxing a car for 45 to 60 minutes

Washing windows or floors for 45 to 60 minutes

Playing volleyball for 45 minutes

Playing touch football for 30 to 45 minutes

Gardening for 30 to 45 minutes

Wheeling self in wheelchair for 30 to 40 minutes

Walking 1 3/4 miles in 35 minutes (20 minutes per mile)

Playing basketball (shooting baskets) for 30 minutes

Bicycling 5 miles in 30 minutes

Dancing fast (social) for 30 minutes

Pushing a stroller 1 1/2 miles in 30 minutes

Raking leaves for 30 minutes

Walking 2 miles in 30 minutes (15 minutes per mile)

Doing water aerobics for 30 minutes

Swimming laps for 20 minutes

Playing wheelchair basketball for 20 minutes

Playing basketball (playing a game) for 15 to 20 minutes

Bicycling 4 miles in 15 minutes

Jumping rope for 15 minutes

Running 1 1/2 miles in 15 minutes (10 minutes per mile)

Shoveling snow for 15 minutes

Stair walking for 25 minutes

Figure 1.5 Examples of moderate amounts of physical activity.

Note: The activities at the top of the list are less intense and therefore require a longer duration to produce benefits. The activities in the lower portion of the list are more intense and therefore require a shorter duration to produce benefits.

Source: U.S. Public Health Service, *Physical Activity and Health: A Report of the Surgeon General: Executive Summary* (Washington, DC: U.S. Department of Health and Human Services, 1996), p. 2.

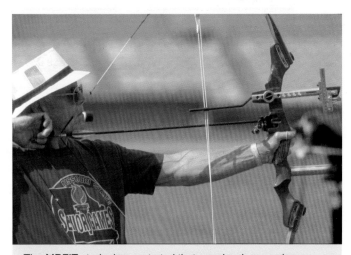

The MRFIT study demonstrated that people who exercise regularly can add years to their life, and life to their years.

Myth and Fact Sheet

Myth	Fact
1. The most important component of overall health is physical health.	**1.** Health consists of more than just physical health. It includes social, emotional, mental, and spiritual health as well. People will value different components of health during different stages of their lives. This tendency is not wrong but simply a matter of shifting values. Who is to say which component of health is more important than another for any individual?
2. Wellness and health are the same.	**2.** Health refers to the degree to which a person has the five components of health. Wellness means having the five components of health in balance. No one component is exaggerated at the expense of any other. Consequently, health and wellness are not synonymous.
3. Someone who is good at basketball is physically fit.	**3.** A person who is skilled at a particular sport may not be physically fit. Someone who can shoot baskets or hit a tennis ball may not be able to run a long distance or may not have upper-body muscular strength or muscular endurance. Further, that individual may not be flexible or agile enough. To be physically fit, a person must work on all fitness components.
4. Because the leading causes of death result from unhealthy lifestyles, the U.S. government can do little to make people healthier.	**4.** The U.S. government developed national health objectives to encourage individuals to adopt healthier lifestyles and thereby live longer, better-quality lives. These health objectives are intended to be achieved by the year 2010, at which time an assessment of progress will be made and national health objectives for the next decade determined.
5. Being physically fit makes you healthier, but you probably won't feel any different about yourself.	**5.** If you become physically fit, you will feel better about yourself and your self-esteem will improve. You will develop more confidence, feel less depressed, and experience a sense of more control in your life. The benefits of physical fitness go well beyond the healthy changes that occur within your body. They include improvements in your mind and your spirit as well.

Self-Esteem and Physical Activity

Physical activity also has the potential of giving you more confidence and making you feel better about yourself. We call this **self-esteem.** A number of research studies support the contention that self-esteem facilitates physical activity among multiethnic women (Felton and Parsons, 1994; Eyler et al., 1998). Mosca et al. (1998) also found this to be true among White women. These benefits occur for several reasons. First, regular exercise helps maintain body weight and develop a positive body image. Feeling good about how your body looks and feels will translate into feeling good about yourself.

Second, physical activity often provides challenges that you can meet and overcome. That aspect is one of the advantages of competitive sports activities. Being successful at these challenges will give you confidence to face other challenges in your life. Yet no one masters all challenges. Physical activity allows you to fail to meet the challenge but recognize that life goes on. You have probably heard someone say that you cannot hit a home run if you do not step up to the plate. When you bat, however, you can also strike out. So what? Striking out, or trying and failing, can be a more effective learning and growth experience than succeeding. After all, if you succeed, by definition you were able to do whatever it was

self-esteem—The regard you hold for yourself, the value you place on yourself.

anyhow. Only when you fail can you learn what you need to adjust to become better.

Lastly, physical activity improves endurance and strength, allowing you to perform activities more effectively and for longer periods. Being able to perform in this way can make you more confident and less likely to avoid events that are physically challenging. The result will be greater self-esteem and, as a result, better emotional health.

Prevalence of Physical Activity

Despite the many benefits of physical activity, a surprisingly large number of Americans are not sufficiently active. As reported in the Behavioral Risk Factor Surveillance System (BRFSS), the prevalence of those who engaged in recommended levels of activity increased slightly from 24.3% in 1990 to 25.4% in 1998. Over the same period, however, the prevalence of those reporting insufficient activity increased slightly from 45.0% to 45.9% (Physical Activity Trends, 2001). Physical inactivity is most prevalent among women, African Americans and Hispanics, older adults, and the less affluent.

In a study conducted by the U.S. government, the National Health Interview Survey (NHIS), researchers found that 38.3% of adults were physically inactive during their leisure time and another 22.7% engaged only in light to moderate physical activity at least 5 days a week (Schoen-born and Barnes, 2002). The most inactive were Hispanic Americans (62.9% engaged in no physical activity during their leisure time), followed by African Americans (57.9%), Whites (44.4%), and Asians and Pacific Islanders (43.3%).

Physical Activity Among Adolescents

Numerous national research studies confirm that physical activity during adolescence has declined substantially, more so for girls than for boys. Whether adolescent girls live in an urban or rural setting (Felton et al., 2002), racial and gender patterns of physical inactivity emerge during their youth that relate directly to later trends in obesity and chronic diseases, such as cardiovascular disease.

The National Heart, Lung, and Blood Institute recently revealed the results of a 10-year longitudinal analysis of the physical activity patterns of 1,213 African American and 1,166 White adolescent females followed from the ages 9 or 10 to the

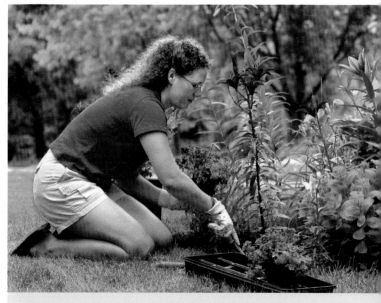

Even gardening can be an effective fitness activity, and can contribute especially to social and spiritual health.

Jim Whitmer Photography

ages of 18 to 19 (Kimm et al., 2002). Based on a self-reported leisure-time physical activity (LTPA) questionnaire, White adolescent females had a higher median activity score than African American females during the initial assessment (30.8 versus 27.3 MET-times per week. One MET is equal to your resting metabolic oxygen consumption rate (VO_2). Intensity of exercise is described as a multiple of this resting rate. If you are exercising at four METS, the intensity is four times greater than resting metabolic rate. Ten years later, the young White females experienced a 64% decline in self-reported LTPA. African American females reported a staggering 100% decline in LTPA during the same 10-year period.

Physical Activity Patterns Among Ethnic Minority Women

Studies examining the lack of routine physical activity among women of color have repeatedly shown that the same racial patterns of inactivity that emerged during adolescent girls persist in women throughout the life cycle (Eyler et al., 2002). Even while enrolled in college, women display racial differences in physical inactivity, with African American and Asian American women reporting less LTPA than do White women (Palaniappan et al., 2002). National studies of adult women further confirm racial differences in physical activity (Banks-Wallace and Conn, 2002). For example, 37% of African American women reported no LTPA in the U.S. Women's Determinants Study (Brownson et al., 2000). Among Hispanic women, the prevalence of no self-reported LTPA ranged from 33% (Brownson et al., 2000) to 44% (Crespo et al., 1999). When Sallis et al. (2001) measured physical activity in Mexican American and White mothers, they found White mothers to have significantly higher levels of vigorous LTPA.

The activity patterns of Asian Americans and Native Americans have been less well documented (King et al., 2000). The U.S. Women's Determinant Study (Brownson et al., 2000) and the Strong Heart Study examined tribal groups in the Dakotas, Oklahoma, and Arizona. Both surveys found that 48% of women reported no LTPA in the previous week (Welty et al., 1995). The national prevalence of physical activity among Asian American women has only recently been evaluated. The Filipino Women's Health Study conducted by Maxwell et al. (2002) is one of few intervention studies assessing physical activity habits within an Asian ethnic group.

Barriers to a Physically Active Lifestyle

The removal of barriers to a physically active lifestyle is of primary importance when designing physical activity interventions. National trends in levels of physical activity have consistently reported men as having a higher level of LTPA than women do within nearly every ethnic minority group (Caspersen and Merritt, 1995). Until the past decade, however, relatively little information was published on the lifestyle risk factors that predispose ethnic minority women of all ages past adolescence to be more sedentary (USDHHS, 1996). Table 1.3 summarizes determinants associated with the level of physical activity among women based on ethnicity as reported in a comprehensive review of research studies conducted in the past two decades (Eyler et al., 2002). The prevalence of such potentially modifiable risk factors warrants consideration for explaining the increased incidence of heart disease in at-risk ethnic minority populations.

Factors Affecting Physical Activity Among Adolescents

Having validated ethnic and gender physical activity patterns during adolescence, researchers have now shifted their focus toward exploring the underlying reasons for this well-documented decline. They have identified a number of those determinants. The NHLBI Growth and Health Study (Kimm et al., 2002) reported several racial differences in the factors associated with the decrease in LTPA among adolescent African American and White females. For example, among White females, determinants of physical inactivity included cigarette smoking and lower levels of parental education. Among African American adolescent females, sedentary lifestyle was related to pregnancy rates and a higher body-mass index. Other studies report excessive TV and video viewing, access to sports equipment, perception of neighborhood safety, parental behavior, and attitudes toward exercise as having a significant effect on physical activity among adolescent males and females (Felton et al., 2002; McGuire et al., 2002; Gordon-Larsen et al., 2002). Given the important role of physical activity with respect to a variety of chronic diseases, greater emphasis at an earlier age should be placed on those determinants considered modifiable.

Determinants of Physical Activity Among Adults

Various factors explain why adults, especially women, from ethnic minority populations are less physically active than adult Caucasians are. In a cross-sectional study conducted among U.S. adults from 1999 to 2000, Brownson et al. (2001) found that the availability of areas for physical activity was generally higher among men than among women. They further stated that the four most commonly reported personal barriers to a physically active lifestyle were lack of time, feeling too tired, obtaining enough exercise at one's job, and having no motivation to exercise. Neighborhood characteristics such as the presence of sidewalks, pleasant scenery, lack of heavy traffic, and hills were positively associated with the level of physical activity. Among some ethnic minorities living in urban areas, residents reported not feeling safe using public exercise facilities (Centers for Disease Control and Prevention, 1999). Seefeldt et al. (2002) and Eyler et al. (2002) reported barriers for African American women such as physical appearance during work hours, unaffordable facilities, unavailable or unaffordable child care, and fear for personal safety because of high crime rates as having a prohibitive effect on their level of LTPA.

TABLE 1.3—Associations With Women's Physical Activity (PA) by Ethnic Group According to Published Reports[a]

Factor	Black (B)	White (W)	Hispanic (H)	American Indian (AI)	Asian (A)	Comments
PERSONAL						
Sociodemographic						
Race	-	-	-	-	-	Possibly confounded by type of PA
Education	+	+	+	+		Different for household or occupational
Age	-	-	0	-		Conflicting for W, B, AI; may be due to age range restrictions
Income	+	+		+		Conflicting reports for W and B
Employment	+	-	-	0		Conflicting reports for W and B
Marital status	0	0	0	0	0	Conflicting reports for W
Urban residence	0	0	0	0		
Rural residence	-	-	-	-		National surveys (including BRFSS)
Biological and health						
Perceived health	+	+	+	+		May not affect household or occupational
Health status	+	++		+		Chronic conditions for women
Body-mass index	0	-		-		
Attempting weight loss	++	++				
Smoking status	0	0		0		Conflicting reports for W and B
Alcohol consumption	00	0				All associations reported for W
Pap smear or breast self-examination	+	+				Infrequent studies of other health behaviors
PSYCHOLOGICAL						
Self-efficacy		++				Little study in ethnically diverse women
Attitudes and beliefs						
Perceived benefits	++	++	+			
Lack of time	-	--		-		May be only a barrier to sport or exercise
Lack of motivation		-				Only for sport or exercise
Fatigue or lack of energy	-	-	-	-		Sample of older W
Self-conscious				-		One study
Positive outcome expected	++	+				Conflicting results in W
Negative outcome expected	--	-				
John Henryism	+	+				
Competitiveness	+	+				One study
Need to excel	0	+				
Type A, hostility	0	0				One study
Enjoyment of exercise	+					One study
Self-esteem	+	+	+			One study
Stress	-	-	-			Stress reported as a barrier
Stress reduction		++				
Knowledge	++	++				
Past PA behavior	+	+	+	+	+	

(continued)

TABLE 1.3 (continued)

Factor	Black (B)	White (W)	Hispanic (H)	American Indian (AI)	Asian (A)	Comments
ENVIRONMENTAL						
Social environment						
Social support (family and friends)	+	++	+	+	+	May be important for sport or exercise
Professional support	+	+				Physicians or other health professionals
Family responsibility	-	--	-	-		Negatively or not associated with household activity
Number of children	-	--	-	-		May be confounded by type of activity
PHYSICAL, ENVIRONMENTAL, AND PUBLIC POLICY						
General physical environment						Qualitative studies
Bad weather	-	--		-		Qualitative studies
Lessened daylight hours	-					
Lack of personal safety, crime	-			-		
Transportation	-					
Lack of public policy						Studies conflict in H
Community resources		-	-			
Work incentives	+					One study
Worksite facilities	+		+	+	+	One study
Provision of child care	+					One study
Monetary cost	-	-		-		
Culture issues						Based on limited number of qualitative studies
Appearance after exercise						
During workday	-					
Importance of relaxation	-					
Already perceived active enough	-			-		
Acculturation			+			
Social stigma				-		Among women with diabetes
Language			-			

[a]++, repeatedly documented positive association with physical activity; +, weak or mixed evidence of positive association with physical activity; 00, repeatedly documented lack of association with physical activity; 0, weak or mixed evidence of no association with physical activity; --, repeatedly documented negative association with physical activity; -, weak or mixed evidence of a negative association with physical activity.

Adapted, from A.E. Eyler et al., 2002, "Correlates of physical activity among women from diverse racial/ethnic groups," *Journal of Women's Health & Gender-Based Medicine* 11(3): 239-253.

Your Personal Physical Fitness Profile

The first step in achieving the benefits of physical fitness is to determine where to begin. What is your current level of physical fitness? Which components of physical fitness do you want to maintain and which do you want to improve?

We help you perform such an assessment in the next chapter. In addition, throughout this book, we include questionnaires, scales, physical tests to evaluate components of fitness, and even measures of psychosocial factors (such as self-esteem) related to decisions to exercise. We also provide lab activities in each chapter designed to help you learn more about yourself and about physical fitness. By the time you finish reading this book, you will have enough information about yourself to plan an effective fitness program, one based on your personal fitness profile that will meet your personal fitness goals.

Summary

Components of Physical Fitness Physical fitness encompasses cardiorespiratory endurance, muscular strength, muscular endurance, flexibility, and body composition. It also includes the motor skills of agility, balance, coordination, power, speed, and reaction time.

Health and Wellness Health consists of five components: physical, social, mental, emotional, and spiritual. Physical fitness is but one component of physical health, albeit an important one.

Wellness is maintaining the components of health in sufficient amounts and in balance with one another. An ideal state of wellness is one in which no one component of health is emphasized at the expense of any other component.

In the past, the conditions causing the deaths of the most people in the United States were passed from one person to another or were the result of unsanitary practices. Tuberculosis and pneumonia are examples. The federal and state governments responded by passing legislation that eliminated these unsafe practices and effectively reduced deaths from these conditions. Today, most deaths result from lifestyle practices such as cigarette smoking, lack of exercise, inadequate sleep, and poor nutrition. Changing those practices is up to the individual; governments cannot legislate those changes.

The federal government, however, has developed national health objectives to publicize and encourage healthier lifestyles and attempt to reduce death and disability from lifestyle diseases and illnesses. Several of these objectives are specific to physical fitness and physical activity, and others are tangentially related.

Health Objectives for the Nation Medical researchers estimate that 50% of the major causes of deaths result from unhealthy lifestyle behaviors. Recognizing the need to encourage the adoption of healthful lifestyles, the surgeon general of the United States developed health goals for the nation. Each decade these national health goals and objectives are updated. Currently, national health goals and objectives are designed to be met in the year 2010. Many of these goals and objectives concern physical fitness and wellness.

What Physical Fitness Can Do for You Physical activity can improve physical health by decreasing LDLs (bad cholesterol) and increasing HDLs (good cholesterol), by preventing or reducing high blood pressure, by helping to maintain desirable weight and lean body mass, and by preventing some cancers.

Physical activity can also improve emotional health by helping to manage stress, enrich spiritual health by focusing on nature and bodily sensations, and enhance social health by exercising with other people. In addition, physical activity can help diminish and postpone the effects of aging and aid in recuperation from illnesses and medical procedures. Further, physical activity can make you feel more confident and thereby improve your self-esteem by helping you maintain recommended body weight and a desirable body image. Physical activity can provide challenges that develop confidence and the realization that even if you do not overcome the challenges, significant learning occurs. Self-esteem also improves when you develop endurance and strength and can perform daily activities effectively and for longer periods.

Prevalence of Physical Activity A variety of national research studies confirm that a substantial decline has occurred in the physical activity patterns of adolescent females. African American adolescent females have markedly lower levels of LTPA than White females. The National Health Interview Study found that 38.3% of adults reported no LTPA and another 22.7% engaged in only light to moderate physical activity at least 5 days a week. Hispanic Americans were the most inactive, followed by African Americans, Whites, and Asians and Pacific Islanders.

Barriers to a Physically Active Lifestyle Barriers to a physically active lifestyle among adolescent females include cigarette smoking, pregnancy, high body-mass index, excessive TV and video viewing, access to sports equipment, and perception of neighborhood safety. Roadblocks to physical activity among adult minority women include time constraints, fatigue, concern for physical appearance during work hours, and lack of motivation. Environmental barriers also include lack of pleasant scenery, traffic, unaffordable facilities, lack of child care, and neighborhood safety. When designing intervention programs for ethnic minority women, such culturally specific variables should be considered to facilitate compliance.

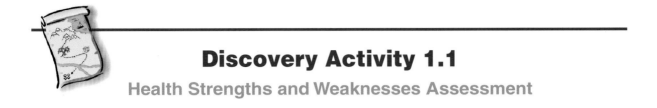

Discovery Activity 1.1

Health Strengths and Weaknesses Assessment

Name _____ **Date** _____

On this chart, list your strengths and weaknesses for each of the five components of health. Once you have done that, develop a plan for maximizing your strengths and minimizing your weaknesses. You should find ways to use your strengths to make them even more influential on your health and to eliminate health weaknesses or decrease their negative effects on your health. Once you put your plan into action, you will become healthier and achieve a higher level of wellness.

Component	Strengths	Weaknesses
Mental health	_____	_____
	_____	_____
	_____	_____
	_____	_____
	_____	_____
Physical health	_____	_____
	_____	_____
	_____	_____
	_____	_____
	_____	_____
Social health	_____	_____
	_____	_____
	_____	_____
	_____	_____
Spiritual health	_____	_____
	_____	_____
	_____	_____
	_____	_____
Emotional health	_____	_____
	_____	_____
	_____	_____
	_____	_____
	_____	_____

From *Physical fitness and wellness, third edition*, by Jerrold S. Greenberg, George B. Dintiman, and Barbee Myers Oakes, 2004, Champaign, IL: Human Kinetics.

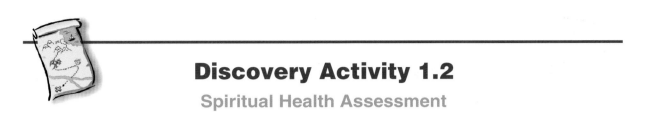

Discovery Activity 1.2
Spiritual Health Assessment

Name _____ **Date** _____

Spiritual health can take many forms. For some people it refers to a feeling of connectedness with those who came before and those who will follow, be they family or humankind in general. For others it is a belief in a Supreme Being. For still others spiritual health is feeling a part of nature and all its wonder. One thing we know about spiritual health is that it is related to forgiveness. Being unable to forgive others or oneself is associated with anger, shame, and other feelings that translate into physiological changes (increased heart rate, blood pressure, and so forth). The result is ill health and less appreciation for life. How is the inability to forgive affecting you, and what can you do about it?

List three people you have had difficulty forgiving:

1. _____

2. _____

3. _____

Identify three negative effects this unforgiving attitude has on you:

1. _____

2. _____

3. _____

With this insight, choose at least two of the three people you listed previously and describe what you will do to forgive them and the date by which you will do it:

1. _____

2. _____

3. _____

From *Physical fitness and wellness, third edition*, by Jerrold S. Greenberg, George B. Dintiman, and Barbee Myers Oakes, 2004, Champaign, IL: Human Kinetics.

Discovery Activity 1.3

Service-Learning for
Physical Fitness, Health, and Wellness

People do not exercise regularly for many reasons. Some people may feel that they are too busy. Some people may not enjoy the feeling associated with exercising. Others may not be aware of the benefits derived from being physically active. You can probably think of many other reasons why people lead sedentary lives.

Yet some people would like to participate in regular fitness activities but encounter barriers they find difficult to overcome. For example, some communities may not have any, or few, places in which to exercise. Parks, community centers, and health clubs may be absent. In some high-crime communities, exercising outdoors may be dangerous. Still other communities may lack qualified staff or adequate equipment for exercise to occur in a healthy manner.

What are the barriers to exercising regularly in your college community? Are adequate facilities and equipment available for your campus community to participate in physical activity in a healthy manner? Are the hours that the facility is available consistent with student, staff, and faculty schedules? Are the facilities reserved for athletic teams or intramurals, thereby depriving adequate access to the majority of students? Are the locker rooms and shower areas conducive to engaging in exercise? What changes can be made in your college community to encourage and facilitate more students to engage in regular physical activity?

With three other students, study the environment and policies related to physical activity and exercise. Interview students and staff. Observe the college community as it exercises. Speak with the fitness facility staff and determine hours of operation.

Inventory available exercise equipment. Identify fitness-related policies on your campus. After studying the issue, prepare a written report recommending changes that would permit more of the campus community to engage in regular exercise. Submit your report to the campus administration.

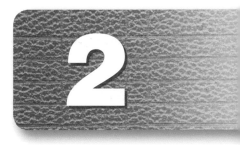

2

Assessing Your Present Level of Fitness

Chapter Objectives

By the end of this chapter, you should be able to

1. indicate when it is appropriate to obtain a medical examination before beginning an exercise program or test;
2. list the components of a good medical evaluation;
3. list the major components of a fitness appraisal;
4. measure and analyze your cardiorespiratory endurance, muscular strength and endurance, flexibility, nutrient intake, and body composition; and
5. explore challenges to assessing physical fitness in physically disabled individuals.

Kim's excuse for avoiding a regular exercise program is one voiced by many university students: "I get enough exercise in my part-time job at the department store and my daily routine. I'm already fit. Why should I use my valuable time exercising more?" Unfortunately, there are few, if any, active occupations, including that of a university student, that develop cardiorespiratory endurance, muscular strength, muscular endurance, and flexibility and that control body weight and fat. One way for Kim to find out if she possesses an adequate level of health-related fitness is to complete the test battery described in this chapter to see whether she scores in the average or above-average category on each item.

Throughout this text, we emphasize the important role of physical activity in determining one's overall health and wellness status, as well as athletic performance capability. Therefore, it is vital that you learn how to make an accurate assessment of your level of fitness. In this chapter, we provide methods to perform every major component of a fitness appraisal and medical evaluation for nondisabled individuals. You will also learn some of the challenges to assessing fitness among physically disabled persons.

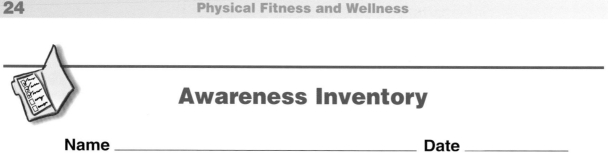

Awareness Inventory

Name _____ **Date** _____

Check the space by the letter T for the statements that you think are true and the space by the letter F for the statements that you think are false. The answers appear following the list of statements. This chapter will present information to clarify these statements for you. As you read the chapter, look for explanations for the reasons why the statements are true or false.

T ___ **F** ___ 1. Every college student should have a complete medical examination before beginning any type of testing or exercise program.

T ___ **F** ___ 2. Most college students know enough about their level of fitness and do not need to be tested.

T ___ **F** ___ 3. A condition referred to as athlete's heart or an enlarged heart muscle resulting from aerobic exercise is dangerous and requires the immediate attention of a physician.

T ___ **F** ___ 4. Aerobic fitness can be measured using tests involving running, step, cycling, or swimming.

T ___ **F** ___ 5. Muscular strength testing isn't necessary because strength is not considered a key component of health-related fitness.

T ___ **F** ___ 6. The best way to determine your abdominal endurance is to complete as many sit-ups as possible.

T ___ **F** ___ 7. Abdominal curls are completed by performing a straight-leg sit-up to right angles.

T ___ **F** ___ 8. A waist-to-hip ratio of more than 0.85 in women and 1.0 in men (waist almost as large as the hips in women or larger than the hips in men) indicates increased risk of heart disease.

T ___ **F** ___ 9. Upper-body strength (arms and shoulders) in most college students is excellent.

T ___ **F** ___ 10. Most college men and women will be capable of bench-pressing an amount equivalent to their body weight.

Answers: 1-F, 2-F, 3-F, 4-T, 5-F, 6-F, 7-F, 8-T, 9-F, 10-F

From *Physical fitness and wellness, third edition*, by Jerrold S. Greenberg, George B. Dintiman, and Barbee Myers Oakes, 2004, Champaign, IL: Human Kinetics.

Analyze Yourself

Assessing Fitness Testing Behavior

Name _____ **Date** _____

Instructions: Indicate how often each of the following occurs in your daily activities and exercise sessions. Respond to each item with a number from 0 to 3, using the following scale:

0 = Never   **1** = Occasionally   **2** = Most of the time   **3** = Always

____ **1.** I regularly complete some type of aerobic fitness test to evaluate my cardiovascular endurance.

____ **2.** I complete an abdominal strength test using some type of modified sit-up at least every several years.

____ **3.** I have a medical examination on a regular basis and annually if I participate in a college sport.

____ **4.** I always follow a preconditioning program for a few weeks before undergoing any type of exercise testing.

____ **5.** I regularly complete at least one upper-body strength test such as the bench press.

____ **6.** I check my range of motion in the major joints in some manner at least once per year.

____ **7.** I regularly use nutritional software to analyze the nutrients in my diet.

____ **8.** I keep my personal medical file with all test results ordered by my physician for future reference and comparison.

____ **9.** I use some form of body-composition analysis (skinfold measurements, hydrostatic weighing, waist-to-hip ratio, BMI) to examine my body-fat content and risk of disease.

____ **10.** I keep a personal record file on my fitness test scores for comparison over the years.

Scoring: Excellent = 25-30

Good = 19-24

Poor = Below 19

From *Physical fitness and wellness, third edition*, by Jerrold S. Greenberg, George B. Dintiman, and Barbee Myers Oakes, 2004, Champaign, IL: Human Kinetics.

Medical Evaluation

An abundance of literature points to the need for medical evaluation before beginning a program of regular exercise. Experts disagree, however, about what components such a medical evaluation should include, who should receive one, and even whether an evaluation is necessary at all. These viewpoints will be presented as objectively as possible to help you make a decision about your need for such an examination.

Need for a Medical Evaluation

Most physicians indicate that a physical examination is necessary for individuals over the age of 46, those with symptoms of heart disease or other medical ailments, and those who have previously been sedentary. Some physicians favor a comprehensive exam; others prefer only general screening.

The recommendations of the American College of Sports Medicine (ACSM) provide sound information related to health, status, and age of the participant (see table 2.1). The ACSM classi-fies individuals who may undergo exercise testing into three categories:

Apparently healthy—those who appear to be in good health and have no major coronary risk factors

Individuals at higher risk—those who have symptoms suggestive of heart disease, pulmonary or metabolic disease, or at least one major coronary risk factor

Individuals with disease—those with known cardiac, pulmonary, or metabolic diseases

The National Heart, Lung, and Blood Institute (NHLBI) advises that most people under 60 years of age do not need a medical examination before beginning a gradual and sensible exercise program. Their rationale is based on the realization that sedentary living is a far more dangerous practice than exercising without a physician's approval, that many people will not take the time to secure an examination, and that a recommended medical exam is nothing more than another excuse to avoid exercise.

TABLE 2.1—ACSM Recommendations for Current Medical Examination* and Exercise Testing Prior to Participation and Physician Supervision of Exercise Tests

	Low risk	Moderate risk	High risk
CURRENT (WITHIN PAST YEAR) MEDICAL EXAMINATION AND EXERCISE TESTING BEFORE PARTICIPATION			
Moderate exercise[a]	Not necessary[b]	Not necessary	Recommended
Vigorous exercise[c]	Not necessary	Recommended	Recommended
PHYSICIAN SUPERVISION OF EXERCISE TESTS			
Submaximal test	Not necessary	Not necessary	Recommended
Maximal test	Not necessary	Recommended[d]	Recommended

*Within the past year.

[a]Absolute moderate exercise is defined as activities that are approximately 3 to 6 METs or the equivalent of brisk walking at 3 to 4 mph for most healthy adults. Nevertheless, a pace of 3 to 4 mph might be considered hard to very hard by some sedentary, older persons. Moderate exercise may alternatively be defined as an intensity well within the individual's capacity, one that can be comfortably sustained for a prolonged period (about 45 min), has a gradual initiation and progression, and is generally noncompetitive. If an individual's exercise capacity is known, relative moderate exercise may be defined by the range of 40 to 60% maximal oxygen uptake.

[b]The designation "Not necessary" reflects the notion that a medical examination, exercise test, and physician supervision of exercise testing would not be essential in the preparticipation screening; however, they should not be viewed as inappropriate.

[c]Vigorous exercise is defined as activities of >6 METs. Vigorous exercise may alternatively be defined as exercise intense enough to represent a substantial cardiorespiratory challenge. If an individual's exercise capacity is known, vigorous exercise may be defined as an intensity of >60% maximal oxygen uptake.

[d]When physician supervision of exercise testing is "Recommended," the physician should be in close proximity and readily available should an emergent need occur.

Reprinted, by permission, from American College of Sports Medicine, *ACSM guidelines to exercise testing and prescription*, 6th ed. (Philadelphia, PA: Lippincott, Williams, and Wilkins), 21.

Certainly, to increase safety and aid in the exercise prescription, it is desirable for everyone to have a complete medical examination before a physical fitness evaluation and the start of a new exercise program. Most experts believe that certain categories of people face some risk when engaging in fitness programs without a medical examination.

Components of the Ideal Medical Evaluation

Although the exact contents of the ideal evaluation depend on the history and symptoms of each person, common areas include a medical history that asks questions about your own and your family's history of diabetes and coronary heart disease and associated risk factors such as hypertension, stress, smoking, eating habits, current activity level, and physical disabilities. If symptoms indicate the need, the examination may also include measurement of blood pressure, listening to the sounds of the heart and lungs, determination of the resting pulse rate, a chest x ray, **blood-lipid analysis,** a resting **electrocardiogram (ECG),** and a **graded exercise test (stress test).**

The examiner should discuss the results of this medical evaluation with the patient and identify at that time any restrictions on physical activity or fitness testing. Remember that the fact that your

blood-lipid analysis—Examination and study of the fats present in the blood.

electrocardiogram (ECG)—A tracing of the electrical currents involved in the cycles of a heartbeat.

graded exercise test (stress test)—Test designed to monitor the electrical activity of the heart; subjects perform it by walking on a treadmill that is slowly elevated to increase the workload.

health-related fitness—An adequate or above-average level of achievement, based on test scores, in components such as cardiorespiratory endurance, muscular strength and endurance, flexibility, and body composition that has been associated with the prevention of certain diseases and disorders, high energy, and a high level of wellness.

physical activity may have limits does not mean you should avoid exercise. This book provides you with a number of sound exercise choices that will meet your fitness needs without endangering your health.

Self-Screening Versus the Medical Examination

Healthy college students and other individuals under the age of 45 can reduce the risk of participation in a testing and fitness program by completing a simple physical activity readiness questionnaire (PAR-Q). Canadian researchers developed the tool to identify the small number of adults who may not be able to complete a fitness testing or exercise program safely.

Take a moment to complete the questionnaire in figure 2.1. If your response to any question is yes, consult your physician before completing a fitness test battery or initiating a new exercise program. If each response is no, you are ready to complete the test battery in this chapter.

Fitness Appraisal

Besides having the medical evaluation, you should also appraise your present level of health-related fitness to monitor your body's response to exercise, to prepare your individualized program, and to monitor your progress.

Specific tests in this section are classified and described according to each component of **health-related fitness:** cardiorespiratory endurance, muscular strength, muscular endurance, flexibility, nutrition, and body composition. Several tests are provided in each area to allow you

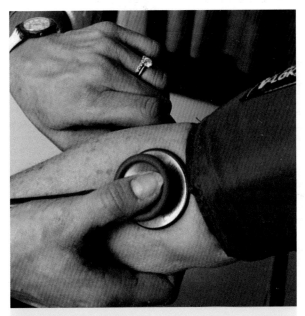

Measuring blood pressure may be part of your medical evaluation before beginning an exercise program.

PhotoDisc

Physical Activity Readiness
Questionnaire - PAR-Q
(revised 2002)

PAR-Q & YOU

(A Questionnaire for People Aged 15 to 69)

Regular physical activity is fun and healthy, and increasingly more people are starting to become more active every day. Being more active is very safe for most people. However, some people should check with their doctor before they start becoming much more physically active.

If you are planning to become much more physically active than you are now, start by answering the seven questions in the box below. If you are between the ages of 15 and 69, the PAR-Q will tell you if you should check with your doctor before you start. If you are over 69 years of age, and you are not used to being very active, check with your doctor.

Common sense is your best guide when you answer these questions. Please read the questions carefully and answer each one honestly: check YES or NO.

YES	NO	
❏	❏	**1. Has your doctor ever said that you have a heart condition <u>and</u> that you should only do physical activity recommended by a doctor?**
❏	❏	**2. Do you feel pain in your chest when you do physical activity?**
❏	❏	**3. In the past month, have you had chest pain when you were not doing physical activity?**
❏	❏	**4. Do you lose your balance because of dizziness or do you ever lose consciousness?**
❏	❏	**5. Do you have a bone or joint problem (for example, back, knee or hip) that could be made worse by a change in your physical activity?**
❏	❏	**6. Is your doctor currently prescribing drugs (for example, water pills) for your blood pressure or heart condition?**
❏	❏	**7. Do you know of <u>any other reason</u> why you should not do physical activity?**

If

you

answered

YES to one or more questions

Talk with your doctor by phone or in person BEFORE you start becoming much more physically active or BEFORE you have a fitness appraisal. Tell your doctor about the PAR-Q and which questions you answered YES.

- You may be able to do any activity you want — as long as you start slowly and build up gradually. Or, you may need to restrict your activities to those which are safe for you. Talk with your doctor about the kinds of activities you wish to participate in and follow his/her advice.
- Find out which community programs are safe and helpful for you.

NO to all questions

If you answered NO honestly to <u>all</u> PAR-Q questions, you can be reasonably sure that you can:

- start becoming much more physically active – begin slowly and build up gradually. This is the safest and easiest way to go.
- take part in a fitness appraisal – this is an excellent way to determine your basic fitness so that you can plan the best way for you to live actively. It is also highly recommended that you have your blood pressure evaluated. If your reading is over 144/94, talk with your doctor before you start becoming much more physically active.

DELAY BECOMING MUCH MORE ACTIVE:

- if you are not feeling well because of a temporary illness such as a cold or a fever – wait until you feel better; or
- if you are or may be pregnant – talk to your doctor before you start becoming more active.

PLEASE NOTE: If your health changes so that you then answer YES to any of the above questions, tell your fitness or health professional. Ask whether you should change your physical activity plan.

<u>Informed Use of the PAR-Q:</u> The Canadian Society for Exercise Physiology, Health Canada, and their agents assume no liability for persons who undertake physical activity, and if in doubt after completing this questionnaire, consult your doctor prior to physical activity.

No changes permitted. You are encouraged to photocopy the PAR-Q but only if you use the entire form.

NOTE: If the PAR-Q is being given to a person before he or she participates in a physical activity program or a fitness appraisal, this section may be used for legal or administrative purposes.

"I have read, understood and completed this questionnaire. Any questions I had were answered to my full satisfaction."

NAME _____

SIGNATURE _____ DATE _____

SIGNATURE OF PARENT _____ WITNESS _____
or GUARDIAN (for participants under the age of majority)

Note: This physical activity clearance is valid for a maximum of 12 months from the date it is completed and becomes invalid if your condition changes so that you would answer YES to any of the seven questions.

 © Canadian Society for Exercise Physiology

Supported by: 🍁 Health   Santé
Canada   Canada

Reprinted from the 1994 revised version of the Physical Activity Readiness Questionnaire (PAR-Q and YOU). The PAR-Q and YOU is a copyrighted, pre-exercise screen, owned by the Canadian Society for Exercise Physiology.

Figure 2.1 PAR-Q and You

to make appropriate choices depending on the facilities and equipment available, your specific likes and dislikes, and physical and emotional factors that may cause you to favor one test over another. For a more comprehensive analysis of your health-related fitness, we recommend taking additional tests. This section also describes the proper techniques to administer each test.

To help you interpret your scores, Discovery Activity 2.1: Your Physical Fitness Profile provides test norms and standards next to where you record your scores. In this lab we have also attempted to provide a health interpretation for your fitness scores based on the various test norm categories in which you fall. Besides comparing your scores to other college students of a similar age, we analyze the health implications of your scores.

During your fitness appraisal, stop any test immediately if you begin to feel chest pains, faintness, or dizziness; develop an excruciating headache; or cannot get enough air. If you notice any other disturbing sensations, do not complete the test. If any of these symptoms appear, consult a physician to determine their causes. Your fitness level may simply be so low that your body cannot handle strenuous activity, or a medical problem may exist. To avoid endangering your health and to eliminate worry, you should have the problem diagnosed.

Cardiorespiratory Assessment

All sound exercise programs place primary emphasis on cardiorespiratory endurance. The publicity surrounding the benefits of exercise in combating the nation's leading killer (heart disease), whether justified or not, is probably responsible for the emphasis on improving the functioning of the heart, circulatory system, and lungs. Exercise that overloads the **oxygen-transport system** (aerobic activity) leads to an increase in cardiorespiratory endurance and the muscular strength and endurance of some large muscle groups.

The aerobic metabolism energy system is used primarily in activities lasting longer than 3 minutes and is the major energy source for daily activities and endurance exercise. The maximal

oxygen-transport system—The ability of the body to take in and use oxygen at the tissue level during physical activity.

aerobic power, or maximal oxygen consumption ($\dot{V}O_2$max), of females is also lower than that of males. Before puberty the $\dot{V}O_2$max of girls and boys is the same. Most researchers estimate that the $\dot{V}O_2$max of women is 15 to 25% lower than that of adult males past 20 years of age. Table 2.2 shows gender differences in $\dot{V}O_2$max. As you can see, from age 20 men have consistently higher $\dot{V}O_2$max values than do women.

Table 2.2 also clearly shows a consistent decline in $\dot{V}O_2$max, or maximal aerobic power, every decade past the age of 20 for both women and men. For both sexes, there is a 25% decline in $\dot{V}O_2$max in the more than 40 years of life after age 20. This decrease in aerobic power is reflected in lesser endurance times among adult athletes.

Women have a lower $\dot{V}O_2$max than men do for several reasons. Because $\dot{V}O_2$max is a product of oxygen delivery to the muscles times the amount of oxygen extracted from the blood by the muscles, several major systems are involved. The cardiorespiratory system is responsible for delivering oxygen to the muscles. In particular, cardiac output determines the amount of oxygen delivered to the muscles. The maximal stroke volume is lower in women than in men because women have smaller hearts than men do. Also, as can be seen in table 2.3 the maximal heart rate is lower in women than in men regardless of age. Thus, the overall output of the heart is lower in women than in men because of a lower number of beats in a given period and a smaller amount of blood pumped by the heart with each beat.

Another factor affecting gender differences in the amount of oxygen delivered to the muscles is the difference in blood volume and amount of hemoglobin in the blood. Women tend to have

TABLE 2.2—Gender Differences in $\dot{V}O_2$max

Age	Males	Females
20-29	40.0	31.1
30-39	37.5	30.3
40-49	36.0	28.0
50-59	33.6	25.7
Over 60	30.0	22.9

(ml O$_2$/kg^{-1}/min^{-1}) (50th percentile)

Data from J.H. Wilmore, M. Pollock, and S.M. Fox, 1978, *Health and fitness through physical activity* (New York: John Wiley & Sons, Inc.).

lower total blood volume than do men. Hemoglobin is responsible for carrying oxygen in the bloodstream to the muscles. Women also have lower concentrations of hemoglobin in the blood than men do. Because both the total amount of blood and its oxygen-carrying capacity are lower in women, the maximal aerobic capacity of women is lower than that of men.

In terms of the amount of oxygen removed from the blood for use by the muscles, women also have less capacity because they have small muscle masses. If you compare the amount of oxygen used per unit of muscle, there is little difference between women and men. But when the total amount of oxygen used by muscles is compared, women have less capacity. For this reason, it is important to learn different ways of expressing the $\dot{V}O_2$max when examining sex differences.

The $\dot{V}O_2$max is highest in women who participate in endurance sports. Table 2.4 shows body composition and $\dot{V}O_2$max data for female athletes of varying ages. As can be seen, women who participate in cross-country skiing have the highest measured $\dot{V}O_2$max. The next highest values occur in women engaging in activities such as the triathlon, track and field, cycling, and cross-country running. Participants in sports that do not require high aerobic capacity, such as golf, have lower $\dot{V}O_2$max values. Note that some of the highest

TABLE 2.3—Gender Differences in Resting and Maximal Heart Rates

Age	RESTING		MAXIMAL	
	Males	Females	Males	Females
20-29	64	67	192	188
30-39	63	68	188	183
40-49	64	68	181	175
50-59	63	68	171	169
Over 60	63	65	159	151

(50th percentile) (in beats/min^{-1})

Data from J.H. Wilmore, M. Pollock, and S.M. Fox, 1978, *Health and fitness through physical activity* (New York: John Wiley & Sons, Inc.).

TABLE 2.4—Body Composition and Maximal $\dot{V}O_2$ Data for Female Athletes of Varying Ages

Athletic group or sport	Age	Height (cm)	Weight (kg)	Relative fat (%)	Maximal $\dot{V}O_2$ (ml/kg^{-1}/min^{-1})
Basketball	19.1	169.1	62.6	20.8	42.9
Bicycling	-	167.7	61.3	15.4	57.4
Dancing, ballet	15.0	161.1	48.4	16.4	48.9
General	21.2	162.7	51.2	20.5	41.5
Golf	33.3	168.9	61.8	24.0	34.2
Gymnastics	15.2	161.1	50.4	13.1	45.2
	19.4	163.0	57.9	23.8	36.3
Pentathlon	21.5	175.4	65.4	11.0	45.9
Racquetball	23.0	173.0	68.0	14.0	-

Athletic group or sport	Age	Height (cm)	Weight (kg)	Relative fat (%)	Maximal $\dot{V}O_2$ (ml/kg^{-1}/min^{-1})
Skating, figure	16.5	158.8	48.6	12.5	48.9
Skiing, alpine	19.5	165.1	58.8	20.6	52.7
Cross country	20.2	163.4	55.9	15.7	61.5
	24.3	163.0	59.1	21.8	68.2
Swimming	19.4	168.0	63.8	26.3	37.6
Distance	-	166.3	60.9	17.1	43.2
Tennis	39.0	163.3	55.7	20.3	44.2
Track and field	19.9	161.3	52.9	19.2	57.5
	32.4	169.4	57.2	15.2	59.1
	43.8	161.5	53.8	18.3	43.4
Sprint	20.1	164.9	56.7	19.3	-
Cross country	15.6	163.3	50.9	15.4	50.8
Discus	21.1	168.1	71.0	25.0	-
Jumping and hurdling	20.3	165.9	59.0	20.7	-
Shot put	21.5	167.6	78.1	28.0	-
Triathlon	-	-	-	12.6	58.7
Volleyball	19.9	172.2	64.1	21.3	43.5
Weightlifting					
Bodybuilding	27.0	160.8	53.8	13.2	-

Reprinted from J.H. Wilmore and D.L. Costill, 1988, *Training for sport and activity: The physiological basis of the conditioning process*, 3rd ed. (Dubuque, IA: Wm. C. Brown Publishers). Reproduced with permission of The McGraw-Hill Companies.

recorded $\dot{V}O_2$max values have been for women older than 30.

Run-Walk Tests

You can assess your cardiorespiratory endurance using a **run-walk test**—either the 1.5-mile run test, 1-mile run, 3-mile walk, 9-minute run test, or 12-minute run test.

The 1-mile run, 1.5-mile run test, and 3-mile walk can be completed indoors or outdoors. Begin by measuring off a 1- to 3-mile course on a track

> **run-walk tests**—Field tests designed to measure cardiorespiratory endurance (aerobic fitness).

or other flat area where you can run or walk. After performing an adequate warm-up consisting of 8 to 12 minutes of walking and jogging followed by 4 to 5 minutes of stretching, your objective is to complete the distance as quickly as possible by running, walking, or combining the two. You can easily time yourself in the 3-mile walk test on the track or an accurately measured grass or sidewalk area. Record your times and ratings in Discovery Activity 2.1 at the end of this chapter.

The 9-minute run test and 12-minute run test are best performed on a 400-meter track or other measured area that allows the tester to determine the exact distance you cover after 9 or 12 minutes. Markers can be placed every 10 to 25 yards on the

Myth and Fact Sheet

Myth	Fact
1. Cardiorespiratory fitness testing is too dangerous	**1.** All of the running tests (1.5-mile run, 9- and 12-minute run tests) are run-walk tests that allow you to go at your own safe pace. You can also stop anytime during the Harvard step test if you have trouble. The tests are not dangerous if performed properly. If you have been inactive for more than a year or have never engaged in aerobic exercise, you have several choices. First, you can skip these tests, assume that your cardiorespiratory fitness rating is poor, and choose a beginner's aerobic exercise program that allows you to progress slowly and safely to higher levels. Second, you can undertake a 2- to 3-week preconditioning program of walking and jogging to prepare yourself for the 1.5-mile run test. Finally, you can choose to stop and walk during any of the tests as long as you give your best effort.
2. Fitness testing will make you too sore to function the next day.	**2.** When sedentary people complete tests that require maximum effort, they do experience considerable soreness the next day. The areas of soreness show which muscles you have not been using. Many college instructors eliminate the problem of soreness by using a 2- to 3-week preconditioning program before having any of their students perform any maximum-effort fitness testing.
3. You know enough about your fitness level already and do not need to be tested.	**3.** You may have a good feel for some aspects of your physical fitness. On the other hand, standardized tests may be just what you need to compare yourself to others of your age and to highlight the areas in which you need the most improvement. Test results often provide strong motivation for individuals to begin an exercise program.
4. You're fit enough—too much exercise will cause "athlete's heart" and jeopardize your health.	**4.** "Athlete's heart," or "sportherz," is a term used by a Swedish researcher who detected enlarged heart muscles among skiers in 1899. As the years passed, the term gained momentum and was used incorrectly to refer to an abnormally large heart brought on by exercise. Because of this myth, some people became concerned that exercise would damage their hearts and result in disability or death. Aerobic exercise does develop the heart muscle more fully and cause it to become heavier and larger. Exercise also causes the heart to pump more blood per beat (stroke volume) and per minute (cardiac output) and to become a more efficient organ. Cardiac changes that occur from aerobic exercise are both natural and healthy, and it is highly unlikely that proper aerobic exercise will cause damage to a healthy heart.
5. Abdominal exercise tests are not necessary because one doesn't have to be capable of performing a high number of sit-ups to be fit.	**5.** Abdominal strength and endurance are important in maintaining posture, protecting the lower back from injury, performing daily chores, and building a positive body image. Although the test may produce some muscle soreness the following day, it will also give you a good indication of the strength and endurance of your midsection.
6. Sit-ups and other abdominal exercises will give me a flat tummy.	**6.** Regular upper and lower abdominal work will strengthen the muscles in that area. A reduced caloric intake that shrinks fat cells, regular aerobic exercise, a high number of repetitions of several types of sit-ups, and 4 to 6 months will be required to move toward a flat midriff. Calorie restriction and aerobic exercise will shrink the fat cells; abdominal exercises will strengthen the abdominal muscles.

course with a spotter assigned to each runner to improve the accuracy of scoring. After warming up and stretching properly, you stand on the starting line and await the signal to run and walk as many laps as possible around the course within the allotted time. When the allotted time expires, the tester blows a whistle, signaling the spotter, who has also been counting laps, to mark the distance to the nearest 10 yards. In the meantime, you should continue to jog or walk for a 4- to 5-minute cool-down period.

Cycling and Swimming Tests

If you prefer to swim or cycle, you can determine your level of cardiorespiratory endurance using a **cycling or swimming test**—either the 12-minute swimming test or the 12-minute cycling test. You should first complete an adequate warm-up consisting of swimming or slow pedaling followed by 4 to 5 minutes of stretching. Both tests are completed in the same manner in a swimming pool or on a premeasured road course with total yards recorded at the point where time expires in the swimming test and total miles recorded (to the nearest 10th) in the cycling test. Scores and rating categories are recorded in Discovery Activity 2.1.

Harvard Step Test

The **Harvard step test** provides an alternative assessment method that accurately identifies your cardiorespiratory fitness level. Because test results are based on accurate resting and exercise heart rates, you should improve your skill in this area by completing Discovery Activity 2.2: Determining Your Resting and Exercise Heart Rate. To complete the test, secure a sturdy 18-inch bench or stool and a wristwatch with a second hand and then follow these procedures:

1. Step on the bench first with one foot and then the other until you are standing erect with the knees unbent. Then step down with one foot followed by the other to return to the starting position.
2. Step at a cadence that will result in 30 such repetitions each minute (1 every 2 seconds) for 4 minutes (females) or 5 minutes (males).
3. At the end of the 4- or 5-minute period, sit down.
4. After waiting exactly 1 minute, take your pulse or have a partner take your pulse for 30 seconds, and record that number.

5. Wait an additional 30 seconds before taking your pulse again for a 30-second period, and record that number.
6. Wait again for 30 seconds and take your pulse a third time for 30 seconds. You will now have taken your pulse between 1 and 1 1/2 minutes, 2 and 2 1/2 minutes, and 3 and 3 1/2 minutes after completing the step test.
7. Using the total of the three pulse counts, compute the following formula:

$$\text{index} = \frac{\text{duration of exercise in seconds} \times 100}{2 \times \text{sum of three pulse counts in recovery}}$$

Again, record your scores in Discovery Activity 2.1 and determine your cardiorespiratory fitness level from table 2.F.

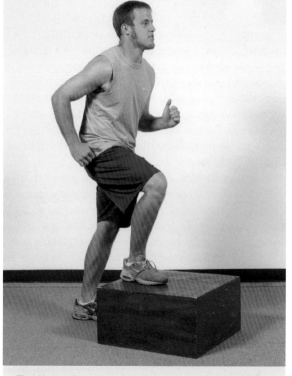

The Harvard step test is one way to determine your cardiorespiratory endurance. The test involves stepping up and down repeatedly and then measuring the pulse rate to determine how fast the heart recovers.

Muscular Strength Assessment

In the laboratory, muscular strength, the absolute maximum force that a muscle can generate, is measured using elaborate and expensive equipment: Dynamometers, cable tensiometers, and force transducers and recorders have all been used this way. One problem with such methods is the need to test numerous muscle groups to obtain an accurate measure in the legs, abdomen, and arms. These muscles, however, cover body parts so diverse that you can safely assume their levels of muscular strength are representative of total body strength.

You can also measure the strength and endurance of practically any muscle group by using free weights or a variety of weight machines. In some cases, you can test yourself; in others, such as **1RM testing** using barbells, you will need a spotter to assist you throughout the movement.

In general, women's muscular strength is about 70% that of men. Part of the explanation for this phenomenon is that people participating in different types of sports use different types of muscle fibers—specifically, **slow-twitch (ST)** and **fast-twitch (FT) fibers.**

Both women and men who participate in endurance sports have a higher percentage of ST fibers. Women and men who participate in anaerobic sports have a higher percentage of FT fibers. Men and women do not differ in percentage of ST fibers. The gender difference appears in the size of the muscle fibers, not the percentage. Female athletes who participate in endurance sports have 66 and 71% of the male FT and ST fiber areas, respectively. This smaller total muscle mass in women accounts for the difference in total muscle strength.

Have you ever wondered why women in a weight-training class do not experience the same degree of muscular **hypertrophy** as men even when they use the same training program? Both women and men will increase in strength with a weight-training program. Women may even achieve a greater percentage increase in strength. Yet women seldom experience the muscular bulkiness seen in men following intense weight-training programs. The primary reason for this is that muscular hypertrophy is controlled by the male sex hormone testosterone. The level of testosterone in the blood is about 10 times higher in men than in women. Because women have lower levels of testosterone, they will experience less muscular development, although they will gain strength from participating in a weight-training program.

1RM (repetition maximum) testing—Free weights are commonly used to determine your 1RM (maximum amount of weight you can lift one time) for a particular muscle group.

slow-twitch (ST) fibers—The type of muscle fibers used in endurance sports; equipped metabolically to meet the demands of aerobic activities of long duration.

fast-twitch (FT) fibers—The type of muscle fibers used in anaerobic, power sports; equipped metabolically to meet the demands of short-duration, high-intensity activities.

hypertrophy—An increase in the size of the muscle.

You should also remember that because women have a smaller total muscle mass than men, they will also have less muscle hypertrophy than men. Finally, because women have more subcutaneous body fat than men do, much of the muscular hypertrophy they experience is masked beneath the layers of fat. As women lose body fat, they will see greater muscle definition, but they need not worry about becoming too "masculine" because of participating in a weight-training program.

The bench press and shoulder press accurately measure the strength of your triceps, pectoralis, and deltoid muscles; the arm curl measures biceps muscle strength; and the leg press determines the strength of the quadriceps muscle group. For each test, you select a weight that you can lift comfortably. You then add additional weight in subsequent trials until you find the weight that you can lift correctly only one time. If you can lift the weight more than once, add weight until you determine a true 1RM. Approximately three trials with a 2- to 3-minute rest interval after each are needed to determine the 1RM for each muscle group. Because the resistance you must overcome in 1RM testing is heavy, you should use one or two spotters to protect you from injury should you be unable to complete the lift. (Chapter 7 discusses the proper technique for these tests.) Record your scores in Discovery Activity 2.1.

Muscular Endurance Assessment

Muscular endurance and muscular strength are far different from one another, so the kinds of tests that apply to these components vary. Strength tests determine the maximum amount of weight that can be moved one time, whereas endurance tests measure continuous work by determining the total number of times a specific weight can be moved.

You can evaluate the muscular endurance of your abdominal area, arms, and shoulders by completing the curl test (men and women) and one of the following: the pull-up (men) or flexed-arm hand test (women) or the push-up (men) or modified push-up test (women).

Abdominal Endurance

Although obtaining a pure, isolated measurement of the abdominal region is difficult, the 1-minute abdominal curl test provides a fairly accurate score. To prepare for the test, place a strip of tape 3 inches wide across a mat (see figure 2.2). Lie on your back with your knees flexed, both feet flat on the floor as close to the hips as possible, and your fingertips at the edge of the strip. On signal, curl forward until your fingertips move forward 3 inches (from the front to the back of the tape), then curl back until both shoulder blades touch the mat. Your shoulder blades should lift from the

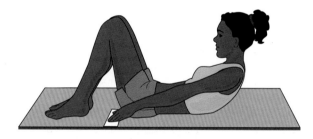

Figure 2.2   Abdominal curls.

mat with each repetition while your lower back and feet remain on the mat. Record the number of curls completed in 1 minute and your rating in Discovery Activity 2.1.

Arm and Shoulder Muscular Endurance

You can complete the pull-up test for men by grasping an adjustable horizontal bar with your palms facing away from your body. Raise your body until your chin clears the top of the bar and then slowly lower yourself to a full hand without any pause as many times as you can (see figure 2.3a). Your body must return to a stretch position (elbows locked) each time. Deliberate swinging, resting, or leg kicking is not permitted. The bench press and shoulder press columns in table 2.G will help you evaluate the strength and endurance of your arms and shoulders.

The modified pull-up test for women closely resembles the pull-up for men. Grasp an adjustable horizontal bar with your palms facing away from your body at a level that is just even with the base of the sternum (breastbone). Place your body under the bar until a 90-degree angle is formed at the point where your arms and chest join. Only your heels support the weight of your lower body (see figure 2.3b). You score 1 point each time you pull your chin over the bar and return your body to the support position with your arms fully extended.

The push-up test for men begins with your arms and back straight and your fingers forward. Lower your chest to the floor until your elbows

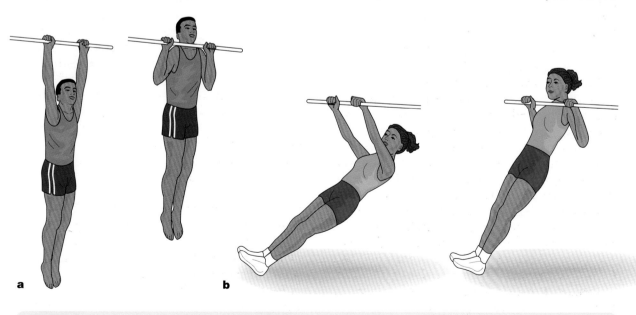

a   b

Figure 2.3   (a) Pull-ups and (b) modified pull-ups.

form a right angle and your upper arms are parallel to the floor (the chest must almost touch the floor) before returning to the starting position (see figure 2.4a). The modified push-up test for women is performed in a similar manner but with the knees rather than the toes supporting the body (see figure 2.4b). Again, record your scores and ratings in Discovery Activity 2.1.

Flexibility Assessment

Flexibility is an important component of fitness. It involves the ability to move the body throughout a range of motion and stretch the muscles and tissues around skeletal joints. The shoulder reach, trunk flexion, and trunk extension tests provide an excellent indication of body flexibility.

Shoulder Reach

You can complete the shoulder reach test by standing against a pole or a projecting corner, raising your right arm, and reaching down behind your back as far as possible. At the same time, reach up from behind with your left hand and try to overlap the palm of your right hand (see figure 2.5a). Have a partner measure, in inches, how much the fingers on your right hand overlap the fingers of your left hand. If you overlap, place a plus sign in front of the amount of overlap in

Discovery Activity 2.1; if the fingers of your right and left hand do not touch, place a minus sign in front of the amount of the gap. If the fingers of one hand just barely touch those of the other, give yourself a score of zero. Repeat this test with your arms reversed; that is, the arm that first reached down over the shoulder will now reach up from behind the back.

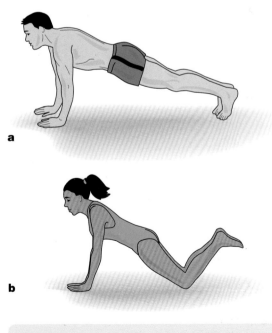

Figure 2.4 (a) Push-ups and (b) modified push-ups.

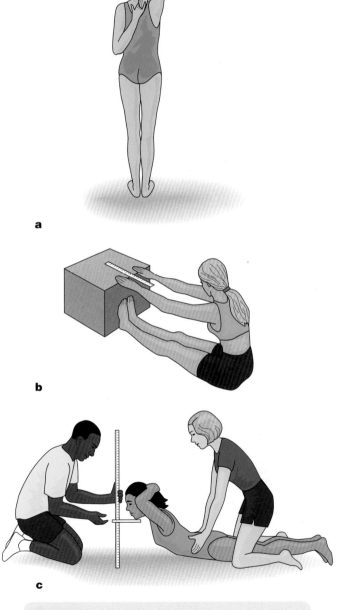

Figure 2.5 Flexibility: (a) shoulder reach test, (b) trunk flexion, (c) trunk extension.

Trunk Flexion

The trunk flexion test measures your ability to flex your trunk and stretch the back of your thigh muscles. To begin, remove your shoes and sit with your legs straight and your feet flat against a box positioned against a wall. Place a ruler on top of the box. Place one hand on top of the other so your middle fingers are together and the same length. While your partner keeps your knees from bending, lean forward and place your hands on top of the box. Slide your hands along the measuring scale as far as possible without bouncing and hold that position for at least 3 seconds (see figure 2.5b). Perform the test two more times and record your highest score to the nearest inch in Discovery Activity 2.1. Your score is the number of inches beyond the edge of the box you can stretch (use a plus sign in front of that value) or the number of inches short of the edge of the box you can reach (use a minus sign in front of that value). If you can reach only to the edge of the box, give yourself a score of zero.

Trunk Extension

To determine the flexibility of your back, complete the trunk extension test. Lie on the floor face down with a partner applying pressure on your upper legs and buttocks. Clasp your hands behind your neck, raise your head and chest off the ground as high as possible, and hold that position for 3 seconds (see figure 2.5c). Ask your partner to measure the distance to the nearest inch between your chin and the floor. Again, enter this value in Discovery Activity 2.1.

Nutritional Assessment

Numerous IBM- and Apple Macintosh-compatible software programs are available to analyze your dietary intake accurately over a 3- to 7-day period. Regardless of the software program you choose, you will need to record your dietary intake (food and drink) carefully over the period, making note of portion sizes, brand names of products when available, specific fast-food products, and other information that you will code later according to the specifications of the software manual.

Body-Composition Assessment

The average adult female is 3 to 4 inches shorter, weighs 25 to 30 pounds less, and has 10 to 15 pounds more fat tissue than the typical adult male does. These differences are usually present even among athletes. The average gender differences in body-fat percentage are shown in table 2.5. In every age category, women have a higher percentage of body fat than men do. For both men and women, the body-fat percentage increases as they get older.

The reason for a higher percentage of body fat in women as compared with men has to do with the types of fat in the body. **Essential fat** is stored in the muscles, heart, lungs, liver, spleen, intestines, kidneys, and bone marrow. **Storage fat** includes **subcutaneous tissue** and fat tissue that protects the internal organs. The higher body-fat level of women compared with men results primarily from women's higher percentage of essential fat. Women need a minimum of 12% body fat to maintain their essential body-fat stores and conduct all the necessary functions for normal body metabolism, whereas men only need 3% body fat. When women reduce their body-fat stores below 12%, menstrual disorders and hormone irregularities are likely to occur.

This higher level of body fat, coupled with a decrease in muscle mass, adversely affects physiological performance in females. Endurance activities are affected the most. In general, a high amount of body fat and a lesser amount of muscle mass will adversely affect any activity that demands that body weight be supported. This is one reason that women tend to have poorer performances in distance-running events.

TABLE 2.5—Gender Differences in Fat Percentage (50th percentile)

Age	Males	Females
20-29	21.6	25.0
30-39	22.4	24.8
40-49	23.4	26.1
50-59	24.1	29.3
Over 60	23.1	28.3

Data from J.H. Wilmore, M. Pollock, and S.M. Fox, 1978, *Health and fitness through physical activity* (New York: John Wiley & Sons, Inc.).

essential fat—The amount of fat required for normal physiological functioning.

storage fat—Fat that is stored in the adipose tissue.

subcutaneous tissue—The layer of adipose tissue directly beneath the skin.

Let's take another look at table 2.4. The wide range of body-fat percentages shown illustrates the diversity among women who participate in different sports. Women who participate in some anaerobic sports have lower body-fat percentages than do women who participate in aerobic sports. Thus, the energy system used is not the primary criterion for estimating body-fat percentage among female athletes. Female athletes tend to manipulate their body-fat percentage to improve performance. The optimal percentage of body fat for the particular sport and the aesthetic value of having a low body-fat percentage are important determinants for female athletes in maintaining a particular body-fat percentage.

Numerous tests are available to measure your body's composition. Height-weight charts, discussed in chapter 8, are perhaps the least accurate method of providing an indication of associated health risks, except for the extremely obese individual. Three practical tests—body-mass index, waist-to-hip ratio, and skinfold measures—provide an accurate assessment of your body composition and the associated health risks.

■ **Body-mass index (BMI).** This test provides a more sensitive indicator of body composition and health risks than body weight does. You can determine your BMI using figure 2.6 by placing a dot at your exact height in inches in the column to the right and another dot at your exact weight in pounds in the column to the left, drawing a straight line to connect the two dots, and recording the number where the line intersects the vertical column in the middle. The following categories are used to interpret BMI scores: underweight (less than 19), desirable (19 to 25), increased health risks (26 to 29), obese (30 to 40), and extremely obese (more than 40). Keep in mind that weights and heights are determined without clothing.

■ **Waist-to-hip ratio.** This test provides an indication of the way you store fat. Obese people who tend to store large amounts of fat in the abdominal area, rather than around the hips and thighs, are at higher risk for coronary heart disease, high blood pressure, congestive heart failure, strokes, and diabetes. To provide an accurate and practical indicator, a panel of scientists appointed by the National Academy of Sciences and the Dietary Guidelines Advisory Council for the U.S. Departments of Agriculture and Health and Human Services devised the waist-to-hip ratio test. The panel recommends weight loss for men with a waist-to-hip ratio of 1.0 or higher and for women with a ratio of 0.85 or higher. For example, John has a 40-inch waist and a 38-inch hip. His ratio of 1.05 (40 divided by 38) is indicative of increased risk for disease.

■ **Skinfold measures.** At various sites on the body, these measures provide an accurate indicator of your percentage of body fat. The four-site skinfold test described in chapter 8 is designed for both college men and college women.

The **body-mass index (BMI)** is not entirely accurate for everyone and must be viewed as only one indicator of obesity or overfatness. A muscular 6-foot-1-inch, 235-pound athlete with only 10% body fat would be considered obese. On the other hand, a 5-foot-9-inch, 175-pound individual would register an acceptable BMI even when he or she has a high degree of body fat, a circumstance that would place the person at much greater risk of cardiovascular disease

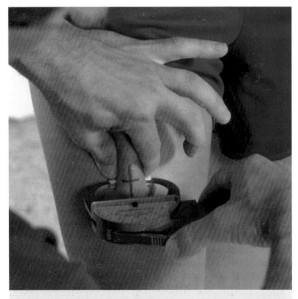

Taking skinfold measurements at several sites on the body is an accurate and easy way to determine a person's percentage of body fat.

body-mass index (BMI)—A method of determining overweight and obesity by dividing body weight (in pounds) by height (in inches) squared; this method is considered superior to height-weight table ranges.

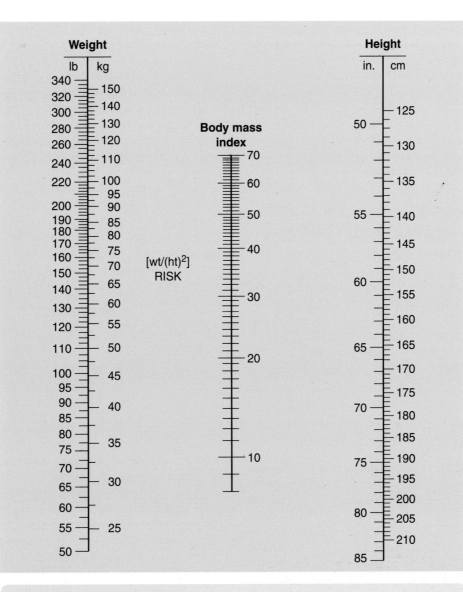

Figure 2.6   Nomogram for BMI.

than the athlete. Height-weight charts have similar limitations.

According to Gaesser (1999), an important question that remains to be answered is whether the proposed link between increased mortality and overweight results in large part from the greater prevalence of physical inactivity and low cardiorespiratory fitness in those individuals in the high BMI strata. Although the answer to this question is still under investigation, we do know that the correlation between sedentary living and high BMI is strong (Walcott-McQuigg et al., 2002 and Sjostrom, 1993).

Putting It All Together

Your fitness profile is complete. You can now evaluate your physical fitness in absolute terms (Are you satisfied with your levels of each component?) or in relative terms (Are you happy with how you compare with others?). Wellness requires information. Where are you now? Where do you want to be? How can you get there? Now that you have identified your current fitness level, you can decide on what goals you need to set for yourself. For example, if you are not satisfied with your cardiorespiratory fitness, read the remainder of this book with a view toward improving that component. You can do the same for muscular strength and endurance, flexibility, or body composition. This book contains the means for you to be successful at enhancing your level of physical fitness. All you need to do is apply them. Always keep in mind that improving one aspect of your health or fitness should not result in the decline of another component. You should strive for balance in all components of physical fitness.

Assessing Physical Fitness in Physically Disabled Individuals

Researchers are now exploring the role of physical activity as an integral factor in the rehabilitation of physically challenged individuals (Kennedy, 2001). The Physical Activity Scale for Individuals with Physical Disabilities (PASIPD) has emerged as a standard assessment tool for evaluating the activity level of those who are disabled (Washburn et al., 2002). We are now learning more about the complications of assessing the fitness level of those who are disabled because of trauma or disease.

In an effort to quantify differences in strength and aerobic work capacity, Van der Woude et al. (2002) studied 68 wheelchair athletes who competed in the World Games and Championships for the Disabled. Collectively, their level of cardiorespiratory fitness was generally high but was also highly variable among and within classified groups. As in nondisabled individuals, a clear gender difference in maximal aerobic fitness level does exist. Yet, accurately assessing fitness functionality for wheelchair athletes is often complicated by their age, the nature of the impairment, training status, coordination, and the talent or expertise of the individual.

Most persons with multiple sclerosis (MS) live 90% of a full life span, which in turn increased their risk for developing chronic conditions as they become older. In a recent study Slawta et al. (2002) studied the activity levels of women who had MS. Women are twice as likely as men to develop this chronic disease, yet many women with MS avoid participation in leisure-time physical activity (LTPA) (Stuifbergen and Roberts, 1997). The researchers reported an inverse association between LTPA and waist circumference. In addition, the higher the level of activity, the better the overall cardiovascular risk factor profile for women with MS. Hence, understanding the limitations to assessing the fitness level of individuals with MS may help

attenuate many of the barriers that prohibit those individuals from participating in structured exercise programs.

Over the past few decades, athletic competitions and sporting events have evolved considerably for individuals with physical disabilities (Steadward and Peterson, 1999). From assessing cardiorespiratory fitness (Chin et al., 2002) and static and dynamic balance in highly active lower-limb amputees (Buckley et al., 2002), to quantifying the role of exercise training in patients who have Parkinson's disease (Reuter and Engelhardt, 2002) or osteoarthritis (Penninx et al., 2001), there is an increasing need to establish a practical approach to evaluating the fitness level of those who are disabled.

Summary

Medical Evaluation   Not all experts agree that everyone starting an exercise program should obtain a medical evaluation. Even when there is agreement in this area, experts may disagree concerning exactly what the examination should entail. We recommend a medical examination after age 45 and at any age when identifiable risk or disease is present. The content of the evaluation depends on the age of the patient and the symptoms present. The evaluation may include taking a medical history, measuring blood pressure, listening to the sound of the heart and lungs, determining resting pulse rate, having a chest x ray, administering a resting ECG and a graded exercise test, and administering blood tests for blood fats and the ratio between high- and low-density lipoproteins. We also believe that you should decide whether you need a medical examination before you start exercise testing and an exercise program based on your knowledge of your personal health, present physical fitness level, and medical history.

Fitness Appraisal   The ideal health-related fitness appraisal should include measures of cardiorespiratory endurance, muscular strength and endurance, flexibility, nutrition, and body composition. This chapter allows you and your instructors to choose from a number of tests in each area depending on individual interest, equipment, and the time available for assessment. Cardiorespiratory endurance can be measured with any one or more of the following tests: the 1-mile, 1.5-mile, or 3-mile run-walk; the 9-minute or 12-minute run; the 12-minute swimming or cycling test; and the Harvard step test. The 1RM (amount

Behavioral Change and Motivational Strategies

Many factors influence adherence to an exercise program, and people offer many excuses for not exercising. Here are some barriers (roadblocks) to exercising and strategies for overcoming them.

Roadblock	Behavioral Change Strategy
You are too busy to exercise. Although your schedule periodically loosens up, it happens irregularly.	The best way to ensure that you exercise regularly is to set aside a certain time of day—the same time each day—that you will devote to exercising. In that way you will schedule events around your exercise time, rather than the other way around. If you use social support—that is, exercise with someone else—and set up an appointment with that person, you will be more likely to maintain your exercise program because you will not want to disappoint your exercise partner.
You feel self-conscious about your body and embarrassed to have others watch you exercise.	You can use self-talk. Remind yourself that other exercisers don't look so great either and that the only way that you will eventually feel better about your body is to exercise and change its shape. If need be, you can exercise by yourself—for example, by walking—or you can arrange a time to exercise at the gym or health club at times when it is least crowded.
Like many other people, you do not like undergoing a medical examination. Consequently, you will do anything to avoid it.	These feelings are natural. Fortunately, there are ways to make the experience less traumatic. You can use chaining to start the process of acquiring a medical exam. In this case, the first link on the chain is to call for an appointment. In addition, you can use the behavior change technique of covert rehearsal. Close your eyes and start by imagining being in the doctor's waiting room waiting for your turn to be called. When you can imagine yourself in this way, reward yourself with a few minutes of imagining a relaxing setting you enjoy—being at the beach, at a lake, in a place you find relaxing. Next, imagine being examined with no pain or discomfort involved. Reward yourself as you did before. Rehearsing your examination in this way will help alleviate anxious feelings.
List roadblocks interfering with your working on improving your body image.	Now cite behavioral change strategies that can help you overcome the roadblocks you just listed. If necessary, refer to chapter 4 for behavioral change and motivational strategies. If you need help, do not hesitate to ask your instructor for assistance.

1. _____

2. _____

3. _____

1. _____

2. _____

3. _____

of weight that can be lifted one time) measures muscular strength through one or more of the following tests: bench press, military press, two-arm curl, and leg press. Muscular endurance is determined through such tests as the abdominal curl, pull-ups (men), or modified pull-ups (women). Flexibility is measured using the shoulder reach, trunk flexion, and trunk extension tests. Tests designed to measure body composition include body-mass index (BMI), waist-to-hip ratio, and skinfold measures (explained in detail in chapter 8). Nutritional analysis is best completed by using software programs that analyze dietary intake over a period of 3 days.

For an accurate evaluation of your health-related fitness, you must give your best effort on each test while staying alert to physical signs of overexertion.

Assessing Physical Fitness in Physically Disabled Individuals   Researchers are studying the role of physical activity and physical fitness with respect to rehabilitating physically disabled persons. Many factors complicate fitness assessment of those who are disabled. For example, assessing functionality for wheelchair athletes is compounded by age, the nature of the impairment, training status, and the talent or expertise of the individual. Likewise, although being physically active is highly correlated with an improved cardiorespiratory risk factor profile among women with MS, we have little understanding of the limitations of assessing such individuals. With the increasing focus of research in this field, we need to establish practical approaches in evaluating the fitness level of those who are disabled.

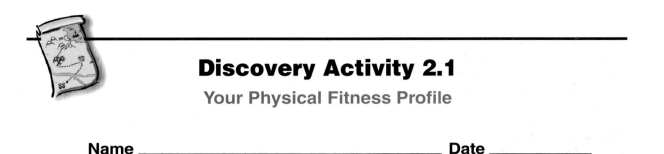

Discovery Activity 2.1

Your Physical Fitness Profile

Name _____ **Date** _____

Instructions: This lab allows you to choose from a number of tests within each of the major areas of health-related fitness. After you complete a test, consult the norm tables or standards and record your rating. Summarize your health-related fitness profile by completing section VII.

I. Cardiorespiratory Fitness

Health interpretation: Scores on any of the tests shown in table 2.6 that place you in the poor or very poor category, near the 5th percentile or below, or below the standards provided for the 3-mile walk and 12-minute swimming or cycling tests are considered unhealthy. You should strive to meet the minimum standards suggested or achieve scores that place you at the 50th percentile or above or that rate you at least average or fair in cardiorespiratory fitness. Scores that place you in the superior or excellent category or at the 95th percentile or above classify you as athletically fit.

TABLE 2.6—Test Scores for Cardiorespiratory Fitness

Test	Test standards (norms)	Score and rating
1-mile run test	See table 2.A on page 44.	Score_____ Rating_____
1.5-mile run test	See table 2.B on page 45.	Score_____ Rating_____
3-mile walk test	See table 2.C on page 45.	Score_____ Rating_____
9-minute run	See table 2.D on page 46.	Score_____ Rating_____
12-minute run	See table 2.E on page 47.	Score_____ Rating_____
Harvard step test	See table 2.F on page 47.	Score_____ Rating_____

(continued)

Discovery Activity 2.1 *(continued)*

TABLE 2.A—Norms for 1-Mile Run (Minutes and Seconds) for Ages 5 Through College

Percentile	AGE (YEARS)													
	5	6	7	8	9	10	11	12	13	14	15	16	17+	College
MALES														
95	9:02	9:06	8:06	7:58	7:17	6:56	6:50	6:27	6:11	5:51	6:01	5:48	6:01	5:30
75	11:32	10:55	9:37	9:14	8:36	8:10	8:00	7:24	6:52	6:36	6:35	6:28	6:36	6:12
50	13:46	12:29	11:25	11:00	9:56	9:19	9:06	8:20	7:27	7:10	7:14	7:11	7:25	6:49
25	16:05	15:10	14:02	13:29	12:00	11:05	11:31	10:00	8:35	8:02	8:04	8:07	8:26	7:32
5	18:25	17:38	17:17	16:19	15:44	14:28	15:25	13:41	10:23	10:32	10:37	10:40	10:56	9:47
FEMALES														
95	9:45	9:18	8:48	8:45	8:24	7:59	7:46	7:26	7:10	7:18	7:39	7:07	7:26	7:02
75	13:09	11:24	10:55	10:35	9:58	9:30	9:12	8:36	8:18	8:13	8:42	9:00	9:03	8:15
50	15:09	13:48	12:30	12:00	11:12	11:06	10:27	9:47	9:27	9:35	10:05	10:45	9:47	9:22
25	17:59	15:27	14:30	14:16	13:18	12:54	12:10	11:35	10:56	11:43	12:21	13:00	11:28	10:41
5	19:00	18:50	17:44	16:58	16:42	17:00	16:56	14:46	14:55	16:59	16:22	15:30	15:24	12:43

Adapted, by permission, from American Alliance of Health, Physical Education, Recreation, and Dance, 1980. Norms for 1-mile run for ages 5-college. In *Health related fitness test manual* (Reston, VA: AAHPERD); and R.R. Pate, 1985, *Norms for college students: Health related physical fitness test* (Reston, VA: AAHPERD).

Discovery Activity 2.1 *(continued)*

TABLE 2.B—Norms for 1.5-Mile Run Test (Minutes) for Ages 13 Through 60 and Older

Fitness category		AGE (YR)					
		13-19	20-29	30-39	40-49	50-59	60+
I. Very poor	Men	>15:31	>16:01	>16:31	>17:31	>19:01	>20:01
	Women	>18:31	>19:01	<19:31	>20:01	>20:31	>21:01
II. Poor	Men	12:11-15:30	14:01-16:00	14:44-16:30	15:36-17:30	17:01-19:00	19:01-20:00
	Women	16:55-18:30	18:31-19:00	19:01-19:30	19:31-20:00	20:01-20:30	21:00-21:31
III. Fair	Men	10:49-12:10	12:01-14:00	12:31-14:45	13:01-15:35	14:31-17:00	16:16-19:00
	Women	14:31-16:54	15:55-18:30	16:31-19:00	17:31-19:30	19:01-20:00	19:31-20:30
IV. Good	Men	9:41-10:48	10:46-12:00	11:01-12:30	11:31-13:00	12:31-14:30	14:00-16:15
	Women	12:30-14:30	13:31-15:54	14:31-16:30	15:56-17:30	16:31-19:00	17:31-19:30
V. Excellent	Men	8:37-9:40	9:45-10:45	10:00-11:00	10:30-11:30	11:00-12:30	11:15-13:59
	Women	11:50-12:29	12:30-13:30	13:00-14:30	13:45-15:55	14:30-16:30	16:30-17:30
VI. Superior	Men	<8:37	<9:45	<10:00	<10:30	<11:00	<11:15
	Women	<11:50	<12:30	<13:00	<13:45	<14:30	<16:30

Note: < means less than; > means more than.

From THE AEROBICS PROGRAM FOR TOTAL WELL BEING by Kenneth H. Cooper M.D., M.P.H., Copyright © 1982 by Kenneth H. Cooper. Used by permission of Bantam Books, a division of Random House, Inc.

TABLE 2.C—Standards for Classification of Good Fitness for 3-Mile Walk, 12-Minute Swimming, and 12-Minute Cycling Tests for Ages 13 Through 60 and Older

Test	AGE (YR)					
	13-19	20-29	30-39	40-49	50-59	≥60
MALES						
3-mile walking (min and sec)	33:00-37:30	34:00-38:30	35:00-40:00	36:30-42:00	39:00-45:00	41:00-48:00
12-minute swimming (yd)	700-799	600-699	550-649	500-599	450-549	400-499
12-minute cycling (mi)	3.75-5.75	4.50-5.49	4.25-5.24	4.00-4.99	3.50-4.49	3.00-3.99
FEMALES						
3-mile walking (min and sec)	35:00-39:30	36:00-40:30	37:30-42:00	39:00-44:00	42:00-47:00	45:00-51:00
12-minute swimming (yd)	600-699	500-599	450-549	400-499	350-449	300-399
12-minute cycling (mi)	3.75-4.74	3.50-4.49	3.25-4.24	3.00-3.99	2.50-3.49	2.00-2.99

Note: Lower times or greater distances place the individual in the excellent fitness category and higher times or lesser distances place the individual in the fair or very poor fitness categories.

From THE AEROBICS PROGRAM FOR TOTAL WELL BEING by Kenneth H. Cooper M.D., M.P.H., Copyright © 1982 by Kenneth H. Cooper. Used by permission of Bantam Books, a division of Random House, Inc.

(continued)

Discovery Activity 2.1 *(continued)*

TABLE 2.D—Norms for 9-Minute Run (Yards) for Ages 5 Through College

Percentile	AGE														
	5	6	7	8	9	10	11	12	13	14	15	16	17+	College
MALES															
95	1,760	1,750	2,020	2,200	2,175	2,250	2,250	2,400	2,402	2,473	2,544	2,615	2,615	2,640
75	1,320	1,469	1,683	1,810	1,835	1,910	1,925	1,975	2,096	2,167	2,238	2,309	2,380	2,349
50	1,170	1,280	1,440	1,595	1,660	1,690	1,725	1,760	1,885	1,956	2,027	2,098	2,169	2,200
25	990	1,090	1,243	1,380	1,440	1,487	1,540	1,500	1,674	1,745	1,816	1,887	1,958	1,945
5	600	816	990	1,053	1,104	1,110	1,170	1,000	1,368	1,439	1,510	1,581	1,652	1,652
FEMALES															
95	1,540	1,700	1,900	1,860	2,050	2,067	2,000	2,175	2,085	2,123	2,161	2,199	2,237	2,230
75	1,300	1,440	1,540	1,540	1,650	1,650	1,723	1,760	1,785	1,823	1,861	1,899	1,937	1,870
50	1,140	1,208	1,344	1,358	1,425	1,460	1,480	1,590	1,577	1,615	1,653	1,691	1,729	1,755
25	950	1,017	1,150	1,225	1,243	1,250	1,345	1,356	1,369	1,407	1,445	1,483	1,521	1,460
5	700	750	860	970	960	940	904	1,000	1,069	1,107	1,145	1,183	1,221	1,101

Adapted, by permission, from American Alliance of Health, Physical Education, Recreation and Dance, 1980. Norms for 1-mile run for ages 5-college. In *Health related fitness test manual* (Reston, VA: AAHPERD); and R.R. Pate, 1985, *Norms for college students: Health related physical fitness test* (Reston, VA: AAHPERD).

Discovery Activity 2.1 *(continued)*

TABLE 2.E—Norms for 12-Minute Run (Yards) for Ages 13 Through 18

Percentile	Males	Females
95	3,297	2,448
75	2,879	2,100
50	2,592	1,861
25	2,305	1,622
5	1,888	1,274

Adapted, by permission, from American Alliance of Health, Physical Education, Recreation, and Dance, 1976, *Youth fitness test manual* (Reston, VA: AAHPERD).

TABLE 2.F—Ratings for Harvard Step Test

Score	Rating
Below 55	Poor
55-64	Low average
65-69	Average
70-89	Good
90 and above	Excellent

II. Muscular Strength

Health interpretation: Scores on the 1RM strength tests shown in table 2.7 are optimal values for your body weight. Your weight-training program should elevate you to these optimal levels within a period of 3 to 6 months. Reaching these levels provides a number of health- and performance-related benefits, such as increased muscle mass, increased basal metabolism (calorie expenditure at rest), more energy, reduced chance of soft-tissue injury (muscles, tendons, ligaments), and improved ease in performance of daily movements (getting out of a car or chair, lifting objects, going up steps). A program that helps you reach and then maintain these values will also help prevent the loss of lean-muscle tissue as you age.

TABLE 2.7—Test Scores for Muscular Strength

Test	Test standards (norms)	Score and rating (above or below optimal rating)
Military press	See table 2.G.	Score_____ Rating_____
Two-arm curl	See table 2.G.	Score_____ Rating_____
Leg press	See table 2.G.	Score_____ Rating_____

TABLE 2.G—Optimal Strength Values for Various Body Weights (Based on 1RM Test)

Body weight (lb)	BENCH PRESS		SHOULDER PRESS		BICEPS CURL		LEG PRESS	
	Male	Female	Male	Female	Male	Female	Male	Female
80	70	60	55	40	40	30	160	120
100	85	70	70	50	50	35	200	150
120	105	85	80	60	60	40	240	180
140	125	100	95	65	70	50	280	210
160	145	115	110	75	80	60	320	240
180	160	125	120	85	90	65	360	270
200	180	140	135	95	100	70	400	300
220	200	155	150	105	110	75	440	330
240	225	170	160	115	120	85	480	360

Note: Data in pounds; obtained on Universal Gym apparatus; applicable ages 17 to 30.

(continued)

Table from HEALTH AND FITNESS THROUGH PHYSICAL ACTIVITY by Michael L. Pollock. Reprinted by permission of Pearson Education, Inc.

Discovery Activity 2.1 *(continued)*

III. Muscular Endurance

Health interpretation: Scores on the muscular endurance tests in table 2.8 have similar health implications as the fitness and strength tests discussed previously. Low scores in the abdominal curl tests may also increase the possibility of lower-back problems in the future. Ratings that place you in the low, very low, poor, or very poor category on any of these tests are considered unhealthy. You should strive to achieve scores that place you in at least the average or moderate category by engaging in regular muscular endurance training (see chapter 7). Ratings of excellent or very high place you in the category of athletically fit.

TABLE 2.8—Test Scores for Muscular Endurance

Test	Test standards (norms)	Score and rating
Abdominal (curls)	See table 2.H.	Score_____ Rating_____
Arm and shoulder (pull-ups)	See table 2.I.	Score_____ Rating_____
Arm and shoulder (push-ups)	See table 2.J.	Score_____ Rating_____

TABLE 2.H—Norms for Abdominal Curls for Ages 18 Through 30

Rating	Males	Females
Excellent	96 and above	89 and above
Good	82-95	76-88
Average	68-81	63-75
Poor	54-67	49-62
Very poor	53 and below	48 and below

Reprinted from Robbins et al., 1991, *A wellness way of life* (Dubuque, IA: Wm. C. Brown Publishers). Reproduced with permission of The McGraw-Hill Companies.

TABLE 2.I—Performance Standards for Pull-Ups and Modified Pull-Ups

Rating	Pull-ups	Modified pull-ups
Excellent	13 or above	30 or above
Good	10-12	25-29
Average	5-9	16-24
Poor	0-4	0-15

TABLE 2.J—Ratings for Push-Ups and Modified Push-Ups

	RATING				
Age	Very high	High	Moderate	Low	Very low
PUSH-UPS					
15-29	Above 54	45-54	35-44	20-34	Below 20
30-39	Above 44	35-44	25-34	15-24	Below 15
40-49	Above 39	30-39	20-29	12-19	Below 12
Over 50	Above 34	25-34	15-24	8-14	Below 8
MODIFIED PUSH-UPS					
15-20	Above 48	34-48	17-33	6-16	Below 6
30-39	Above 39	25-39	12-24	4-11	Below 4
40-49	Above 34	20-34	8-19	3-7	Below 3
Over 50	Above 29	15-29	6-14	2-5	Below 2

Discovery Activity 2.1 *(continued)*

IV. Flexibility

Health interpretation: Scores on the flexibility tests in table 2.9 have numerous health implications in terms of injury prevention, lower-back pain, and the ease with which people of all ages perform routine tasks such as dressing, tying shoes, bending, lifting, and even moving efficiently. Scores that place you in the category of below average are considered unhealthy. You can easily improve your range of motion by following one of the flexibility-training programs discussed in chapter 6. You should strive to reach at least the average category shown in table 2.K. Scores 10 to 20% higher than the above-average rating place you in the category of athletically fit.

TABLE 2.9—Test Scores for Muscular Endurance

Test	Test standards (norms)	Score and rating
Shoulder reach	See table 2.K.	Score_____ Rating_____
Trunk flexion	See table 2.K.	Score_____ Rating_____
Trunk extension	See table 2.K.	Score_____ Rating_____

TABLE 2.K—Flexibility Interpretations

Rating	Shoulder reach (RUP/LUP)	Trunk flexion	Trunk extension
MEN			
Above average	6+/3+	11+	15+
Average	4-5/0-2	7-10	8-14
Below average	Below 4/below 0	Below 7	Below 8
WOMEN			
Above average	7+/6+	12+	23+
Average	5-6/0-5	7-11	15-22
Below average	Below 5/below 0	Below 7	Below 15

V. Body Composition

Health interpretation: Body-composition scores have numerous health-related implications. Unacceptable BMI scores, waist-to-hip ratio scores, and skinfold measures (percentage of body fat) are associated with a higher risk of atherosclerosis, hypertension, diabetes, heart and lung difficulties, early heart attack and stroke, numerous other chronic and degenerative disorders, some types of cancer, and higher death rates at all ages. Scores on any of the following tests in table 2.10 that place you in categories such as severe overweight or morbid obesity (BMI test), higher waist-to-hip ratios, and very high fat or obese (skinfold measures) are considered unhealthy. You should strive for so-called normal levels of body fat—average or ideal. The literature does not support the notion of increased health benefits by achieving the very low levels found in some endurance athletes. In fact, the essential fat in the human body is approximately 3 to 4% for men and 12 to 14% for women. Achieving fat levels below those levels is unrealistic and potentially unhealthy.

TABLE 2.10—Test Scores for Body Composition

Test	Test standards (norms)	Score and rating
Body-mass index	See table 2.L on page 50.	Score_____ Rating_____
Waist-to-hip ratio	See table 2.M on page 50.	Score_____ Rating_____
Skinfold measures	See table 8.A on page 218.	Score_____ Rating_____

(continued)

Discovery Activity 2.1 *(continued)*

TABLE 2.L—BMI Values for Men and Women

	Men	Women
Underweight	<20.7	<19.1
Acceptable weight	20.7 to 27.8	19.1 to 27.3
Overweight	27.8	27.3
Severe overweight	31.1	32.3
Morbid obesity	45.4	44.8

Reprinted from *Journal of the American Dietetic Association,* vol. 85, B.T. Burton and W.R. Fosters, Health implication of obesity, pgs. 1117-1121. Copyright 1983, with permission from American Dietetic Association.

TABLE 2.M—Waist-to-Hip Ratio Scores

	Ratio	Recommendation
Men	1.0 or higher	Weight loss
Women	0.85 or higher	Weight loss

VI. Nutrition

The best procedure for determining the status of your dietary intake is to keep careful records of all food and fluid intake for 3 to 4 days (2 to 3 weekdays and 1 weekend day) by carefully recording this information on the forms accompanying the nutritional analysis software available at your school's health and physical education department. Chapter 10 also provides less accurate methods of identifying some obvious shortcomings in your diet. Careful record keeping and nutritional analysis software can often identify nutrient deficiencies that can be corrected before symptoms develop.

1. List the deficient areas identified:

   a. _____

   b. _____

   c. _____

   d. _____

   e. _____

   f. _____

   g. _____

2. List a plan of action and specific food and fluid items that will help correct deficiencies:

   a. _____

   b. _____

   c. _____

   d. _____

   e. _____

   f. _____

   g. _____

Discovery Activity 2.1 *(continued)*

VII. Summary

List in the appropriate category how you performed in the various components of health-related fitness:

1. Above average or superior

    a. _____

    b. _____

    c. _____

    d. _____

    e. _____

2. Average

    a. _____

    b. _____

    c. _____

    d. _____

    e. _____

3. Poor or very poor (unhealthy)

    a. _____

    b. _____

    c. _____

    d. _____

    e. _____

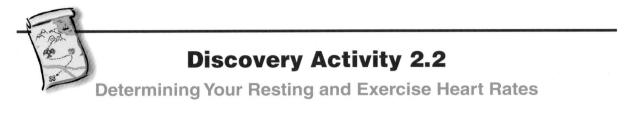

Discovery Activity 2.2

Determining Your Resting and Exercise Heart Rates

Name _____ **Date** _____

Instructions: Resting and exercise heart rates can often provide useful information about your fitness level and training method. You can learn how to obtain accurate measures by using these steps.

1. Lie down for 15 minutes in a comfortable place. Be sure not to eat or drink for at least 3 hours before starting this activity. If you have not given up smoking, do not smoke for at least 30 minutes before starting this activity.

2. After the rest period and while you are still lying down, take your pulse at the carotid artery on either side of the neck or use the radial pulse at the thumb side of your wrist. Because your thumb has its own pulse and will cause inaccurate readings, use only the fingers to find and count the pulse. Count for an entire minute. The resulting number is your resting heart rate.

3. To determine your postexercise heart rate, stop at the end of your next aerobic workout and take your carotid or radial pulse for only 6 seconds. Add a zero to determine the number of beats per minute. The 30- and 60-second pulse count should not be used at the end of a workout because the heart slows down rapidly during that lengthy period.

4. Record your resting and postexercise pulse in the following list.

Date _____   Date _____

Resting heat rate _____   Resting heart rate _____

Postexercise heart rate _____   Postexercise heart rate _____

Date _____   Date _____

Resting heart rate _____   Resting heart rate _____

Postexercise heart rate _____   Postexercise heart rate _____

5. Repeat this activity each month to measure your progress. Your resting heart rate will continue to decline as you become more aerobically fit. This decrease is a direct result of an increase in both stroke volume (more blood pumped per beat) and cardiac output (more blood pumped per minute). Later you can use the postexercise method to determine whether your aerobic workout is elevating your heart rate above the target level.

Discovery Activity 2.3

Service-Learning for Assessing Physical Fitness Levels

If more people were aware of their level of physical fitness, they might be more motivated to improve it. You can help your college community become more fit by organizing and conducting a physical fitness awareness fair. Spring is a good time of year to conduct the fair because people are apt to be outdoors, and beach and bathing suit season is approaching. This fair might include physical fitness assessments such as those presented in this chapter, organized fitness activities such as a fitness walk, and booths staffed by local merchants who sell fitness-related equipment. Involve the physical education or kinesiology department and the health education department. They may be able to provide faculty or knowledgeable graduate students to answer participants' questions—perhaps using the doctor-is-in format. Make sure to have an evaluation form for participants to complete. In this way, the next time the physical fitness awareness fair is offered, it can be even more responsive to participants' needs and interests.

The interesting aspect of service-learning is that you learn more by participating in the service than you might otherwise. By organizing and conducting the physical fitness awareness fair, you will learn more about physical fitness because you are interacting with people who are experts in the field, observing fitness activities, and becoming aware of fitness-related products.

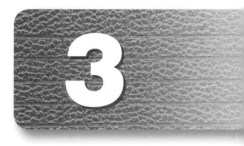

Principles of Exercise

Chapter Objectives

By the end of this chapter, you should be able to

1. identify the key components of a complete fitness program;

2. apply the progressive resistance exercise (PRE) principle to your specific workout program;

3. design formal warm-up and cool-down sessions for your exercise program;

4. identify your target heart rate range and determine whether your exercise program is intense enough to elevate and maintain your heart rate within that range;

5. examine exercise guidelines for special groups, including pregnant women and individuals with certain chronic diseases or physical disabilities; and

6. evaluate various exercise programs in terms of their effectiveness in developing aerobic fitness, muscular strength, muscular endurance, and flexibility and in lowering body fat and improving lean body mass.

For the past year, I have seen Maya in the university gymnasium almost every time I work out. No matter what time I choose to exercise, she always seems to be there exercising. Finally, I couldn't resist asking her about her exercise habits and was not surprised to learn that she trains seven times a week for 2 to 3 hours each session in a combination of formal aerobic classes, weight training, jogging, and stationary cycling. Nor was I surprised to hear that she has recovered from a number of overuse injuries, is tired most of the time, and suffers from aching muscles and sore knees.

Although Maya is doing many things correctly, she is obviously overdoing the training and does not thoroughly understand the basic principles of exercise such as the PRE principle, cross-training, alternation between light and heavy workouts, and other key concepts that protect the body from injury and ensure safe progression to higher levels of fitness.

You may know someone like Maya. Her situation is a common one that people can avoid by applying the exercise principles discussed in this chapter. Once you decide to begin a fitness program, you are ready to master the principles that will help you achieve a higher level of aerobic (cardiorespiratory) fitness; increase muscular strength, muscular endurance, and flexibility; and help you lose or maintain body weight and fat. Keep in mind that participation in an exercise program or a sport is no guarantee that your fitness level will improve unless you apply to your routine the exercise principles discussed in this chapter.

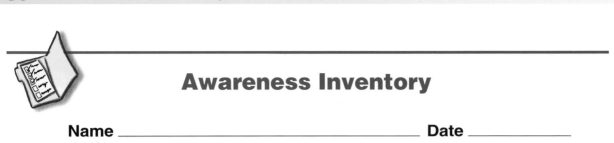

Awareness Inventory

Name _____ **Date** _____

Check the space by the letter T for the statements that you think are true and the space by the letter F by the statements that you think are false. The answers appear following the list of statements. This chapter will present information to clarify these statements for you. As you read the chapter, look for explanations for the reasons why the statements are true or false.

T ___ F ___ 1. The single most important component of health-related fitness is aerobic or cardiovascular fitness.

T ___ F ___ 2. Strength training and the addition of muscle mass will increase metabolism and help me control body weight.

T ___ F ___ 3. Previously sedentary individuals who begin an exercise program can easily complete 20 to 30 minutes of continuous exercise at or above their target heart rate in the first workout.

T ___ F ___ 4. The volume of blood pumped by the heart per minute of exercise is referred to as stroke volume.

T ___ F ___ 5. Running or walking 2 miles on each of 2 consecutive days burns more calories than one 4-mile walk or run.

T ___ F ___ 6. Studies show that 70 to 75% of our nation's adult population exercises in a manner that meets the surgeon general's recommendation of three times weekly at the target heart rate for 20 to 30 minutes.

T ___ F ___ 7. Alternating step classes with jogging and swimming is a sound approach to exercise referred to as cross-training.

T ___ F ___ 8. All-out exercise efforts such as a 200-meter dash or 10 to 15 40-yard dashes at 30-second intervals are examples of anaerobic training.

T ___ F ___ 9. The key to body-fat loss through exercise is intensity, not volume; short, highly intense workouts burn more calories than long, sustained efforts.

T ___ F ___ 10. Elderly men and women over the age of 70 should engage in a regular strength-training program (weight training).

Answers: 1-T, 2-T, 3-F, 4-F, 5-T, 6-F, 7-T, 8-T, 9-F, 10-T

From *Physical fitness and wellness, third edition,* by Jerrold S. Greenberg, George B. Dintiman, and Barbee Myers Oakes, 2004, Champaign, IL: Human Kinetics.

Analyze Yourself

Assessing Your Exercise Workout Behavior

Name _____ **Date** _____

Instructions: Indicate how often each of the following occurs in your daily activities and exercise sessions. Respond to each item with a number from 0 to 3, using the following scale:

0 = Never   **1** = Occasionally   **2** = Most of the time   **3** = Always

____ **1.** I use a general warm-up that produces perspiration, followed by a stretching session before beginning the workout.

____ **2.** I engage in aerobic exercise and complete 20 to 30 minutes of continuous, uninterrupted activity or total 60 minutes of activity by the end of the day three to four times each week.

____ **3.** I engage in a strength-training (weight-training) program at least three times weekly.

____ **4.** To avoid repetitive motion injuries, I use two or more different types of aerobic exercise each week such as jogging, step, cycling, and swimming.

____ **5.** Each workout includes a cool-down period that tapers off to allow my body to return slowly to its resting state.

____ **6.** I follow the progressive resistance principle in my workouts and keep records to make sure I do more work each training session.

____ **7.** I take my pulse during or immediately after activity and know that I am in my target heart rate zone throughout the aerobic workout.

____ **8.** I am careful to alternate light and heavy workouts in my exercise program.

____ **9.** I exercise on soft surfaces such as grass, synthetic track, or mats whenever possible.

____ **10.** I keep some records weekly to monitor my progress, frequency of exercise, fatigue level, and injuries.

Scoring: Excellent = 25-30

Good = 19-24

Poor = Below 19

From *Physical fitness and wellness, third edition,* by Jerrold S. Greenberg, George B. Dintiman, and Barbee Myers Oakes, 2004, Champaign, IL: Human Kinetics.

The Ideal Exercise Program

The following principles can be applied to most exercise choices to develop the five key components of health-related fitness: (1) cardiorespiratory endurance, (2) muscular strength, (3) muscular endurance (4) flexibility, and (5) body composition (fat, muscle, and bone). Programs that improve these components also provide the health benefits discussed in chapter 1. Because motor skill–related areas such as agility, explosive power, balance, coordination, and speed are important to competitive athletes but have little to do with health-related fitness, this chapter does not address those components.

Cardiorespiratory Function

Cardiorespiratory function, or aerobic fitness, is the most important health-related fitness component and should be the foundation of your complete program. You should choose at least one aerobic exercise activity that requires 20 to 30 minutes of continuous, uninterrupted exercise. Walking (4 miles per hour or faster), jogging, running, cycling, lap swimming, aerobic dance, aerobic exercise, and conditioning classes all are excellent aerobic choices. If you choose the sports approach to aerobic fitness, you may want to consider racquetball or squash (singles with a player of similar skill), tennis or handball (singles), soccer, rugby, lacrosse, or full-court basketball. These activities can help prevent heart disease and other disorders and can contribute significantly to fat and weight loss and maintenance.

Muscular Strength, Muscular Endurance, and Flexibility

Strength training will increase the strength and size of your muscles. The additional muscle mass also elevates metabolic rate (calories burned at rest over a 24-hour period) and assists you in losing fat and maintaining body weight. And by improving the ratio of muscle mass to body fat, you can exercise longer and more intensely and efficiently.

Improved muscular endurance enables you to exercise for longer periods and is critical to participants in sports requiring short, all-out efforts such as sprinting, football, field hockey, and soccer. Depending on the design of your weight-training program (see chapter 7), you will develop muscular endurance and strength simultaneously.

For the adult population and the elderly, strength and endurance training is even more important. Studies of the elderly who engage in weight training report a number of significant findings that have implications for improved quality of life. For example, evidence shows that weight training among the elderly increases muscular strength, endurance, bone mass, walking and stair-climbing ability, and reduces the risk of falls and fractures (Vincent et al., 2002). Improvement in strength and endurance also increases the ability to perform daily functions such as getting out of a chair or automobile, dressing, and other movements. The point is, you are never too old to improve muscular strength and endurance. The loss of lean-muscle tissue that occurs with aging among the sedentary population can be prevented, and additional muscle tissue can be added. Even as few as two strength-training workouts per week can produce positive results.

Now complete Discovery Activity 3.1: Choosing and Committing to an Exercise Program at the end of this chapter, keeping in mind the importance of the five key components of health-related fitness discussed in this section.

Improved flexibility may help reduce the incidence of both home- and exercise-related injuries and allow you to perform various activities more efficiently and effectively.

Body Composition

Aerobic exercise burns more calories than do other exercises. Activities such as walking, jogging, cycling, and lap swimming allow you to exercise for longer periods of time (20 to 60 or more minutes) than do activities requiring higher intensity such as sprinting and full-court basketball. The key to fat loss through exercise is volume, not intensity. The longer you can continue to exercise, the more calories you burn and the more your fat cells shrink. To reduce body fat, lower your weight, and improve your appearance, you need only three ingredients: (1) reduced caloric intake to put yourself into a negative daily caloric balance; (2) daily aerobic exercise to burn calories and tone the body; and (3) flexibility, strength, and endurance training to add muscle mass and eliminate skin sagging. Chapters 6 and 7 discuss these ingredients in detail.

Fitness Concepts

This section discusses in detail the specific components of a proper exercise program. Study them carefully so that you can apply each concept to your specific exercise choice.

Begin With a Preconditioning Program

You will need a minimum of 6 to 8 weeks to improve your aerobic fitness. Avoid attempting to move quickly from one fitness level to another in the early stages of your program. Too much too soon can produce muscle soreness, increase the chances of soft-tissue injury (see chapter 13), and cause you to quit long before results are noticeable.

The first 2 to 3 weeks of your new program should be considered a **preconditioning period** during which you progress slowly and enjoy each workout session. Although preconditioning will help reduce residual muscle soreness, you can expect some delayed soreness following an exercise session that involves unconditioned muscles. The time between the exercise session and the highest soreness level depends somewhat on your age—the older you are, the longer it takes to experience the soreness. Even when using a preconditioning period, maximum-effort fitness tests may result in severe muscle soreness the following day.

Apply the Progressive Resistance Exercise (PRE) Principle

The **progressive resistance exercise (PRE)** principle is simple to understand and has fascinating implications when correctly applied. If you gradually overload one of the body's systems (muscular, circulatory, or respiratory), it will develop addi-

> **preconditioning period**—A period of several weeks taken to prepare the body gradually for maximum-effort testing or engagement in a vigorous activity or sport.
>
> **progressive resistance exercise (PRE)**—The theory of gradually increasing the amount of resistance to be overcome or the number of repetitions in each workout.
>
> **stroke volume**—The amount of blood ejected per beat.
>
> **cardiac output**—The volume of blood pumped by the heart per minute.

tional capacity. When you repeatedly perform more strenuous exercise, the body repairs itself through elaborate cellular changes to prepare for more challenging exercise demands.

Application of the PRE principle produces dramatic changes in the heart and circulatory system. Regular exercise places stress on the heart, causing it to become larger and stronger and improving **stroke volume** (by pumping more blood each beat). A trained heart muscle with improved **cardiac output** pumps considerably more blood per beat and per minute, allowing the heart to slow down, beat fewer times per minute, and rest longer between beats. As the heart muscle adapts to the stress of exercise, the arteries that supply it also enlarge.

Although everyone starts at a different conditioning level, we can generalize about what happens to your body when you begin an exercise program (see figure 3.1). You start the program

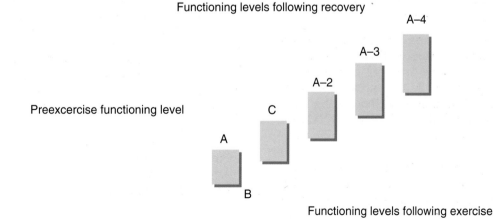

Functioning levels following recovery

Preexcercise functioning level

Functioning levels following exercise

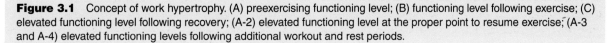

Figure 3.1 Concept of work hypertrophy. (A) preexercising functioning level; (B) functioning level following exercise; (C) elevated functioning level following recovery; (A-2) elevated functioning level at the proper point to resume exercise; (A-3 and A-4) elevated functioning levels following additional workout and rest periods.

at a certain functioning, or conditioning, level (level A in figure 3.1). During and immediately after your first workout, this conditioning level temporarily declines to point B. You are now actually in worse shape, in terms of physical capacity to exercise, than you were before the workout. During the recovery phase, however, tissue will rebuild beyond your original level of conditioning to level C. You are now able to perform more work than you could before you began your exercise program, but with no more effort. You are also in better physical condition 24 hours later than you were before you completed your first workout.

Repetition of this simple process will lead to continued improvement of conditioning levels—A-2, A-3, then A-4—provided you follow certain basic guidelines:

- Keep exercise sufficiently strenuous to cause an initial decrease in the conditioning level; the depth of the valley (A to B) and the corresponding increase (B to C) in figure 3.1 is in proportion to the intensity and duration of your workout.

- Allow sufficient time for recovery; improvement will not occur and conditioning will suffer if you perform your second workout before the recovery phase is complete (48 hours for strength training and 18 to 24 hours for aerobic and other workouts). Failure to follow this principle of recuperation can lead to overuse injuries and reduce the benefits of your workout.

- Conduct your next workout within 24 to 48 hours; a greater time lapse will cause your conditioning level to decline.

If you apply this concept to any training program, improved conditioning is guaranteed. Even strength training (see chapter 7) uses this approach to acquire muscle mass and increase strength and endurance.

The resistance principle also applies to the skeletal system. Gradual stress to the bones stimulates the accumulation of calcium and other minerals. In the adult years, **osteoporosis** can occur, especially among postmenopausal women. When you walk, jog, run, or perform other aerobic exercise, the force of your feet hitting the ground sends an important signal to your body to maintain bone density. At this point, more of the calcium consumed in your diet reaches the orthopedic system.

Exercise Four Times a Week for 30 Minutes at Your Target Heart Rate (THR)

Although results can be attained without lengthy workouts, there are no shortcuts. Ten-second contractions, massages, mechanical devices, steam baths, 3-minute slimnastic programs, and other such approaches range from slightly effective to worthless.

To receive the health-related benefits of exercise, you must apply the FIT principle:

Frequency—3 to 4 days per week

Intensity—at or above your target heart rate

Time—20 to 30 minutes of continuous exercise

Frequency of exercise is the key to the success of your program. Exercising three to five times per week rather than undergoing one hard workout per week will greatly increase the chances of meeting your training objectives. Frequency is also strongly related to weight and fat loss, cardiovascular development, and disease prevention. One 30-minute session will not transform you into a lean, mean, muscle machine, but three to four sessions weekly for 6 to 12 months will do wonders. Regularity is also a critical factor in changing the way your body handles fats (cholesterol and triglycerides).

Intensity (work per unit of time) is the aspect of your training that determines whether you are receiving any cardiorespiratory (heart-lung) benefits. Researchers have developed simple formulas to determine how much your heart rate must increase during exercise and how long you need to keep it elevated (20 to 30 minutes) to improve cardiovascular fitness. In the early stages of your newly started program, you will need to work up to 20 to 30 minutes of continuous activity slowly, over 4 to 6 weeks, rather than attempt to maintain high intensity in early workout sessions. To locate your THR, complete Discovery Activity 3.2: Finding Your Target Heart Rate at the end of this chapter.

Time (the duration of your workout) is the final aspect of the complete cardiorespiratory exercise session. Intensity affects exercise duration. Obviously, you cannot sprint at near-maximum effort for 20 minutes. If aerobic conditioning is your goal, the session should maintain your THR for 20 to 30 minutes. If the purpose of your program is cosmetic—to lose weight and fat and to improve your appearance—duration is the key. In general, the longer you exercise, the more calories you burn and the more fat you use as fuel. If weight loss is your primary objective, keep in mind that walking 3 miles burns only slightly fewer calories than running 3 miles. The longer you walk or run, the more calories you use. Thus, you might want to exercise longer and slow down your walking, pedaling, running, rope jumping, and so on. To exercise longer, it is important to stay near the lower portion of your THR range. Providing that you reach your THR, you are not only burning a high number of calories but improving your cardiovascular system as well.

Running or walking 3 miles on each of 2 successive days also burns more calories than one 6-mile run. This disparity occurs because the body burns an extra 60 to 150 calories as a result of metabolic rate increases (calories burned while the body is at rest) following the exercise period. In other words, two short exercise sessions burn more calories than one long session, because the metabolic rate will become, and remain, elevated for several hours after each session. The extra calorie usage after exercise ceases is called **afterburn.** If you walk or run too far in a day and are unable to exercise the next day, you will eliminate one afterburn period and forfeit the burning of 60 to 150 calories. Late afternoon, when metabolic rates begin to slow in most people, may be one of the best times to exercise. You then burn calories while exercising and activate a faster metabolic rate for 2 to 4 hours at a time in the day when metabolic rate normally slows down.

If you follow the FIT principle, the evidence is strong that you will receive considerable health benefits from your exercise program. Not everyone agrees, however, that more is better. According to the Centers for Disease Control and Prevention, a brisk daily 2-mile walk will provide most of the health benefits that can be derived from physical activity. But a 1996 report from the surgeon general counters that engaging in physical activity of more vigorous intensity or longer duration will bring about greater health benefits (U.S. Public Health Service, 1996). Higher levels of regular physical activity, according to this report, are associated with lower mortality rates for both older and younger adults. Men who exceeded the levels of the FIT principle have been found to have greater levels of the protective HDL cholesterol, less body fat, lower triglyceride levels, and a better ratio of good to bad cholesterol. And the more both men and women exercised, the more benefits they received. The report also recommends that people supplement cardiorespiratory endurance activity with strength-developing exercises at least twice per week.

Unfortunately, only half of the nation's young people ages 12 to 21 and 37% of adults currently meet the lower standard; proposing a standard that is even more demanding could produce negative results.

Apply the Principle of Specificity

The effect of training is unique to an activity or sport. Football or field hockey players who have just completed their seasons, for example, will find that they are not capable of meeting the physical demands of wrestling or basketball. The scientific basis for this is that training occurs, in part, within the muscles themselves and that training is specific to the energy system being used. Thus, complete training transfer, regardless of the similarity of the activities, is not possible.

Training a particular muscle group is referred to as **neuromuscular specificity;** training one of the energy systems is called **metabolic specificity.** If your main training objective is to improve aerobic fitness, you must include activities such as jogging, running, cycling, aerobic dancing, and distance swimming. Although gains in cardiorespiratory fitness will occur from each of these activities, a specific activity that closely simulates the movement of the sport for which you are training provides the most transfer. In other words, swimming is the preferred training method to improve distance swimming, running is the preferred training method for 10K races, and so on.

> **osteoporosis**—An abnormal decalcification of bones causing loss of bone density.
>
> **afterburn**—The period following exercise when resting metabolism remains elevated.
>
> **neuromuscular specificity**—Training a specific muscle group.
>
> **metabolic specificity**—Training a specific energy system (citric acid cycle or glycolysis cycle).

Alternate Light and Heavy Workouts

The body responds best to training programs that alternate light and heavy workouts. This approach reduces the risk of injury, provides several emotionally relaxing workouts each week, and allows the body time to recover. In other words, it helps you receive maximum benefits from a fitness program. Thus, you should consider never training extremely hard on consecutive days; training hard no more than three times a week; scheduling one extra-hard, all-out workout once a week; and knowing your body and allowing it to direct you. For instance, you should stop exercising if pain continues or worsens or if you get heavy legged, regardless of whether it is a light- or heavy-workout day. Apply the PRE principle by increasing the volume or intensity on the heavy-workout days.

Warm Up Properly
Before Each Workout

A **warm-up** is almost universally used at the beginning of an exercise or activity session to improve performance and prevent injury. The theory behind the warm-up is that muscular contractions depend on temperature. Because increased muscle temperature improves work capacity and a warm-up increases muscle temperature, we assume that a warm-up is necessary. The amount of knee fluid also increases with a warm-up, oxygen intake improves, and the amount of oxygen needed for exercise declines. Nerve messages also travel faster at higher temperatures.

Suggestions that can be drawn from the findings of well-controlled studies on the warm-up include the following:

- Warm up for 10 to 15 minutes before the actual workout or exercise session. You need a longer period in a cold environment to allow the body to reach the desired temperature before activity.
- Warm up until you begin to sweat. The main purpose of a warm-up is to elevate core temperature by 1 to 2°F before engaging in stretching exercises or explosive muscular movements; you will generally reach this point at the same time your warm-up routine causes sweating.
- Let only a few minutes elapse from completion of the warm-up until the start of activity.
- Remember that warming up will not cause early fatigue or hinder performance.

Warm-up methods fall into four categories:

1. Formal methods involve the skill or act that you will use in competition or in your workout, such as running before performing a 100-meter dash, jogging before doing a 3-mile run, or shooting a basketball and jumping before playing a basketball game.
2. Informal methods involve a general warm-up, such as calisthenics or other activity unrelated to the workout routine to follow.
3. Passive methods involve applying heat to various body parts.
4. Overload methods involve simulating the activity for which you are using the warm-up by increasing the load or resistance, such as swinging two bats before hitting a baseball.

Each of these methods has been shown by some researchers to be helpful and by other researchers to be of little value. A formal warm-up appears to be superior to informal procedures. When body temperature is elevated and sweating occurs,

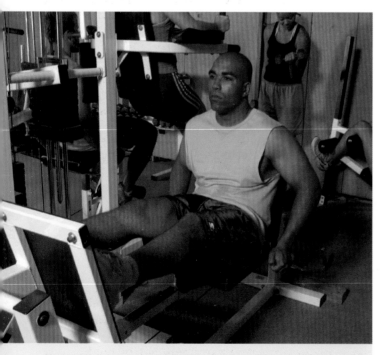

Alternating light and heavy workouts reduces the risk of injury and gives the muscles time to recover.

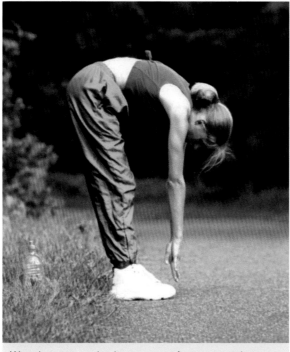

Warming up muscles improves performance and prevents injuries.

PhotoDisc

> **warm-up**—The preparation of the body for vigorous activity through stretching, calisthenics, running, and specific sport movements designed to raise core temperature.
>
> **cool-down**—The use of 3 to 10 minutes of very light exercise movements at the end of a vigorous workout designed to cool the body slowly to near-normal core temperature.
>
> **norepinephrine**—An end product of some of the secretions of the adrenal gland; influences nervous system activity, constricts blood vessels, and increases blood pressure.
>
> **postexercise peril**—Illness, dizziness, nausea, and sudden death following vigorous exercise, particularly when a cool-down period is not used.

your muscles are ready for a brief stretching or flexibility session (see chapter 6).

How long you decide to engage in warm-up activities is also important. The temperature of your muscles will rise in about 5 minutes and continue to rise for 25 to 30 minutes. If you stop exercising and become inactive, your muscle temperature will decline significantly, and you may need an additional warm-up period. The best advice is to use a 10- to 15-minute warm-up period that ends in an all-out effort and causes you to perspire. You should plan to complete your warm-up period about 5 minutes before an exercise session or competition begins. Find the magic combination for you and your activity and stay with it.

Cool Down Properly at the End of Each Workout

The justification for a **cool-down** period following a vigorous workout is simple. Blood returns to the heart through a system of vessels called veins. Heart contractions push the blood along, and muscle contractions during exercise assist the veins' milking action. Veins contract, or squeeze, and move the blood forward against gravity, while valves prevent the blood from backing up. If you stop exercising suddenly, this milking action will stop, and blood return will drop quickly and may cause blood pooling (blood remaining in the same area) in the legs, leading to shock or deep breathing, which may in turn lower carbon dioxide levels and produce muscle cramps.

At this point, blood pressure can also drop precipitously and cause trouble. The body compensates for the unexpected drop in pressure by secreting as much as 100 times the normal amount of **norepinephrine.** This high level of norepinephrine can cause cardiac problems for some individuals during the recovery phase of vigorous exercise, such as a marathon or a triathlon.

Postexercise peril can occur in some individuals immediately after strenuous exercise, particularly the elderly, the nonfat, and those who fail to use a cool-down period. The least desirable postexercise behavior is standing. Lying down flat is acceptable; the preferred activity, however, is walking or jogging for 4 to 5 minutes (light exercise).

You should also cool down following a long aerobic exercise session. A general routine might consist of walking or jogging a quarter mile to a mile at a pace of 3 to 4 minutes per quarter mile, covering each quarter mile slower than you did the previous one. The ideal cool-down routine should take place in the same environment as the workout (except in extremely hot or cold weather), last at least 5 minutes, and be followed by a brief stretching period.

Be Aware of the Variation in Individual Response to Exercise

Individuals respond differently to a given exercise or training program. Some men and women develop strength, add muscle mass, increase their aerobic fitness, or enhance their range of motion faster than others do. An individual may also respond quickly to one training program and slowly to another. Numerous factors are responsible for these individual differences:

- Heredity—physique and physiological makeup.
- Stage of growth and development—preadolescent boys and girls respond poorly to strength training, and the point of development plays a role in the response to other exercise programs.
- Nutrition, rest, and sleep—highly individual factors that affect energy levels for a workout and the training effect.
- Illness and injury—imposes demands on the body that alter the response to training.
- Level of fitness—progress is usually marked for those with a low level of fitness and much more difficult to detect in the highly fit.
- Motivation—determines the amount of effort one puts into a workout, which alters the effect that the workout produces.

If you apply the conditioning principles discussed in this chapter to your exercise program, your fitness level will continue to improve until you eventually reach your desired goals. At that point, you may choose to switch to a maintenance program merely to hold your present level of strength, flexibility, and aerobic fitness by completing two or three carefully designed workouts per week.

Dress Appropriately for Ease of Movement and Heart Regulation

What you wear depends on your exercise program and the weather. The general rule is to have good shoes and to wear as little clothing as conditions permit.

Shoes

To avoid injuries, quality shoes are essential for most aerobic activities. The primary criteria are fit, comfort, and quality. Most activities require a specialized shoe, and although they often look identical, the various styles have different effects. Specialty stores are more likely to provide sound advice about the shoe best suited to your aerobic goals. Because fit is so important, wear the same style of socks you use for exercising when you are selecting a shoe.

Clothes

For indoor and warm-weather outdoor exercise, wear the least clothing possible. The cooling process requires air to pass over the skin and evaporate; clothing must allow this process to take place. Some individuals mistakenly feel that they will lose weight by wearing multiple layers of clothes to increase fluid loss. It is the total calories expended, however, not the total sweat count, that determines weight and fat loss.

When you are exercising outside during the winter, do not overdress or underdress. Like summer clothing, winter attire must allow the skin to breathe. Windbreakers and other nylon garments are therefore not recommended. Combining a T-shirt with a wool sweater, a hat, and gloves is usually sufficient for protection down to temperatures below 32°F (0°C). Under extremely cold conditions, however, frostbite is a real danger, particularly to exposed skin. Creams and jellies can protect the skin, but only to a degree. Men, for example, must protect the penis and testicles from frostbite. Nylon shorts are of little value, and frostbite can occur without warning. Appendix D provides additional information on the prevention and treatment of hypothermia and heat-related disorders.

Take Special Precautions When Exercising Outdoors

Weather is not your only concern when you exercise outside. Pollution, particularly lack of clear air, is a danger worth paying attention to. Although the benefits of exercise overshadow the dangers of unclean air, workouts during smog alerts and in high traffic areas should be avoided. Motor vehicles and even bicycles can present life-threatening situations to runners and others who exercise outside. Give vehicles and bicycles the right-of-way, no matter what the law indicates. Run or walk toward traffic and wear reflective gear at night. Do not be aggressive because you are no match for a vehicle that weighs several thousand pounds.

Dogs tend to have considerable bark and little bite, but the exceptions can produce disaster.

Because dogs can be territorial, it is wise to avoid crossing property lines. For the occasional dog that comes after you, the best action is to stop, face the dog, and assume a passive posture before slowly backing away. As you vacate the property, the animal generally becomes less aggressive. Two-legged animals are far more dangerous than any of the four-legged varieties. Women in particular must be alert to dangerous situations and take care to exercise with others, avoid outside exercise at night, ignore taunts, and always remain alert.

Choose Soft Surfaces Whenever Possible

Although exercise involves some risk of injury (see chapter 13), choice of surface can reduce the risk. Generally, the harder the surface, the greater the injury potential. A surface that is too soft or uneven also increases the risk of certain types of exercise injuries. A soft, uneven surface, such as a beach, can cause ankle and knee injuries. Dirt and gravel paths and trails covered with wood chips are best for walking and running, but the isolated nature of most trails increases the chances of assault. Fitness courses in public parks usually provide relatively safe, soft places to exercise. Avoid exercising on concrete floors, sidewalks, hard tennis courts, and gymnasium floors when possible. Daily activity on such surfaces is almost certain to produce injury.

Use Cross-Training in the Aerobic Component of Your Program

Repetitive motion syndrome can produce both injury and loss of interest in exercise. A daily step class or 5-mile run, for example, engages the same motion, movement, muscles, and joints repeatedly and is almost certain to result in injury over time. Many individuals use **cross-training** and avoid these dangers by varying their exercise choices weekly. Runners may choose to ride a stationary cycle or swim once or twice a week. Aerobic dancers cycle, walk, swim, or play racket sports. Such an approach provides a more complete workout and eliminates exercise boredom and burnout.

Use a Maintenance Approach After Reaching Your Desired Level of Fitness

It is possible to alter your exercise program to maintain the level of conditioning you have acquired. You can maintain considerable strength, for example, by completing one or two hard weight-training workouts weekly. Maintaining your cardiorespiratory endurance may require two to three workouts weekly. When you are unable to exercise daily, you may choose to alter your routine by increasing the intensity and duration of the workouts you complete.

Monitor Your Progress Carefully

Records can be a source of motivation besides aiding in the prevention of injury. Keeping records of resting heart rate, miles walked or run, laps swum, weight lifted, and workouts completed can provide the needed incentive to continue an exercise program. Record keeping also helps you apply the PRE principle to guarantee continued improvement. Improving and working harder today is difficult when you are not aware of the intensity and duration of your previous workouts.

If an overuse injury occurs, a perusal of records can aid in determining its cause and help you set a course toward recovery. Unfortunately, records can also lead to compulsive behavior known as negative addiction. To the addicted, records are made to be broken, more is better, and the record rather than the fitness benefit becomes the goal. Such individuals experience frequent injury intermixed with emotional stress in attempting to maintain or break records.

The daily log in figure 3.2 can help you apply many of the exercise concepts discussed in this chapter. The log information should include the time spent in aerobic activity, the distance covered, and rest intervals between repetitions, if applicable. Your log should also note weather, water temperature, heart rate, positive impressions, particular problems that indicate the possibility of future injury, number and type of activities completed, and (for weight training) the weight and number of repetitions for each exercise. You should also periodically monitor your aerobic exercise choices.

cross-training—The practice of alternating exercise choices throughout the week to avoid overuse injuries from repetitive movements.

Name_____   Date_____

Weight_____   Starting date_____

                                              Time of day_____

Cardiorespiratory activities _____

Weight training:

Exercises	Starting weight	Repetitions	Sets
_____	_____	_____	_____
_____	_____	_____	_____
_____	_____	_____	_____
_____	_____	_____	_____
_____	_____	_____	_____
_____	_____	_____	_____
_____	_____	_____	_____
_____	_____	_____	_____

Intensity:

Heart rate _____   Repetitions _____ Rest interval _____

Distance covered _____   Pace _____

Duration:

Total exercise time _____

Positive impressions of the workout: _____

_____

_____

_____

_____

Unusual feelings or problems during workout: _____

_____

_____

_____

_____

Figure 3.2   Daily exercise log.

From *Physical Fitness and Wellness*, third edition, by Jerrold S. Greenberg, George B. Dintiman, and Barbee Myers Oakes, 2004, Champaign IL: Human Kinetics.

New Exercise Guidelines for Children, Adults, and the Elderly

A September 2002 report from the Institute of Medicine of the National Academy of Sciences recommends that adults and children engage in physical activity (aerobic exercise, walking, jogging, or different types of activities that use major muscle groups, at moderate to moderately high intensity) for a total of 60 minutes daily. This figure represents twice the amount of both our current recommendation and the 1996 recommendation of the U.S. surgeon general (30 minutes three to four times weekly). The 936-page report also encourages high and low consumption levels for carbohydrates, fats and fatty acids, protein, amino acids, fiber, and other so-called macronutrients and links regular exercise and sound nutrition in an attempt to reduce the increasing rates of chronic conditions such as obesity, cardiovascular disease, diabetes, and cancer in the United States.

The need for greater physical activity among the elderly was also the subject of a position statement released by the World Health Organization (WHO) in September 2002. The WHO's Guidelines for the Promotion of Physical Activity for Older Persons is based on evidence that suggests that most elderly persons can benefit from a physically active lifestyle involving aerobic exercise, flexibility, and strength training.

The new exercise and nutrition recommendations for children, adults, and the elderly are a step in the right direction and provide more flexibility in eating and exercising than the earlier guidelines did. The intent is not to promote jogging, swimming, or cycling for an hour each day but to suggest that people should move at a moderately intense level, equal to the rate of a brisk walk or a climb up the stairs, for a total of 60 minutes throughout the day. Because the exercise portion of the report was calibrated based on a brisk walk, you can accomplish the goal in less time through more vigorous activity such as a 30-minute jog four to seven times weekly. Four 15-minute walks with your dog or an accumulation of 60 minutes through a number of activities also meets the criteria. The new guidelines do not change our recommendation of performing more intense aerobic exercise four times weekly for 30 minutes at your target heart rate. The ideal program for all age groups also includes regular stretching exercises (after a general warm-up and before each workout) and two to three weight-training sessions weekly.

Exercise Guidelines for Special Groups

Scientific studies continue to support the physical and emotional benefits of aerobic exercise and strength training for individuals of all ages and with varying degrees of disease and physical disability. Regular aerobic exercise, strength, and flexibility training slow the decline in aerobic capacity, cardiovascular fitness, flexibility, and loss of muscle mass that occurs based on a variety of physical conditions, many of which are exacerbated by aging. Hence, we shall examine guidelines for improving fitness for individuals belonging to a number of special groups.

Exercise During Pregnancy and the Postpartum Period

As exercising during pregnancy has become an increasingly common practice, the American College of Obstetrics and Gynecology (ACOG) has continually updated their guidelines over the past few decades to promote the safety of both the mother and the fetus. From early research studies, we know that athletes tend to have fewer complications of pregnancy than do nonathletes. Also, exercisers who remain active during pregnancy weigh less, gain less weight during pregnancy, and deliver smaller babies than do nonexercising mothers. Exercising women generally have shorter labor and appear to tolerate labor pain better when compared with nonexercising women. Athletes may have fewer cesarean sections than nonathletes do. Although all women decrease their amount of total work as the pregnancy progresses, many remain active up to the day of delivery.

Recommendations for exercise and pregnancy published in 1994 by the ACOG were updated in 2002 to reflect an increased promotion of the overall health benefits to be derived by women who maintain exercise programs during and after pregnancy (ACOG, 1994, 2002). In addition to being more flexible concerning exercise intensity and type, the primary difference in the recommendations is that those in 1994 emphasized the safeness of healthy women who chose to exercise during pregnancy, whereas the 2002 guidelines suggest that all healthy women should exercise during pregnancy and lactation (News Brief, 2002).

Myth and Fact Sheet

Myth	Fact
1. You can achieve aerobic development in half the time by doubling the workout intensity.	**1.** Short, high-intensity workouts will improve anaerobic, not aerobic, fitness. There are no shortcuts to aerobic development.
2. The more I exercise, the more health benefits I achieve.	**2.** This statement is partially true. Numerous studies have provided guidelines for health-related fitness, such as the number of minutes you need to exercise each session and each week for protection from heart disease, stroke, and other illnesses. In many cases, these guidelines identify the minimum level needed. A 3-mile daily run or walk will provide more health benefits (weight and fat loss, prevention from certain chronic and degenerative diseases, and so on) than a 1-mile walk will. More is better unless you reach the point of producing overuse injuries and illnesses that are sure to occur when you become overenthusiastic and fail to apply the training principles in this chapter.
3. Muscle soreness is caused by intense exercise that produces lactic acid.	**3.** Lactic acid buildup during anaerobic exercise is removed before soreness develops. The main culprit is unaccustomed exercise or higher than usual exercise intensity and swelling from microtrauma to muscles and connective tissue.
4. "No pain, no gain" means that you must train until it hurts to reap the benefits.	**4.** Exercise can be difficult, particularly on your heavy workout every other day, but it should never hurt. If you experience anything worse than discomfort, reduce the intensity of the workout to prevent injury to soft tissue and burnout, which in a few weeks or months can cause you to discontinue exercising. Discomfort is necessary to reach higher levels of fitness. Some degree of distress is safe and common during heavy lifting in weight training, intense anaerobic or speed endurance training, and long-distance training.
5. You should wear a hat when exercising.	**5.** Although extremely popular in tennis, baseball, and some other activities, the value of a hat depends on the type you choose. Hats help keep the sun off the face, reduce glare, and allow you to see better. You should use a hat with an open top (visor) in hot, humid weather because considerable heat loss and cooling occur through the head. In cold weather, a full hat will prevent heat loss.
6. Because the main source of energy (fuel) in aerobic exercise is fat, aerobic workouts are the best activity for weight and fat loss.	**6.** A calorie is a calorie is a calorie. To lose weight, your caloric intake must be less than your caloric expenditure, regardless of the type of fuel used. As the intensity of a workout increases from a resting state (when two-thirds of energy used comes from stored fat) to low or moderate aerobic activity (when fat is still the main fuel) to more intense, anaerobic activity, the percentage of fat used decreases and glycogen (stored glucose) provides much more fuel. After exercise ceases, regardless of the fuel used (fat or glucose), the internal calorie count is what matters. If you burn up more calories than you consume on a particular day, you will lose weight. The main advantage of aerobic activity (walking, slow jogging, cycling, dancing, swimming laps) for weight and body-fat loss is that you are likely to continue exercising for longer periods when the intensity is low. You therefore will burn more total calories each workout. You also receive considerable health benefits that anaerobic exercise does not provide.

General Exercise Guidelines During Pregnancy

Women should always receive a thorough clinical evaluation whether they are beginning or maintaining an exercise program during pregnancy. Women who are in good physical condition before pregnancy and accustomed to exercise, however, are unlikely to experience any negative effects on fetal outcome. In addition, exercise offers many benefits to the physical and emotional well-being of the expecting mother. For the first time, exercise during pregnancy is promoted for its potential role in the prevention of gestational diabetes.

In general, in the absence of complications (see figure 3.3), pregnant women are encouraged to exercise as long as they observe the following precautions. When modifying their usual exercise routines as medically indicated, pregnant women should exercise at moderate intensity for at least 30 minutes daily, rather than three to four times each week. Pregnant women should also avoid motionless standing and exercising in the supine position after the first trimester. Both positions have adverse effects on cardiac output that could result in fainting. In terms of recreational activities, pregnant women should beware of those endeavors that have high potential for contact, increased risk of falling, or inherently high risk for trauma. Women engaging in competitive events should be cautious of the potential effect of strenuous training and competition on both the mother and the fetus and maintain close supervision by a physician. Finally, we still know little about the effect of exercise on core temperature during pregnancy. Therefore, pregnant women should be especially careful to avoid overheating while exercising.

General Exercise Guidelines During the Postpartum Period

Although many of the changes occurring during pregnancy persist 4 to 6 weeks after delivery, once the physician determines it to be medically safe, the 2002 guidelines note that there are no known contraindications to returning to training during the postpartum period for the female athlete. Postpartum exercise enhances cardiorespiratory fitness and facilitates weight reduction. Weight loss after delivery is a desirable benefit. Note that when moderate weight loss occurs during the nursing period, neonatal weight gain has not been found to be compromised. Weight loss after delivery has also been related to a decline in

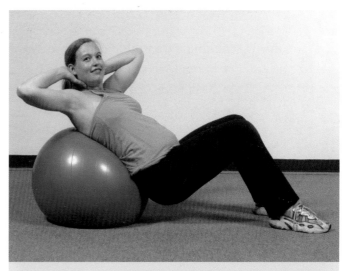

More and more women remain physically active longer into their pregnancies as research has shown that exercising while pregnant results in many benefits for mother and child.

low back pain. This effect may last at least three years postpartum (Noren et al., 2002). An additional desirable effect is the decreased incidence of postpartum depression when women engage in stress-relieving rather than stress-provoking exercise. Naturally, the importance of considering individual differences cannot be overstated here.

Ringdahl (2002) also reported a number of perceived barriers to postpartum exercise. For many women, physiological changes during pregnancy may result in deconditioning and a higher risk of injury because of increased joint laxity. For others, time constraints are prohibitive because of the myriad demands of being a new mother. Fears about the safety of premature weight reduction during breastfeeding have discouraged many women from exercising after delivery. Although aerobic exercise does not have negative effects on lactation, infants may prefer preexercise milk because postexercise milk has increased levels of lactic acid (Carey et al., 1997). Stress incontinence occurs more frequently in women who have had multiple deliveries; hence, low-impact activities are recommended to minimize incontinence until bladder control is restored.

Exercise Guidelines for Senior Adults

Maintaining a physically active lifestyle by exercising regularly ranks among the healthiest habits older adults can practice because exercise helps them both sustain and partly restore aerobic

Absolute Contraindications to Aerobic Exercise During Pregnancy

- Hemodynamically significant heart disease
- Restrictive lung disease
- Incompetent cervix, cerclage
- Multiple gestation at risk for premature labor
- Persistent second- or third-trimester bleeding
- Placenta previa after 26 weeks of gestation
- Premature labor during the current pregnancy
- Ruptured membranes
- Preeclampsia or pregnancy-induced hypertension

Relative Contraindications to Aerobic Exercise During Pregnancy

- Severe anemia
- Unevaluated maternal cardiac arrhythmia
- Chronic bronchitis
- Poorly controlled type 1 diabetes
- Extreme morbid obesity
- Extreme underweight (BMI < 12)
- History of extremely sedentary lifestyle
- Intrauterine growth restriction in current pregnancy
- Poorly controlled hypertension
- Orthopedic limitations
- Poorly controlled seizure disorder
- Poorly controlled hyperthyroidism
- Heavy smoker

Warning Signs to Terminate Exercise While Pregnant

- Vaginal bleeding
- Dyspnea before exertion
- Dizziness
- Headache
- Chest pain
- Muscle weakness
- Calf pain or swelling (need to rule out thrombophlebitis)
- Preterm labor
- Decreased fetal movement
- Amniotic fluid leakage

Figure 3.3 2002 ACOG recommendations for exercise during pregnancy and the postpartum period.

capacity, flexibility, strength, and musculoskeletal function. Many older individuals are at particular risk for leading sedentary lives because disease or disability limits their activity or they are reluctant to engage in exercise programs for other reasons.

Benefits of habitual exercise include slowing the decline in aerobic capacity, cardiovascular fitness, flexibility, and loss of muscle mass that inevitably occur with aging. In addition, exercise decreases blood pressure, produces favorable changes in blood lipids, helps prevent osteoporosis, improves glucose tolerance, increases bone density and decreases the chances of a bone break, and maintains strength, endurance, and flexibility in the legs and arms. These physiological changes foster continued independence in performing normal activities of daily living (ADL), while also slowing the progression of disability. Therefore, even if older adults are not interested in pursuing sports, they often find that it is easier to carry groceries, climb stairs, or even play with young children if they maintain muscular strength. Likewise, as seniors focus on improving their balance, they will be less susceptible to falling down.

Many ethnic minority women get their physical activity from the types of activities that classic physical activity questionnaires do not typically include. For example, the Navajo Health and Nutrition Examination Survey found women to have higher than expected levels of activity. The primary reason was that many of the women hunted and gathered and chopped wood. LTPA was also reported to be extremely low in a sample of middle-aged Hispanic women. Yet these women reported moderate to high levels of activity based on activities such as lifting, carrying, housework, and conducting chores. Older African American women also report higher levels of activity from engaging in housework, doing yard work, gardening, being caregivers, and from performing their occupations than they do when asked about their involvement in LTPA (Eyler et al., 2002). Consequently, physical activity intervention programs should integrate specific ethnic and cultural activity patterns to produce accurate assessments of total energy expenditures among nonmajority populations.

We propose that seniors regularly participate for 30 minutes daily, at least three to five times each week, in moderately intense activities such as climbing stairs, walking, yard work or gardening, cycling, and heavy housework. Most research studies recommend that men over age 40 and women over age 50 obtain medical consent before exercising. Figure 3.4 summarizes other guidelines for seniors about obtaining consent before participating in an exercise program.

Exercise Guidelines for Individuals With Diseases and Disabilities

In this section we provide some exercise guidelines and precautions that can be applied to individuals with various chronic diseases or physical disabilities. In chapter 14 you will learn more specific guidelines and precautions for individuals with chronic conditions associated with cardiovascular disease. Exercise guidelines for diseased or disabled persons are discussed simultaneously for several reasons. Many seniors discover that their ability to recover from certain chronic diseases is complicated by their inability to exercise because of limitations imposed by other disabilities associated with aging, such as arthritis. Although both chronic disease and physical disability are positively associated with sedentary living (Penninx et al., 2001), it is important to note that having a disability may limit participation in exercise programs but is not necessarily synonymous with a poorer overall quality of life.

Orthopedic problems, diabetes, asthma and exercise-induced asthma, arthritis, high blood pressure, chronic low back pain, chronic obstructive pulmonary disease, and cardiovascular disease, to name a few, all require special care and adherence to the guidelines prescribed by a physician. In summary, whether you are a recreational exerciser or an athlete of any age, you can more easily obtain a high level of physical fitness when you execute an exercise program according to the limitations imposed by your state of disease or disability.

Once considered an issue only among older adults, many of these debilitating conditions we now know to be prevalent among adolescents. As an example, asthma and exercise-induced asthma often manifest during childhood. Studies have repeatedly shown, however, that participation in an exercise program of moderate intensity enhances the ability to cope with asthma while also increasing the level of fitness (Van Valdhoven et al., 2001). Because we know the important role of physical activity in improving the risk factor profile of those with chronic diseases as well as its effect on disabilities, we must place greater

Older adults should obtain their doctors' approval before beginning an exercise program if they have any of the following conditions:

Circulatory Conditions

- Severe shortness of breath
- Irregular, rapid, or fluttery heartbeat
- Chest pain
- High blood pressure
- Foot or ankle sores that will not heal (especially if they have diabetes mellitus)
- A blood clot
- An abdominal aortic aneurysm (a weakening in the wall of the heart's major outgoing blood vessel)
- Aortic stenosis (a narrowing of one of the heart valves)

Musculoskeletal Conditions

- Chronic low back pain
- Joint swelling
- Knee pain
- Hip repair or hip replacement surgery
- Persistent pain or problems walking after a fall (potentially indicates a fracture)
- Osteoarthritis
- Rheumatoid arthritis

Other General Medical Conditions

- Any new, undiagnosed symptom
- Ongoing, significant, and undiagnosed weight loss
- Morbid obesity
- Any acute infection, such as pneumonia, accompanied by fever (can cause a rapid heartbeat and dehydration)
- A hernia that is causing symptoms such as pain and discomfort
- Eye conditions such as bleeding in the retina or a detached retina, especially after a cataract removal, lens implant, laser treatment, or other eye surgery
- Heavy smokers (more than one pack per day)

Figure 3.4 Guidelines for seniors who should obtain medical approval before engaging in an exercise program.

emphasis on understanding the complex factors that mediate exercise participation in disabled and nondisabled adolescents and young adults.

An increasing number of people of all ages have reported orthopedic problems, such as knee pain or back pain, that are correlated to a decline in their level of physical activity in their senior years. Exercise programs for these individuals must take into account many factors. For example, low back pain (LBP) is one of the most common conditions managed in medicine today. Surprisingly, the occurrence of nonspecific low back pain in 14- to 16-year-old adolescents is nearly the same as it is in adults (Ebbehoj et al., 2002), due largely to extremes in exercise participation among youths today. In other words, young people at either end of the continuum from sedentary living to participating in activities with high physical impact have increased risk of developing LBP.

Osteoarthritis (OA) is another debilitating culprit that contributes to sedentary living among older individuals. Many studies, however, have measured the beneficial role of exercise on ADL among older individuals with OA. Typical of these studies, Penninx et al. (2001) reported that the lowest ADL disability risks were found for participants with the highest compliance to participating in an aerobic and resistance-training exercise program. In particular, the debilitating effects of knee OA declined markedly after 18 months of exercise training at low to moderate intensity. Because knee pain, whether due to OA, cartilage damage, fluid retention, congenital anomaly, or injury, adversely affects physical activity habits in many older individuals, this particular exercise benefit is noteworthy.

Although exercise is advised, elevated risk is associated with exercising among seniors who have had hip repair or replacement surgery. These individuals should always check with their physicians before doing lower-body exercises. They should also avoid crossing their legs or bending their hips farther than a 90-degree angle. Finally, they should avoid locking the joints in their legs into a strained position. In most cases, a modified exercise program can be prepared within the limits of that kind of medical condition. Adhering to safe and appropriate exercise guidelines is vital to maintaining fitness and autonomy for diseased or disabled individuals of all ages.

In the future, greater emphasis should be placed on identifying exercise facilities that are appropriately designed to foster adherence to an exercise program for the disabled. After all, being labeled wheelchair accessible is not necessarily the same as being wheelchair friendly. The National Center on Physical Activity and Disability (NCPAD) recently began publishing a monthly electronic newsletter. In a current issue (NCPAD News, 2002), they provided a number of tips for evaluating a potential exercise facility for people with disabilities (see figure 3.5). Introducing some of these modifications in exercise facilities may attenuate many of the perceived

- Does the facility have automatic entrance doors and accessible parking (wide spaces to accommodate vans and lifts)?
- Are aisles between machines wide enough for wheelchairs, walkers, and other assistive devices?
- Is there an accessible elevator?
- Is the staff trained in sensitivity to disabilities and assistive technology?
- Are staffers willing and competent to help adjust equipment or assist with transfers?
- Is adaptive exercise equipment available, such as roll-in strength-training machines, hand cycles, underwater exercise equipment, and so on?
- Are classes offered that are tailored to disabled patrons, such as wheelchair aerobics, aqua yoga, martial arts for persons who are physically challenged, and so on?
- Are the machines with cables and pulleys adjustable for people of different height?
- Do locker rooms have accessible rest rooms, showers with benches, lockers and sinks at appropriate height, accessible hooks, lowered blow dryers for hair and hands?
- Are floor materials nonskid?
- Do the whirlpool and pool have ramp entry? Is a submersible wheelchair available for water entry?
- If services such as massage, tanning, and spa treatments are available, do they have accessible beds?

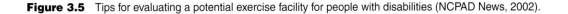

Figure 3.5 Tips for evaluating a potential exercise facility for people with disabilities (NCPAD News, 2002).

barriers that frequently prohibit disabled adults from participating in traditional, structured exercise programs.

The comprehensive exploration of the role of physical activity intervention among ethnic minority individuals with disability should be another integral component of future research. Myriad scientific studies have correlated sedentary living with racial ethnicity, aging, being economically disadvantaged, having lower educational levels, and having concurrent chronic diseases and physical disability (Taylor et al., 1998). Therefore, maximally effective exercise interventions will only emerge as we define and understand correlates of physical activity for at-risk populations such as these.

Making the Right Exercise Choices

A good exercise program should have four components: aerobics, muscular strength, muscular endurance, and flexibility. The **aerobic** component will provide the health-related benefits in addition to controlling and maintaining body weight and fat. A sound weight-training program will improve muscle tone, strength, and endurance; prevent the loss of lean-muscle mass; add muscle mass; and help control body weight and fat by increasing metabolism. Flexibility training will help maintain and improve range of motion and prevent joint stiffness.

Choosing an Aerobic Program

You should select a program that is effective in developing the cardiorespiratory system and is compatible with your training objectives, time available, and interests. Table 3.1 compares aerobic exercise choices based on the characteristics of the ideal program. Study this table carefully before making your selection. You may wish to sample different approaches to find activities that you enjoy for use in cross-training later.

If you are interested in the sports approach to aerobic fitness, study table 3.2 before making your selections. As you are now aware, the term aerobic means "with oxygen" and describes extended vigorous exercise that stimulates heart and lung activity enough to produce a training effect. This result occurs when you reach your target heart rate and maintain it for 20 minutes or longer. Many sports are more anaerobic than

> **aerobic**—Activity performed in the presence of oxygen, using fat as the major source of fuel.
>
> **anaerobic**—High-intensity activity, such as sprinting, performed in the absence of oxygen, using glucose as the major source of fuel.
>
> **oxygen debt**—The difference between the exact amount of oxygen needed for an exercise task and the amount actually taken in.

aerobic and fail to improve heart-lung endurance or provide the health benefits you desire. Aerobic exercises should produce some changes within 3 to 4 weeks.

Anaerobic means "without oxygen" and describes short, all-out exercise efforts such as the 100-, 200-, or 400-meter dash and sports such as football and baseball. Anaerobic metabolism occurs when the oxygen you breathe in is insufficient to supply active muscles, **oxygen debt** occurs, and you begin to breathe heavily. After you stop exercising, oxygen debt is repaid and normal breathing returns. Unfortunately, you cannot sustain anaerobic activities for long periods. Consequently, you burn fewer calories and fail to achieve some important health benefits. Improving your aerobic fitness only through participation in a sport is difficult, and we recommend that you supplement such participation with a minimum of two aerobic workouts weekly.

Choosing Muscular Strength and Endurance Programs

Chapter 7 describes numerous choices for increasing your muscular strength and endurance effectively. Your choice of workout routine depends on your training objectives, which also help you decide between free weights and the other types of exercise equipment.

Selecting an Appropriate Flexibility Training Program

Although a simple, static stretching routine is the wisest choice for effectively improving your flexibility, specific exercise choices depend on your objectives, including that of the particular activity for which you are training. The detailed information in chapter 6 will help you make the right decision. In less than 10 minutes daily, you can maintain and even improve range of motion in your major joints.

TABLE 3.1—Evaluation of Exercise Programs

Characteristics of ideal program	Aerobic exercise and dance	Anaerobics	Calisthenics	Cycling	Rope jumping	Running programs	Sports[a]	Walking	Swimming (laps)	Weight training
Easily adaptable to individual's exercise tolerance	P	Y	Y	Y	Y	Y	P	Y	Y	Y
Applies the progressive resistance principle	Y	Y	Y	Y	Y	Y	P	Y	Y	Y
Provides for self-evaluation	Y	Y	P	Y	Y	Y	P	Y	Y	Y
Practical for use throughout life	Y	N	N	Y	Y	Y	P	Y	Y	Y
Scientifically developed	Y	Y	P	Y	Y	Y	U	Y	Y	Y
Involves minimum time	Y	P	N	N	Y	Y	N	N	Y	Y
Involves little or no equipment	P	Y	Y	N	Y	Y	N	Y	Y	N
Performed easily at home	N	N	Y	Y	Y	Y	N	Y	Y	N
Widely publicized	Y	N	N	Y	Y	Y	Y	Y	Y	Y
Accepted and valued	Y	P	N	Y	Y	Y	P	Y	Y	Y
Offers challenge	Y	Y	N	Y	Y	Y	Y	Y	Y	Y
Firms body	Y	Y	Y	Y	Y	P	P	Y	Y	Y
Develops flexibility[b]	Y	N	Y	N	N	Y	Y	N	P	N
Develops muscular endurance	Y	Y	Y	Y	Y	Y	Y	Y	Y	Y
Develops cardiovascular endurance and prevents heart disease	Y	N	N	Y	Y	Y	Y	P	Y	P
Develops strength	P	P	Y	P	P	Y	Y	P	P	Y
Expends many calories and helps with weight loss	Y	P	P	Y	Y	P	Y	Y	Y	N

Note: Y = yes, P = partially, N = no provision, U = unknown (referring to meeting ideal characteristics).

[a]The value of the sports approach depends on the activity and the level of competition.

[b]Flexibility can be improved only if the complete range of movement is performed in each exercise applying static pressure at the extreme range of motion before returning to starting position.

From J. Unitas and G.B. Dintiman, 1979, *Improving health and fitness in the athlete* (Englewood Cliffs, NJ: Prentice-Hall), 180. Reprinted by permission of author.

TABLE 3.2—Ratings of Sports

Sport	Type	Cardiovascular	Caloric expenditure	Legs	Abdomen	Arms and shoulder	Age range recommended
Archery	Anaerobic	L	L	L	L	L	Age 10 and up
Backpacking	50% aerobic	M-H	H	H	M	L	All ages
Badminton	40% aerobic	M-H	H	H	L	M	Age 7 and up
Baseball or softball	Anaerobic	L	L	M	L	L	All ages
Basketball	25% aerobic	M	H	H	L	L	Age 7 to 60
Bicycling (competitive)	Aerobic	H	H	H	L	M	All ages
Bowling	Anaerobic	L	L	L	L	L	All ages
Dance (aerobic)	Aerobic	M-H	M-H	M	M	M	All ages
Canoeing or rowing (recreational)	Anaerobic	L	M	L	L	M	Age 12 and up
Canoeing or rowing (competitive)	Aerobic	H	H	M	M	H	Age 12 to 40
Fencing	Anaerobic	L-M	M	M	L	M	Age 12 and up
Field hockey	40% aerobic	M-H	M-H	H	L	M	Age 7 and up
Golf—motor cart	Anaerobic	L	L	L	L	L	All ages
Golf—walking	Aerobic	L	M	M	L	L	All ages
Handball, racquetball, or squash (singles)	40% aerobic	M-H	H	H	L	H	All ages
Hiking	Aerobic	L-M	M	H	L	L	All ages
Hunting	Aerobic	L-M	M	M	L	L	All ages
Ice or roller skating—speed	Anaerobic	L-M	M	H	L	L	Under age 50

Ice or roller skating—figure	Aerobic	L-M	H	H	M	M	All ages
Jogging	Aerobic	M-H	H	H	L	L	Age 7 and up
Lacrosse	40% aerobic	M-H	H	H	M	M	Under age 45
Orienteering	50% aerobic	M-H	H	H	M	L	All ages
Rugby	60% aerobic	H	H	H	L	H	Under age 45
Skiing (cross-country)	Aerobic	H	H	H	H	H	Under age 65
Skin and scuba diving	Aerobic	M	M	M	M	L	All ages
Soccer	50% aerobic	H	H	H	L	H	Under age 55
Surfing	Anaerobic	L	M	H	M	L	Age 7 and up
Swimming	Aerobic	M	H	M	L	H	Age 7 and up
Tennis (singles)	40% aerobic	M	M	H	L	L	All ages
Touch football	Anaerobic	L	L-M	H	L	L	Under age 55
Volleyball	Anaerobic	L	L	M-H	L	M	All ages
Walking	Aerobic	L-M	M	H	L	L	All ages
Water skiing	Anaerobic	L-M	M	H	L	M	All ages
Weight training	Anaerobic	L	L	H	H	H	All ages
Wrestling	30% aerobic	M	H	H	H	H	Under age 45

Note: H = high, M = medium, L = low.

Behavioral Change and Motivational Strategies

Many things can interfere with your application of sound exercise principles. Here are some typical barriers (roadblocks) and strategies for overcoming them.

Roadblock

Exercise just isn't fun anymore, and you no longer look forward to your afternoon workout session. Even if you do get into the workout, you are not motivated to put forth much effort.

Behavioral Change Strategy

You may be experiencing some of the emotional and physical effects of overtraining or exercising too often. To renew your interest, try one or more of the following approaches:

- Change aerobic activities every other day as a cross-training technique. If you are jogging or using step daily, for example, substitute cycling, lap swimming, aerobic dance, or a sports activity two to three times weekly.
- Change the time you exercise. Try early mornings, noon, or just before bedtime to see if your mood improves.
- Apply the light-heavy concept discussed in this chapter and avoid two consecutive workouts of the same level of difficulty.
- Add one or two fun workouts weekly and exercise with a group of friends.

Your muscles are sore the following morning, making your day unpleasant. Sitting, standing, and moving around on the job are somewhat painful.

A number of factors may be causing the problem. You may be exercising untrained muscles; training much too hard; not consuming enough fluids before, during, and after your workout; or stretching improperly or not at all. Try some of these remedies for at least a week:

- Hydrate 15 to 30 minutes before your workout by drinking three or four 8-ounce glasses of water.
- Record the amount of water and other fluids you consume daily, making certain to drink at least eight glasses of water.
- Alternate light- and heavy-workout days.
- Warm up for a longer period than you normally do and then stretch carefully for at least 10 minutes.
- At the end of your workout, cool down properly and end with a mild 5-minute stretching session.

Although you have been exercising daily for a month, you don't seem to be losing weight and fat.

To lose body fat and weight, you need to change your exercise emphasis and reduce your caloric intake. Don't give up. Be certain that you do the following:

- Monitor both your exercise sessions and your food intake by keeping accurate records of total exercise volume and daily calories consumed.
- Increase the duration of your workout and exercise every day. If you are walking, try to walk continuously for at least 1 hour. Reduce the intensity of your workout and continue exercising longer each workout.
- Schedule your workout about 2 hours before mealtime or 2 hours after your evening meal to help control hunger and the temptation to overeat or snack.

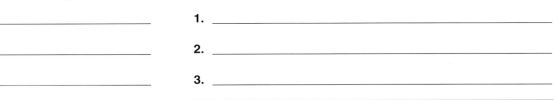

List other roadblocks that you are experiencing that seem to be reducing the effectiveness of your program and limiting your success.

1. _____

2. _____

3. _____

Now list behavioral change strategies that can help you overcome the roadblocks you listed. If necessary, refer to chapter 4 for behavioral change and motivational strategies.

1. _____

2. _____

3. _____

Summary

The Ideal Exercise Program   A complete exercise program should bring about improvement in five key health-related fitness areas: cardiorespiratory endurance, muscular strength, muscular endurance, flexibility, and body composition. Aerobic exercise is the most important component and should form the foundation of the ideal program. To guarantee continued improvement, you must apply the principles of exercise specifically to your workout choice.

New Exercise Guidelines for Children, Adults, and the Elderly   College students should engage in an aerobic activity at moderate to moderately high intensity for a total of 60 minutes throughout the day (four 15-minute walks or an accumulation of 60 minutes through a number of different activities) or 30 minutes of continuous aerobic exercise at the target heart rate four to seven times weekly. The ideal complete program also includes regular stretching exercises after the warm-up and before the workout and two to three weight-training sessions weekly.

Fitness Concepts   A preconditioning period may be necessary before you begin a new exercise program, particularly if you have previously been inactive. This 3- to 4-week period will prepare you for workouts that are more vigorous and allow you to reach and maintain your THR for 20 to 30 minutes safely.

The PRE principle can easily be adapted to aerobic, muscular strength and endurance, and flexibility training to ensure steady progress and improvement in these areas. To train for a specific sport or activity, you must apply the principle of specificity by using movements and exercises that closely simulate those performed in the sport. Using a warm-up and cool-down period, applying FIT to your aerobic workout, alternating light- and heavy-workout days, dressing appropriately for the weather, monitoring your progress with record keeping, and cross-training will improve the benefits of each workout, keep you emotionally and physically healthy, and eliminate boredom and overtraining.

Making the Right Exercise Choices   Select aerobic activities that you enjoy, that are effective, and that meet your training objectives. The sports approach to aerobic fitness requires special care in selecting activities that are primarily aerobic in nature, such as soccer, rugby, field hockey, and racquetball (singles). Anaerobic activity choices will provide little in the way of health-related benefits. Two to three additional workouts weekly in an aerobic activity are also recommended.

Guidelines for Special Groups   Pregnant women, the elderly, and those suffering from various illnesses and disabilities may need to modify their approach to exercise. Pregnancy does not prevent most women from engaging in regular mild or moderate exercise three or more times weekly. Suggested changes involve consuming an additional 300 calories per day, avoiding exercise in the supine position after the first trimester, reducing intensity according to maternal symptoms, stopping when fatigued, avoiding exercise that may produce even mild abdominal trauma, hydrating properly, and avoiding extreme heat conditions. The elderly should also continue regular aerobic, strength, and flexibility exercise with restrictions depending on fitness levels and medical limitations. A number of diseases and disabilities require special precautions and guidelines that only a physician can provide. For the healthy man or woman, regular exercise should continue, with some modifications, throughout life.

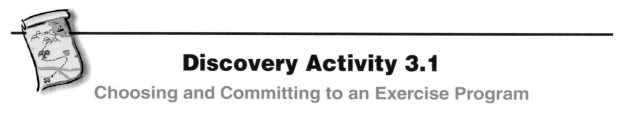

Discovery Activity 3.1

Choosing and Committing to an Exercise Program

Name _____ **Date** _____

Instructions: This lab will assist you in identifying specific times, dates, and places to exercise in activities you enjoy that also produce significant health benefits.

1. Determine the best time and days for you to exercise. Prepare a schedule of your daily routine Monday through Sunday. Include your class, study, work, mealtime, church, and other activities.

	Monday	Tuesday	Wednesday	Thursday	Friday	Saturday	Sunday
7-8							
8-9							
9-10							
10-11							
11-12							
12-1							
1-2							
2-3							
3-4							
4-5							
5-6							
6-7							
7-8							
8-9							
9-10							

Now choose a block of time (at least 1 hour, ideally 1 1/2 hours) on 3 separate days, avoiding 2 days in succession. You may want to exercise early in the morning (which has been shown to boost metabolic and energy levels), keep exercise as a reward at the end of the day, or take advantage of a lull between classes to break up your day. Whatever your choice, force yourself to adhere to the schedule for at least a month.

Weekly exercise days and time _____

Discovery Activity 3.1 *(continued)*

2. List the three most important outcomes you expect from your exercise program.

   a. _____

   b. _____

   c. _____

3. Determine the type of exercise you are most likely to enjoy. Review table 3.1 and select several activities you can try in your newly chosen exercise time slot that develop a moderate to high level of cardiorespiratory fitness. You may want to use the sports approach and play tennis, handball, racquetball, squash, badminton, basketball, soccer, or some other sport that is convenient and enjoyable for you, or you might prefer to take an aerobic approach and join an exercise class, walk, cycle, or swim. Each of these activities and many others can provide significant health benefits over time. Try several activities until you discover a cardiorespiratory workout that you really enjoy. If your schedule allows, consider using two weight-training workout sessions per week for 20 to 30 minutes following your cardiorespiratory exercise. Go to the university weight room and ask for help in setting up a program that meets your needs. Make certain that your exercise choices are capable of producing the desired outcomes you identified in step 2.

4. Keep a record of each workout using a form like the one in figure 3.2. By monitoring your progress and recording your feelings, you are more likely to avoid overuse and other injuries and remain motivated enough to stay with your program. After a month, you should begin to feel better and have more energy.

5. Sign the exercise contract on page 82 to confirm your commitment to a month of regular exercise 3 to 4 days per week.

From *Physical fitness and wellness, third edition,* by Jerrold S. Greenberg, George B. Dintiman, and Barbee Myers Oakes, 2004, Champaign, IL: Human Kinetics.

Contract to Increase My Physical Activity Level

During the next 4 weeks, from _____ to _____, I hereby agree to work as hard as possible at achieving the following:

1. Physical activity goals for increasing my energy use during occupational time:
   a. I will park my car or leave public transportation and walk ___ additional minutes per day.
   b. I will spend ___ minutes daily standing instead of sitting while I work.
   c. I will walk up ___ flights of stairs each working day.
   d. I will walk around my work area ___ minutes every day.
   e. I will spend ___ minutes during each coffee break standing instead of sitting.
   f. I will spend ___ minutes during each lunch break walking outdoors.

2. Physical activity goals for increasing my energy use during recreational time:
   a. I will spend ___ minutes daily doing stretching activities to increase my flexibility.
   b. I will spend ___ minutes at least three times per week doing aerobic activities to improve my endurance.
   c. I will spend ___ minutes at least three times per week doing strength activities.
   d. I will spend ___ minutes Saturday and Sunday in active recreational activities.

3. I agree to do one of the following as my reward when I achieve my daily goals in increased activity:
   a. _____
   b. _____
   c. _____
   d. _____
   e. _____
   f. _____

4. I agree to do one of the following as my consequence when I do not achieve my daily goals:
   a. _____
   b. _____

5. I will reward myself every week with one of the following when I achieve my weekly exercise goals:
   a. _____
   b. _____
   c. _____
   d. _____
   e. _____
   f. _____

6. When I do not achieve my weekly goals, I agree to do the following:
   a. _____
   b. _____

I agree to follow this contract until I reach my goals.

Signed _____   Date _____

Witnessed _____

From *Physical fitness and wellness, third edition*, by Jerrold S. Greenberg, George B. Dintiman, and Barbee Myers Oakes, 2004, Champaign, IL: Human Kinetics.

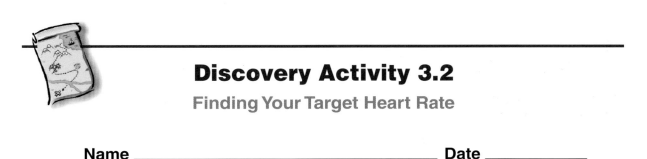

Discovery Activity 3.2
Finding Your Target Heart Rate

Name _____ **Date** _____

Instructions: The target heart rate (THR) is the range of heart rate that will produce training effects on the heart if it is maintained for a sufficient length of time (usually 20 to 30 minutes) at least three times per week. This kind of exercise is commonly known as aerobic exercise. The purpose of this lab is to determine your THR, or exercise benefit zone (EBZ).

1. Determine your resting heart rate (RHR)—the lowest heart rate you experience anytime during your waking hours, day or evening. Check it several times during the day when you feel relaxed. (Refer to steps 1 and 2 of Discovery Activity 2.2 on page 52 for specific instructions on finding your RHR.)

2. Use the following formula to compute your 60%, 70%, and 85% target heart rates. You should stay in this zone during aerobic exercise.

60% THR

220 – _____ (subtract age) – _____ (subtract RHR) × .60 + _____ (add RHR) = _____

70% THR

220 – _____ (subtract age) – _____ (subtract RHR) × .70 + _____ (add RHR) = _____

85% THR

220 – _____ (subtract age) – _____ (subtract RHR) × .85 + _____ (add RHR) = _____

From *Physical fitness and wellness, third edition,* by Jerrold S. Greenberg, George B. Dintiman, and Barbee Myers Oakes, 2004, Champaign, IL: Human Kinetics.

Discovery Activity 3.3

Service-Learning for Principles of Exercise

Many fitness clubs, YMCAs, Jewish Community Centers, and other community centers encourage program participants to become physically fit by offering ongoing fitness programs or organizing fitness clubs. You can volunteer to conduct one of these programs. One possibility is to conduct a "Walk to the Beach (or Lake)" fitness program that has participants log the number of miles they work out during each session with the goal of accumulating the number of miles required to travel to the beach or lake. Beginning these programs in spring, when people are thinking about fitting into last year's bathing suits, may make recruiting participants easier. Staff at these organizations can help you translate various workouts—such as walking on a treadmill—into approximate miles of exercise. Before the first session of the program, you can conduct a workshop on principles of exercise. Periodically distributing handouts on the principles of exercise will reinforce their use by the exercisers. In this way, program participants will be encouraged to work out in a safe, healthy way, with greater likelihood that they will benefit from the program.

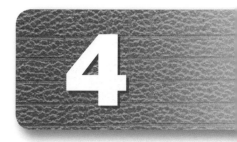

Behavioral Change and Motivational Techniques

Chapter Objectives

By the end of this chapter, you should be able to

1. discuss the importance of psychosocial lifestyle factors such as locus of control, social support, and self-esteem in deciding on a fitness program;
2. describe several techniques that researchers have demonstrated to be effective in helping people achieve their fitness goals;
3. list several means of improving the chances of maintaining a physical fitness program once one has been started; and
4. modify a physical fitness program in the face of obstacles so that it need not be interrupted.

The comedian Henny Youngman tells of a man who told his psychiatrist, "Doc, I have a guilt complex," to which his doctor replied, "You ought to be ashamed of yourself!" We do not want to shame you into regularly engaging in physical activity. That approach would be dysfunctional, somewhat like the method of a physical education instructor who makes physical activity so distasteful that students are repelled by exercise for the remainder of their lives. Instead, we want you to appreciate the benefits of being physically fit and then decide for yourself whether to engage in regular exercise. If you decide to do that, we can show you how to begin a program and continue participating in it over an extended period.

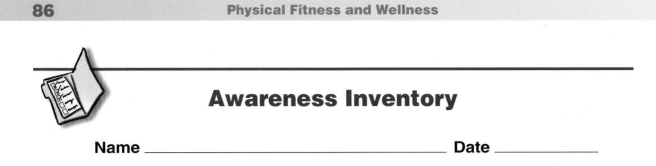

Awareness Inventory

Name _____ **Date** _____

Check the space by the letter T for the statements that you think are true and the space by the letter F for the statements that you think are false. The answers appear following the list of statements. This chapter will present information to clarify these statements for you. As you read the chapter, look for explanations for the reasons why the statements are true or false.

T___ **F**___ 1. Locus of control refers to how much control you have over events that affect your life.

T___ **F**___ 2. If you are socially isolated you are more likely to exercise regularly.

T___ **F**___ 3. Body cathexis refers to how highly you regard your physical self.

T___ **F**___ 4. When you write a contract to encourage the adoption of a regular program of exercise, the punishments that you will apply if you do not exercise will be more effective than the rewards that you will apply if you do exercise.

T___ **F**___ 5. In planning your exercise program you should increase your performance goals gradually.

T___ **F**___ 6. Just thinking about exercising can help you to begin exercising regularly.

T___ **F**___ 7. Behavioral change theories are useful for explaining why you do or do not exercise, but they are not useful in helping you begin to exercise in the first place.

T___ **F**___ 8. If you believe that you are susceptible to a serious illness or disease if you are physically inactive, you will most likely exercise regularly.

T___ **F**___ 9. Monitoring your exercise behavior and progress, such as how much weight you can lift, is too compulsive and may interfere with your achieving your exercise goals when you become discouraged about not improving quickly enough.

T___ **F**___ 10. Because you can conduct isometric and isotonic contractions in a limited space, the activity is a good one to perform in your dormitory room or apartment.

Answers: 1-F, 2-F, 3-T, 4-F, 5-T, 6-T, 7-F, 8-F, 9-F, 10-T

From *Physical fitness and wellness, third edition*, by Jerrold S. Greenberg, George B. Dintiman, and Barbee Myers Oakes, 2004, Champaign, IL: Human Kinetics.

Analyze Yourself

Assessing Your Locus of Control

Name _____ **Date** _____

Instructions: For each pair of statements, circle the item that best describes your beliefs.

1. **a.** Grades are a function of the amount of work students do.
   b. Grades depend on the kindness of the instructor.
2. **a.** Promotions are earned by hard work.
   b. Promotions are a result of being in the right place at the right time.
3. **a.** Meeting someone to love is a matter of luck.
   b. Meeting someone to love depends on going out often to meet many people.
4. **a.** Living a long life is a function of heredity.
   b. Living a long life is a function of adopting healthy habits.
5. **a.** Being overweight is determined by the number of fat cells you were born with or developed early in life.
   b. Being overweight depends on what and how much food you eat.
6. **a.** People who exercise regularly set up their schedules to do so.
   b. Some people simply don't have time for regular exercise.
7. **a.** Winning at poker depends on betting correctly.
   b. Winning at poker is a matter of being lucky.
8. **a.** Staying married depends on working at the marriage.
   b. Marital breakup is a matter of being unlucky in choosing the wrong marriage partner.
9. **a.** Citizens can have some influence on their governments.
   b. Citizens can do nothing to affect governmental functioning.
10. **a.** Those skilled at sports are born well coordinated.
    b. Those skilled at sports work hard learning the skills.
11. **a.** People with close friends are lucky to have met people with whom to be intimate.
    b. Developing close friendships takes hard work.
12. **a.** Your future depends on whom you meet and on chance.
    b. Your future is up to you.
13. **a.** Most people are so sure of their opinions that nothing can change their minds.
    b. A logical argument can convince most people.
14. **a.** People decide the direction of their lives.
    b. For the most part, we have little control over our future.
15. **a.** People who do not like you simply do not understand you.
    b. You can be liked by anyone you choose to have like you.
16. **a.** You can make your life a happy one.
    b. Happiness is a matter of fate.
17. **a.** You evaluate feedback and make decisions based on it.

(continued)

    b. You tend to be easily influenced by others.

18. **a.** If voters studied candidates' records, they could elect honest politicians.

    b. Politics and politicians are corrupt by nature.

19. **a.** Parents, teachers, and bosses have a great deal to say about your happiness and self-satisfaction.

    b. Whether you are happy depends on you.

20. **a.** Air pollution can be controlled if citizens become angry about it.

    b. Air pollution is an inevitable result of technological progress.

Scoring

To determine your locus of control, give yourself 1 point for each listed response:

1-a, 2-a, 3-b, 4-b, 5-b, 6-a, 7-a, 8-a, 9-a, 10-b, 11-b,
12-b, 13-b, 14-a, 15-b, 16-a, 17-a, 18-a, 19-b, 20-a

Scores of 10 or above indicate that you believe you are generally in control of events that affect your life (an internal locus of control). Scores below 10 indicate that you believe you generally do not have control of events that affect your life (an external locus of control).

From *Physical fitness and wellness, third edition,* by Jerrold S. Greenberg, George B. Dintiman, and Barbee Myers Oakes, 2004, Champaign, IL: Human Kinetics.

Psychosocial Factors to Consider

The fact that women in the United States are less likely than men to adhere to recommended guidelines for physical activity is verified by a plethora of scientific studies such as the survey conducted by the 1996 surgeon general's report on physical activity and health. Furthermore, despite several decades of warnings about the potentially negative health consequences of a sedentary life, ethnic minority women are less likely than white women are to participate in leisure-time physical activity, regardless of age, occupation, and socioeconomic status (Kimm et al., 2002). Thus, greater understanding of the modifiable factors that can pose barriers to an exercise program would likely prove valuable for public health officials.

To plan an exercise program, you need to know something about yourself: your motivations, your perceptions of the amount of control you have over your life, the degree to which you associate with other people, and the confidence you have in yourself. This chapter makes the importance of this information clear.

Locus of Control

Some people believe that they can control events in their lives. This construct is called one's locus of control. People who believe in this construct possess an internal locus of control, or internality. People who do not believe in the construct possess an external locus of control, or externality.

Externals believe that the course of their lives is a matter of luck, fate, chance, or the actions of powerful others. The distinction between externality and internality is more than academic. If you do not believe that you control events in your life, you are apt to adopt a laissez-faire attitude. Relative to physical fitness, you might believe that whether you are in good shape or not is a function of luck or genetic makeup. Engaging in an exercise program makes no sense if you do not control your fitness level.

Internals believe that what they get is, for the most part, a result of what they do. Therefore, internals will probably learn a good deal about exercise and physical fitness and plan a program in which they can participate. An internal locus of control is important if you are serious about becoming physically fit and maintaining that level of fitness.

If you scored as an external in the Analyze Yourself exercise that opened this chapter, make a list of the parts of your life that you influence. Then read that list daily to change your focus. In addition, take some measures before beginning an exercise program (for example, your pulse rate and weight) and measure those variables again after engaging in exercise for several weeks. Observing a change will reinforce the notion that you can influence your body rather than resign yourself to being a victim of your habits or your genetic makeup.

Social Isolation

Friends change as Life changes.

We all need to interact with other people. Researchers have found that the social support we have helps prevent us from getting ill and enhances the quality of our lives. Conversely, not having significant others with whom to share our joys and sorrows causes ill health or **social isolation.**

If you find that you need to improve your social network, structure your fitness program accordingly. Consider joining an exercise club, a health spa, the YMCA, or the Jewish Community Center. You might meet people there with whom you can become friendly. Participation in organized sports (at levels suited to your skill and experience) can also provide an opportunity to meet people. Playing in leagues and tournaments (team as well as individual) is another avenue for alleviating social isolation. You should not ignore your social self when structuring your fitness program. To do so is to endanger your health and wellness.

Self-Esteem

How you feel about yourself.

What you think of yourself, whether that perception is accurate or not, influences your fitness, health, and wellness. If you do not think highly of yourself, you might not believe that you can become fit. You may lack confidence, see yourself as genetically inferior, or think you have so far to go that beginning a fitness program is futile.

In particular, what you think of your body, your bodily self-esteem—sometimes called **body cathexis**—will affect your health and fitness.

You may be satisfied with parts of your body and dissatisfied with other parts. Be proud of those parts about which you are satisfied and do not fret about those parts about which you are dissatisfied. You can improve them, at least many of them, and thereby feel better about yourself.

locus of control—The degree to which you believe you are in control of events in your life.

social isolation—The lack of other people with whom to discuss important matters relevant to your life.

body cathexis—Physical self-esteem; how highly you regard your physical self.

External LOC- B/C of someone else

Internal LOC- B/C of myself

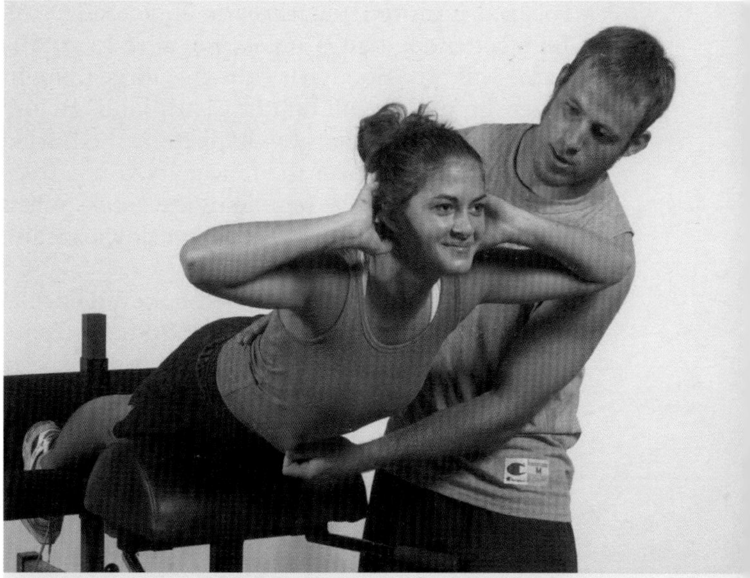

Having friends who encourage you can be an important part of achieving your fitness goals.

For example, if you are dissatisfied with your waist, you can do exercises to strengthen the muscles in your waist. We discuss those in chapter 7, which covers weight training and body shaping. Useful strategies are available to deal with those body parts you are dissatisfied with that cannot be changed, such as your nose. You need to become more accepting of those body parts. One effective way of doing this is to recognize that things could be worse. Volunteering for an organization that caters to the needs of the physically challenged or the socioeconomically disadvantaged can help you put your concern about your nose, for example, in proper perspective.

Strategies for Achieving Your Fitness Goals

A good deal of research identifies effective ways of achieving your fitness goals. Before you can apply the appropriate techniques, however, you must identify the goals.

Goal Setting

In determining your fitness goals, it is important to set realistic goals and to assess your progress periodically.

Jorge was playing tennis with a friend one pleasant summer day. The sun was out, the birds were chirping, and the water in the creek alongside the tennis court was gently caressing the rocks as it moved downstream. You couldn't ask for a better day, that is, unless you were Jorge. His game was off. "Enough is enough," Jorge thought when he netted still another backhand. Before anyone realized what was happening, he hurled his tennis racket over the fence, above the trees beyond, and into the middle of the creek. When last seen, the racket was heading downstream, never again to be used.

Some of you may know a Jorge or even be one. The problem is in being realistic. Some of us are has-been athletes expecting to perform at the level we could when we were younger and practiced daily. Others of us are never-beens with grand delusions and dreams that we will never fulfill. Do not fall into either trap when setting your fitness goals. Be realistic in what you can attain and how long it will take you to attain it. If your goals are unobtainable, you will become frustrated and give up on physical fitness altogether.

In the beginning it is wise to set goals that are easy to achieve. In that way, when you attain them you will reinforce fitness behavior and be more likely to achieve subsequent goals.

Periodically Assess — *to see how fast you do something or how much you lift*

Once you decide on your fitness goals, periodically assess how you are meeting them. If you conclude that you are making progress in an appropriate amount of time, keep doing what you are doing. If your assessment indicates problems meeting your goals, make adjustments. Maybe you need to exercise longer, more intensely, or more frequently. Without periodically assessing your program, you will not identify needed changes to help you achieve your fitness goals.

Behavioral Change Techniques

For sedentary individuals, making a lifelong commitment to integrate habitual exercise into their routines can be challenging. As we learn more about why certain individuals tend to be more successful than others, we will be more effective in designing intervention strategies.

Among the more effective techniques you can employ in meeting your fitness goals are the use of social support, contracting, reminder systems, gradual programming, tailoring, chaining, and covert techniques.

Social Support

Using social support is just another way of saying that you need other people to encourage and help you. Social support for engaging in an exercise program is the most commonly studied psychosocial determinant of physical activity. As hypothesized, scientific studies examining exercise correlates among sedentary, ethnically diverse women indicate that having strong social support from family, friends, and spouses improves adherence to a fitness program (Walcott-McQuigg et al., 2001; Nies et al., 1999; Eyler et al., 1998, 1999; Mosca et al., 1998). Likewise, not having an exercise partner was reported to be a barrier to physical activity among women of varying ethnicities (Nies et al., 1999; Conn, 1998; Moore, 1996; Kaplan et al., 1991; Johnson et al., 1990). Among the many predictors of long-term exercise compliance among older adult women, social support appears to be an overwhelmingly positive determinant of physical activity for women of all ethnicities (Litt et al., 2002; Kaplan et al., 2001; Troped and Saunders, 1998).

Adopting a habit of regular exercise, or any habit for that matter, is much easier if others encourage you. If you can persuade someone to exercise with you, to ask you daily whether you have exercised, or to buy you a piece of exercise clothing or equipment periodically, you will be more apt to stick with your regimen. To begin, make a list of people who you think would be willing to assist you and discuss with them how they can help.

Contracting

One way to use social support is to develop a contract to achieve a certain exercise goal and have someone else witness it. If that person then helps you periodically to assess your progress, you will be more likely to be successful. Figure 4.1 shows a sample contract that identifies the behavior goal, the date when it should be achieved (and assessed), the reward for achieving the goal, and the punishment for not achieving it. Rewards can be going to the movies, buying something you have wanted for a long time, or taking a night off from schoolwork. Punishments might include not watching television for a week or not eating your favorite snack for several days. Although rewards are more effective than punishments in controlling behavior, punishments have a place as well. And although contracts have been found to work best when witnessed, they can be effective if you merely contract with yourself.

One reviewer of this book related a story of how one student monitored her behavior as part of her behavioral change contract. Her goal was to eliminate swearing. To do so, she devised a

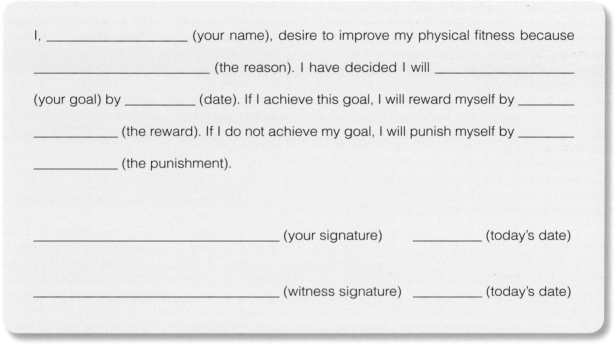

I, _____ (your name), desire to improve my physical fitness because

_____ (the reason). I have decided I will _____

(your goal) by _____ (date). If I achieve this goal, I will reward myself by _____

_____ (the reward). If I do not achieve my goal, I will punish myself by _____

_____ (the punishment).

_____ (your signature)   _____ (today's date)

_____ (witness signature)   _____ (today's date)

Figure 4.1 Fitness contract.

From *Physical Fitness and wellness*, by Jerrold S. Greenberg, George B. Dintiman, and Barbee Myers Oakes, 2004, Champaign, IL: Human Kinetics.

system whereby she started with a bunch of pennies in her right pocket. Every time she swore, she transferred a penny from the right pocket to the left pocket. At the end of the day, she could easily tally the number of times she swore that day. Such ingenuity can go a long way toward helping you achieve your behavioral change goals.

Reminder Systems

One way to remember things is to make a note of them. Reminder notes will help you remember to exercise, especially if you leave the notes in places where you cannot miss them—for example, on refrigerator doors or bathroom mirrors. You can also use notes in appointment books and calendars as reminders, as well as make computer reminders on Microsoft® Outlook or on handheld computers and Palm Pilots.

Gradual Programming

Too often, people who have never exercised regularly or who have not done so for some time expect to be able to run a mile in under 4 minutes. Less obvious, but no less unrealistic for many people, is the goal of exercising every other day when they have been sedentary for years or of exercising intensely when they have not done so for a while. Giving up the sedentary life cold turkey can be extremely difficult. If it is, do not fret. Instead, use

a graduated plan in which you start slowly and gradually increase both frequency and intensity. In fact, to prevent injury, fitness experts recommend graduated plans even for those who are already highly fit. For example, runners should not increase their distance by more than 10% a week, and weight trainers should not increase the weight they lift by more than 5%. Annesi (2002) further revealed the importance of this concept by correlating the feeling-state changes induced in new exercisers by moderate bouts of aerobic exercise. Both adult men and women were less motivated to maintain an exercise program when they were physically exhausted at the conclusion of their workouts. You can even use graduated plans to study more, to change your eating habits, or to alter other behaviors you have been meaning to change.

Tailoring

No two people are alike. This declaration is not the most provocative of statements, yet we sometimes act as though we do not know this simple fact. When you adopt a wholesale exercise program designed for a group without adjusting it to your own needs and circumstances, you are increasing the likelihood that you will soon stop exercising regularly. Some people are free to exercise in the mornings, others in the evenings. Some people are in better physical condition than others. People vary in their choice of mealtimes. Some are more committed to exercise than others. We could go on and on, but the point is that any program of regular exercise must be tailored to the individual. We will present exercise activities in later chapters, but for now you should know that for your program to be successful, you must choose which ones to do, when, how frequently, and how intensely.

Tailoring has proven to be effective among individuals across the lifespan and from a variety of cultures (Seefeldt et al., 2002). Individuals have the highest rates of compliance with exercise programs when they are tailored to their individual needs, account for individual fitness levels, allow individuals to dictate the type of activity, and provide social support. For example, when an exercise intervention program for older Filipino American women was tailored to incorporate their capabilities, cultural beliefs, and needs, adherence was high during the entire 3-month program (Maxwell et al., 2002). In studies of employed African American women, sweating and messing up their hair limited their participation in an exercise program during the workday (Carter-Nolan et al., 1996; Airhihenbuwa et al., 1995). Although individuals of myriad ethnically diverse populations share many correlates of physical activity, each minority group may have unique barriers that need to be identified when designing exercise programs (Banks-Wallace and Conn, 2002; Wilcox et al., 2002). Many studies such as these reveal the importance of modifying both the intervention delivery as well as the intervention content when designing fitness programs for individuals, particularly for new exercisers.

Chaining

In chaining, one behavior is linked to a previous one, and that to a previous one, and so on, like links in a chain. You can use chaining to help you achieve your fitness goals. To adopt a behavior, such as exercising regularly, you want to have as few links as possible between deciding to exercise and actually engaging in a fitness activity. To demonstrate, let us look at two people, Pat and Alex.

Pat decides to exercise at about 5:30 in the afternoon, rushes home, and starts gathering exercise clothes. In one drawer are gym shorts and socks, in another a shirt, and under the bed

in another room sneakers. Then Pat looks for the car keys for the drive to the track to jog. The track is 10 minutes away. On the way there, Pat realizes the car needs gas and stops to get some. Finally, Pat arrives at the track and is ready to exercise.

Alex decides to exercise at the same time of day. But Alex prepares beforehand. All the clothes needed for later are on the bed in the morning. Alex decides to run around the neighborhood instead of the track so that all that is required at 5:30 is to come home, dress, step outside the front door, and exercise.

If we consider each behavior needed to exercise as a link in a chain, we see that Pat has many more links. The more links, the more difficult it is to exercise, and the more likely it is not to happen. The trick is to decrease the links for a behavior you want to adopt and to increase the links for a behavior you want to give up (for example, cigarette smoking).

Covert Techniques

Some people are so inactive or busy that it is difficult for them to engage in regular exercise. Yet research has shown that one's awareness of the exercise habits of others has been a positive stimulant in terms of encouraging them to adopt an activity program. For example, King et al. (2000) found that frequently seeing other individuals exercise was positively associated with physical activity among a group of African American women. Three covert techniques can help people, perhaps like these women, initially change behavior without requiring them to do anything physically:

1. **Covert rehearsal.** This procedure requires that you imagine yourself exercising regularly. Your image must be extremely vivid; that is, you must notice all the details (your outfit, the weather, the location), smell the atmosphere, feel the bodily sensations, and so on. Being able to imagine yourself exercising makes it more likely that you will actually exercise. You will have desensitized yourself to the image of you exercising so that seeing yourself exercising will not seem foreign to you.

2. **Covert modeling.** For some of us, even imagining ourselves exercising is difficult. If that is the case with you, there is still hope. First, identify someone else you can envision exercising. Once that image is clear in your mind,

substitute yourself for that person. Model the image of you exercising after the image of that person exercising. After a while, it will be easier for you to think of yourself as a potentially regular exerciser, and you will be more likely to become one.

3. **Covert reinforcement.** With this technique, you imagine yourself exercising and then reward yourself for it with another image. Usually, a pleasant image serves as a reward (a day at the beach, a calm lake), and you allow it to surface and focus on it only after you have successfully accomplished the goal image.

Behavioral Change Theories and Exercise

Theories can help explain behavior or help change behavior. These two purposes of theory are interrelated. That is, if we can explain why a behavior is adopted or not adopted, we can intervene and control, or change, that behavior. This process will become clear as we discuss specific theories that you can use to take charge of your exercise behavior. Space limitations dictate a discussion of only two theories, but you can use many others to take charge of your exercise behavior. A good source to consult if you want to learn about other theories of behavior is the book *Health Behavior and Health Education,* by Karen Glanz, Frances Marcus Lewis, and Barbara K. Rimer (eds.), San Francisco: Jossey-Bass, 1990.

Stages of Change Theory

Researchers theorize that people are at different points in motivation, or readiness, to change a behavior. Five stages of the stages of change theory differentiate one's readiness to change (Prochaska, DiClemente, and Norcross, 1992).

1. **Precontemplation.** One is unaware of the problem or the need to change. Consequently, the person will not even contemplate action to change. For example, if you didn't know the benefits of exercise, you might not even be thinking about engaging in regular physical activity.

2. **Contemplation.** One is thinking about changing a behavior but has not taken any action to do so. For example, you might know that exercise is healthy and are think-

ing about starting an exercise program, but not soon.

3. **Decision and determination.** One actually starts planning to change the behavior. For example, you might start researching health clubs in your area and buy exercise clothing.

4. **Action.** One implements an exercise program and does so regularly. For example, you might start jogging every other day or weight train several days a week.

5. **Maintenance.** One continues the changed behavior over time. For example, you exercise at a health club throughout the year.

Evidence for the validity of the stages of change theory abounds. For example, Lee et al. (2001) found that adolescents reported less exercise when they were in the earlier stage of change. Woods et al. (2002) found that introducing a simple intervention based on the stages of change theory positively affected the activity habits of sedentary undergraduate college students. Studies of older adult men and women reported that readiness for change was the primary reason many of them initially adopted exercise programs (Litt et al., 2002; Bull et al., 2001; Faulkner and Biddle, 2001; Mullineaux et al. 2001).

Recognizing your current stage of change will help you strategize to take charge of your exercise behavior. If you are at the precontemplation level, you might need to begin by reading about the benefits of exercise to motivate you to move toward exercising regularly. If you are at the contemplation stage, you might realize that you value exercise and know that you need to start planning to do so. Perhaps the first step is to speak with someone who is knowledgeable about physical fitness, such as your instructor. If you are ready for the action phase, you will need to make concrete plans to exercise regularly. Write down the steps you will take and the dates by which you will take them. Again, your instructor might be a good resource to help you develop your plan. If you are at the action level, make sure you are engaging in exercise you find enjoyable. You may want to exercise with a friend. Keep a journal to monitor improvements in your strength, endurance, and other fitness components. Finally, if you have been exercising regularly and are at the maintenance stage of change, schedule your exercise time in your date book or place reminders to exercise on your refrigerator.

Health Belief Model

Another model warranting further examination theorizes that health behavior, such as exercising, is a result of factors other than those suggested by the stages of change theory. The health belief model suggests that the following factors are significant determinants of activity in adults, especially among ethnically diverse individuals (Glanz and Rimer, 1997):

- **Perceived susceptibility**—one's opinion of the chances of developing an undesirable condition. For example, if you didn't think that living a sedentary lifestyle would result in an unhealthy state, you might not be motivated to exercise regularly. But if you believed that not engaging in physical activity would make you susceptible to a state of ill health, you might be motivated to exercise.

   Research conducted to identify constraints to motivating African American women to exercise often contends that those who successfully maintained an activity program for at least a year were those who began exercising because they perceived themselves to be susceptible to health concerns, weight control, and stress reduction (Young et al., 2001; Fischer et al., 1999; Harnack et al., 1999; Kaplan et al., 1991). These findings are important from the perspective of prevention because several other research studies found that African American, Hispanic, Asian, and Native American women were less physically active when they had already developed chronic health conditions (Eyler et al., 2002; Eyler et al., 1998). Several studies additionally found that illness was a significant predictor of noncompliance to an exercise program among White men and women (Norman et al., 2002; Conn, 1998; Kaplan et al., 1991).

- **Perceived severity**—one's opinion of the severity of the resulting undesirable condition. For example, if you believed that living a sedentary lifestyle would result only in being a few pounds overweight, you might not engage in physical activity. On the other hand, if you believed that not engaging in physical activity would result in heart disease or stroke, you might be more motivated to exercise.

- **Perceived benefits**—one's opinion of the positive results to be expected by engaging in the healthy behavior. Even if you believed that you were susceptible to a serious condition, you might not be motivated to exercise if you didn't think that exercising would likely prevent that serious condition. On the other hand, if you thought exercise would help you prevent a serious condition, you might be more motivated to be physically active.

   Many studies among Hispanic, African American, and White women confirm that women who perceive greater benefits from being physically active are more likely to engage in exercise programs (Nies et al., 1999; Scharff et al., 1999; Sternfeld et al., 1999). Rich and Rogers (2001) also reported health benefits of exercise as being the most important factor in the decision of older men and women to become active.

- **Perceived barriers**—one's opinion of the costs of engaging in the behavior. If you thought that the time devoted to exercise, the money needed to buy exercise clothing or to join a health club, or the embarrassment of exercising in front of others was too high a price to pay for the benefits of exercise, you might be less likely to be physically active. The many factors that induce individuals to adopt and maintain exercise programs are typically divided into those that are invariable, such as age, race, and gender, and those that are presumably modifiable, including psychosocial factors, environmental circumstances, and community settings. Because the prevalence of obesity and inactivity continues to rise, especially among racial and ethnic minorities, we face the daunting challenge of learning more about the barriers, both perceived and real, that decrease exercise adherence among individuals of all ages. An assessment of the barriers and supports to exercise among Native American children (Thompson et al., 2001) revealed that barriers to activity during school hours included a lack of facilities, equipment, and staff trained in teaching physical education. Weather, neighborhood safety issues, and homework or household chores affected participation in leisure-time activity. In a number of ethnic minority groups, the removal of barriers such as these is of primary importance.

- **Self-efficacy**—one's confidence in one's ability to engage in the healthy behavior. Body cathexis is synonymous with physical self-esteem or how highly one thinks of one's physical self. Self-efficacy is different. Self-efficacy is how much confidence one has in one's ability to perform a behavior (such as giving up cigarette smoking or exercising regularly). If you believed that exercising regularly would prevent a serious condition but didn't think you could ever manage to exercise correctly or regularly, you might be discouraged from even beginning an exercise program. For example, Barnett et al. (2002) conducted a 5-year longitudinal study of physical activity compliance correlates in a cohort of nearly 2,000 inner-city schoolchildren. They concluded that low physical activity self-efficacy played a major role in predicting the decline in physical activity among both the boys and the girls. Hagger et al. (2001) studied 1,152 young adolescents and found them more likely to form intentions to become physically active when they had positive attitudes and high self-efficacy. Other researchers have discovered the significant role of physical activity self-efficacy in White, African American, and Taiwanese adolescents (Felton et al., 2002; Pender et al., 2002; Wu and Pender, 2002). Self-efficacy is also an important predictor of attenuating and maintaining exercise habits among women with young children (Miller et al., 2002), young adults with chronic illnesses such as diabetes mellitus (Johnston-Brooks, Lewis, and Garg, 2002), young adults with physical disability (Bent et al., 2001), and Korean adults with chronic diseases (Shin, Jang, and Pender, 2001). Self-efficacy and social support were also significant contributors with respect to adherence to aerobic and strength-training programs among older adults (Resnick, 2002; Norcross et al., 2002; Ronda, Van Assema, and Brug, 2001; Rhodes et al., 2001). In at-risk populations, such as older ethnic minorities, stage of change and self-efficacy theories have been suggested as being the most promising approaches to promoting the adoption and maintenance of exercise programs (Clark, 1997), yet this construct has currently had surprisingly little study in ethnically diverse women (Sternfeld et al. 1999; Skelly et al., 1995).

To use the health belief model to begin and maintain a regular program of exercise, you must pay attention to all the theory's components. You should learn about the likelihood of contracting a serious condition by living a sedentary lifestyle (perceived susceptibility). Study health statistics provided in this book and available on the Internet at government Web sites that describe the relationship between exercise and conditions such as heart disease, stroke, depression, and others (perceived severity). Next, recall our discussions in earlier chapters about the research findings showing that exercise can prevent, and even rehabilitate, precursors to these serious conditions (perceived benefits). Once you have done that, you are motivated to engage in regular physical activity, and you should identify factors that interfere with your starting or maintaining an exercise program (perceived barriers). Then you should come up with strategies to overcome those barriers. For example, if you are usually busy without much time to exercise, prioritize it by scheduling an exercise session into your date book at a regular time so that you become accustomed to devoting that time to physical activity. In contrast, if you are too tired to exercise after school or work, schedule your exercise sessions early in the morning or with a friend so that you feel committed to show up.

Maintaining Your Fitness Program

Once you have begun a regular program of exercise, the trick is to maintain it. Annesi (2002) found that both adult men and women were more highly motivated to maintain a moderately intense aerobic exercise regimen because exercise induced feelings of positive engagement, revitalization, and tranquility. In a number of reports, African American women who successfully participated in a long-term exercise program explained that the key reasons they continued exercising included feeling good, having improved self-esteem, and having a significantly higher energy level (Young et al., 2001; Nies et al., 1999). Besides the methods already described, here are additional suggestions for keeping at it.

- **Material Reinforcement**—Behavior that is rewarded tends to be repeated. Consequently, if you want to exercise regularly, reward yourself when you do. Material rewards can take many forms. For example, you might treat yourself to a trip to the beach to show off your newly toned body. Alternatively, you might buy yourself an article of clothing you have been eyeing for some time.

- **Social Reinforcement**—Peer-group pressure need not be limited to negative influences. We can use such pressure to encourage and reward desirable behavior. Take a moment to list five people whose opinions you value. Then enlist them as social reinforcers to inquire about your exercise behavior and to pat you on the back if you report exercising regularly. After a while, exercise will become part of your lifestyle, and you will no longer need to receive rewards for continuing.

- **Joining a Group**—One of the reasons Weight Watchers is so effective in helping people lose weight is that it employs group support and positive peer pressure. Accomplishing your goals is often easier if you are working with others. You can join a health club, a local YMCA, or a Jewish Community Center, or you can organize a group of friends to exercise together at a predetermined time. You can enroll in an exercise class at a local university or community college or in a community program. Any group involvement will increase the likelihood of your maintaining a fitness program.

- **Boasting**—Many people, while they are students, have two tests returned the same day, one on which they did well and the other on which they did not. They complain about the poor grade for days while ignoring the test on which they did well. Many of us react this way. We relive negative experiences by repeatedly thinking about them, by being embarrassed about them, or by feeling inadequate in other ways. For positive experiences, such as receiving an A on a test, we exhibit false modesty and say, "It was nothing." We would do better to learn from our mistakes and let them go. We could relive our positive experiences and even boast about them. Of course, you do not want to be obnoxious or conceited. But if you run 3 miles daily and someone asks how far you usually run, rather than say, "Only 3 miles," you might say, "I'm proud to say that I run 3 miles regularly." Boasting in this way will help reinforce your exercise behavior.

- **Self-Monitoring**—Another effective method is self-monitoring—the process of observing and recording your own behavior. It is helpful to know that your fitness program is having a positive effect, that it is moving you toward your goal. Remember not to expect immediate dramatic results. Assuming that your exercise goal is realistic, accept small gains. Do not expect more rapid change than is warranted by the general effects of exercise and training on the body. Eventually, with persistence, you will attain your goal. When you see slow but steady progress toward your goal, you will be encouraged to maintain the program.

- **Making It Fun**—If the fitness program you designed is not fun, you selected the wrong activities. If it is not fun at least most of the time, you will not continue it for long. We present so many options in this book that you should be able to find activities that accomplish your goals while providing enjoyment. All you need to do is be selective. Think about your choices carefully and seek help from others when necessary.

Exercising Under Difficult Circumstances

If you maintain a fitness program long enough, you will undoubtedly encounter obstacles. If you are serious about training, obstacles need not interrupt your program. We demonstrate here how you can overcome five such obstacles—traveling, being confined to a limited space, being injured, being busy, and having visitors.

Traveling

If you travel often, you should consider that circumstance when you develop your program. For example, rather than joining a local health club, you would be wise to join one with facilities throughout the country so that you can exercise when you are in other cities. YMCAs, Jewish Community Centers, and some nationally franchised health clubs have facilities throughout the United States. In addition, select activities that you can more easily perform when you are away from home. You would be better off jogging, for example, than playing tennis. Jogging involves little in the way of equipment or facilities and does not require a partner. So, if you travel often, consider equipment, facilities, and dependence on other people in formulating your exercise program.

Being Confined to a Limited Space

If you are sometimes confined to a limited space (for example, if you are a student studying for final examinations and seldom leave your dormitory room), you need not abandon your physical fitness program. If you have access to an exercise room, you might have treadmills, stair steppers, ski machines, stationary bikes, or rowers at your disposal. But you can exercise without leaving your office or room. For example, you can run around the room, which can fill your need for cardiorespiratory endurance. If you do, be sure not to run in one place because that might cause too much strain on your legs and knees. Of course, the confines of the room will limit the speed you generate, and you will have to be careful not to bump into walls. Alternatively, you can buy a jump rope and use it in your room. You can do some of the flexibility exercises described in chapter 6 or perform isometric muscular strength activities.

Isometric contractions involve exerting a force that is equal to, or less than, that required to move an object. Therefore, the object does not move, the joint does not move, and the length of the muscle does not change. For example, pushing against a wall is an isometric contraction. You can also do isotonic activities. **Isotonic contractions** consist of movement at the joint and changes in the length of the muscle. For example, if you lift weights, you are engaged in isotonic contractions. You need not use a barbell or other weight-lifting equipment. Lifting any object of sufficient weight to offer resistance will suffice. You might be able to find someone else who also feels confined to exercise with you. For example, rather than pushing against a wall, you might be able to push against each other and thereby create the resistance you require (see figure 4.2).

Being Injured

If you exercise long enough, you will inevitably experience an injury of some sort. As with any other obstacle, you can always use such an injury as an excuse not to exercise. On the other hand, you can usually find a way to exercise around the injury. For example, a leg injury may preclude jogging but not swimming. A shoulder injury may eliminate a regular racquetball game but not jogging. For most injuries, common sense will dictate what you can and cannot do. For fitness injuries that are more serious, however, consult a professional for advice. By doing so, you might prevent further damage or prolonged recovery.

isometric contraction—Force applied to an immovable object that does not result in muscle shortening.

isotonic contraction—Shortening of the muscle in the positive phase and lengthening during the negative phase of an action.

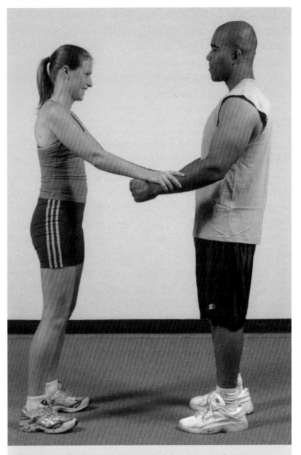

Figure 4.2 You don't need elaborate equipment to accomplish fitness goals. Here, partners help each other improve muscular strength. The man on the right attempts to lift his arms upward while the woman on the left provides resistance by pressing downward on her partner's forearms.

Being Busy

"I don't have time to exercise. I'm too busy," is a battle cry people often use. Dissection of busy schedules, however, often reveals that enough time is available for participation in fitness activities. The problem is that people decide to use this time for other activities, such as watching television, partying, or talking on the telephone. Using your time in that way is your decision to make, and as with all decisions, you can change it if you so choose.

It seems self-destructive to say that you value health and fitness but take a long lunch instead of a short lunch and a short workout, or to meet your friends at the local watering hole instead of exercising. You can find time to exercise if you really value health and fitness. Exercise can rejuvenate you, make you more efficient, and provide just the break you need, both physically and mentally.

We do not mean to imply that no adjustments are necessary during particularly busy times. The operative word here, however, is adjustment. With proper adjustment, you can maintain your program and resume your normal activities when the busy period passes.

Having Visitors

Suppose that someone comes to stay with you. What happens to your fitness program? Although visits from friends or relatives can encourage fitness, especially if they also exercise regularly, such visits usually interfere with your exercise program. You can use several strategies to maintain training during visits. If visitors are regular exercisers, you have no problem. If your visitors are not regular exercisers, help them organize short trips to take while you exercise. Sightseeing trips are ideal. If relatives or friends are nearby, perhaps they can entertain your visitors while you exercise. What is required is some ingenuity, not interruption of your training.

Summary

Psychosocial Factors to Consider   To plan a fitness program, you need to know certain things about yourself. These include your locus of control, the degree to which you feel socially isolated, and your level of self-esteem (in particular, your bodily self-esteem).

Locus of control is your perception of the amount of control you exert over events in your life. If you believe that you have a great deal of control, you have an internal locus of control. If you believe that you have little control, you have an external locus of control.

Socially isolated people are susceptible to illness and disease. Fitness programs can be organized to respond to social needs as well as to physical ones.

What you think of yourself and your body has significant influence on your health and wellness. Body cathexis is the esteem in which you hold your body and bodily functions. Fitness programs can improve self-esteem while they improve more traditional fitness components.

Strategies for Achieving Your Fitness Goals   Among the more effective strategies for achieving your fitness goals are goal setting and behavioral change techniques. When you are determining fitness goals, be realistic about what is possible and periodically assess your progress toward meeting your goals. Behavioral change techniques that you can use to help you achieve your fitness goals include developing social support, contracting with yourself and others, using reminder systems, programming gradually, tailoring, chaining, and practicing the covert techniques of rehearsal, modeling, and reinforcement.

Behavioral Change Theories and Exercise   Behavioral change theories both explain behavior and provide guidance for controlling behavior. The stages of change theory postulates that people are at different stages of motivation, or readiness, for change and therefore strategies to facilitate a change in behavior should be made specific to the stage of change at which people are located. Stages of readiness include precontemplation, contemplation, decision or determination, action, and maintenance. Another theory, the health belief model, identifies several components associated with changing or controlling a behavior. The components of the health belief model include perceived susceptibility, perceived severity, perceived benefits, perceived barriers, and self-efficacy. To change a behavior, such as exercise, a person should believe that a sedentary lifestyle is conducive to the development of a serious condition (such as heart disease), that exercise

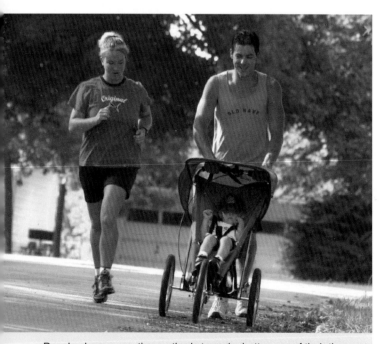

People choose creative methods to make better use of their time. The jogging stroller is a recent innovation that allows fitness-minded parents to exercise while taking babies out in the fresh air.

Myth and Fact Sheet

Myth	Fact
1. Everyone should develop an internal locus of control, because people really can control all aspects of their lives.	**1.** Although most people can take charge of more parts of their lives than they believe they can, that does not mean that we all can take control of all aspects of our lives. Parts of all of our lives are simply beyond our control. But we can always take control of our feelings and reactions. In other words, we are neither masters nor victims of our futures. We participate in developing our lives and can decide to become and remain physically fit and achieve high-level wellness if we choose to.
2. The best way to become fit is simply to make up your mind that you will do it.	**2.** Motivation is certainly an important factor in developing fitness, but by itself it is usually not enough. Deciding to exercise is similar to deciding to diet or to give up smoking cigarettes. People have honorable intentions that may serve them well for a time, but all too frequently they revert to the behavior they were trying to avoid. This chapter provides you with many behavioral change techniques that should accompany your motivation to be fit. Using those techniques will maximize the probability of your achieving that goal.
3. People do not achieve their fitness goals because they do not work long enough.	**3.** Even if you are motivated to achieve a fitness goal, you may not be successful. You may use all the behavioral change techniques outlined in this book and come up short. In that case, you may have selected an unrealistic or unobtainable goal. Try as you might, you will not achieve your goal. Therefore, the first thing you should do in deciding on your fitness goal is to determine whether you are likely to achieve it. If not, choose a more realistic goal. Perhaps you can work your way up to your ultimate goal after first achieving more obtainable ones.
4. When trying to change a behavior, it is best to work at changing by yourself so that you do not embarrass yourself in front of other people.	**4.** In fact, the opposite is true. Involving other people can help you change a behavior because they can provide you with support and peer pressure to encourage you to be successful. Unfortunately, studies show that people hesitate to join health and fitness clubs because the ads for these clubs usually show members with fantastic bodies, in brightly colored leotards, engaged in strenuous exercises. People think they will be embarrassed by not being able to lift as much weight, run as fast on the treadmill, or look as good in spandex. As a result, they refrain from joining a club. That situation is unfortunate because exercising with other people is often the best way to develop recommended levels of fitness and wellness.

is effective in preventing the early onset of that condition, that he or she can overcome impediments to exercising with particular strategies, and that he or she is capable of exercising regularly.

Maintaining Your Fitness Program Strategies to use to maintain your fitness program include getting material and social reinforcement, joining a group, boasting, self-monitoring, and making your program fun.

Exercising Under Difficult Circumstances Periodically, you will face obstacles to maintaining your fitness program. Among these are traveling, being confined to a limited space, being injured, being busy, and having visitors. To overcome these and other obstacles, you can make adjustments to prevent interruption of your program. All that is required is a little ingenuity and determination to continue exercising.

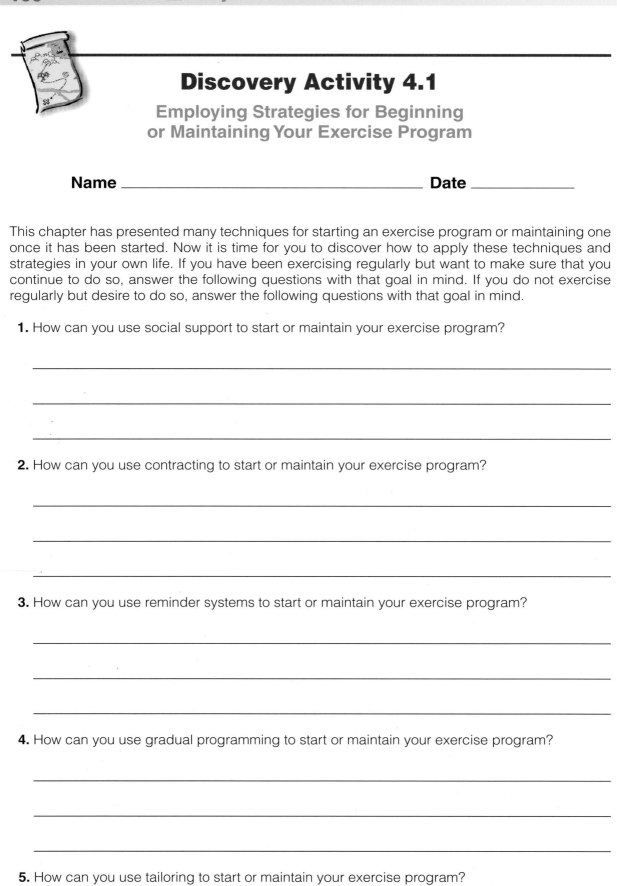

Discovery Activity 4.1

Employing Strategies for Beginning or Maintaining Your Exercise Program

Name _____ **Date** _____

This chapter has presented many techniques for starting an exercise program or maintaining one once it has been started. Now it is time for you to discover how to apply these techniques and strategies in your own life. If you have been exercising regularly but want to make sure that you continue to do so, answer the following questions with that goal in mind. If you do not exercise regularly but desire to do so, answer the following questions with that goal in mind.

1. How can you use social support to start or maintain your exercise program?

_____

_____

_____

2. How can you use contracting to start or maintain your exercise program?

_____

_____

_____

3. How can you use reminder systems to start or maintain your exercise program?

_____

_____

_____

4. How can you use gradual programming to start or maintain your exercise program?

_____

_____

_____

5. How can you use tailoring to start or maintain your exercise program?

_____

Discovery Activity 4.3

Service-Learning Behavioral Change and Motivation Techniques

You can learn more about theories of behavior change if you apply these theories, and you can help people in your community at the same time. Volunteer at a community center, YMCA, or Jewish Community Center by offering to conduct a workshop to help people engage in a physical fitness program. Although you might not be an expert in physical fitness or in helping people exercise in a healthy manner, you can work with staff at the agency at which you volunteer who are experts in these areas. In that way, you could work in a safe manner with various populations such as senior citizens, youth, or those who have traditionally been inactive. What you could bring to this setting is the knowledge of how to use behavioral change theories to help people achieve their fitness goals. For example, you could develop a questionnaire that identifies the program participants' stage of change and design appropriate interventions. Participants who have not thought about adopting regular physical activity (precontemplation) could be mailed flyers detailing the benefits of being active, or you could conduct a class session to present that material. For those who have thought about exercising regularly (contemplation), you could help move them to the next stage (decision or determination) by working with them to develop a plan for exercising. Even those who have been exercising regularly (maintenance) can benefit by your assisting them in organizing a group that exercises together at set times and days.

How else can you use the information you learned in this chapter to help those in your community be more physically fit and achieve higher levels of wellness?

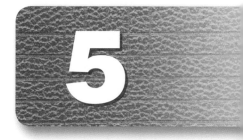

Cardiorespiratory Fitness

Chapter Objectives

By the end of this chapter, you should be able to

1. discuss the difference between aerobic and anaerobic exercise,
2. describe benefits to be derived from participating in a cardiorespiratory conditioning program,
3. describe maximal oxygen uptake ($\dot{V}O_2$max) and show different ways of expressing it,
4. assess your $\dot{V}O_2$max and determine your cardiorespiratory fitness,
5. explain guidelines for safely beginning and progressing in an aerobic fitness program, and
6. compare the energy costs associated with various types of cardiorespiratory activity.

Recently, two women were shopping in a department store. Ms. Green, a professional, 40-year-old, single female, was buying exercise clothing and accidentally bumped into Mrs. Taylor, a 45-year-old, lower-income woman, who was buying clothing for her grandchildren. As the two women struck up a conversation, Ms. Green explained that she had just enrolled in the new Billy Blanks TaeBo class at the local health club. She asked Mrs. Taylor if she had considered joining the class because TaeBo combines aerobic dance steps, self-defense, and boxing to provide an energized workout. Mrs. Taylor responded, "Well, you know, I'm so busy moving boxes on my job that I just don't have the time or the energy to join an exercise class!"

Unfortunately, the cardiorespiratory exercise boom has not reached all segments of the U.S. population for various reasons. Many obstacles, such as increased time demands, may make exercise seem impossible. As your time management skills improve, however, finding time to exercise will not be as difficult as it may seem. Also, many people mistakenly believe, as Mrs. Taylor does, that participating in an exercise class will fatigue them further. The opposite is true. Improved cardiorespiratory fitness often increases your energy level. Many other benefits result from participating in an aerobic conditioning program.

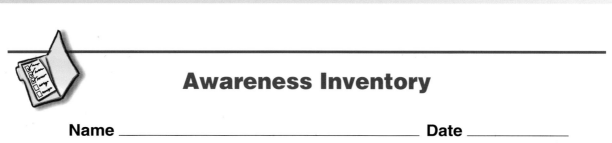

Awareness Inventory

Name _____ **Date** _____

Check the space by the letter T for the statements that you think are true and the space by the letter F for the statements that you think are false. The answers appear following the list of statements. This chapter will present information to clarify these statements for you. As you read the chapter, look for explanations for the reasons why the statements are true or false.

T___ **F___** 1. Physical fitness is having the ability to carry out daily tasks with alertness and vigor, without undue fatigue, and with enough energy reserve to meet emergencies or enjoy leisure-time pursuits.

T___ **F___** 2. To perform work, the muscles directly use the energy released when food is broken down in the body.

T___ **F___** 3. Increased cardiorespiratory fitness results in higher maximal oxygen consumption because of a higher submaximal exercise heart rate and lower stroke volume.

T___ **F___** 4. Fat is the major energy source used for sustained physical activity, and it can only be burned through aerobic metabolic processes.

T___ **F___** 5. As your body adapts to an aerobic fitness program, you will feel more alert and less fatigued throughout the day.

T___ **F___** 6. Typically, the amount of muscle mass used in a sport or activity of sustained duration has little effect on the maximal oxygen uptake obtained from a training program.

T___ **F___** 7. Your maximal oxygen uptake can be measured directly with submaximal field tests such as the 1-mile walking test or the 12-minute run test.

T___ **F___** 8. If you are presently in the poor or fair fitness category, you should begin with any of a variety of more strenuous aerobic activities so that you can quickly reach a higher level of aerobic fitness.

T___ **F___** 9. When you engage in a walking program, you should use your target heart rate (THR) as a measure of your exercise intensity rather than a particular walking speed.

T___ **F___** 10. Using principles of cross-training often promotes compliance with an aerobic conditioning program.

Answers: 1-T, 2-F, 3-F, 4-T, 5-T, 6-F, 7-F, 8-F, 9-T, 10-T

From Physical fitness and wellness, third edition, by Jerrold S. Greenberg, George B. Dintiman, and Barbee Myers Oakes, 2004, Champaign, IL: Human Kinetics.

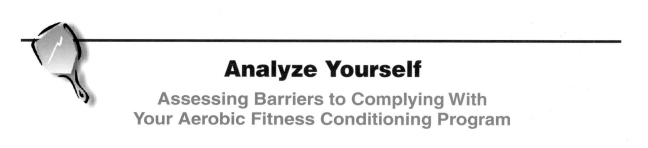

Analyze Yourself

Assessing Barriers to Complying With Your Aerobic Fitness Conditioning Program

Name _____ **Date** _____

Instruction: Indicate how often each of the following occurs in your aerobic exercise program. Respond to each item with a number from 0 to 3, using the following scale:

0 = Never   **1** = Occasionally   **2** = Most of the time   **3** = Always

____ **1.** I have developed a support system by enlisting significant others in my life to exercise with me on a regular basis.

____ **2.** My exercise program is based on a variety of aerobic fitness activities to accommodate my variable workout schedule and help me maintain my motivation, enjoyment, and interest.

____ **3.** I set aside a regular time for exercise and give my workout sessions the highest priority in my weekly planner.

____ **4.** I refuse to allow unexpected events to keep me from reducing the total work I accomplish each week through my exercise program.

____ **5.** When I feel too tired to exercise, I call my exercise partners and enlist their support instead of postponing my workout until the next day.

____ **6.** If I have a lot of work to do, I exercise by walking the stairs or walking throughout the building so that I can still get in a workout.

____ **7.** If I am concerned about having time to maintain my physical appearance after exercise, I schedule my exercise workouts at the beginning of the day or later in the evening.

____ **8.** If travel, holiday, or vacation plans threaten to interrupt my exercise program, I make changes in the type of activities and the amount of time I spend exercising that will allow me to maintain my level of fitness until I can return to my regular schedule.

____ **9.** When unfavorable weather conditions occur, I engage in any of a wide variety of inside aerobic activities instead of taking a break from my regular exercise routine.

____ **10.** I keep a record of my exercise sessions and review it on a monthly basis to monitor my progress. Then I compare my exercise record with the goals I established.

Scoring: Excellent = 25-30

               Good = 19-24

               Poor = Below 19

From *Physical fitness and wellness, third edition,* by Jerrold S. Greenberg, George B. Dintiman, and Barbee Myers Oakes, 2004, Champaign, IL: Human Kinetics.

Understanding the Difference Between Anaerobic and Aerobic Exercise

Physical fitness can be defined in many ways. Here we define the concept from a health perspective as having the ability to carry out daily tasks with alertness and vigor, without undue fatigue, and with enough reserve to meet emergencies or to enjoy leisure-time pursuits. Being physically fit depends on your ability to provide energy for high-intensity, short-duration activities (anaerobic exercise), as well as activities that you sustain over an extended period (aerobic exercise).

To perform work, the muscles do not directly use the energy released when food is broken down in the body. Instead, the body uses food to manufacture a substance called **adenosine triphosphate (ATP),** the primary energy molecule of the body. ATP is either stored in small amounts in the muscles or manufactured through the process of metabolism. Only when energy is liberated from the breakdown of ATP can the cells of the body perform work. The major ATP-producing or energy-producing systems in the body are the anaerobic and aerobic metabolism systems. When ATP is generated by the process of using oxygen, we refer to metabolism as being aerobic.

Anaerobic Exercise

With anaerobic exercise, ATP is needed quickly to perform an activity. Anaerobic activities do not depend on oxygen metabolism at all because the exercise intensity is high and the duration is less than 2 or 3 minutes. Anaerobic energy systems are of two major types. The immediate energy system is used for high-intensity activities that last less than 30 seconds, such as running the 100-meter dash or lifting heavy weights. Here, the muscles use ATP and **creatine phosphate (CP)** supplies that are already stored in the muscles.

The lactic acid system is a second source of energy for anaerobic activities. This system generates ATP for high-intensity activities lasting from 30 seconds to 3 minutes, such as the 400-meter or 800-meter run. In general, events or activities that require a combination of speed and power over a short time rely heavily on the lactic acid energy system.

Research has shown that the muscular concentrations of ATP and CP are similar in women and men. But women tend to have a smaller total muscle mass because of differences in physical stature, so their total amount of ATP and CP is less than that of the average male. When we evaluate the capacities of ATP, CP, and lactic acid systems, women have less total anaerobic capacity than the average male does. The effect on performance is that women have less power and less explosive capability when compared with men. This partially explains the difference in world-record performances for most weight-lifting and track and field events, such as sprint races or the shot put.

Aerobic Exercise

Increasing your level of aerobic or cardiorespiratory fitness is probably the most important component of a physical fitness program. Again, we refer to exercises as being aerobic when they depend on oxygen metabolism or oxygen utilization to generate the necessary amount of ATP to perform the activity. Activities must last a minimum of 3 to 5 continuous minutes to generate most of the energy from aerobic energy systems. When you exercise for prolonged periods, the muscles need vast quantities of energy. Therefore, as your aerobic exercise capacity increases, so does your total work capacity.

Aerobic fitness is often used interchangeably with terms such as *aerobic power, cardiorespiratory fitness,* **cardiorespiratory endurance,** and *maximal oxygen consumption,* and is defined as the ability of the heart, blood vessels, and the lungs to deliver oxygen to the exercising muscles in amounts sufficient to meet the demands of the workload. **Endurance** is the ability to perform prolonged bouts of work without experiencing fatigue or exhaustion. As your cardiorespiratory endurance level increases, so does your ability to engage in sustained physical activity. By the end of several months of cardiorespiratory activity, you will be able to exercise for long periods without experiencing prolonged fatigue.

Benefits of Cardiorespiratory Fitness

Many benefits result from participating in a cardiorespiratory endurance training program. As we examine some of the benefits, we will also explore a variety of physiological changes that occur after an individual participates in an aerobic training program for an extended period. Although the list of physiological changes in figure 5.1 may seem overwhelming at first, all these changes can be reduced to one primary benefit—increased aerobic power, or volume of oxygen consumption ($\dot{V}O_2$).

Increased Maximal Oxygen Consumption ($\dot{V}O_2$max)

Maximal oxygen consumption, $\dot{V}O_2$max, is regarded as the single best indicator of cardiorespiratory endurance or aerobic fitness. A high $\dot{V}O_2$max indicates a large capacity of the heart to pump blood, of the lungs to fill with larger volumes of air, of the arteries and blood vessels to deliver oxygen through the blood, and of the muscle cells to use the oxygen and remove the waste products produced during the process of **aerobic metabolism.** The two primary factors influencing maximal aerobic power are (1) the ability of the **cardiorespiratory system** to deliver oxygen to the muscles and (2) the ability of the muscles to extract oxygen from the blood. From figure 5.1 you see that as a person engages in an aerobic training program, the capacity to deliver oxygen to the muscles during exercise increases. This improvement occurs because aerobic fitness leads to positive changes in the entire cardiorespiratory system (heart, blood vessels, and lungs).

When you inhale, oxygen-rich blood travels from the lungs, enters the bloodstream by combining with hemoglobin molecules, and is transported into the heart and on to the muscles. Increased lung capacity resulting from aerobic training allows you to inhale a larger quantity of oxygen with each breath. With aerobic training, your hemoglobin level also increases, enabling you to carry more oxygen to the muscles. Simultaneously, the total output of the heart, the cardiac output, increases significantly. Cardiac output is determined by the heart rate (number of beats per minute) multiplied by the **stroke volume** (volume of blood pumped per beat).

Cardiac output = heart rate × stroke volume

As you engage in an aerobic fitness program, your heart muscle (myocardium) becomes stronger, allowing you to pump a larger amount of blood with each stroke. In addition, you develop a greater number of capillaries, tiny blood vessels, in the muscles. All these changes allow you to transport a greater volume of blood to the muscle tissue during exercise.

Changes also occur within the muscle when you engage in an aerobic fitness program. These musculoskeletal changes are all designed to increase your ability to extract or remove oxygen from the bloodstream and use it to pro-

adenosine triphosphate (ATP)—The basic substrate used by the muscle to provide energy for muscle contraction.

creatine phosphate (CP)—A substrate present in muscle tissue that is broken down into its component parts (creatine and phosphate) to provide phosphates for the production of ATP.

cardiorespiratory endurance—The ability of the heart, blood vessels, and lungs to deliver oxygen to the exercising muscles in amounts sufficient to meet the demands of the workload.

endurance—The ability to work a long time without experiencing fatigue or exhaustion.

maximal oxygen consumption ($\dot{V}O_2$max)—The optimal capacity of the heart to pump blood, of the lungs to fill with larger volumes of air, and of the muscle cells to use oxygen and remove waste products produced during the process of aerobic metabolism.

aerobic metabolism—The process of breaking down energy nutrients such as carbohydrates and fats in the presence of oxygen to yield energy in the form of ATP.

cardiorespiratory system—Joint functioning of the respiratory system (the lungs and airway passages) and the circulatory system (the heart and blood vessels).

stroke volume—The amount of blood pumped per beat of the heart, usually expressed in units of milliliters per beat.

duce energy for exercise. For example, ATP is produced in the mitochondria, which are often referred to as the powerhouse of the muscle cell. Because the number and the size of mitochondria increase after participation in an aerobic training program, the capacity to produce energy also improves. Likewise, the increased concentration of fat-burning enzymes allows you to exercise longer before the onset of fatigue by facilitating the aerobic production of energy. Collectively, as you are able to deliver more oxygen to the muscles while also using more of the oxygen within the muscle, your exercise duration and exercise intensity increase. Hence, your maximal exercise capacity also increases.

Improved Submaximal Exercise Efficiency

After you participate in an aerobic training program for several months, the physiological changes shown in figure 5.1 will make exercise at workloads below maximum feel much easier.

Changes that improve overall functioning of the cardiorespiratory system

- Higher maximal oxygen uptake ($\dot{V}O_2$max)
- Lower resting heart rate
- Lower exercise heart rate
- Stronger heart muscles
- Lower resting blood pressure in hypertensive individuals
- Greater lung capacity
- Greater ability to burn fat for energy
- Lower levels of stress hormones

Changes that increase the amount of oxygen delivered to the muscles during exercise

- Higher maximal cardiac output
- Higher stroke volume
- Larger number of capillaries in muscles
- Higher total blood volume
- Higher hemoglobin level (carries oxygen to the muscles)

Changes that increase the amount of oxygen used by the muscles during exercise

- Increased number and size of mitochondria
- Higher muscle glycogen stores
- Higher ATP and creatine phosphate stores
- Higher concentration of fat-burning enzymes

Immediate postexercise changes

- Faster recovery time
- Decreased amount of lactic acid buildup
- Blood-lipid profile changes
- Higher level of high-density lipoprotein (HDL) cholesterol
- Lower level of low-density lipoprotein (LDL) cholesterol
- Lower level of triglycerides (fats)

Musculoskeletal changes

- Stronger bones (greater bone density)
- Stronger cartilage, tendons, and ligaments
- Greater muscular endurance
- Increased flexibility

Body-composition changes

- Lower percentage of body fat
- Greater muscle mass

Figure 5.1 Overview of physiological changes that occur after participating in an aerobic training program.

One reason is that your exercise heart rate will be lower when you perform the same submaximal activity. Your lower heart rate will occur in part because your total blood volume increases and your myocardium becomes stronger, creating a more forceful pump, thereby increasing the amount of blood pumped each beat (the stroke volume) as your level of fitness rises. Ultimately, the longer you participate in aerobic conditioning programs, the greater your efficiency because your body does not work as hard to produce the same amount of energy. You will find that you are not only less exhausted when performing the same workout regimen but also have more energy when engaging in activities of daily living.

Faster Recovery From an Aerobic Exercise Session

As your fitness level increases, you will produce more energy through aerobic systems, rather than anaerobic energy systems. This transformation is advantageous because the lactic acid anaerobic energy system causes large amounts of lactic acid to accumulate in the muscles after exercise. The result is muscle soreness until the lactic acid is finally removed from the muscle. The removal of lactic acid occurs faster when you engage in an active cool-down period. We will provide some guidelines for cooling down later in the text. Naturally, the faster you recover from an aerobic training session, the more alert and energetic you feel.

Improved Blood-Lipid Profile

We will discuss changes in your blood-lipid profiles that result from participating in a chronic aerobic exercise program more fully in chapter 14. Here, we simply note that most individuals who engage in cardiorespiratory endurance conditioning programs experience an improved blood-lipid profile. In general, the level of fats such as triglycerides and LDL (bad) cholesterol fall dramatically. On the other hand, the level of HDL (good) cholesterol increases. These changes are linked to a decreased risk of coronary heart disease, atherosclerosis (hardening of the arteries), hypertension, and related chronic diseases.

Enhanced Body Composition

Although many individuals participate in aerobic exercise programs primarily to enhance their cardiorespiratory fitness, experiencing a reduction in your body-fat percentage is another welcome benefit. Fat is the major energy source used for sustained physical activity, and it can be burned only through aerobic processes. Consequently, the higher your level of aerobic fitness, the more fat you can burn during an exercise session. Eventually, your body becomes leaner, and you experience an increase in muscle tone and strength.

Increased Bone Density and Greater Joint Integrity

Bone density reaches its peak around age 25, regardless of your level of activity. Individuals who maintain a high level of aerobic fitness, however, can slow the rate of bone-density decline, often delaying the onset of osteoporosis and other related diseases. In addition, older adults report having greater strength, flexibility, and agility when they participate in an aerobic conditioning program. They report fewer injuries and tend to be less susceptible to falls as their level of fitness increases. Many of these benefits occur because aerobic exercise strengthens bones, cartilage, tendons, and ligaments, while also increasing flexibility.

Enhanced Ability to Cope With Stress

We will explore a variety of stress-management techniques in chapter 12. Myriad research studies report a marked reduction in the presence of stress hormones in the bloodstream after an aerobic exercise session. Furthermore, individuals tend to respond more favorably to mental stress when they maintain an active lifestyle. Reducing a person's level of stress has an especially positive effect on hypertensive individuals. As their bodies adapt to an aerobic conditioning program, many individuals also report feeling much more alert and less fatigued throughout the day. Additional benefits such as the improved self-esteem and self-satisfaction that most people derive from participation in aerobic fitness programs inspire them to sustain an active lifestyle through their senior years.

Reduced Susceptibility to and Severity of Chronic Diseases

Many life-threatening chronic diseases such as hypertension, cardiovascular disease, stroke, and cancer are related to sedentary living. A high level of cardiorespiratory endurance can help postpone or delay many of these chronic diseases. Recent research (which will be detailed more thoroughly in chapters 14 and 15) has shown that people with high levels of aerobic fitness are less prone to cardiorespiratory and metabolic diseases, and even to be less susceptible to cancer, than are sedentary individuals. In addition, exercisers are less prone to developing crippling diseases such as osteoporosis in adult years than are nonexercisers. Because several of these chronic debilitating illnesses are among the leading causes of death and disability in the United States today, it is especially important for you to maintain a healthy cardiorespiratory system and an active lifestyle. If you have not been involved in an exercise program, start today.

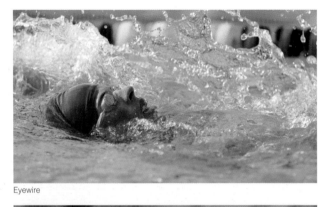

Eyewire

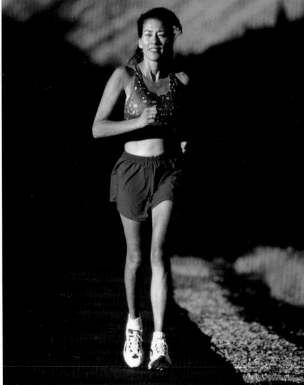

Endurance is greater when you exercise by using large-muscle groups through participation in such activities as swimming and jogging.

PhotoDisc

Measuring Cardiorespiratory Fitness

Factors such as age, gender, genetic background, and physical training influence $\dot{V}O_2$max. Typically, as you become older, your maximal level of aerobic power declines. After age 30, sedentary individuals experience a decrease in $\dot{V}O_2$max of about 1% per year. The rate of decline is much slower among active individuals. Men tend to have a higher level of aerobic power than women of similar ages do, primarily because of men's larger body size and greater amount of lean-muscle tissue.

Some people are born with a genetic predisposition to be elite endurance athletes. They inherit larger and stronger hearts, greater lung capacity, better blood supply in their muscles, larger quantities of red blood cells, and a higher percentage of slow-twitch muscle fibers, which are found in greater percentages in the muscles used in aerobic exercise. These muscle fibers contain energy foodstuffs and enzymes that enhance aerobic metabolism and promote exercise of longer duration. As shown in figure 5.1, aerobic training also leads to many of the same changes. Thus, even if you are not born an elite marathon runner, you can become a good one by engaging in a prolonged aerobic conditioning program.

The $\dot{V}O_2$max, or aerobic power, of an individual is expressed in volume (in liters) per unit of time (in minutes). Scores ranging from 3 to 4 liters per minute are common for the average healthy individual who exercises three to four times per week. Highly trained endurance athletes, however, may have a $\dot{V}O_2$max ranging from 5 to 6 liters per minute. Usually, the greater the amount of muscle mass used in a sport or activity, the higher the maximal oxygen uptake obtained through training. Thus, people who engage in activities such as running, cross-country skiing, and cycling often have the highest measured $\dot{V}O_2$max.

Assessing Maximal Aerobic Fitness

Directly measuring $\dot{V}O_2$max during a maximal exercise test on a treadmill, cycle ergometer, or other mode of testing provides the most accurate assessment of one's optimum cardiorespiratory fitness capacity. Yet direct measurement of $\dot{V}O_2$max requires expensive specialized equipment and a trained staff. In addition, according to the American College of Sports Medicine, a physician must be present for all maximal exercise tests conducted on apparently healthy men over the age of 40 and women past the age of 50. Guidelines such as these are provided because certain individuals may be at risk due to the potential onset of chronic illnesses typically associated with aging.

For these reasons, the direct measurement of $\dot{V}O_2$max is not always practical. Instead, we recommend using submaximal tests, or field tests, to estimate or categorize aerobic fitness when testing large groups or those older individuals mentioned earlier. A wide variety of field tests have been developed that provide an accurate estimate of $\dot{V}O_2$max without the risk, time, or expense associated with direct assessment. Some of these indirect measures are based on maximal performance by the individual, whereas others are based on the prediction of $\dot{V}O_2$max from a submaximal performance. Among the most representative, accurate, and commonly used field tests for the prediction of $\dot{V}O_2$max are the 1-mile walking test, the 1.5-mile run test, the 12-minute run test, the 12-minute swimming test, and the Åstrand-Rhyming cycle ergometer test.

Interpreting the Results of Your $\dot{V}O_2$max Test

We have provided two tests designed to assess your $\dot{V}O_2$max in this text. Remember when choosing a field test, be sure to consider the accuracy of the test, the population on which the test was developed, and your estimated fitness level at the time of testing. If you are just beginning your aerobic exercise program, we recommend that you assess your maximal oxygen uptake by completing the 1-mile walking test in Discovery Activity 5.1: Assessing Your Level of Aerobic Fitness by the 1-Mile Walking Test at the end of this chapter. This test provides an excellent means of assessing aerobic fitness with low risk of injury for someone who is just beginning an exercise program or who may be slightly overweight. If you have already been in a physical conditioning program, you may elect to complete the 12-minute run test found in Discovery Activity 5.2.

Once you complete either of these discovery activities, use table 5.1 to determine your current fitness classification based on your gender and age. Find the section of the chart with the $\dot{V}O_2$max values listed for those in your age and gender group. Your present fitness classification is based on the highest level of $\dot{V}O_2$ you reached during the field test. In table 5.1 you will note that although there is a gradual decline in $\dot{V}O_2$max for both women and men as they become older, men have higher $\dot{V}O_2$max values when compared with women at all ages and in every fitness category.

For example, a 21-year-old woman with a $\dot{V}O_2$max of 42 milliliters per kilogram per minute would be classified as having a good level of aerobic fitness, whereas a 21-year-old man with the same $\dot{V}O_2$max would be classified as having only an average level of aerobic fitness.

We caution that if you are presently in the poor or fair fitness category, consider beginning with any of a wide variety of less strenuous aerobic activities until you reach a higher level of aerobic fitness. If you are in the good or excellent fitness category, consider beginning with an intermediate or advanced level of the aerobic conditioning program of your choice. We will present guidelines that are more specific, as well as options for aerobic exercise choices, later in this chapter.

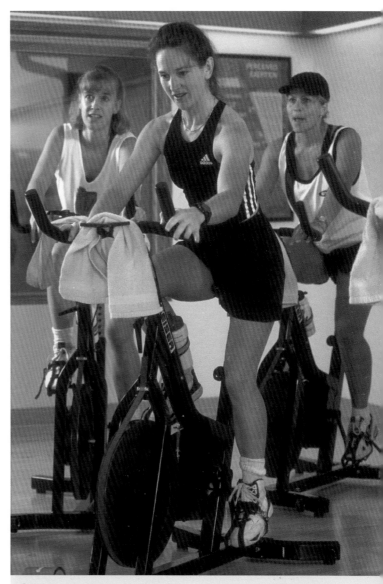

Spinning is a popular fitness program that allows people to work out vigorously in the winter months.

Need to Know!

TABLE 5.1—Cardiorespiratory Fitness Classification for Women and Men Based on Maximal Oxygen Uptake ($\dot{V}O_2$max) in ml/kg/min and METS

			FITNESS CLASSIFICATION			
Gender	Age		Fair	Average	Good	Excellent
Women	<30	(ml/kg/min)	24-30	31-37	38-48	>48
		(METS)	7-8.5	9-10.5	11-14	>14
	30s	(ml/kg/min)	20-27	28-33	34-44	>44
		(METS)	6-7.5	8-9.5	10-12.5	>12.5
	40s	(ml/kg/min)	17-23	24-30	31-41	>41
		(METS)	5-6.5	7-8.5	9-12	>12
	50s	(ml/kg/min)	15-21	22-33	34-40	>40
		(METS)	4.5-6	6.5-9.5	10-11.5	>11.5
	60s	(ml/kg/min)	13-20	21-32	33-36	>36
		(METS)	4-5.5	6-9	9.5-10	>10
	≥70	(ml/kg/min)	12-19	20-30	31-34	>34
		(METS)	3.5-5	5.5-8.5	9-10	>10
Men	<30	(ml/kg/min)	25-33	34-42	43-52	>52
		(METS)	7-9.5	10-12	12-15	>15
	30s	(ml/kg/min)	23-30	31-38	39-48	>48
		(METS)	6.5-8.5	9-11	11-14	>14
	40s	(ml/kg/min)	20-26	27-35	36-44	>44
		(METS)	5.5-7	7.5-10	10-12.5	>12.5
	50s	(ml/kg/min)	18-24	25-37	38-42	>42
		(METS)	5-7	7-10.5	11-12	>12
	60s	(ml/kg/min)	16-22	23-35	36-40	>40
		(METS)	4.5-6.5	6.5-10	10-11.5	>11.5
	≥70	(ml/kg/min)	13-20	21-32	33-37	>37
		(METS)	4-5.5	6-9	9.5-10.5	>10.5

MET = metabolic equivalent; 1 MET = 3.5 ml/kg/min oxygen uptake or the rate of energy expenditure at rest. For example, a 10 MET activity requires a 10-fold increase in the resting energy requirement, or 35 ml/kg/min. METS are often used as an alternative method for describing the exercise intensity of an activity.

Sample Starter Programs

In this section, we offer guidelines for starting aerobic conditioning programs including walking, jogging, cycling, swimming, or rope skipping. Although many aerobic exercise options are available, the guidelines offered through these sample programs can be adapted to accommodate most forms of aerobic exercise.

You can maintain an active lifestyle by including variety in your exercise regimen. Hence, using principles of cross-training often promotes compliance to an aerobic conditioning program. If you enjoy participating in outdoor activities during

Myth and Fact Sheet

Myth	Fact
1. Most Americans are getting enough aerobic exercise to reduce their risk of developing heart disease.	**1.** Heart disease remains a national crisis. More than 60% of adults do not achieve the recommended amount of regular physical activity, and 25% of adults are not active at all. Even more distressing is that nearly half of young people (ages 12 to 21) are not vigorously active on a regular basis.
2. Younger individuals have less need to stretch before exercising compared with older people.	**2.** Whatever your age, being flexible helps you use your muscles more effectively and efficiently. When you have complete range of motion, you tend to perform better in your workout activity, with decreased risk of muscle injury. Other benefits of stretching include less muscle fatigue, less soreness after exercise, better posture, and reduced risk of lower-back pain.
3. You should exercise every day to increase your level of cardiorespiratory fitness.	**3.** When you begin an exercise program, you should not exercise every day because you will increase the risk of being injured. Exercising on alternate days allows adequate time for recovery. After you reach your maximal level of aerobic fitness, you can exercise daily because your risk of injury will be lower after a long period of training.
4. You are more likely to stick with an exercise program if you maintain the same exercise program each workout.	**4.** Many individuals find that their motivation tends to decrease when engaging in the same routine for weeks or months. Cross-training is a way to put the pizzazz back in your workout. Switching activities once or twice a week may provide the variety you need to stay motivated over the long haul. Cross-training can also help you prevent injuries caused by overtraining. By alternating high- and low-impact activities or routines that involve different parts of your body, you give overstressed muscles a chance to heal without interrupting your training.

the spring and summer seasons, consider adding in-line skating or water exercises to your walking or jogging routine. In addition, consider hiking or canoeing with your family and friends occasionally to enjoy nature while also getting in a strenuous physical workout. Recreational sports such as soccer, kickball, water polo, and tennis are also great options as cross-training activities designed to promote aerobic fitness. Try enrolling in a TaeBo class or a spinning class, also referred to as indoor cycling, during the fall and winter months to provide variety to your program. If you are not interested in participating in structured exercise programs such as these, or if you have other time restrictions, begin climbing stairs at work or in your home, rather than avoiding them, as many individuals do. The main thing is to find an enjoyable activity that provides a suitable cardiorespiratory workout that you can perform safely given your present level of fitness, and start today!

Sample Walking Program

In recent years walking has become one of the most popular of all aerobic activities. One reason for its popularity is that it does not require any specialized skills and is both safe and painless when participants follow some basic guidelines. You can walk almost anywhere, at any time, and at little cost. Many people choose walking over activities like jogging because walking puts less stress on the hips, knees, and ankles and presents reduced risk of orthopedic injuries. In addition, exercisers have found walking to be an excellent means of reducing body weight and lowering body-fat percentage.

We covered the basic principles of beginning an exercise program earlier, so we limit our discussion here to special considerations for beginning and advanced walkers. Follow the guidelines in figure 5.2 when you begin your walking program.

- Maintain good postural alignment to avoid tension in the neck, back, and shoulders.
- Hold your head high to help maintain good posture.
- Use full, deep abdominal breathing to enhance relaxation and monitor your walking pace.
- Hold your arms in a relaxed position with the elbows flexed at a 90-degree angle.
- Form a slightly clenched, relaxed fist with your hands.
- Swing your arms naturally back and forth to add power to each stride.
- Begin each stride with a slight forward lean of your body at the ankles.
- Make contact on the outer edge of your heel as your foot contacts the surface.
- Roll your foot smoothly forward on contacting the surface, with most of your body weight distributed along the outer edge of the foot, and then transfer the weight to the ball of the foot and on to the toes for the pushoff.
- Walk at a pace of 3 to 3.5 miles per hour for a comfortable workout.
- Walk at a pace of 3.75 miles per hour for a vigorous workout.
- Walk faster than 4 miles per hour if you are an advanced walker.
- Walk on dirt trails or grass rather than on concrete sidewalks for a more comfortable workout.
- Be cautious when walking on uneven surfaces such as grass or dirt because of the increased risk of ankle sprains.
- Walk in shoes with a comfortable fit, a cushioned sole, and good arch support.
- Wear loose-fitting clothing to allow freedom of movement and dissipation of heat.
- Wear several layers of clothing in cold weather to slow the rate of heat loss.
- Wear a cap in cold weather to avoid heat loss through the scalp.
- Wear cotton socks to avoid getting blisters and to absorb perspiration.
- Warm up before each walking session and cool down afterward.

Figure 5.2 Guidelines for a walking program.

Duration

During the initial phase of a walking program, you should walk 10 to 15 minutes at a pace that is comfortable to you. After 1 or 2 weeks, you can advance to 30-minute sessions. Continue walking for 30 minutes per session for at least 4 weeks to decrease your risk of injury and minimize fatigue. After approximately 6 weeks, you can increase the exercise period to 45 minutes. Advanced walkers typically progress to a 60-minute walking session.

Intensity

The first step in regulating exercise intensity is to forget the familiar saying "no pain, no gain." Calculate your target heart rate (THR) as instructed in Discovery Activity 3.2. Begin your walking program at 50 to 60% of that rate. Once you advance to 30-minute walking sessions, you can increase your exercise intensity to 60 to 65% of your THR. As you advance to 45- to 60-minute exercise sessions, remember to stay within your THR.

Your THR is a better measure of intensity than a particular walking speed is because your THR gives you the best measure of the cardiorespiratory benefits of your workout. During the initial phase of your walking program, check your exercise heart rate every 5 minutes. Use a 10-second pulse count while walking and multiply the result by six to determine your heart rate per minute. At the end of your exercise session, if you have walked at a comfortable pace, your heart rate should drop below 100 beats per minute following a 10-minute cool-down period.

A great way of monitoring exercise intensity while walking without counting your pulse is to use the talk test. If you are walking with a partner and your breathing rate is so fast that you cannot carry on a conversation, you are probably walking too fast. Beginning to feel winded is an instant indication that you should slow the pace.

Remember that exercise intensity is inversely related to exercise duration. If your exercise heart rate is too high, you will tire more quickly, exercise for shorter periods, and increase your risk of becoming injured.

Frequency

At the beginning of your exercise program, you should walk every other day up to a maximum of 3 to 4 days per week. After the first 6 weeks, you can increase your frequency to 4 to 5 days per week. Limit your exercise frequency to a maximum of 5 days per week to allow a few days for recovery, thereby minimizing your risk of injury.

Sample Jogging or Running Program

After you complete an advanced walking program, you may be ready for a jogging program.

For purposes of changing body composition, increasing muscular endurance, and improving cardiorespiratory endurance, jogging is one of the most effective activities. For a given distance, the energy costs of running are greater than those of walking. Thus, if you have reached a moderate to high level of fitness and want to increase your caloric expenditure but are unable to increase the amount of time you exercise, you should increase the exercise intensity by jogging instead of walking.

Complete the most advanced level of a walking program before you begin a jogging program. This approach will allow adequate time for you to develop your cardiorespiratory system and strengthen your ligaments and tendons to reduce the risk of injury. Many options are available in beginning a jogging program, depending on your initial level of fitness and prior exercise experience. Here are a few guidelines for jogging.

Duration

In the initial phase of a jogging program, exercise for 15 to 30 minutes. During the session, alternate brief periods of slow jogging (approximately 5 to 6 miles per hour) with intervals of walking. Gradually increase the time you spend jogging and decrease the walking time until you reach a level of fitness in which you can jog continuously for 30 minutes within your THR. As you reach an advanced level of running, exercise sessions may last as long as 60 minutes. Most people jog 2 to 3 miles per exercise session during the first 10 weeks of a jogging or running program. When you can jog 3 miles comfortably within 27 to 30 minutes, you are probably ready to advance to a running program. Advanced runners can cover 5 miles per session within 35 to 40 minutes.

Intensity

An important factor in a jogging or running program is monitoring your exercise heart rate. During the initial phase of your program, stay in the 60 to 75% THR zone. As you reach a higher level of fitness, you may increase exercise intensity to 70 to 85%. Remember, however, that as your exercise intensity increases, you tend to exercise for a shorter time because fatigue occurs earlier. Keep your THR in the moderate range to reap the double benefits of improving cardiorespiratory fitness and increasing the percentage of fat calories used. You will see changes in body-fat percentage more quickly by exercising at moderate intensity (60 to 75% THR zone).

Frequency

The optimal frequency for jogging is every other day. If you want to exercise every day, use walking as a form of exercise on alternate days to decrease the amount of stress on your hips and the joints of the legs and feet. Even runners who participate in road races seldom exercise 7 days per week. They recognize the need to allow a rest period between workouts. If you want to increase total work done on a weekly basis, it is better to increase exercise duration gradually and maintain moderate exercise intensity with a frequency of 4 to 5 days per week instead of jogging 7 days per week.

Sample Swimming Program

Swimming is an excellent aerobic activity. Patients in cardiac rehabilitation programs and in physical therapy often use a pool as their primary means of aerobic conditioning because exercising in water decreases stress on hips, knees, and ankles. In addition, the warm water in a pool is therapeutic for arthritic patients. Further, because water offers support to body weight, obese persons have fewer injuries while exercising in water. Consequently, a growing number of people are choosing aquatic exercise, or aquatherapy, as their primary mode of fitness. Because the cardiorespiratory benefits derived from water exercises are similar to those derived from jogging and cycling, consider including water exercises as part of your training program.

Aquatherapy

Water aerobics are highly touted by exercise physiologists because they have virtually no adverse effects on the muscles and the skeletal system and are safe for people of all ages regardless of health status.

For years, people avoided water exercises because it was believed that water provided insufficient resistance to stimulate cardiorespiratory endurance. We now know that the resistance of the water is sufficient to challenge even elite ath-

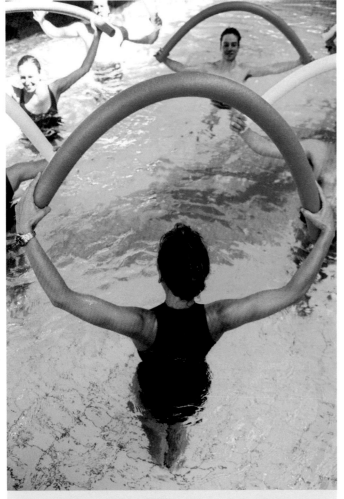

Water exercise places less stress on the body than many other exercises do and is a great way for people of all ages to improve their cardiorespiratory fitness.

Sport The Library

letes. Participating in water exercises can unquestionably increase cardiorespiratory fitness.

An added benefit is that this cushioned medium promotes a virtually injury-free environment. The density of water gives almost any object placed in it some buoyancy. Your body will weigh less in water because of buoyancy, so it undergoes less stress when you exercise in water. Obese people may especially enjoy exercising in water because they can more easily dissipate heat. One advantage water aerobics provides over jogging is that jogging does nothing to work the upper body, but water increases strength and endurance in the upper body as well as in the lower body. Figure 5.3 provides guidelines to follow when you begin a water aerobic exercise program.

Duration

Start at a comfortable level, which will vary depending on your initial level of fitness. If you are a swimmer but have been inactive for a long time, you may need to spend a few weeks walking across the width of the pool in chest-deep water until you can complete two 10-minute intervals at your THR. Gradually alternate walking and jogging across the pool until you can complete four 5-minute intervals of jogging at your THR. As you progress, you can jog across the pool and swim back. Repeat this pattern until you can jog and swim for 20 to 30 minutes. As your level of fitness increases, spend more time swimming and less time jogging until you can swim continuously for 20 to 30 minutes in each exercise session.

Intensity

Research has shown that a person's maximal heart rate is approximately 10 beats lower in the water than it is on land. Thus, when calculating your THR for water activities, use the formula 210 (rather than 220) minus your age to determine your maximal heart rate. From there, follow the standard formula for calculating your THR. During the initial phase of your swimming program, begin at a pace that keeps your heart rate at 50% of your THR zone. Gradually increase exercise duration and intensity as level of fitness increases, but be careful to remain within your heart rate zone.

Frequency

As with other forms of aerobic exercise, you should swim 3 to 4 days per week. If you have trouble tolerating chlorinated pools, you can

- Always exercise in a supervised environment. You can get muscle cramps in water, especially if you swim too soon after eating a meal. If you are exercising in chest-deep water, you could be in danger.

- Exercise in water 2 or 3 inches above the waist. The depth of the water determines the amount of resistance that you experience. When the water is too shallow, you place more stress on the lower extremities. Conversely, when the water level is too high, buoyancy increases, which reduces resistance and makes the exercises less effective.

- To minimize the risk of injury, avoid excessive twisting in the water.

- If the surface of the pool is rough, wear cotton socks to avoid scratching the soles of your feet.

- Stand with your knees slightly bent and avoid locking your joints.

- Keep your arms in the water to generate more resistance. This position helps raise the heart rate into the THR zone.

- Cup your hands to increase resistance.

- Use ankle weights to increase the intensity of lower-body workouts.

- Use a stride stance (one foot forward, the other behind) to improve your balance in the water.

- Use hand paddles, fins, pull buoys, or wrist weights to increase resistance.

- Keep your pelvis tilted upward when you are doing lower-body exercises to help support the lower back.

- Include warm-up exercises before your water workout and do cool-down exercises afterward.

Figure 5.3 Guidelines for a water aerobic exercise program.

alternate swimming with other forms of aerobic exercise. You can also wear swimming goggles to protect your eyes from irritation.

Sample Cycling Program

Bicycling, or cycling, has become an increasingly popular aerobic activity especially for those who have joint problems or those who are overweight. For them, cycling is ideal because the bicycle supports their weight. Consequently, they often can exercise for longer periods. Cycling has high energy expenditure per minute and can produce tremendous increases in cardiorespiratory endurance, muscular strength, and muscular endurance.

Duration

Each cycling session should last approximately 30 to 45 minutes. When you can cycle several miles within a 30-minute period, you have reached a high level of cardiorespiratory fitness. Examine figure 5.4 for guidelines to reduce your risk of injury when cycling.

Intensity

When you are at the beginning of your cycling program, you may have to exercise below your THR to cycle 1 to 2 miles. After a few weeks of cycling that distance, however, you should be able to exercise at 60% of your THR zone. As you progress to cycling 3 to 5 miles, you may increase your exercise intensity to as high as 70 to 75%. Be careful to limit the intensity so that you can maintain your endurance. Once you reach a maximal level of fitness and can cycle 10 to 15 miles, you may increase your exercise intensity to 80% of your THR zone. A word of caution to those using stationary bikes: Periodically check your resistance setting because the workload tends to shift when you ride for long periods. Figure 5.5

- Adjust the handlebars and the seat height to fit properly! Set the seat height so that your knee has a slight bend when your foot is at the bottom of a pedal swing. This position prevents your body from swaying as you cycle while giving you maximum power without creating stress on your spine.
- Wear appropriate shoes and clothing. To avoid an accident, be sure to keep your shoestrings tied. To facilitate heat loss, wear lightweight clothing that does not restrict movement or reduce airflow.
- Use toe clips when possible to keep your feet from sliding and to assist you in maintaining equal force on the pedals through the entire range of motion.
- Wear cycling shorts padded with soft chamois sewn in the seat to increase cushioning and reduce friction. Shorts should be long enough to prevent the skin from rubbing against the seat.
- Take precautions against saddle soreness. Saddle soreness occurs because of chafing caused by friction on the skin of the buttocks or increased pressure on the genital area and the buttocks that causes pain and numbness. To avoid or minimize saddle soreness, use cornstarch or talcum powder. You may also consider buying a larger seat for the bicycle.

Figure 5.4 Guidelines for reduced injury risk when cycling.

- Wear a properly fitting helmet that is certified by either the American National Standards Institute or the Snell Memorial Foundation.
- Adhere to all traffic rules when you are cycling outdoors. Observe traffic lights and stop signs, just as motorists do.
- Use hand signals to alert other riders and motorists of any intended directional changes.
- Yield to turning motorists and to vehicles that are backing up because you may not be clearly visible to the driver.
- To reduce risk of accidents, do not ride beside another cyclist.
- When possible, avoid residential areas, parks, and other recreational areas when small children are present.
- Beware of dogs when cycling through residential neighborhoods.
- Be careful to avoid potholes, ditches, or other areas of the road that can increase your risk of having an accident.

Figure 5.5 Safety rules for road cyclists.

contains precautions to observe when you are cycling on the road.

Frequency

As with other forms of cardiorespiratory exercise, you should cycle 3 to 5 days per week. Cycle on alternate days to allow adequate rest. During the first phase of a cycling program, ride a maximum of 3 days per week. Because cycling is not a familiar exercise to many people, they may experience more muscle soreness initially than they would with activities such as walking.

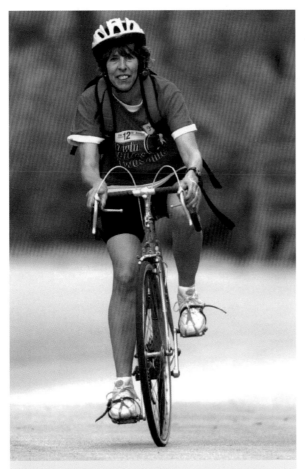

Begin a cycling exercise regimen by riding approximately 1 to 2 miles per session, increasing to 3 to 5 miles after several weeks.

Sample Rope-Skipping Program

On days when you cannot do outdoor aerobic activities or when you want to try a different form of aerobic conditioning, rope skipping is an excellent alternative. One factor that deters many exercisers from using rope skipping as their primary form of exercise is the amount of skill involved in turning and jumping. With practice, however, even a novice can become a good rope skipper.

You must be sure to buy a rope of the correct length. The rope should be long enough to reach from armpit to armpit while passing under both feet. In addition, you need a good pair of exercise shoes because of the stress that jumping places on the balls of your feet.

Duration

Most beginners use an interval program consisting of brief periods of skipping followed by periods of rest. Unless you are already involved in a physical-conditioning program, start with a beginning-level walking program to improve your level of fitness and strengthen your joints, tendons, and ligaments before you begin rope skipping.

Intensity

During the initial phase of a rope-skipping program, you should exercise at an intensity below your THR zone. Do not push too hard too soon. As your level of fitness increases, you will be able to exercise at 65 to 75% of your THR. Avoid exercising at high intensity while rope skipping because of the stress it places on your hips, knees, ankles, and feet.

Frequency

As with other forms of aerobic exercise, skip rope no more than 3 days per week on alternate days. Because rope skipping places a lot of stress on the lower parts of the body, you may choose to alternate rope skipping with other forms of exercise to reduce the risk of injury. Water exercises are an especially good alternative because of the lack of stress to the joints.

Comparison of Energy Expenditure From Various Types of Aerobic Exercise

In chapter 3 we provided some recommendations for making the right exercise choices. Table 3.1 contains 10 types of exercise programs evaluated on various criteria including whether or not the program facilitates weight loss through the expenditure of a large number of calories. Table 3.2 provides a rating of 32 sports and includes the intensity of caloric expenditure achieved while engaging in those activities. Numerical estimates of energy expenditure are not included in either table because caloric expenditure depends on the weight of the individual for most aerobic sports or activities.

Table 5.2 compares the estimated number of calories typically burned during a 1-hour aerobic exercise session, depending on body weight and type of physical activity performed. Let's take a closer look at the amount of energy expended to perform aerobic activity at different intensities. Walking at a speed of 3 miles per hour is categorized as moderately intense aerobic activity. A walking speed of 4 or 5 miles per hour is considered fast-paced walking. As walking speed increases, so do the number of calories expended and the distance covered during a given period.

TABLE 5.2—Approximate Energy Expenditure of Various Activities per Hour

Activity	Weight in pounds											
	90	110	130	150	170	190	210	230	250	270	290	310
Baseball												
Player	162	204	246	282	318	354	396	438	480	522	564	606
Pitcher	210	258	306	354	402	444	492	540	588	636	684	732
Badminton (singles)	246	294	342	396	450	498	554	612	672	732	796	860
Basketball (full court)	450	474	486	564	636	714	765	798	822	840	864	888
Half court	174	198	234	270	306	342	389	432	474	501	546	588
Bowling	162	188	210	246	276	312	342	378	420	462	504	546
Boxing	546	666	786	906	1,026	1,146	1,272	1,372	1,512	1,632	1,752	1,872
Calisthenics	162	216	268	306	348	374	423	462	510	546	582	618
Carpentry (general)	126	156	186	210	240	270	294	318	342	366	390	414
Circuit training	414	558	654	756	852	954	1,056	1,128	1,200	1,272	1,344	1,404
Cycling												
Leisure 5.5 mph	168	192	228	264	300	330	368	402	438	480	522	564
Leisure 9.5 mph	246	299	355	410	465	519	576	636	696	768	822	876
Racing	420	510	600	690	780	870	966	1,062	1,158	1,254	1,350	1,446
Canoeing or kayaking												
Leisure	108	132	156	180	204	228	253	276	300	324	348	372
Racing	258	312	366	420	474	534	590	642	696	750	804	858
Dance (vigorous aerobic)	330	402	474	546	618	690	744	798	852	906	950	1,014
Square	246	300	354	408	462	516	570	624	678	732	786	840
Digging trenches	360	438	516	594	642	750	828	906	996	1,086	1,176	1,266
Electrical work	144	174	204	234	270	300	330	360	390	420	450	480

Activity												
Farming												
Cleaning stalls	336	408	480	552	624	696	768	840	912	984	1,056	1,128
Driving tractor	96	120	144	162	186	204	228	252	276	300	324	348
Feeding cattle	168	198	228	264	300	336	372	408	444	480	516	552
Shoveling grain	216	258	300	348	390	438	486	534	588	638	684	732
Fencing												
Moderate	174	216	258	300	342	378	420	462	504	546	588	630
Vigorous	378	438	522	582	684	762	846	930	1,014	1,098	1,182	1,266
Field hockey	330	402	474	546	618	690	762	834	906	978	1,050	1,122
Football (touch)	326	396	468	540	612	684	753	816	882	948	1,014	1,080
Forestry												
Ax chopping (fast)	732	894	1,050	1,212	1,374	1,530	1,692	2,010	2,208	2,406	2,604	2,862
Sawing by hand	300	366	432	498	564	630	696	762	828	894	960	1,026
Sawing (power)	192	228	264	306	348	390	426	462	498	540	582	624
Gardening												
Digging	312	378	444	516	582	648	720	792	864	936	1,008	1,080
Hedging	198	234	270	312	354	396	438	480	522	564	606	642
Mowing	276	336	396	456	516	576	636	696	756	816	876	936
Raking	132	162	198	222	252	276	306	336	366	396	426	456
Golf (walking)	216	258	300	348	390	438	486	534	588	636	684	726
Handball or racquetball												
Competitive	522	636	750	864	978	1,092	1,211	1,332	1,452	1,572	1,692	1,812

(continued)

TABLE 5.2 (continued)

Activity	Weight in pounds											
	90	110	130	150	170	190	210	230	250	270	290	310
Horseback riding												
Walk	102	126	150	174	198	222	246	270	294	318	342	366
Sitting to trot	140	180	210	246	276	312	342	372	402	432	462	492
Basting to trot	222	276	330	384	432	486	534	582	630	678	726	774
Gallop	290	370	450	522	588	660	732	804	876	948	1,020	1,092
Horseshoes	138	168	198	228	258	288	318	348	378	408	438	468
Hiking (pack, 3 mph)	246	300	354	408	462	516	570	624	678	732	786	840
Ice hockey	354	438	522	600	684	762	846	930	1,014	1,098	1,182	1,356
Ice skating (9 mph)	210	276	342	384	432	486	534	582	630	678	726	774
Judo or karate	486	588	690	796	900	1,008	1,115	1,224	1,332	1,440	1,548	1,620
Jogging or running												
5 mph	348	432	516	594	612	750	828	906	984	1,062	1,140	1,218
6 mph	414	510	606	696	786	882	972	1,062	1,152	1,242	1,320	1,410
7 mph	504	588	640	798	906	1,008	1,116	1,224	1,332	1,440	1,548	1,638
8 mph	576	666	786	906	1,026	1,146	1,266	1,326	1,446	1,566	1,688	1,806
9 mph	630	738	876	1,068	1,146	1,278	1,410	1,542	1,674	1,806	1,932	2,058
Painting (inside)	84	102	120	138	156	174	192	210	228	246	264	294
Outside	198	234	312	354	396	438	480	522	564	606	648	690
Plastering	192	0234	318	360	402	444	486	528	570	612	654	696
Rope jumping												
Slow	368	450	534	612	696	780	858	936	1,014	1,092	1,164	1,236
Fast	462	552	654	750	852	954	1,050	1,146	1,242	1,338	1,500	1,596
Scraping paint	162	192	222	258	294	324	348	396	432	468	504	549

Sedentary activities	54	66	78	90	102	114	126	138	150	162	179	186
Lying down	54	66	78	90	102	114	126	138	150	162	179	186
Sitting	66	84	102	114	132	144	162	186	198	216	234	253
Standing	150	180	210	246	276	312	342	372	402	432	462	492
Skating												
In-line (13 mph)	564	654	744	858	972	1,086	1,200	1,314	1,428	1,542	1,656	1,770
Roller (9 mph)	242	276	330	384	432	486	534	582	630	678	726	774
Skiing (cross-country)												
4 mph	352	432	510	594	672	774	828	882	936	990	1,044	1,098
5 mph	412	504	600	690	786	882	972	1,062	1,152	1,242	1,332	1,416
Skiing (downhill)	380	432	510	594	672	750	828	906	984	1,062	1,140	1,218
Soccer or rugby	324	395	468	540	612	684	756	824	900	972	1,044	1,116
Squash (competitive)	384	504	624	690	786	882	972	1,062	1,152	1,242	1,332	1,410
Stair climbing and descending												
1 stair—25 trips/min	246	294	360	408	462	509	576	624	660	708	756	792
1 stair—30 trips/min	282	318	396	444	498	558	624	378	726	774	822	870
1 stair—35 trips/min	312	360	450	510	570	635	714	774	834	894	954	1,014
3 stairs—12 trips/min	294	342	426	486	540	599	678	732	786	840	894	948
3 stairs—15 trips/min	364	414	516	588	654	727	816	888	960	1,032	1,104	1,176
Stock clerk	132	162	192	222	252	276	306	336	366	396	426	456

(continued)

TABLE 5.2 (continued)

Activity	Weight in pounds											
	90	110	130	150	170	190	210	230	250	270	290	310
Swimming												
Backstroke	420	510	600	690	780	870	966	1,062	1,164	1,260	1,356	1,452
Breaststroke	404	486	576	660	750	934	927	1,020	1,113	1,206	1,299	1,392
Sidestroke	296	366	432	498	564	630	698	765	833	900	967	1,044
Crawl (slow)	306	396	486	522	612	660	732	804	876	948	1,020	1,092
Crawl (fast)	384	468	552	636	720	804	892	979	1,067	1,154	1,242	1,330
Table tennis	190	228	270	312	354	396	438	480	522	564	606	648
Tennis singles	276	330	384	444	504	564	626	686	746	806	866	926
Doubles	192	228	270	312	354	396	438	480	522	564	606	648
Typing (computer)	72	84	96	108	126	138	156	174	192	210	228	246
Volleybal	120	150	180	204	234	258	288	318	348	378	408	426
Walking												
3 mph	144	168	192	222	252	282	312	342	372	402	432	462
4 mph	212	246	288	336	378	430	468	516	558	600	642	684
5 mph	314	396	468	540	612	684	756	824	900	972	1,044	1,116
Wall papering	120	144	198	222	246	276	306	336	366	396	426	456
Water skiing	270	330	390	450	510	570	636	702	768	834	900	966
Weight training	274	340	408	468	534	594	660	732	798	864	930	996
Wrestling	462	558	990	768	870	972	1,074	1,176	1,278	1,380	1,482	1,524

Note: The approximate figures in the table include resting energy expenditure (the kcal you would have expended during this period while at rest) and the kcal expended by the activity. The chart does not account for the additional caloric expenditure occurring from metabolism remaining above baseline for 20 minutes to several hours after exercise ceases (afterburn). Calculations are only approximate and include only the time you are actually performing the activity. Small differences do exist between males and females in kcal expended, but the difference is not significant in the total kcal expended for most activities.

Not all body weights are listed. Use the closest weight shown to determine the approximate number of kcal expended.

For optimum weight and fat loss, choose an activity that expends a minimum of 2,000 kcal per week in four to five workouts, or 400 to 500 kcal per exercise session.

From G.B. Dintiman and R. Ward, 1999, *The Mannatech exercise program* (Cappell, TX), 8 and 9. By permission of G.B. Dintiman.

Behavioral Change and Motivational Strategies

Many factors might interfere with your ability to improve your cardiorespiratory fitness. Here are some barriers (roadblocks) and strategies for overcoming them.

Roadblock	Behavioral Change Strategy
You have been involved in an aerobic exercise program for 4 months and find that your motivation has decreased. You also have been walking the same exercise path for weeks and feel that you need something new.	The simple answer is cross-training. Cross-training can help put the pizzazz back in your workout if you find your interest slipping after a few weeks or a few months. Many regular exercisers use cross-training to target different parts of their bodies or add variety. Because cross-training is an important motivation tool, you should base it on your individual needs and preferences. Some factors to consider when selecting activities are the following: ■ Impact. Choose complementary workouts that provide different levels of impact to reduce risk of injury. ■ Intensity. Alternate low- and high-intensity workouts. You may consider a walking or cycling program. ■ Location. Choose activities that take you to a variety of locations or alternate working out in a health club and at a local public park. ■ Weather. Consider choosing at least one indoor activity so that periods of inclement weather will not force you to alter your workout schedule. ■ Social support. Find an activity that you can participate in with a partner. Most people find the buddy system helpful in increasing motivation. ■ Regularity. Always remember that it is OK to take a break from your workout routine periodically. You are more likely to enjoy yourself when your body and your mind are refreshed and relaxed.
You recently joined a health club but are dismayed because you find it difficult to gain access to the equipment. It seems as if the regulars have taken over and aren't too willing to accept a newcomer.	Health clubs are busy places, especially during peak hours (early mornings, noon, and early evenings). Most clubs post written rules about using the facility and the equipment. Unwritten rules for behavior simply boil down to one simple principle: Be considerate of others. To observe health club etiquette, follow these guidelines: ■ Put towels where they belong. ■ Use only one locker unless plenty are available. ■ Limit your shower to 5 minutes when others are waiting. ■ Follow the flow of other exercisers when possible. ■ Be considerate of the time of other exercisers. Do not monopolize certain pieces of equipment. Remember: Your favorite is probably theirs, too. ■ Don't interrupt exercisers while they are in the middle of a routine. Wait until they take a break. ■ Respect personal space. Learn to read body language. If someone doesn't want to be disturbed, choose someone else to chat with.
You have been a regular aerobic exerciser for several years and find that exercise seems to consume your life. You have tried to decrease your time commitment but cannot seem to stop. Secretly, you fear that things are getting out of control.	You may be a victim of exercise addiction. If that is the case, consider seeking professional advice. Exercise addiction involves three classic characteristics: dependence, tolerance, and withdrawal. Signals of exercise addiction include ■ devoting less attention to interpersonal relationships, ■ having greater interest in the gains you make in your training program than you do in work and other issues, and ■ exhibiting a pattern in which your feelings about your body and the euphoria from exercise become more important than anything else.

(continued)

List other roadblocks preventing you from participating in a cardiorespiratory fitness program or factors hindering your progress in your current program.

Now cite behavioral change strategies that can help you overcome these roadblocks. If necessary, refer to chapter 4 for behavioral change and motivational strategies.

1. _____

1. _____

2. _____

2. _____

3. _____

3. _____

The calorie costs of walking for an hour, regardless of the pace, and jogging for an hour are not the same. For example, walking at a speed of 3 miles per hour requires less than half the energy of jogging at 6 miles per hour. The disparity occurs because you require more energy to lift your body from the ground when you are running than you do when you are moving your body forward on a horizontal plane when walking.

Table 5.2 compares the caloric expenditure of cycling at a leisurely pace of 5.5 miles per hour versus traveling at 9.5 miles per hour. Again, energy expenditure doubles at the faster pace because the cyclist covers a greater distance during the fixed time span. Rope skipping expends more energy than walking or cycling does. As we stated earlier, however, use caution when choosing this form of exercise because of the increased susceptibility to injury.

The calorie costs associated with swimming are also provided in table 5.2. Note, however, that skill level can affect caloric expenditure during swimming nearly as much as body weight does because the efficiency of the stroke varies so much from one person to the next. Unskilled swimmers often experience fatigue much more quickly than experienced swimmers do because they tend to fight the water and waste a lot of energy during each stroke. Nonetheless, swimming is an excellent mode of cardiorespiratory exercise because it results in a high level of energy expenditure.

For each of the aerobic activities listed in table 5.2, you will notice that the number of calories expended during an exercise session is higher for heavier individuals. This information is especially important to those participating in an aerobic conditioning program with the combined objective of enhancing fitness and losing weight. When you begin an aerobic exercise program, you may initially lose weight rapidly providing you also create a negative daily calorie balance. But as you continue the same exercise and diet regimen, you will probably find it more difficult to keep losing weight at the initial rate of loss.

The decline in the rate of weight loss can be partially explained by the fact that you burn fewer calories while performing the same total amount of work as your body weight decreases. To continue losing weight, you must increase your total caloric expenditure by exercising for longer periods, increasing the number of days per week that you exercise, or exercising at higher intensity. Making these progressive changes to your total workout program in proportion to the increase in your cardiorespiratory fitness level should be one of your fitness goals. We will explore the relationship between exercise and diet in more detail in chapter 8.

Summary

Understanding the Difference Between Anaerobic and Aerobic Exercise   The major ATP-producing or energy-producing systems in the body are the anaerobic and aerobic metabolism systems. When ATP is generated by the process of using oxygen, we refer to metabolism as being aerobic. When ATP is generated without the use of oxygen, we refer to metabolism as being anaerobic. The two major types of anaerobic energy systems are the immediate energy system and the lactic acid system. The immediate energy system provides energy for high-intensity activities that last less than 30 seconds. The lactic acid anaerobic system generates energy for high-intensity activities lasting up to 2 or 3 minutes.

Aerobic activities depend on oxygen metabolism to generate the ATP necessary to perform the activity. Aerobic fitness is used interchangeably with the terms *aerobic power, cardiorespiratory fitness, cardiorespiratory endurance,* and *maximal oxygen consumption.* As your cardiorespiratory endurance increases, so does your ability to engage in sustained physical activity.

Benefits of Cardiorespiratory Fitness Many benefits result from participating in a cardiorespiratory endurance conditioning program. A major reason for participating in an aerobic fitness program is to increase the maximal oxygen consumption ($\dot{V}O_2$max). $\dot{V}O_2$max, the single best indicator of cardiorespiratory fitness, is influenced primarily by (1) the ability of the cardiorespiratory system to deliver oxygen to the muscles and (2) the ability of the muscles to extract or remove oxygen from the blood to be used in the production of ATP.

Besides increasing your maximal aerobic capacity, an aerobic conditioning program makes exercise easier at workloads below maximum. As your stroke volume and blood volume increase, in addition to other physiological changes, you are able to exercise at lower heart rates. Ultimately, the longer you participate in an aerobic conditioning program, the greater your level of efficiency because your body does not work as hard to produce the same amount of energy.

You will also experience faster recovery from aerobic exercise as your level of fitness improves. Susceptibility to chronic debilitating diseases decreases because your blood-lipid profile becomes more positive through a reduction of fats and certain forms of cholesterol in the bloodstream. Your agility improves as you experience a reduction in body fat while simultaneously increasing bone density and strengthening your joints. Finally, exercisers tend to respond more favorably to mental stress when maintaining an active lifestyle.

Measuring Cardiorespiratory Fitness Factors such as age, gender, genetic background, and physical training influence $\dot{V}O_2$max. Typically, as you become older, your maximal level of aerobic fitness declines. The $\dot{V}O_2$max of an individual is expressed in volume (in liters) per unit of time (in minutes). Scores ranging from 3 to 4 liters per minute are common for the average healthy individual who exercises three to four times per week. Usually, the greater the muscle mass used in a sport or activity, the higher the maximal oxygen uptake obtained through training.

Direct measurement of $\dot{V}O_2$max during a maximal exercise test on a treadmill, cycle ergometer, or other mode of testing provides the most accurate assessment. Because of risks associated with maximal exercise testing in older individuals, specialized costly equipment, and the time required for testing large groups, submaximal or field tests that predict $\dot{V}O_2$max are frequently recommended. When choosing a field test to assess maximal cardiorespiratory capacity, consider the accuracy of the test, the population on which the test was developed, and your present level of fitness.

Sample Starter Programs Walking is one of the most popular aerobic activities because it does not require any specialized skills. Gradually increase your rate of progression until you reach a distance of 5 miles.

Complete the advanced walking program before beginning a jogging or running program. Gradually increase the amount of time spent jogging until you can jog continuously for 30 to 45 minutes. To prevent injury, we recommend that you increase your distance before you increase your speed.

Swimming and water aerobics have increased in popularity because of the high rate of musculoskeletal injuries associated with other aerobic activities. If you are not a strong swimmer, begin with a walking program and spend more time doing water exercises.

Cycling is also a great aerobic activity because the bicycle supports your body weight. Begin cycling a distance of 1 or 2 miles, even if you are exercising below your THR zone.

Aerobic exercisers often avoid rope skipping because of the skill needed and the high impact involved. Begin with brief periods of jumping followed by periods of rest to reduce risk of injury while increasing your fitness level.

Comparison of Energy Expenditure From Various Types of Aerobic Exercise The caloric expenditure from aerobic activities generally depends on the body weight of the individual and the intensity of the activity. A heavier person will burn more calories performing an activity for a given period than will an individual who weighs less. As you progress in an aerobic conditioning program, you may experience a decline in the rate of weight loss because your caloric expenditure decreases as your weight decreases.

As walking speed increases, so does the number of calories expended during the same period. Caloric expenditure also increases significantly for jogging compared with walking because of the vertical lift component in jogging. The calorie cost of swimming is difficult to assess because of the effect of the swimmer's skill.

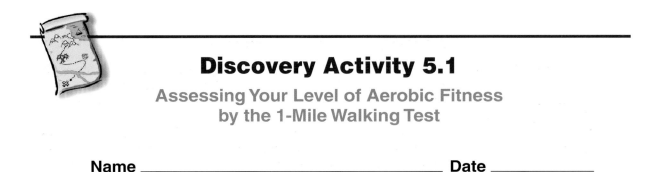

Discovery Activity 5.1

Assessing Your Level of Aerobic Fitness by the 1-Mile Walking Test

Name _____ Date _____

Instructions: This test is designed for older adults or for those who are just beginning an aerobic conditioning program. The time of the walk and the postexercise heart rate value are used to predict the subject's maximal oxygen consumption.

Step 1: Pretest Screening

- If you are over age 35, seek the advice of your physician before taking this test.
- Do not eat or drink anything except water for at least 3 hours before taking the test.
- Avoid using any type of tobacco, including cigarettes and chewing tobacco, for at least 3 hours before taking the test.
- Avoid heavy physical activity on the day of the test.
- If you are on medication, report it to your instructor before you begin this test.
- Wear loose-fitting clothes, such as shorts and a T-shirt, and running shoes.

Step 2: Administration of the Test

1. Participants divide into two groups.
2. Each participant in the first group should choose a partner from the other group.
3. Those taking the test first complete a thorough warm-up session and slowly walk one lap around the track.
4. The partners maintain a scorecard that records time in minutes and seconds and keeps track of the number of laps walked.
5. The instructor explains the procedures (such as the fact that the faster participants walk, the higher their level of cardiorespiratory fitness will be) and tells the first group to begin.
6. The students walk the mile as fast as they can. Only walking is allowed.
7. As walkers complete each lap, the partners let them know how many laps remain and encourage them to maintain a steady pace.
8. The instructor periodically calls out the time in minutes and seconds.
9. The partners write the final time on the scorecard.
10. The partners immediately take the walkers' 10-second heart rate. Instruct the walkers that they should complete the heart rate count within 15 seconds after the end of the mile walk. Any further time delay will overestimate maximal oxygen consumption.
11. After all walkers in the first group finish, the walkers in the second group take the test while those in the first group act as partners.

Step 3: Interpretation of the Results

- Tables 5.A and 5.B contain the estimated maximal oxygen uptake (milliliters per kilogram per minute) for women and men ages 20 to 39 based on the 1-mile walk test. Use these tables with table 5.1 to obtain an estimate of your maximal aerobic power based on your performance in this walk test.

Discovery Activity 5.1 *(continued)*

■ To use the tables, find the section that pertains to your age and sex. On the horizontal line across the top, find the length of time (to the nearest minute) it took you to walk a mile. In the vertical column, find the point of intersection for your walking time and your postexercise heart rate (listed in the far left column). The number where the postexercise heart rate and the 1-mile time intersect is your maximal oxygen consumption expressed in milliliters per kilogram per minute. For example, a 34-year-old woman who walked the mile in 17 minutes and had a postexercise heart rate of 170 would have an estimated oxygen consumption of 27.6 milliliters per kilogram per minute. According to Table 5.1, she would be between the fair and average fitness categories.

Step 4: Cardiorespiratory Endurance Record

Name _____   Date _____

Age _____ Sex _____ Body weight _____

Walking time _____ Fitness category _____

Maximal $\dot{V}O_2$ (milliliters per kilogram per minute) _____

TABLE 5.A—Estimated Maximal Oxygen Uptake (ml/kg/min) for Women, 20 to 39 Years Old

Heart rate	MIN/MILE										
	10	11	12	13	14	15	16	17	18	19	20
WOMEN (20-29)											
120	62.1	58.9	55.6	52.3	49.1	45.8	42.5	39.3	36.0	32.7	29.5
130	60.6	57.3	54.0	50.8	47.5	44.2	41.0	37.7	34.4	31.2	27.9
140	59.0	55.7	52.5	49.2	45.9	42.7	39.4	36.1	32.9	29.6	26.3
150	57.4	54.2	50.9	47.6	44.4	41.1	37.8	34.6	31.3	28.0	24.8
160	55.9	52.6	49.3	46.1	42.8	39.5	36.3	33.0	29.7	26.5	23.2
170	54.3	51.0	47.8	44.5	41.2	38.0	34.7	31.4	28.2	24.9	21.6
180	52.7	49.5	46.2	42.9	39.7	36.4	33.1	29.9	26.6	23.3	20.1
190	51.2	47.9	44.6	41.4	38.1	34.8	31.6	28.3	25.0	21.8	18.5
200	49.6	46.3	43.1	39.8	36.5	33.3	30.0	26.7	23.5	20.2	16.9
WOMEN (30-39)											
120	58.2	55.0	51.7	48.4	45.2	41.9	38.7	35.4	32.1	28.9	25.6
130	56.7	53.4	50.1	46.9	43.6	40.4	37.1	33.8	30.6	27.3	24.0
140	55.1	51.8	48.6	45.3	42.1	38.8	35.5	32.3	29.0	25.7	22.5
150	53.5	50.3	47.0	43.8	40.5	37.2	34.0	30.7	27.4	24.2	20.9
160	52.0	48.7	45.4	42.2	38.9	35.7	32.4	29.1	25.9	22.6	19.3
170	50.4	47.1	43.9	40.6	37.4	34.1	30.8	27.6	24.3	21.0	17.8
180	48.8	45.6	42.3	39.1	35.8	32.5	29.3	26.0	22.7	19.5	16.2
190	47.3	44.0	40.8	37.5	34.2	31.0	27.7	24.4	21.2	17.9	14.6

Calculations assume a body weight of 125 lb for women. For each 15 lb beyond 125 lb, subtract 1 ml from the estimated maximal oxygen uptake given in the table.

Reprinted, by permission, from B.D. Franks and E.T. Howley, 1998, *Fitness leader's handbook*, 2nd ed. (Champaign, IL: Human Kinetics), 76.

From *Physical fitness and wellness, third edition*, by Jerrold S. Greenberg, George B. Dintiman, and Barbee Myers Oakes, 2004, Champaign, IL: Human Kinetics.

(continued)

Discovery Activity 5.1 *(continued)*

TABLE 5.B—Estimated Maximal Oxygen Uptake (ml/kg/min) for Men, 20 to 39 Years Old

Heart rate	MIN/MILE										
	10	11	12	13	14	15	16	17	18	19	20
MEN (20-29)											
120	65.0	61.7	58.4	55.2	51.9	48.6	45.4	42.1	38.9	35.6	32.3
130	63.4	60.1	56.9	53.6	50.4	47.1	43.8	40.6	37.3	34.0	30.8
140	61.8	58.6	55.3	52.0	48.8	45.5	42.2	39.0	35.7	32.5	29.2
150	60.3	57.0	53.7	50.5	47.2	43.9	40.7	37.4	34.2	30.9	27.6
160	58.7	55.4	52.2	48.9	45.6	42.4	39.1	35.9	32.6	29.3	26.1
170	57.1	53.9	50.6	47.3	44.1	40.8	37.6	34.3	31.0	27.8	24.5
180	55.6	52.3	49.0	45.8	42.5	39.3	36.0	32.7	29.5	26.2	22.9
190	54.0	50.7	47.5	44.2	41.0	37.7	34.4	31.2	27.9	24.6	21.4
200	52.4	49.2	45.9	42.7	39.4	36.1	32.9	29.6	26.3	23.1	19.8
MEN (30-39)											
120	61.1	57.8	54.6	51.3	48.0	44.8	41.5	38.2	35.0	31.7	28.4
130	59.5	56.3	53.0	49.7	46.5	43.2	39.9	36.7	33.4	30.1	26.9
140	58.0	54.7	51.4	48.2	44.9	41.6	38.4	35.1	31.8	28.6	25.3
150	56.4	53.1	49.9	46.6	43.3	40.1	36.8	33.5	30.3	27.0	23.8
160	54.8	51.6	48.3	45.0	41.8	38.5	35.2	32.0	28.7	25.5	22.2
170	53.3	50.0	46.7	43.5	40.2	36.9	33.7	30.4	27.1	23.9	20.6
180	51.7	48.4	45.2	41.9	38.6	35.4	32.1	28.8	25.6	22.3	19.1
190	50.1	46.9	43.6	40.3	37.1	33.8	30.5	27.3	24.0	20.8	17.5

Calculations assume a body weight of 170 lb for men. For each 15 lb beyond 170 lb, subtract 1 ml from the estimated maximal oxygen uptake given in the table.

Reprinted, by permission, from B.D. Franks and E.T. Howley, 1998, *Fitness leader's handbook*, 2nd ed. (Champaign, IL: Human Kinetics), 76.

Discovery Activity 5.2

Assessing Your Level of Aerobic Fitness by the 12-Minute Run Test

Name _____ **Date** _____

Instructions: The objective of the test is to cover the greatest possible distance in a 12-minute period. Participants should perform it on a track or other accurately measured course.

Step 1: Pretest Screening

- If you are over 35 years of age, seek the advice of your physician before taking this test.
- Do not eat or drink anything except water for at least 3 hours before taking the test.
- Avoid using any type of tobacco, including cigarettes and chewing tobacco, for at least 3 hours before taking the test.
- Avoid heavy physical activity on the day of the test.
- If you are on medication, report it to your instructor before you begin the test.
- Wear loose-fitting clothes, such as shorts and a T-shirt, and running shoes.

Step 2: Administration of the Test

1. Participants divide into two groups.
2. Each participant in the first group should choose a partner from the other group.
3. Those taking the test first complete a thorough warm-up session and slowly walk one lap around the track.
4. The partners maintain a scorecard that records the distance covered during the 12-minute period.
5. The instructor explains the procedures again and tells the first group to begin.
6. As runners complete each lap, the partners let them know how much time remains and encourage them to maintain a steady pace.
7. The instructor uses a stopwatch or wristwatch to time a 12-minute period accurately.
8. The instructor periodically calls out the time in minutes and seconds.
9. The partners write the distance run in 12 minutes in fractions of a mile.
10. After all individuals in the first group finish, those in the second group take the test while those in the first group act as partners.

Step 3: Interpreting the Results

- Table 5.C contains five fitness classifications based on age and sex.
- To use the table, find on the horizontal line the age of the individual and the distance covered in 12 minutes. Then locate on the vertical column the fitness category, according to sex.
- For example, if you are an 18-year-old female and you covered 1.5 miles in 12 minutes, you are in the high-performance category.

Discovery Activity 5.2 *(continued)*

TABLE 5.C—Fitness Classification for Men and Women, Ages 17-50+

MEN (AGE)				
Classification	**17-26**	**27-39**	**40-49**	**50+**
High-performance zone	>1.80	>1.60	>1.50	>1.40
Good fitness zone	1.55-1.79	1.45-1.59	1.40-1.49	1.25-1.39
Marginal zone	1.35-1.54	1.30-1.44	1.25-1.39	1.10-1.24
Low zone	<1.35	<1.30	<1.25	<1.10
WOMEN (AGE)				
Classification	**17-26**	**27-39**	**40-49**	**50+**
High-performance zone	>1.45	>1.35	>1.25	>1.15
Good fitness zone	1.25-1.44	1.20-1.34	1.15-1.24	1.05-1.14
Marginal zone	1.15-1.24	1.05-1.19	1.00-1.14	0.95-1.04
Low zone	<1.15	<1.05	<1.00	<0.94

Step 4: Cardiorespiratory Endurance Record

Name _____ Date _____

Age _____ Sex _____ Body weight _____

Distance covered _____ Fitness category _____

From *Physical fitness and wellness, third edition,* by Jerrold S. Greenberg, George B. Dintiman, and Barbee Myers Oakes, 2004, Champaign, IL: Human Kinetics.

Discovery Activity 5.3

Service-Learning for Cardiorespiratory Fitness

People who have heart problems of various types often enroll in cardiac rehabilitation or physical therapy programs. Working with people with these conditions requires an educated and experienced staff of professionals. Of course, you do not have that background. But you could assist program staff by helping identify or produce handouts describing various exercises or offering information that would contribute to the health of the participants. That task might require a review of literature from companies who produce patient education materials, government brochures, and other sources recommended by program staff. You might also want to develop a questionnaire for program participants to obtain their feedback regarding the educational materials currently used in the program. Is that material easily comprehended, is it helpful, and is it produced in a manner that encourages reading it? (For example, is it in large enough type, or is it colorful?) Which materials currently used should be maintained, and which should be replaced? Although you may feel that your experience and skills are limited, with the assistance of program staff you can contribute to the health of program participants.

From *Physical fitness and wellness, third edition,* by Jerrold S. Greenberg, George B. Dintiman, and Barbee Myers Oakes, 2004, Champaign, IL: Human Kinetics.

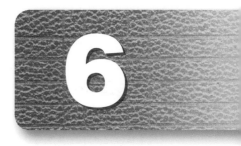

Flexibility Training

Chapter Objectives

By the end of this chapter, you should be able to

1. identify the factors that directly or indirectly affect range of motion in various joints,
2. cite the advantages of acquiring and maintaining adequate lifelong flexibility,
3. describe the role of flexibility in the prevention of injuries,
4. self-administer a series of tests that evaluate your flexibility,
5. design a personalized flexibility-training program that applies sound training principles, and
6. complete a flexibility routine using one of the methods described in this chapter.

Jamil is proud of the fact that he is muscular and athletic, although his lack of flexibility troubles him. In the past he thought that limited flexibility was a normal part of developing muscles and becoming strong. He now realizes that his inflexibility is interfering with his ability to enjoy recreational activities and competitive sports and to perform daily tasks such as picking up an object, tying his shoes, and even getting up out of a chair. Unfortunately, Jamil does not know what to do to improve his range of motion and correct the problem.

Flexibility is the range of motion around a joint. Of the five components of health-related physical fitness, flexibility is the aspect most neglected by the exercising population, by athletes, and by health care professionals and practitioners. Like Jamil, few individuals understand the importance of developing and maintaining acceptable levels of joint flexibility, yet the health, injury, and performance consequences of doing so are evident.

In this chapter, we will provide solutions to all of Jamil's problems and examine the many aspects of joint flexibility, such as the factors affecting range of motion, its importance, assessment techniques, sound training principles, and choice of specific stretching exercises to help evaluate range of motion and devise a program that meets your specific health and fitness needs.

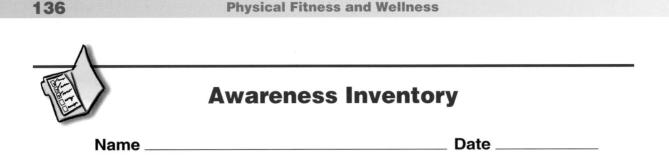

Awareness Inventory

Name _____ **Date** _____

Check the space by the letter T for the statements that you think are true and the space by the letter F for the statements that you think are false. The answers appear following the list of statements. This chapter will present information to clarify these statements for you. As you read the chapter, look for explanations for the reasons why the statements are true or false.

T___ F___   1. The major cause of lower-back pain in young adults is bulging disks.

T___ F___   2. According to orthopedic surgeons, the best treatment for the sudden onset of lower-back pain is complete bed rest for 5 to 7 days.

T___ F___   3. Sleeping while lying flat on your back with no pillows improves a condition called swayback.

T___ F___   4. Using a rocking chair will rest the back by changing the muscle groups used.

T___ F___   5. Before each exercise session, the first thing you should do is stretch.

T___ F___   6. Among athletes, some orthopedics feel that there is an increase in joint and soft tissue injuries due to overstretching and attempts to become too flexible.

T___ F___   7. Ballistic stretching is the most effective technique to increase range of motion.

T___ F___   8. When using static stretching exercise, the hold period at the extreme range of motion must be at least 30 seconds.

T___ F___   9. Maintaining flexibility throughout life is next to impossible because of the continuous loss of range of motion with aging.

T___ F___ 10. Adding a second stretching session at the end of your workout during the cool-down period is sound practice.

Answers: 1-F, 2-F, 3 –F, 4-T, 5-F, 6-T, 7-F, 8-F, 9-T, 10-T

Analyze Yourself

Assessing Your Flexibility Behavior in Exercise and Everyday Activity

Name _____ **Date** _____

Instructions: Indicate how often each of the following occurs in your daily activities and exercise sessions. Respond to each item with a number from 0 to 3, using the scale below:

0 = Never   **1** = Occasionally   **2** = Most of the time   **3** = Always

____ **1.** I can tie my shoes and put on socks with little difficulty.

____ **2.** I sleep on a firm mattress and avoid sleeping facedown on my front.

____ **3.** I keep the car driver's seat in a position where I can maintain an erect back and do not have to reach for the pedals.

____ **4.** When I sleep on my back, I place a pillow under both knees for proper support.

____ **5.** When I am forced to sit for a long period to study, work, read, or watch TV, I protect my back by using a straight, hard chair, throw my head back, tighten my abdominal muscles and sit upright with both feet on a footrest.

____ **6.** When lifting a light or heavy object from the floor, I bend at the knees and hips, not at the waist.

____ **7.** I warm up and stretch before every exercise session.

____ **8.** I use a general warm-up routine and make certain that I am perspiring before stretching any muscle group.

____ **9.** I avoid bouncing movements at the extreme range of motion during my stretching routine.

____ **10.** I avoid the following potentially dangerous stretching exercises: yoga plow (rocking back and bringing both feet overhead from a sitting position), straight-leg toe touch, straight-leg sit-up, duck walk, deep knee bends, squat jumps, hurdler's stretch, and straight-leg raise.

Scoring: Excellent = 25-30

Good = 19-24

Poor = Below 19

From *Physical fitness and wellness, third edition,* by Jerrold S. Greenberg, George B. Dintiman, and Barbee Myers Oakes, 2004, Champaign, IL: Human Kinetics.

Factors Affecting Flexibility

Because flexibility is specific to each joint, having good hip flexibility is no guarantee that you will be flexible in the shoulders, back, neck, or ankles. Depending on your stretching routine and choice of exercises, you may become highly flexible in some joints and remain inflexible in others. A number of factors combine to determine the range of motion around each joint.

Joint structure determines the limits of our range of motion (ROM) in all our joints, and we cannot alter it. Ball-and-socket joints, such as the hip and shoulder, allow the greatest ROM; ellipsoidal joints, such as in the wrist, are among the least flexible, with an ROM of only 80 degrees. Hinge joints, such as the knee and elbow, have an ROM of 130 degrees. We cannot force joints to extend movement beyond the limitations imposed by their structure.

Age and gender advantages also clearly exist—the young are more flexible than older people, and females are more flexible than males. Older adults undergo a process called **fibrosis** that causes some muscle fibers to degenerate and be replaced with a less elastic fibrous connective tissue. Females may be more flexible than males because of anatomical differences and differences in the type and extent of activities they perform throughout life.

Muscle bulk, involving a large increase in muscle mass, can limit movement in a number of joints. Extremely large biceps and deltoids, for example, can make it difficult to stretch the triceps. A change in weight-training routine could reduce the amount of bulk, but this approach is unadvisable for power athletes such as interior linemen in football, some positions in rugby, shot-putters, discus and hammer throwers in track and field, and athletes in other sports in which muscle bulk, push weight, and power are important.

Connective tissue (tendons, ligaments, fascial sheaths) and even the skin may limit ROM. Changes in the **elasticity** (ability to return to the original form) and **plasticity** (inability to return to original form) of connective tissue occur with age and injury and may restrict ROM.

Improper weight-training techniques involving high-volume resistance training with limited ROM (as in bodybuilding) can restrict ROM in various joints. Exercises that overdevelop one muscle group while neglecting opposing groups produce an imbalance that restricts flexibility.

Individuals who perform each weight-training exercise by going through the full ROM (see chapter 7) for both the agonist and antagonist muscles (such as the biceps and triceps when performing barbell curls) do not suffer loss of flexibility and can actually increase their ROM. For example, in a research study, women past the age of 62 who engaged in a 10-week comprehensive resistance-training program and did not perform any flexibility exercises achieved an average 13% increase in total flexibility (Barbosa et al., 2002). Similarly, inactive men past the age of 65 have experienced dramatic increases in flexibility by participating in strength-training programs focusing on total joint range of motion (Fatouros et al., 2002). Hence, strengthening muscles through the full ROM can increase flexibility even in elderly adults.

Improper stretching procedures also play a role in the decrease in ROM. Maximum benefits occur when each training session begins with a general warm-up period and 8 to 12 minutes of stretching and concludes with another 4 to 5 minutes of stretching.

Activity levels also affect ROM throughout life. Active individuals are considerably more flexible than inactive ones. A sedentary lifestyle can lead to shortening of muscles and ligaments and restricted ROM. Poor posture, long periods of sitting or standing, or immobilization of a limb can have a similar effect.

Finally, excessive body fat can reduce ROM by increasing resistance to movement and creating premature contact between adjoining body surfaces.

Fortunately, everyone is capable of increasing ROM in particular joints. Regular stretching routines cause permanent lengthening of ligaments and tendons. Muscle tissue undergoes only temporary lengthening following a warm-up and stretching routine as **muscle extensibility** increases. Muscle temperature changes alone, attained through proper warm-up, can increase flexibility by 20%.

Importance of Flexibility

A regular stretching routine will help increase ROM, improve performance in some activities, help prevent soft-tissue injuries, aid muscle relaxation, and help you cool down at the end of a workout. Stretching is a valuable part of a complete exercise program, and it provides some benefits to everyone.

Increased Range of Motion and Improved Performance

Because we have established the fact that ROM is joint specific, a well-rounded flexibility program must devote attention to all the body's major joints: neck, shoulders, back, hips, knees, wrists, and ankles. You can increase your ROM in each of these major joints in 6 to 8 weeks by following one of the recommended stretching techniques discussed in this chapter.

In sports such as gymnastics, diving, skiing, swimming, and hurdling and in other activities requiring a high level of flexibility, a stretching routine that focuses on the key joints can also help improve performance. Although little scientific evidence is available, the association between flexibility and sports performance is almost universally accepted.

Injury Prevention

Regular stretching routines may help reduce the incidence of injury during exercise for athletes and others. Continuous exercise such as jogging, running, cycling, and aerobics tightens and shortens muscles, and tight muscles are more vulnerable to injury from the explosive movements common in sports. A brief warm-up period followed by stretching will not only increase range of motion but also provide some protection from common soft-tissue injuries such as strains, sprains, and tears. Striving to maintain a full, normal ROM in each joint with adequate strength, endurance, and power throughout the range will reduce your chances of experiencing an exercise-induced injury.

Lower-Back Pain

Pain in the lower back occurs as frequently in our society as the common cold. This 20th-century plague affects an estimated 8 to 10 million people in the United States, who lose over 200 million workdays each year. Informal surveys of middle and high school athletes indicate that as many as 40% have experienced back problems severe enough to result in missed practice time.

In fact, the occurrence of nonspecific lower-back pain (LBP) in 14- to 16-year-old adolescents has almost reached the level experienced by adults because of earlier onset of sedentary lifestyles among children, intensive sports, genetics, psychosocial factors, smoking, and participation in high impact leisure-time physical activity (Ebbehoj et al., 2002). Injuries to the

fibrosis—A condition in which muscle fibers degenerate with age and are replaced by fibrous connective tissue.

elasticity—The ability of connective tissue to return to its original form.

plasticity—The inability of connective tissue to return to its original form.

muscle extensibility—The ability of muscle tissue to stretch.

vertebrae—The 33 bones of the spinal column, some of which are normally fused together (sacral and coccygeal vertebrae).

sciatica—Pain along the course of the great sciatic nerve (hip, thigh, leg, foot).

lower back are also common among both amateur and professional athletes in sports such as golf (Grimshaw et al., 2002).

Although back pain affects all age groups, the elderly are the most vulnerable. The older you are, the more likely you are to have problems with your lower back. No one seems to be immune.

A brief description of your spinal column will help you understand why the back is so vulnerable to injury (see figure 6.1). The human body has 33 **vertebrae** that extend from the base of the skull to the tailbone. The vertebrae form a double-S, reverse curve to ensure proper balance and weight bearing. If the vertebrae were placed directly on top of one another, the back would be only 5% as strong as it is, and one step would produce enough trauma and brain jolt to cause concussion. Shock absorbers, known as discs, are located between vertebrae. These capsules of gelatinous matter contain approximately 90% water in young people but only 70% in older individuals. With loss of water comes a loss of compressibility and increased vulnerability to injury, often referred to as a slipped, ruptured, or herniated disc. Ruptured disc material may bulge through the rear portion of the outer ring and pressure nerves, thereby producing pain in the lower back that may radiate down into the legs and feet (**sciatica**).

Not all sufferers of LBP have bone or disc disorders. The problem for most people involves muscle, tendons, or ligaments. No one cause can be identified as the trigger that causes an episode of back pain. Some of the more common factors include physical injury, hard sneezing or coughing, improper lifting or bending, standing

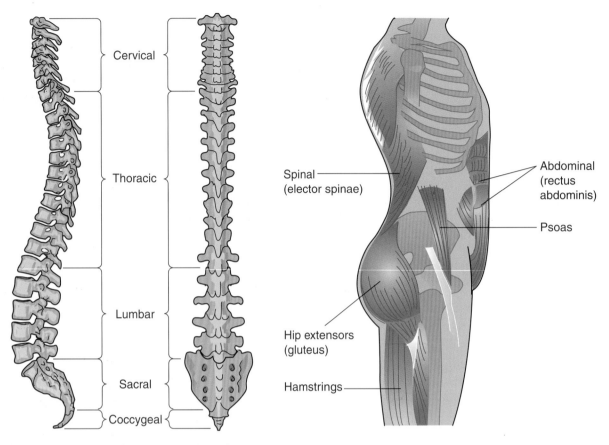

Figure 6.1   The vertebral column and muscle support.

or sitting for long hours, sitting slumped in an overstuffed chair or automobile seat, tension, anxiety, depression, obesity, and disease (for example, arthritis and tumors). Some individuals simply have a genetically weak back involving 1 or more of the approximately 140 muscles that provide support to the back and control its movements. Typically, a muscle, ligament, or tendon strain or sprain causes nearby muscles to spasm to help support the back. Inflexible and weak muscles due to the improper alignment of the spinal column and pelvic girdle cause about 7 out of 10 back problems.

The exact cause of most LBP, however, remains something of a mystery. Blaming back pain on pressure against a spinal nerve caused by one of the bulging spongy discs may be erroneous. Magnetic resonance imaging scans show that about one-third of young adults and practically all older adults who have no back pain have some bulging disks. A so-called normal back without some degree of bulging may be the exception. Other theories suggest that lower-back muscles

spasm or that arthritic spurs or bony overgrowth compress spinal nerve roots.

Prospective research studies that focus on the multifactor causes of LBP are rare. Stevenson et al. (2001) conducted a longitudinal study of industrial workers who initially reported no chronic LBP. Because these workers lifted 5,000 kilograms per shift, they were generally considered highly susceptible to developing LBP. Indeed, the results of the study confirmed that age, quadriceps muscle strength and endurance, level of physical fitness, social support, and the number of medications the workers were currently taking predicted the development of LBP with 75% accuracy.

You can also reduce your chances of developing LBP by changing the way you stand, bend, lift objects, sit, rest, sleep, and exercise. The "Your Back and How to Care for It" box summarizes the key factors for taking good care of your back. Study this box carefully to make sure you are practicing correct sitting, standing, and sleeping posture.

Your Back and How to Care for It

Whatever the cause of low back pain, part of its treatment is the correction of faulty posture. But good posture is not simply a matter of "standing tall." It refers to correctly using the body at all times. For the body to function in the best of health, you must use it so that you put no strain on muscles, joints, bones, and ligaments. To prevent low back pain, avoiding strain must become a way of life, practiced while lying, sitting, standing, walking, working, and exercising. When body position is correct, internal organs have enough room to function normally and blood circulates more freely.

With the help of this guide, you can begin to correct the positions and movements that bring on or aggravate backache. Pay particular attention to the positions recommended for resting, because it is possible to strain the muscles of the back and neck even while lying in bed. By learning to live with good posture under all circumstances, you will gradually develop the proper carriage and stronger muscles needed to protect and support your hard-working back.

How to Stay on Your Feet Without Tiring Your Back

To prevent strain and pain in everyday activities, it is restful to change from one task to another before fatigue sets in. Homemakers can lie down between chores; others should check body position frequently, drawing in the abdomen, flattening the back, and bending the knees slightly.

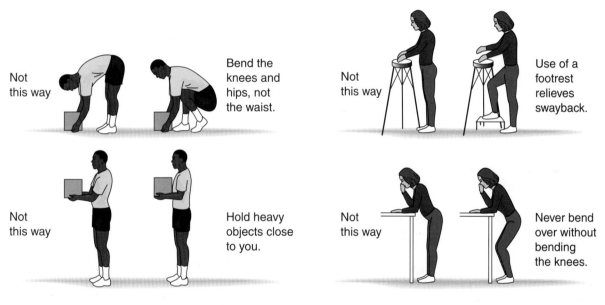

Not this way | Bend the knees and hips, not the waist.

Not this way | Use of a footrest relieves swayback.

Not this way | Hold heavy objects close to you.

Not this way | Never bend over without bending the knees.

Check Your Carriage Here

In correct, fully erect posture, a line dropped from the ear will go through the tip of the shoulder, middle of hip, back of kneecaps, and front of anklebone.

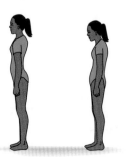

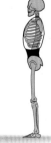

Incorrect: Lower back is arched or hollow.

Incorrect: Upper back is stooped, lower back is arched, abdomen sags.

Incorrect: Note how, in strained position, pelvis tilts forward, chin is out, and ribs are down, crowding internal organs.

Correct: In correct position, chin is in, head is up, back is flattened, pelvis held straight.

(continued)

Your Back and How to Care for It *(continued)*

To Find the Correct Standing Position

Stand 12 inches away from a wall. Now sit against the wall, bending the knees slightly. Tighten the abdomen and buttock muscles. This position will tilt the pelvis back and flatten the lower spine. Holding this position, inch up the wall to a standing position by straightening the legs. Now walk around the room, maintaining the same posture. Place your back against the wall again to see if you have held it.

How to Sit Correctly

A back's best friend is a straight, hard chair. If you can't get to the chair you prefer, learn to sit properly on whatever chair you have. To correct your sitting position from a forward slump, throw your head well back and then bend it forward to pull in the chin. This action will straighten the back. Now tighten the abdominal muscles to raise the chest. Check your position frequently.

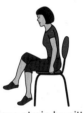

Relieve strain by sitting well forward, flatten back by tightening abdominal muscles, and cross knees.

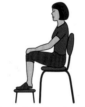

Use of footrest relieves swayback. Aim is to have knees higher than hips.

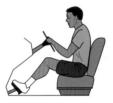

Correct way to sit while driving, close to pedals. Use seat belt or hard backrest, available commercially.

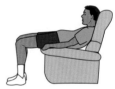

TV slump leads to "dowager's hump," strains neck and shoulders.

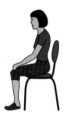

If chair is too high, swayback is increased.

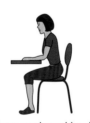

Keep neck and back in as straight a line as possible with the spine. Bend forward from the hips.

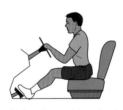

Driver's seat too far from pedals emphasizes curve in lower back.

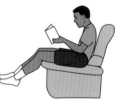

Strained reading position. Forward thrusting strains muscles of neck and head.

How to Put Your Back to Bed

For proper bed posture, a firm mattress is essential. Bed boards, sold commercially or devised at home, may be used with soft mattresses. Bed boards should be made of 3/4-inch plywood. Faulty sleeping positions intensify swayback and result not only in backache but also in numbness, tingling, and pain in arms and legs.

Your Back and How to Care for It *(continued)*

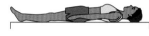

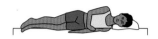

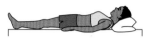

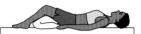

Incorrect:
Lying flat on back makes swayback worse.

Correct:
Lying on side with knees bent effectively flattens the back. Flat pillow may be used to support neck, especially when shoulders are broad.

Incorrect:
Use of high pillow strains neck, arms, shoulders.

Correct:
Sleeping on back is restful and correct when knees are properly supported.

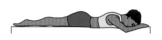

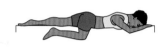

Incorrect:
Sleeping face down exaggerates swayback, strains neck and shoulders.

Correct:
Raise the foot of the mattress eight inches to discourage sleeping on the abdomen.

Incorrect:
Bending one hip and knee does not relieve swayback.

Correct:
Proper arrangement of pillows for resting or reading in bed.

When Doing Nothing, Do It Right

Rest is the first rule for the tired, painful back. The following three positions relieve pain by taking all pressure and weight off the back and legs. Note the pillows placed under the knees to relieve strain on the spine. For complete relief and relaxing effect, you should maintain these positions for 5 to 25 minutes.

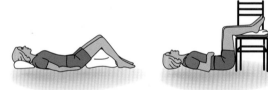

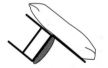

A straight-back chair used behind a pillow makes a serviceable backrest.

Exercise—Without Getting Out of Bed

Exercises performed while lying in bed aim not so much at strengthening muscles as at teaching correct positioning. Muscles used correctly, however, become stronger and in time are able to support the body with the least amount of effort.

Do all exercises in this position. Legs should not be straightened.

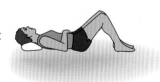

Bring knee to chest. Lower slowly but do not straighten leg. Relax.

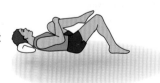

Exercise—Without Attracting Attention

Use these inconspicuous exercises whenever you have a spare moment during the day, both to relax tension and improve the tone of important muscle groups.

- Rotate shoulders forward and backward.
- Turn your head slowly side to side.

(continued)

Your Back and How to Care for It *(continued)*

- Watch an imaginary plane take off, just below the right shoulder. Stretch your neck, follow the plane as it slowly moves up, around, and down, disappearing below the other shoulder. Repeat, starting on the left.

- Slowly, slowly, touch your left ear to your left shoulder. Touch your right ear to your right shoulder. Raise both shoulders to touch your ears and then drop your shoulders as far as possible.

- At any pause in the day—waiting for an elevator to arrive, for a traffic light to change—pull in the abdominal muscles, tighten, and hold for the count of eight without breathing. Relax slowly. Increase the count gradually after the first week. Practice breathing normally with the abdomen held flat and contracted. Do this sitting, standing, and walking.

This exercise gently stretches the shortened muscles of the lower back, while strengthening abdominal muscles. Lying on the floor, bring both knees slowly up to the chest. Tighten the muscles of the abdomen, pressing your back flat against the floor. Hold your knees to your chest for 20 seconds. Then lower slowly. Relax. Repeat five times. Clasp the knees, bringing them up to the chest while coming to a sitting position. Rock back and forth.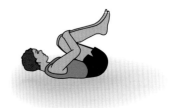

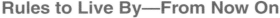

Rules to Live By—From Now On

- Never bend from the waist only; bend from the hips and knees.

- Never lift a heavy object higher than your waist.

- Always turn and face the object you wish to lift.

- Avoid carrying unbalanced loads; hold heavy objects close to your body.

- Never carry anything heavier than you can manage with ease.

- Never lift or move heavy furniture. Have someone who knows the principles of leverage do it.

- Avoid sudden movements, sudden overloading of muscles. Learn to move deliberately, swinging legs from the hips.

- Learn to keep the head in line with the spine when standing, sitting, and lying in bed.

- Put soft chairs and deep couches on your "don't sit" list. During prolonged sitting, cross your legs to rest your back.

- Your doctor is the only one who can determine when low back pain is due to faulty posture. She or he is the best judge of when you may do general exercises for physical fitness. When you do, omit any exercise that arches or overstrains the lower back, such as backward or forward bends and touching the toes with the knees straight.

- Wear shoes with moderate heels, all about the same height. Avoid changing from high to low heels.

- Put a foot rail under the desk and a footrest under the crib.

- Diaper a baby by sitting next to him or her on the bed.

- Don't stoop and stretch to hang the wash; raise the clothesbasket and lower the wash line.

- Beg or buy a rocking chair. Rocking rests the back by changing the muscle groups you use.

- Train yourself vigorously to use your abdominal muscles to flatten your lower abdomen. In time, this muscle contraction will become habitual, making you the envied owner of a youthful body profile!

- Don't strain to open windows or doors.

- For good posture, concentrate on strengthening "nature's corset"—the abdominal and buttock muscles. The pelvic roll exercise is especially recommended to correct the postural relation between the pelvis and spine.

In the past, treatment for LBP has involved a little bit of everything, from major surgery to traction, bed rest, and enzyme injections. Experts now feel that for most people who experience the sudden onset of lower-back pain, the best treatment may be no treatment at all. Like the common cold, chances are good that the condition will improve quickly. Existing evidence indicates that bed rest is not an effective therapy (Quittan, 2002; Van Tulder, 2001). On the contrary, research supports the use of early activity and exercise in the treatment of both acute and chronic LBP (Lively, 2002; Manniche et al., 2002). Tritilanunt and Wajanavisit (2001) assessed the efficacy of an aerobic exercise program in the treatment of chronic LBP and found that the exercisers experienced a significant improvement of pain score compared with those who simply participated in a lumbar flexion exercise program. Existing evidence also supports the use of early exercise in the treatment of LBP among athletes (George and Delitto, 2002).

The use of a firm mattress, moderate application of heat and cold, and gentle massage until muscle spasms are eliminated or significantly reduced will prepare you for a series of daily exercises designed to strengthen the four key muscle groups supporting your back and the important abdominal muscles (refer to the "Your Back and How to Care for It" section for more details). Three other components may help your rehabilitation and prevention program: (1) exercising more, (2) decreasing your abdominal fat by reducing your caloric intake, and (3) continuing to do lower-back exercises daily in addition to 30 minutes of aerobic activity 3 to 4 days per week after recovery. Only rarely is surgery needed to correct lower-back problems.

Other Benefits of Stretching

Among the other benefits of regular stretching are that it

- warms deep muscle fibers, joint fluids, lubricants, and synovial fluids to provide more efficient joint movement;
- prepares you mentally for vigorous activity;
- helps maintain joint flexibility and reduces pain as you age; and
- helps prevent loss of function and inability to perform certain chores, such as dressing, tying shoes, putting on socks, and so forth in the elderly.

Cool-Down Phase

As we discussed in chapter 3, the final 3 to 8 minutes of a workout should be a period of slowly diminishing intensity through the use of a slow jog or walk followed by a brief stretching period. By stretching at the end of your workout as the final phase of the cool-down, you are helping fatigued muscles return to their normal resting length and to a more relaxed state.

Assessment of Flexibility

Because range of motion is joint specific, no one test provides an accurate assessment of overall flexibility. Instead, each joint must be evaluated. This difficulty explains why so few physical fitness batteries employ a flexibility test. Only recently have test developers begun to include flexibility as part of health-related, physical fitness test batteries. Unfortunately, modern tests generally include only the **sit-and-reach test,** which measures only lower-back and hamstring (the large muscle group located on the back of the upper leg) flexibility. Although this test is valuable and accurate, primarily because it involves some of the muscle groups associated with lower-back pain, a more thorough test is also needed. Take a moment to complete Discovery Activity 6.1: Measuring Lower-Back and Hamstring Flexibility at the end of this chapter. Evaluate your performance using the sit-and-reach standards identified in the lab and determine your flexibility rating. Repeat this test after 6 to 8 weeks of stretching to determine the effectiveness of your flexibility-training program.

A quick evaluation of your overall flexibility level, using a less objective approach, may be even more valuable in determining your needs and the effectiveness of your stretching program. You can do this by completing the seven subjective tests described in Discovery Activity 6.2: Determining Your Total Body Flexibility at the end of the chapter. If you check yes in any test, your flexibility is good in that joint. Strive to improve your flexibility in the areas where you checked no. Repeat this series of tests after you have followed a stretching routine for 6 to 8 weeks. You will discover how easy it is to achieve a substantial increase in your range of motion.

sit-and-reach test—A test designed to measure the flexibility of the lower-back and hamstring muscles.

Myth and Fact Sheet

Myth	Fact
1. Stretching exercises are an excellent warm-up activity.	**1.** Stretching exercises are only one part of a sound routine to warm up the body. To prevent injury and muscle soreness, avoid stretching cold muscles. Begin with a general warm-up routine that involves large-muscle groups, such as walking or jogging, for at least 5 minutes or until sweating is evident; then follow with 5 to 10 minutes of stretching to complete the warm-up phase.
2. Stretching is needed only before vigorous activity.	**2.** Stretch before any workout. Stretching is also an excellent cool-down activity at the end of a workout, particularly after strength training.
3. Using your body's weight to bounce into the stretch helps increase flexibility.	**3.** Ballistic stretching (bouncing) causes the muscle to shorten by stimulating a muscle spindle. The technique is unsound and may result in joint injury.
4. Stretching will keep you from injury.	**4.** This statement is only partially true. Too much flexibility may increase the likelihood of ligament injury and joint separation and dislocation. Excessive stretching and flexibility may also lead to hypermobility and loose joints, leading to injury or premature development of osteoarthritis. You must stretch correctly, avoid dangerous exercises, and back off if pain is present, if you were recently injured, or if inflammation or infection is present around the joint.
5. Lost flexibility is an inevitable part of aging.	**5.** Some changes with age affect flexibility: increased calcium deposits, increased dehydration in connective tissues, adhesions, change in the chemical structure of tissues, and the replacement of muscle fibers with fatty and fibrous (collagen) fibers. Inactivity, however, causes much more loss of flexibility than aging does. Keep in mind also that people can develop flexibility at any age and that activity can prevent loss of ROM in all joints.
6. Strength training decreases flexibility.	**6.** Acquiring muscle mass does not automatically decrease joint movement. When you perform weight-training exercises correctly through the full range of motion, flexibility improves.

What Stretching Technique to Use

Numerous approaches to stretching have been shown to increase range of motion (ROM): dynamic stretching, static stretching, PNF stretching, ballistic stretching, and passive stretching. We discuss here the advantages and disadvantages of each method. Your choice depends mainly on your training objectives and safety. For each exercise, concentrate on two unique phases of stretching: easy stretching in which you move slowly into the stretch and apply mild tension with a steady, light pressure or execute a movement at slow speed, and developmental stretching in which you increase the intensity for an inch or less, easing off the stretch if the tension does not diminish, or increase the speed of the movement from low to medium to high speed. Breathe normally and avoid holding your breath.

Dynamic Stretching

Dynamic stretching exercises involve sport-specific movements such as high knee lifts while running in place. This technique involves the ability to use the range of joint movement during physical activity progressing from low to normal to high speed. Stretching movements are nearly identical to a specific activity such as jogging, sprinting, jumping, or movements in a sport and have the highest correlation to sport performance. Movements of a sport or activity are performed with the limbs moving to near full ROM at a slow, safe speed and progressing to the high speed used in the sport or activity. This progression is important because flexibility training should also be velocity specific to the activity for which you are training. Unlike ballistic stretching, dynamic stretching does not involve bouncing or jerky movements at the extreme range of motion and is less likely to result in injury. Some experts recommend using a dynamic stretching routine immediately after the warm-up session and a static routine during the cool-down period at the end of the workout.

Static Stretching

While performing each exercise, you can concentrate on three unique phases of **static stretching** (see figure 6.2): (1) easy stretching, in which you move slowly into the stretch and apply only a steady, light pressure; (2) developmental stretching, in which you increase the intensity of the pressure and continue in a "stretch by feel" phase; and (3) drastic stretching, in which you increase the pressure further and hold for 10 to 30 seconds to the point of some discomfort. In phase 3, if pain occurs, simply release the pressure and return to phase 2 for the remainder of the hold. For each exercise, move slowly from the starting position into the stretch, staying relaxed and breathing normally throughout and continuing until you feel a stretching of the muscle. From the easy stretch, move to the developmental stretch by increasing the intensity for 10 to 15 seconds without bouncing. Move to the drastic stretch for the final 10 seconds of the 30-second stretch, decreasing the intensity and returning to the developmental stretch if you feel pain.

The major disadvantage of static stretching is the lack of specificity and inability to mimic the movements used in a sport or activity. Because most activities and movements are dynamic, you should combine static stretching with dynamic stretching rather than use static stretching as your sole method.

Proprioceptive Neuromuscular Facilitation (PNF) Stretching

A two-person technique that combines alternating contraction and relaxation of the agonist and antagonist muscles is known as **proprioceptive neuromuscular facilitation (PNF) stretching.** The interaction of the agonist and antagonist muscles results in decreased resistance and increased ROM when stretching a particular

dynamic stretching—Involves the specific movements of an activity or sport through the range of motion, progressing from low to medium to high speed.

static stretching—Flexibility exercises in which a position is held steady for a designated time at the extreme range of motion.

proprioceptive neuromuscular facilitation (PNF) stretching—A two-person stretching technique involving the application of steady pressure by a partner at the extreme range of motion for a particular exercise and steady resistance to the pressure.

muscle. Both proprioceptive neuromuscular facilitation (PNF) and static stretching techniques will increase your ROM. Some studies have indicated that PNF techniques produce greater improvement. The main difference in the two techniques is that static stretching requires relaxation of the agonist muscle (the muscle being stretched) whereas PNF uses relaxation and isometric or concentric contraction of the agonist and relaxation of the antagonist muscle (the muscle not being stretched). The main disadvantage of PNF stretching is the need for an experienced partner and for supervision to eliminate horseplay and avoid injury because of overstretching.

Three unique types of PNF are used in the hold-relax technique. Your partner performs an easy stretch of your right hamstring (see figure 6.2). With the command "push," you exert a 3- to 4-second isometric contraction of your hamstring (your partner does not allow your leg to move), followed by a 10-second easy stretch on the command "relax" (your partner pushes backward on your right leg). Complete three to five repetitions without lowering your leg before repeating the exercise on your other leg.

The contraction-relax technique (see figure 6.2) begins in the same starting position with your partner providing an easy 4- to 6-second stretch before giving the signal "back" for you to contract your hip flexors and push forward for 4 to 6 seconds as your partner continues to push your leg forward. On the command "relax," your partner provides another easy stretch against your hamstring for 10 seconds. You then lower your leg to the starting position. Complete three to five repetitions with each leg.

The reversal-hold-relax technique (see figure 6.2) begins in the same starting position, with your partner performing an easy stretch until you experience slight discomfort. Your partner now tells you to push against the hand for 6 to 10 seconds

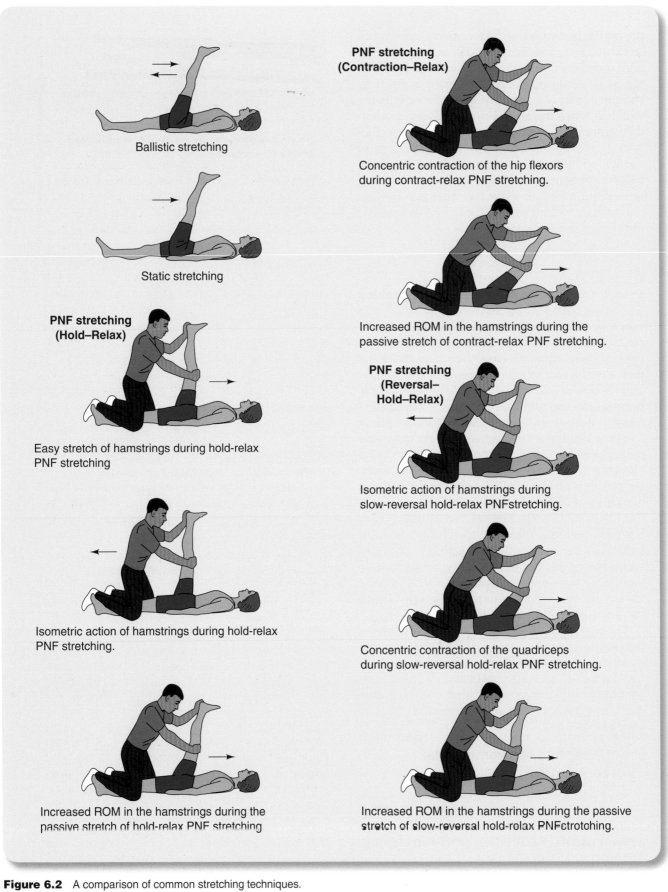

Ballistic stretching

Static stretching

PNF stretching (Contraction–Relax)

Concentric contraction of the hip flexors during contract-relax PNF stretching.

Increased ROM in the hamstrings during the passive stretch of contract-relax PNF stretching.

PNF stretching (Hold–Relax)

Easy stretch of hamstrings during hold-relax PNF stretching

Isometric action of hamstrings during hold-relax PNF stretching.

Increased ROM in the hamstrings during the passive stretch of hold-relax PNF stretching

PNF stretching (Reversal– Hold–Relax)

Isometric action of hamstrings during slow-reversal hold-relax PNFstretching.

Concentric contraction of the quadriceps during slow-reversal hold-relax PNF stretching.

Increased ROM in the hamstrings during the passive stretch of slow-reversal hold-relax PNFstretching.

Figure 6.2 A comparison of common stretching techniques.

(isometric action of the hamstring against an immovable object—the hand). Near the end of the 10-second period, your partner gives the command "back" to signal you to contract your quadriceps and hip flexors in an attempt to pull your leg back and lift the heel of your right foot off the hand. Your partner simultaneously pushes against your straight leg. At this point, with your quadriceps contracted, your hamstrings are relaxed and the ROM of the stretch is increased. Continue to contract your muscles until your partner says "relax," at which time a 10-second easy push is applied. Complete two to three repetitions before moving to your other leg.

Ballistic Stretching

The **ballistic stretching** technique (see figure 6.2) employs bouncing or bobbing at the extreme ROM or point of discomfort. When stretching the hamstring muscles, for example, individuals bounce vigorously three or four times as they reach for their toes in an attempt to aid the stretch forcefully. This method has several disadvantages. A muscle stretched too far and too fast in this manner may actually contract and create an opposing force, causing soft-tissue injury. An injury may also occur if the force generated by the jerking motions becomes greater than the extensibility of the tissues. Ballistic stretching is also likely to result in muscle soreness the following day.

Passive Stretching

The **passive stretching** technique (see figure 6.2) generally involves a partner or special equipment that carefully moves the joints through their range of motion with no contribution by the participant. The technique is commonly used during rehabilitation with the range of motion for each exercise completed in the absence of pain.

Flexibility-Training Principles

The flexibility-training principles discussed in the following sections will help you receive maximum benefit from your stretching routine.

Who Should Stretch

Some individuals need to stretch more than others do. People with lean body types and a high ROM may need very little stretching, whereas stocky, more powerfully built athletes with limited motion need 10 to 15 minutes of flexibility exercise before they make any radical moves such as bending over to touch the toes, jumping

> **ballistic stretching**—Flexibility exercises employing bouncing and jerking movements at the extreme range of motion or point of discomfort.
>
> **passive stretching**—Use of a partner or special equipment to move body parts carefully and safely through the range of motion.

explosively, or sprinting. Almost every healthy individual of any age or level of fitness can benefit from a regular stretching routine. Even older individuals who live relatively sedentary lives can benefit from initiating a flexibility-training program. Numerous scientific studies conducted on older adults past age 70 report that both men and women experienced significant improvements in their balance, gait, and flexibility despite their initial low level of fitness on these components (King et al., 2002; Burbank et al., 2002; Marom-Klibansky and Drory, 2002). As in these research studies, routines can be gentle, easy, relaxing, and safe or extremely vigorous. Daily stretching will help maintain flexibility throughout life and help prevent joint stiffness.

When to Stretch

Stretching exercises are used as part of a warm-up routine to prepare the body for vigorous activity, during the cool-down phase of a workout to help muscles return to a normal relaxed state, as a way to improve ROM in key joints, and as an aid to rehabilitation after injury.

Warm-Up and Cool-Down

Flexibility (stretching) exercises are often too closely associated with warming up. Consequently, most individuals make the mistake of stretching cold muscles before beginning a workout rather than first warming the body up with large-muscle activity such as walking or jogging for 5 to 8 minutes or until perspiration is evident. At this point, body temperature has increased 2 to 4°F, and muscles can be safely stretched.

Keep in mind that you warm up to stretch; you do not stretch to warm up. Table 6.1 provides a suggested order for stretching for those who engage in jogging, walking, cycling, swimming, racket and team sports, and strength training. Most organized aerobics classes follow a similar routine that involves a slow, gentle warm-up to cause sweating, followed by careful stretching, vigorous aerobics, and a cool-down period. Joggers and runners may choose to cover the first half mile or so at a slow pace, then do stretching exercises before completing the run, as opposed to the more

TABLE 6.1—Suggested Order for a Typical Exercise Session

Program	Workout order	Explanation
3 MI JOG (OR RUN, CYCLE, OR SWIM)		
Slow jog (1/2 mi)	1	Jogging will elevate body temperature, produce some sweating, and warm the muscles around the joints for stretching.
Stretch (8-12 min)	2	Muscles can now be safely stretched.
Fast jog (2 mi)	3	The pace can now be increased to elevate the heart rate above the target level for the aerobic portion of the workout.
Cool-down jog (slow 1/2 mi)	4	This final portion of the run helps the body slowly return to the preexercise state.
Cool-down stretch (4-5 min)	5	This concentrated, slow, stretching session will help prevent muscle soreness and improve range of motion.
RACKET SPORTS (OR TEAM SPORTS OR STRENGTH TRAINING)		
Slow, deliberate strokes	1	Movements specific to the sport elevate body temperature and produce sweating.
Stretch (5 min)	2	Muscles can now be safely stretched using sport-specific flexibility exercises.
Actual play or workout	3	Muscles are now ready for vigorous, explosive movement.
Cool-down (5 min)	4	This final portion of the workout should involve a return to slow, deliberate stroking or movements.
Cool-down stretch (4-5 min)	5	This concentrated, slow stretching session will help prevent muscle soreness and improve range of motion.

common routine of stretching cold muscles before the jog or run. Ideally, the majority of a stretching routine should follow the jog, run, cycle, swim, or strength-training or aerobics session and take place at the end of a workout during the cool-down phase. Stretching at the end of your workout when muscle-tissue temperature is high may effectively improve range of motion and reduce the incidence of muscle soreness the following day.

Stretching to Improve Range of Motion

If your main purpose is to improve body flexibility, you can safely stretch anytime you desire—early in the morning, at work, after sitting or standing for long periods, when you feel stiff, after an exercise session, or while you are engaged in passive activities such as watching television or listening to music. Remember, you must first elevate body temperature and produce some sweating by engaging in large-muscle-group activity before you stretch.

Rehabilitation From Injury

When you are recovering from soft-tissue injuries, focus attention on reducing pain and swelling, returning to normal strength, and achieving full, unrestricted range of motion. Unless you begin regular stretching as soon as pain and swelling

have subsided, some loss of flexibility in the injured joint is almost certain to occur.

How Much Intensity to Use

Stretching should involve a slow, relaxed, controlled, and pain-free movement. Disregard the "no pain, no gain" mentality because improvement occurs without undue pain. Too much pain or discomfort is a sign that you are overloading soft tissue and are at risk of injury. You should perform static stretching at a low intensity of 30 to 40% of your maximum exertion. You will learn to judge each exercise by the "stretch and feel" method, easing off the push if pain is too intense. This type of stretching also helps injured tissue recover and breaks down scar tissue between muscles and tendons.

How Long to Stretch

Depending on the stretching technique you choose, the number of repetitions or the length of time you hold each repetition in the stretched position will determine the length of your workout. If your main purpose for stretching is to prepare your body for vigorous exercise and to maintain the existing ROM in the major joints, 10 to 15 minutes is sufficient. For athletes and others striving to increase their ROM in the major joints, 15 to 30 minutes of careful stretching may be necessary. You may want to perform several different stretching exercises for each joint.

How Long to Hold Each Stretch

To improve flexibility, you must remain in the hold position (static technique) at the end of the stretch for a minimum of 30 seconds for the stretch to progress from the middle of the muscle belly to the tendons. Shorter holds will not increase range of motion. You should progress from 15 seconds at first to 30 seconds after 1 to 2 months of regular stretching. A 30- to 60-second stretch appears to increase the benefits only slightly and may be impractical because of the additional time required to complete your routine. In early workouts, you should count the seconds until you learn to stretch by the way it feels without having to count. With dynamic stretching, you should complete at least three sets —one at low speed, one at medium speed, and one at high speed—for each exercise.

How Often to Stretch

Those who are just beginning a flexibility-training program should do their routines three to four times a week. Those who need to produce large increases in ROM may need a minimum of five to seven stretching sessions weekly, stretching twice in some workouts. Adults should stretch at least once daily 3 to 5 days per week to maintain flexibility. Serious athletes may need two or three sessions per day 6 or 7 days per week to obtain desired results.

How Flexible to Become

Just how much flexibility someone needs depends on the individual. Gymnasts, ballet dancers, and hurdlers must be more flexible than people who merely want to maintain a level sufficient to reap the health benefits, perform daily activities, and engage in regular exercise.

Some of the increase in injury cases may be associated with excessive stretching and attempts to acquire high levels of flexibility. The cause may be related to renewed interest in stretching and the popularity of various forms of yoga and aerobics that tend to overemphasize flexibility or use questionable stretching exercises.

Flexibility Exercises

Those who stretch should choose at least one stretching exercise for each of the major muscle groups and apply exercises equally to both sides of the body. Although hundreds of different stretches are in use, many are unsafe and should be avoided. This section identifies the proper way to stretch, some commonly used exercises that have been shown to be potentially harmful, and some safe alternatives.

What Exercises to Use

Each of the stretching techniques described in this chapter will increase ROM. Ballistic stretching is not recommended because of the possibility of injury and an increase in muscle soreness a day or so after the workout. Passive stretching is a safe method of maintaining and reacquiring lost movement following an injury. PNF stretching is also effective but requires a partner. The best two choices for most individuals are dynamic and static stretching. You can complete a dynamic routine using five or six exercises at slow speed immediately following the general warm-up session. Complete five to eight repetitions of each exercise at slow speed before repeating each exercise at medium speed and then at high speed. A static stretching session can immediately follow the dynamic exercises or come at the end of your workout during the cool-down period. You should complete each static exercise slowly, beginning with a 10- to 15-second hold and adding 2 or 3 seconds each workout until you can comfortably maintain the hold position at the extreme ROM for 30 seconds. You can begin with the neck and progress downward to the shoulders and chest, trunk and lower back, groin, hips, abdomen, and upper and lower legs. See figure 6.2 for specific stretching exercises.

What Exercises to Avoid

As we pointed out previously, stretching can be harmful when the routine is too vigorous or too lengthy or when bouncing at the extreme ROM. The wrong choice of exercises also imposes serious risk of injury to joints. In fact, many popular stretching exercises used in the past are potentially harmful. Unfortunately, most people acquire their stretching knowledge by watching others. This informal, copycat approach has spawned a series of popular but dangerous exercises capable of damaging the knees, neck, spinal column, ankles, and lower back. Figure 6.3 identifies a "hit list" of nine popular stretching exercises that should be avoided and offers safe substitutes that will effectively stretch the same muscle groups.

Old Method

Neck roll (circling)

Danger: Drawing the head backward could damage the disks in the neck area, and may even precipitate arthritis.

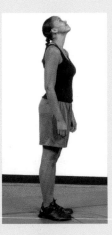

New Method

Forward neck roll

Description: Bend forward at the waist with the hands on the knees. Gently roll the head.

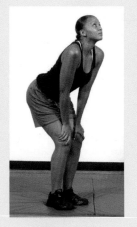

Quadriceps stretch

Danger: If the ankle is pulled too hard, muscle, ligament, and cartilage damage may occur.

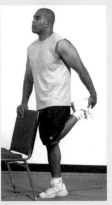

Opposite leg pull

Description: Grasp one ankle with your opposite hand. Instead of pulling attempt to straighten the leg you are stretching.

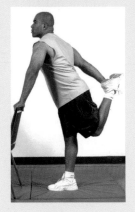

Hurdler's stretch

Danger: Hip, knee, and ankle are subjected to abnormal stress.

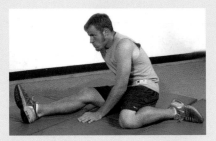

Everted hurdler's stretch

Description: Bend the left leg at the knee and slide the foot next to the right knee. Pull yourself forward slowly by using a towel, or by grasping the toe.

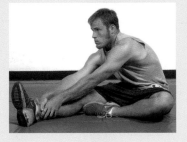

Deep knee bend (or any exercise that bends the knee beyond a right angle)

Danger: Excessive stress is placed on ligament, tendon, and cartilage tissue.

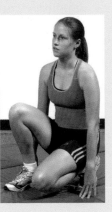

Single-knee lunge

Description: Place one leg in front of your body and extend the other behind. Bend forward at the trunk as you bend the lead leg to right angles.

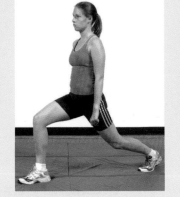

Figure 6.3 Dangerous popular stretching exercises and suggested replacements.

Old Method

Yoga plow

Danger: This exercise could overstretch muscles and ligaments, injure spinal disks, or cause fainting.

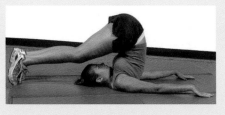

Straight-let sit up

Danger: Produces back strain and sciatic nerve elongation. It also moves the hip flexor muscles and does not flatten the abdomen.

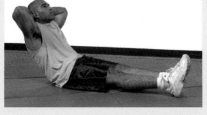

Double leg raise

Danger: Stretches the sciatic nerve beyond its normal limits and places too much stress on ligaments, muscles, and disks.

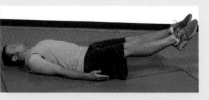

Prone arch

Danger: Hyperextension of the lower back places extreme pressure on spinal disks.

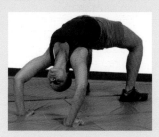

Back bends

Danger: Spinal disks can easily be damaged.

New Method

Extended one-leg stretch

Description: Lead leg extended and slightly bent at the knee. With your foot on the floor, draw the knee of the other leg toward your chest. Bend forward at the trunk as far as possible.

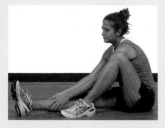

Bent-knee sit up

Description: Cross both hands on your chest, with the knees slightly bent. Raise the upper body slightly to about 25° on each repetition.

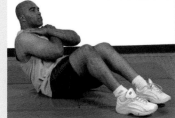

Knee-to-chest stretch

Description: Clasp both hands behind the neck. Draw the knee toward the chest, and hold that position of maximum stretch for 15-30 seconds.

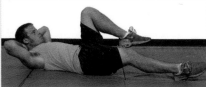

Belly push-up

Description: Lie flat on your belly, resting on your elbows. Push slowly to raise the upper body as the lower torso remains pressured against the floor.

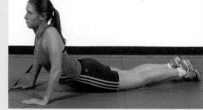

No alternative exercise has been approved.

Behavioral Change and Motivational Strategies

A number of barriers may interfere with your flexibility-training progress. Here are some of these roadblocks and strategies for overcoming them to keep you moving toward your training goals.

Roadblock	Behavioral Change Strategy
You are aware of your need to engage in flexibility training but just can't seem to stay interested long enough to avoid skipping workouts.	The first month of any exercise program is the most difficult. If you are beginning a new exercise program, it is normal to feel overloaded and anxious to complete the workout. At this point, you feel that 5 to 10 minutes of stretching takes valuable time and you are unable to see its benefits. Try some of the following techniques to get past this critical period. ▪ Arrive at the exercise site early with plenty of time to enjoy your workout. ▪ After you walk or jog a few minutes, take 5 or 10 minutes to relax, wind down, and enjoy stretching the major joints. ▪ Keep a log of how far beyond your toes you can reach, how difficult it is to reach behind your back and touch both hands, or how far forward you are able to move when stretching your calf muscles. Having these notes will help make you aware of improvement in future workouts. ▪ Force yourself to stretch carefully before every workout until it becomes habit and you discover the benefits of stretching.
At the end of a workout, your calves feel tight and are sometimes sore.	A feeling of tightness or even some mild soreness should only occur after your first three or four workouts. If it continues, examine every phase of your program. Are you properly warmed up before beginning your stretching session? Are you using static or PNF stretching exercises rather than ballistic movements? Are you stretching for 3 to 5 minutes at the end of your workout? Are you performing the correct exercises? Are you stretching both the calf muscles and the Achilles tendon? You should find the answer to the problem in one or more of these questions.
You find that you are quite inflexible and it hurts when you stretch. Given this feeling, you decide that you will never be comfortable stretching.	You can use covert modeling to copy the stretching behavior of a friend who stretches regularly. Identify someone you know who stretches before and after a workout. Imagine that person stretching and feeling good. The image should be vivid. That is, imagine what that person is feeling, what that person is wearing, the sights and sounds present, and so forth. When you can imagine this person stretching, substitute yourself for that person. Imagine yourself wearing what that person is wearing, feeling what that person is feeling, and experiencing the sights and sounds that person is experiencing. Just imagining yourself in this manner will help motivate you to stretch more regularly.
List other roadblocks you are experiencing that seem to be limiting the effectiveness of your flexibility-training program.	Now list the behavioral change strategies that can help you overcome the roadblocks. If necessary, refer back to chapter 4 for behavioral change and motivational strategies.

1. _____ _____

2. _____

3. _____

1. _____

2. _____

3. _____

Summary

Factors Affecting Flexibility   A number of factors combine to limit the degree of flexibility you attain. After age, sex, heredity, and injury, your choice of lifestyle has the greatest influence on ROM in your joints. By engaging in a regular aerobic exercise program, stretching before and after your workout, and maintaining normal body weight and fat, you can remain relatively flexible throughout your life.

Importance of Flexibility   Regular involvement in stretching exercises two to three times a week will increase joint flexibility, help improve performance in sports, aid in the prevention of soft-tissue injuries, help you prevent and recover from lower-back problems, and assist your muscles in returning to a relaxed status following a workout. Stretching can provide some benefit to almost everyone and make daily chores at home and at work easier and safer.

Assessment of Flexibility   To evaluate your body's flexibility properly, you should use a test for each of the major joints. Although the sit-and-reach test is one of the most common and accurate, it measures only hamstring and lower-back flexibility. Tests are also needed to measure ROM in the neck, elbows, wrists, groin, trunk, hips, and shoulders.

Comparison of Five Stretching Techniques   Each of the common methods of stretching (dynamic, static, ballistic, PNF, passive) will improve joint ROM. Ballistic and PNF stretching are more likely to result in injury and muscle soreness than the other techniques are. Dynamic stretching exercises are specific to the movements used in your activity or sport and may be the best choice. You can use dynamic stretching in combination with static stretching by completing the dynamic exercises immediately after your warm-up and performing static movements during the cool-down period at the end of the workout. Passive stretching is ideal for the rehabilitation of injured joints.

Flexibility-Training Principles   Two to three sessions a week in addition to the stretching routine you normally perform before an aerobic workout will improve your flexibility. You should stretch for 5 or 10 minutes before every workout but only after your body temperature has increased, as indicated by the presence of perspiration following some large-muscle activity such as jogging. You must avoid stretching cold muscles. Perform a more concentrated 10- to 15-minute session during the cool-down phase of a workout.

All four of the most common methods of stretching (dynamic, ballistic, static, and PNF) have been shown to be equally effective in improving joint ROM. Ballistic and PNF methods are more likely to result in injury and muscle soreness than static stretching is.

Stretching should produce only mild discomfort. Pain is an indication of risk of injury from overextending soft tissue. Stretching for too long a period in an attempt to obtain an extremely high degree of flexibility may also result in injury. Extreme flexibility is unimportant for most individuals, and you should avoid yoga-style contortions.

Effective stretching involves warming up, stretching before and after exercise, and stretching slowly and gently.

Flexibility Exercises   A sound program requires at least one exercise for each major joint and emphasis on both sides of the body. You can choose exercises that focus on particular joints you identify as inflexible or important to your personal life, job, sport, or activity. Although not everyone who uses so-called banned stretching exercises will suffer an injury, it is wise to avoid those known to have the potential to damage a joint.

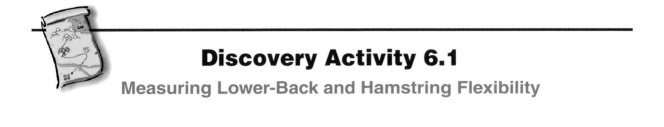

Discovery Activity 6.1
Measuring Lower-Back and Hamstring Flexibility

Name _____ **Date** _____

Instructions: The sit-and-reach test is used to determine the flexibility of your back and hamstring muscles. If a sit-and-reach box is not available, you can build one by placing a yardstick on top of a 12-inch-high box (see figure 6.4). To complete the test, follow these steps carefully:

1. Warm up properly before the first trial by walking or jogging for one-quarter to one-half mile or until you are perspiring. Now complete your warm-up by twice performing the hamstring and quadriceps exercises shown in figure 6.3 and the lower-back exercises shown in the "Your Back and How to Care for It" section (pages 141-144). Maintain the hold position for 30 seconds.

2. Remove your shoes and sit on the floor with your hips, back, and head against a wall and both legs fully extended, feet contacting the sit-and-reach box.

3. Place one hand on top of the other so that the middle fingers are together.

4. Lean forward slowly as far as possible and without bouncing slide your hands along the measuring scale on top of the box. Repeat this movement three times, stretching forward as far as possible a third time and holding that position for 2 seconds.

5. Complete two trials and record the average as your final score.

6. Determine your hamstring- and back-flexibility rating from table 6.A.

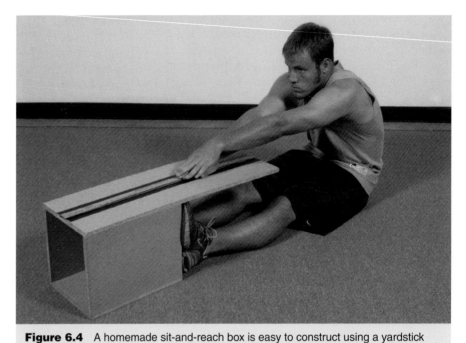

Figure 6.4 A homemade sit-and-reach box is easy to construct using a yardstick and a 12-inch-high box.

TABLE 6.A—Sit-and-Reach Standards

Performance standards	College females (in.)	College males (in.)
Excellent	8 or above	7 or above
Good	5-7	4-6
Average	1-4	1-3
Poor	0 or negative	0 or negative

From *Physical fitness and wellness, third edition,* by Jerrold S. Greenberg, George B. Dintiman, and Barbee Myers Oakes, 2004, Champaign, IL: Human Kinetics.

Discovery Activity 6.2

Determining Your Total-Body Flexibility

Name _____ **Date** _____

Instructions: You can subjectively test aspects of your flexibility alone or with a partner. The only equipment needed is a straight-backed chair and a ruler. Score each test by checking yes or no, depending on whether you can meet the standard cited.

	Yes	No
1. Neck. Lower your chin to sandwich your flattened hand against your chest.	___	___
2. Elbow and wrist. Hold your arms out straight with palms up and little fingers higher than your thumbs.		
Right arm and wrist	___	___
Left arm and wrist	___	___
3. Groin. While standing on one leg, raise the other leg to the side as high as possible. You should be able to achieve a 90-degree angle between your legs.		
Right leg	___	___
Left leg	___	___
While you are sitting on the floor, put the soles of your feet together and draw your heels as close to your body as possible. Try to touch your knees to the floor or to press your upright fists to the floor using your knees.	___	___
4. Trunk. While sitting in a straight chair with your feet wrapped around the front legs, twist your body 90 degrees without allowing your hips to move.		
Right twist	___	___
Left twist	___	___
5. Hip. While standing, hold a yardstick or broom handle with your hands shoulder-width apart. Without losing your grasp, bend down, step over the stick (with both feet, one at a time), and then step back again.	___	___
6. Shoulder. In a standing position, attempt to clasp your hands behind your back by reaching over the shoulder with one arm and upward from behind with the other. Repeat, reversing the arm positions.		
Right arm top	___	___
Left arm top	___	___

Discovery Activity 6.3
Service-Learning for Flexibility

Back pain is one of the most prevalent conditions experienced by adults. Because many adults are working on your campus, you can contribute to their back health by producing a booklet based upon the back pain prevention material appearing in this chapter. Contact your campus health center and work with them to produce the booklet. Then research the causes of back pain, how to prevent it, and what to do about it should it occur. Once the booklet is written, the health center can reproduce it and distribute it to all staff and faculty on your campus. If the cost of reproducing the booklet is more than the health center can afford, a local photocopy store (such as Kinko's) may be willing to either donate that service or provide it at reduced cost. If they do, make sure to highlight their contribution within the booklet.

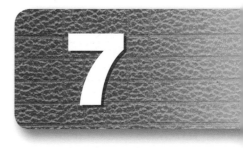

Weight Training and Body Shaping

Chapter Objectives

By the end of this chapter, you should be able to

1. identify the factors that directly or indirectly affect muscular strength and endurance,

2. cite the advantages of acquiring and maintaining adequate muscular strength and endurance throughout life,

3. design a personalized strength-development program using weights that applies sound training principles and meets your fitness objectives,

4. design a personalized muscular endurance training program without weights that applies sound training principles and meets your fitness objectives,

5. complete a strength and endurance routine using one of the methods described in this chapter.

6. design a sound girth-control program to flatten your abdomen, and

7. design a body-shaping program involving aerobic exercise, dietary restriction, and weight training that will reduce body fat, add muscle mass and definition, and change the way you look.

Esther has been interested in trying some form of strength training for years to firm her muscles and improve her appearance. She is also interested in it because she has heard that this type of training aids weight and fat loss. Some of her friends who use the weight room at the gym seem to have improved their bodies and are looking good. Esther wants to get started, too, but she has many questions and concerns. What type of program should she choose? How often should she work out? Should she use heavy or light weights? Will she add too much muscle and lose her femininity?

This chapter includes the answers to these and many more questions to help Esther and you implement sound strength-training programs designed to meet your personal objectives.

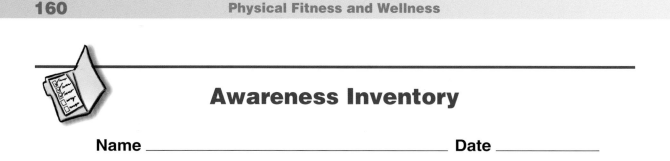

Awareness Inventory

Name _____ **Date** _____

Check the space by the letter T for the statements that you think are true and the space by the letter F for the statements that you think are false. The answers appear following the list of statements. This chapter will present information to clarify these statements for you. As you read the chapter, look for explanations for the reasons why the statements are true or false.

T___ **F**___ 1. Weight training burns few calories and does not help you lose weight.

T___ **F**___ 2. Regular weight training will change your fatty tissue to muscle tissue.

T___ **F**___ 3. Fibrous bands that attach some muscles to the bones to allow movement when muscles contract are called tendons.

T___ **F**___ 4. Using heavy weight, low repetitions, and multiple sets is an excellent way to improve your muscular endurance.

T___ **F**___ 5. You can easily add 4 to 7 pounds of muscle to your body each month through weight training.

T___ **F**___ 6. One of the problems with strength training is that muscle will turn to fat when you stop training.

T___ **F**___ 7. Anyone can develop a flat midriff by using a sound upper and lower abdominal exercise program daily.

T___ **F**___ 8. One acceptable breathing technique is to exhale during the exertion or lifting phase and inhale during the relaxation phase.

T___ **F**___ 9. You can completely reshape your body in 2 to 3 months through weight training.

T___ **F**___ 10. Approximately 48 hours (2 days) of rest is recommended between weight-training workouts to allow full recovery and receive the full benefits of a workout.

Answers: 1-F, 2-F, 3-T, 4-F, 5-F, 6-F, 7-F, 8-T, 9-F, 10-T

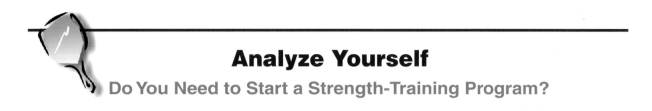

Analyze Yourself

Do You Need to Start a Strength-Training Program?

Name _____ **Date** _____

Instructions: Answer each question with a yes or no before reading the interpretation section to find out how badly you are in need of a strength-training program.

Yes **No**

1. ___ ___ Have you been on a diet within the past 6 to 12 months?

2. ___ ___ Have you ever lost, then regained, 8 to 10 pounds in the same year?

3. ___ ___ Do you find it difficult to control your body weight?

4. ___ ___ Do you have excess, sagging skin on the back of your upper arms, thighs, back of the legs, abdomen, or other body part?

5. ___ ___ Are you interested in changing your appearance by adding muscle and reducing the size of fat deposits?

6. ___ ___ Would a firmer, more muscular body help your body image, how you feel about yourself, and how you think others feel about you?

7. ___ ___ Would additional strength or endurance improve performance in any sports or exercise activity?

8. ___ ___ Would additional strength or muscular endurance help performance on the job or at home?

9. ___ ___ Would you like to strengthen any specific muscle groups in your body?

10. ___ ___ Have you sustained a soft-tissue (muscle, tendon, ligament) injury within the past 12 months, such as an ankle sprain, pulled muscle, or contusion?

Interpretation

If you answered yes to two or more of the questions, you need a strength-training program.

Questions 1 through 3 are concerned with body weight and fat. Strength training can help your skin fit better, help you focus on your body, help you shrink fat cells, and add muscle mass.

Questions 4 through 6 are concerned with body image and your interest in improving your appearance through strength training.

Questions 7 through 9 are concerned with the need for additional strength to aid performance on the job, at home, and in recreational activities.

Question 10 is concerned with the prevention of job, home, and exercise-related injuries.

From *Physical fitness and wellness, third edition,* by Jerrold S. Greenberg, George B. Dintiman, and Barbee Myers Oakes, 2004, Champaign, IL: Human Kinetics.

Although muscular strength and endurance are closely related, it is important to differentiate between the two. Muscular strength is the amount of force or weight a muscle or group of muscles can exert for one repetition. Strength is generally measured by a single maximal contraction. The amount of weight you can bench-press overhead one time, for example, measures the strength of the triceps muscle. You can measure the strength of other muscle groups the same way with specific tests (see chapter 2). Muscular endurance is the capacity of a muscle group to complete an uninterrupted series of repetitions as often as possible with lighter weights. The total number of bench presses you can complete with one-half of your maximum weight on the barbell, for example, measures the endurance of the triceps and pectoralis muscles. Depending on the desired outcome, you can manipulate the training variables (choice of equipment and exercises, amount of resistance or weight, number of repetitions and sets, length of rest intervals) to make your program strength- or endurance-oriented or a balance of the two.

This chapter addresses the key components in the development of strength and endurance, losing body fat, adding muscle mass, and changing the shape of your body, including importance, influencing factors, training principles, specific exercises, equipment, girth control, and body building.

Importance of Strength and Endurance

The improvement of muscular strength and endurance will affect almost every phase of your life. Some of the benefits, such as loss of body fat and improved self-concept, have been overlooked in the past because of overemphasis on adding muscle mass and improving performance. A closer look at the true value of strength and endurance training makes it clear that a sound program can help to improve both physical and mental health. Complete the Analyze Yourself activity, and you will know whether you need to begin a strength-training program.

Management of Body Weight and Fat

Although strength training is generally associated with muscle-weight gain and not with body weight and fat loss, it is a critical part of a total weight-control program. Unfortunately, metabolism slows with age and the amount of calories (cal) we consume does not. As a result, body

basal metabolism—The minimum energy the body needs to support ongoing cellular activity when the body is at rest; work that goes on continuously without your awareness.

weight and fat increase and the amount of lean muscle mass decreases.

Basal metabolism goes down about 3% per decade, mainly because of the loss of muscle mass. Inactive adults lose about a half pound of muscle mass per year and gain about a half pound of fat. From age 20 to 60, a decrease in resting metabolism of 12% or more occurs. This decline is a major contributor to weight and fat gain. The typical 60-year-old, for example, burns approximately 280 fewer calories daily at rest than he or she burned at age 20. This calorie differential is equivalent to 1 pound of fat (3,500 calories = 1 pound of fat) every 12 or 13 days, nearly 3 pounds per month, and over 30 pounds per year. As you can see, even small decreases in metabolism produce large increases in body weight and fat. A 5% slowing of resting metabolism can add 6 to 9 pounds of body fat in just 1 year depending on a person's weight and size at the time (see chapters 8 and 10 for details on resting metabolism and weight loss). A comparison of two individuals identical in weight, one with 10 pounds more muscle than the other, clearly shows that the resting metabolism is significantly higher in the more muscled individual. According to some experts, resting metabolism increases by approximately 30 to 40 calories per day for every pound of muscle weight added. In other words, you burn enough extra calories at rest to lose 3 to 4 pounds per year for every pound of muscle mass you add.

Experts are fairly certain that by age 60 the amount of body fat you possess is directly related to the amount of time you spend exercising. The more active you are, the leaner you will be at any age. Thus, training with weights is crucial for both men and women as they age. Even as few as two weight-training sessions per week can significantly improve muscle mass and bone health. When you engage in weight training three times per week, the number of calories needed to maintain your weight increases by about 15%. The ideal exercise program for the management of body weight and fat throughout life would include aerobic exercise three to four times per week and a half-hour strength-training session every other day, coupled with sound nutrition.

Improved Appearance, Body Image, and Self-Concept

Muscular strength and endurance training can improve your physical appearance. By reducing your caloric intake, losing body fat and weight, improving muscle tone, and adding muscle weight, you will look and feel better.

When you lose weight too rapidly, particularly without exercise, your skin gives the appearance of not fitting your body well. Sagging skin on the back of the arms, for example, is often an indication of weight loss that occurs too rapidly or in too large an amount. With reduced caloric intake, fat cells shrink, but the skin does not keep pace to provide a tight fit. One way to improve your appearance and help your skin fit better during and after weight loss is to include strength training as part of your total program. As fat cells shrink in the back of your arms, for example, strength training can enlarge the triceps muscle tissue and reduce sagging skin.

Keep in mind that these changes will not occur overnight. Depending on your age and current physical state, you may need 12 months or more of regular aerobic exercise, strength and endurance training, and dietary management of calories to decrease your total body fat significantly, add 5 to 10 pounds of muscle weight, tone your entire body, give your skin sufficient time to rebound to a tight fit, and adjust to your new body. These changes will alter both the way you perceive yourself and the way you feel others perceive you. Practically everyone who stays with a program experiences improved body image and self-concept that positively affects their personal and professional lives. But patience is necessary; proper nutrition and exercise, rather than diets, should be lifetime activities.

Increased Strength and Endurance for Work and Daily Activities

Each of the training programs discussed in this chapter will effectively increase both muscular strength and endurance in the relatively short period of 8 to 12 weeks. For example, if you are in the process of moving or helping a friend move, you will notice an improvement in your ability to lift furniture and other heavy objects without undue fatigue. Additional strength and endurance will also help you perform daily personal and work activities more efficiently and provide you with the extra strength needed to cope with unexpected emergencies in life.

Increased Bone-Mineral Content

Recent studies suggest that regular strength training aids in optimal bone development by improving bone-mineral content. The use of strength training in addition to weight-bearing exercise, such as walking, jogging, racket sports, and aerobic dance, may help women reach menopause with more bone-mineral mass, an important factor in the prevention or delay of osteoporosis (see chapter 10).

Heart Health

The American Heart Association (AHA) supports the value of weight training and indicates that it is also good for the heart. For healthy adults and some cardiac patients, the AHA says that weight training will not only increase muscle strength and endurance but also improve heart and lung function, enhance glucose metabolism, reduce coronary-disease risk factors, and boost well-being. When muscles are stronger, less demand is placed on the heart. More muscle also means a higher metabolic rate and less body fat. Although blood pressure rises during a workout, research indicates that weight training can reduce blood pressure by 3 points in resting systolic and diastolic blood pressure.

According to the American Institute of Cancer research, weight training also improves the ratio of LDL (bad cholesterol) to HDL (good cholesterol).

Other Health Benefits

Many health benefits are associated with musculoskeletal fitness, such as reduced cardiovascular risk factors, less low back pain, increased bone-mineral density, increased flexibility and balance, less tendency to develop osteoarthritis and obesity, lower risk of developing diabetes, geriatric vigor, and greater success in completion of activities of daily living. Resistance exercise training also helps reduce falls, bone fractures, and the need for institutional care among elderly individuals. Circuit training, which combines aerobics and resistance exercise, has been identified as a method of training that is effective in improving functional capacity, lean body mass, muscular strength, and glycemic control in older individuals with type 2 diabetes (Dunstan et al., 2002) and moderate-risk patients with coronary artery disease (Santa-Clara et al., 2002). Resistance training can enhance bone density, even among women aged 60 and over. The National

Kidney Foundation has approved resistance training as a safe method of increasing strength and functional capacity in some patients with renal disease (Headley et al., 2002).

Improved musculoskeletal fitness (developed through resistance training combined with stretching, for example) also decreases the severity of a number of debilitating conditions and physical disabilities. For example, recent studies have shown that older adults can make significant improvements in aerobic capacity by participating in resistance exercise programs. Sedentary older women have proved to be susceptible to eccentric exercise-induced muscle dysfunction, but resistance training reduces this susceptibility. Other scientific studies indicate that anaerobic capacity, enhanced by resistance exercise, is important in wheelchair propulsion among disabled athletes. Likewise, research has shown that resistance training improves motor ability in some individuals diagnosed as being in the earlier stages of Parkinson's disease (Reuter and Engelhardt, 2002). Recent studies also conclude that with physician approval, breast cancer survivors should be encouraged to participate in a resistance-training program. They caution, however, that women should wear a compression sleeve on the arm of the affected side when conducting upper-body exercises (Courneya, Mackey, and McKenzie, 2002). In studies of older adults experiencing chronic knee pain from osteoarthritis, increased muscular strength played a significant role in maintaining balance and slowing the decline in loss of mobility. As evidenced by these studies, maintaining musculoskeletal fitness can increase overall quality of life for individuals of all ages and levels of ability.

Benefits for College Men and Women

Strength training, particularly in its most popular form of weight training, has traditionally been a man's activity at all age levels. Unfortunately, boys, girls, and adult men and women of all ages are equally in need of this important aspect of a complete fitness program. Weight training should be a regular component of the exercise program of every male and female. As indicated previously, weight training will add muscle mass, improve appearance and self-concept, increase metabolism, improve sports performance, and prevent sports-related and work-related injuries. College-age women will receive the full benefits of a sound weight-training program including taking on a more healthy, feminine look.

Benefits for Young Boys and Girls

Studies continue to indicate that both girls and boys of elementary school age are extremely weak in the upper body and the abdominal area. A recent survey of 18,857 public school students at 187 schools revealed that 40% of boys ages 6 to 12 and 70% of girls in that age group could not do more than one pull-up, and 45% of boys ages 6 to 14 and 55% of girls in that age group could not hold their chins over a raised bar for more than 10 seconds. The Power Lifting Federation suggests that boys begin weight training at around age 14 and girls begin at a slightly younger age. Because every child is different, age is not a solid guide for determining physical and mental readiness. Parents should consult their physical education instructor, a professional trainer, or a physician for help in determining the physical maturity level and readiness for weight training. Preadolescent children who show no signs of developmental changes will benefit little from weight training and could injure joints and soft tissue. A regular calisthenics program that uses one's own body weight can effectively strengthen the upper body (shoulders, arms, and abdomen). For early adolescents or those age 14 and older, weight training should involve only light weight, high repetitions, short workouts of 30 minutes or less no more than three times weekly, and careful supervision at all times.

Benefits for the Elderly

For decades, studies have indicated the need for weight training among the elderly (65 to 90 years of age). A 2000 Johns Hopkins University School of Medicine study of people over 60, for example, uncovered the following physical limitations attributed to old age rather than a specific condition: 31% had trouble dressing, 25% had trouble walking half a mile, 16% had trouble cutting their toenails, 14% had trouble getting in and out of a car, and 14% had trouble climbing stairs. The Centers for Disease Control (September, 2001) studies the function of the noninstitutionalized elderly, 70 and older, in two areas: activities of daily living (ADL, the ability to perform essential daily tasks such as eating and bathing) and instrumental activities of daily living (IADL, more complex tasks such as cooking or cleaning). Findings revealed that 8.7% were unable to perform at least one ADL and 19.1% were unable to perform at least one IADL. The percentages increase among those 85 and older.

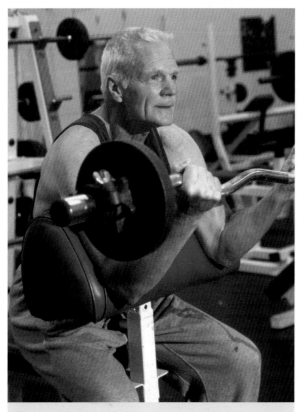

The need for weight training among people over 60 has long been known. Weight training is valuable for the elderly just as it is for younger adults.

Raw Talent

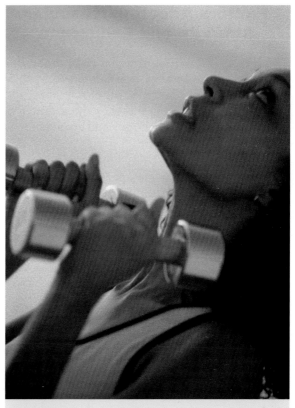

A common misconception is that women who weight train bulk up and lose their femininity. Well-planned weight training allows a woman to achieve a multitude of goals.

Eyewire

Improved Performance in Sports and Recreational Activities

Children and adults often lack strength and endurance in the upper body (arms and shoulders) and in the abdominal area. Many studies also show that most women are weak in the arms and shoulders because they think that strength training will cause a loss of femininity—an unfounded fear. Individualized, safe weight-training programs can be designed for both sexes at all ages. These programs will improve muscular strength and endurance in the upper body, abdomen, lower back, and other areas with little or no health risk or change in femininity. Increased upper-body and abdominal strength and endurance also help improve physical appearance and self-concept. Weight training helps children and young adults perform better in sports such as tumbling, gymnastics, baseball, basketball, field hockey, touch football, and soccer. You will also notice a difference when you participate in an aerobics exercise or dance class, a conditioning class, or your favorite recreational activity. The

tendon—The fibrous band that attaches some muscles to the bones so that they move when the muscles contract.

additional strength and endurance will delay fatigue and make free movement easier.

Decreased Incidence of Sports- and Work-Related Injuries

Improved muscle strength surrounding the joints helps prevent injuries to your muscles, **tendons,** and ligaments. With regular training, bones and connective tissue become stronger and denser. These changes make you less vulnerable to muscle strain, sprains, contusions, and tears (see chapter 13 for more details). Improved strength and flexibility in the abdominal and back extensor muscles can even prevent lower-back pain.

Strength training is also an important part of recovery following certain injuries. A return to normal range of motion and strength following soft-tissue injuries occurs more rapidly and completely with rehabilitative strength training.

Factors Affecting Muscular Strength and Endurance

The extent to which you develop muscular strength and endurance depends on individual muscle structure, the types of muscle fiber, and how well your training matches the manner in which muscles become larger and stronger.

Muscle Structure

A cross section of various parts of a muscle is shown in figure 7.1. Each muscle contains bundles of tissue composed of cells known as **muscle fibers.** A muscle fiber is composed of contractile units called **myofibrils.**

The entire muscle, consisting of the bundles and the muscle fibers, is covered and bound together by layers of connective tissue that blend together to form the tendon. When you contract your biceps, for example, the muscle shortens with the force moving through the tendon to the bones to bend the elbow.

Types of Muscle Fibers

The three types of muscle fibers contained in each muscle in the body can be classified by two

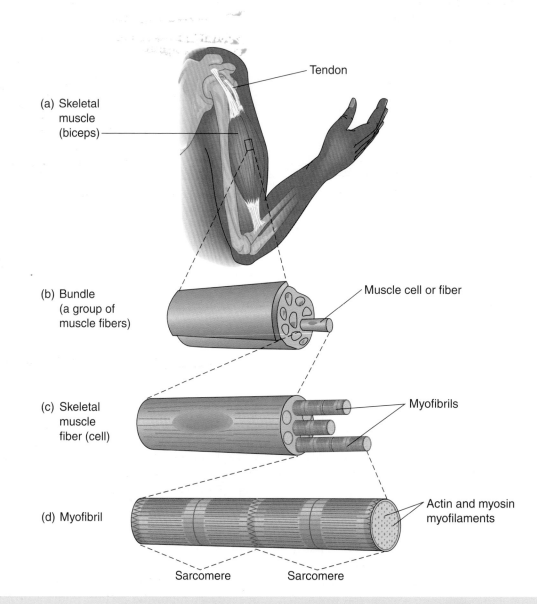

(a) Skeletal muscle (biceps)

Tendon

(b) Bundle (a group of muscle fibers)

Muscle cell or fiber

(c) Skeletal muscle fiber (cell)

Myofibrils

(d) Myofibril

Actin and myosin myofilaments

Sarcomere   Sarcomere

Figure 7.1 The structure of muscle. The whole muscle (a) is composed of separate bundles of individual muscle fibers (b). Each fiber is composed of numerous myofibrils (c), each of which contains thin protein filaments (d) arranged so that they can slide by one another to cause muscle shortening or lengthening. Various layers of connective tissue surround the muscle fibers, bundles, and whole muscles, which eventually bind together to form the tendon.

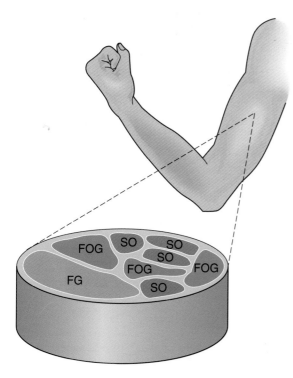

Figure 7.2 Muscle fiber types. SO is the slow-twitch, oxidative fiber; FOG is the fast-twitch, oxidative, glycolytic fiber; and FG is the fast-twitch, glycolytic fiber.

muscle fibers—Bundles of tissue composed of cells.

myofibrils—Thin protein filaments that interact and slide by one another during a muscle contraction.

slow-twitch, oxidative muscle fiber—Red muscle fiber used in aerobic activity that contracts and tires slowly.

fast-twitch, glycolytic muscle fiber—White muscle fiber used in anaerobic activity that contracts rapidly and explosively but tires quickly because it has a poor blood supply.

fast-twitch, oxidative, glycolytic muscle fiber—An intermediate fiber that can be used in both anaerobic and aerobic activity.

set—A group of repetitions for a particular exercise

repetitions—The number of times a specific exercise is completed.

factors: (1) the speed with which they contract and (2) their main energy system (see figure 7.2). **Slow-twitch, oxidative muscle fiber** is used primarily in aerobic endurance activities such as jogging, marathon running, and cycling. These fibers contract slowly but are slow to fatigue because of their tremendous vascular supply. **Fast-twitch, glycolytic muscle fiber** is used primarily for explosive anaerobic movements such as sprinting, jumping, and throwing. These fibers contract explosively and tire rapidly. **Fast-twitch, oxidative, glycolytic muscle fiber** contracts faster than slow-twitch, oxidative fiber but slower than fast-twitch, glycolytic fiber. Fatigue occurs much more slowly than it does with the fast-twitch, glycolytic fiber.

How Muscles Become Larger and Stronger

The capability of a muscle or muscle group to generate force for one maximum repetition depends on such factors as size, type, number of muscle fibers activated, and ability of the nervous systems to activate these fibers. Although genetics and the number and size of fast-twitch fibers limit your strength potential, everyone can improve strength with proper training. As training progresses, muscle cells will increase in size

(particularly the fast-twitch fibers), the myofibrils in each cell may increase in number, and the connective tissue around muscle fibers and bundles of muscle may also thicken. These three factors will significantly increase the size of a muscle in 8 to 10 weeks. Women generally progress at almost the same rate as men do, and they will experience significant increases in cell size after engaging in a sound weight-training program.

You can improve your muscular endurance by training both types of fast-twitch fibers by increasing the number of repetitions and by using lower weight. As training progresses, you will be capable of performing a greater number of repetitions for each exercise.

Strength-Training Principles

The training principles discussed in this section will help you design a program to meet your specific needs. First, consult table 7.1 and choose a primary training objective. This table allows you to approximate the weight and number of **sets** and **repetitions** needed to fit your training objectives. The following basic principles apply to any strength-training program:

- Using heavy weight and low repetitions (three to six) develops considerably more strength and muscle mass than endurance. Your starting weight for each exercise should be about 80% of your 1RM (maximum amount of weight you can lift one time). For example, if your maximum lift on the bench press is 100 pounds, your starting weight is 80 pounds (100 × .80).

TABLE 7.1—Weight-Training Objectives and Variable Control

Desired outcome	Intensity (weight)	Repetitions	Sets (volume)	Contraction speed	Rest (recovery)
Strength and endurance—general body development	40-80% 8RM	6-10	3	Moderate	2-3 min
Maximal strength	75-100% 3RM	3-8	5-10	Slow to explosive	1-4 min
Strength endurance	30-60% 15RM	15-30	3-6	Fast	3-5 min
Speed and strength	30-85% 6RM	1-3 (85%) 3-5 (80%) 5-8 (75%) 8-15 (70%)	3-7	Explosive, maximal	2-8 min
Rehabilitation from injury	20-60% 15RM	15-25	1-5	Slow, pain-free through full range of motion	3-5 min
Muscle mass, bulk	80-100% 5RM	1-10	5-15	Slow to moderate	1-3 min
Body sculpting*	10RM	10-12	3-5	Slow to moderate	1-3 min

*Use of large numbers of different exercises for each muscle group, progressing from a single exercise per muscle group, 10 to 12 repetitions, and two to three workouts weekly (standard program) to three to four exercises per muscle group, four to five sets of 10 to 12 repetitions, and a five- or six-day-per-week regimen (advanced program).

- The closer you work to the 1RM, the greater the strength gains. Unfortunately, the chance of injury increases with added weight, so this approach is somewhat impractical.
- Heavy weight, a moderate number of repetitions (three to five), and multiple sets are more effective in adding muscle weight (mass).
- Light weights and a high number of repetitions develop muscular endurance more than strength.
- From a health standpoint, using 6RM as the starting weight and progressing to nine repetitions is ideal for general body development and the improvement of muscular strength and endurance.
- Regardless of your training objective, you should be able to complete the final repetition in each set with perfect form.

Types of Training

The three most commonly used strength- and endurance-training methods are isotonics, **isokinetics,** and isometrics, each with a number of variations and each requiring special equipment. During an isotonic contraction, such as the execution of an arm curl with free weights or Universal or Nautilus machines, the muscle shortens (posi-

isokinetic—A type of dynamic (concentric) muscular contraction that occurs at a constant velocity through the range of motion as controlled by an ergometer.

positive phase of muscle contraction (concentric exercise)—The phase of exercise when the muscle shortens rather than lengthens during muscular tension; the upward phase, or the phase of an exercise when weight is being lifted.

negative phase of muscle contraction (eccentric exercise)—The phase of exercise when a muscle lengthens rather than shortens during muscular tension; the downward phase, or the phase of an exercise when weight is being lowered.

tive phase) as the lifter brings the weight toward the body and lengthens (**negative phase**) as the lifter returns the weight to the starting position. Inertia helps move the weight during the positive phase, and the lifter slowly lowers the weight under control during the negative phase. During an isokinetic arm curl with special equipment, the muscle also shortens and lengthens during the positive and negative phases, but maximal resistance is provided throughout the full range of movement in both phases. Without the benefit of inertia or gravity to allow a weight to drop, the routine would be considerably more difficult. In an isometric contraction, the exercised muscle contracts, but its overall length remains unchanged.

You perform isotonic contractions when you use free weights or Universal, Nautilus, Cam II, Polaris, and other similar equipment. New Life Cycle equipment has found a way to eliminate cheating and take full advantage of the negative phase of contraction. During the negative phase of each repetition, the weight automatically increases by 25%. This equipment makes it nearly impossible to drop the weight and cheat as you return to the starting position in the negative phase or to use inertia to help during the positive phase.

The Mini-Gym uses the isokinetic, or accommodating resistance, principle to overload the muscle group maximally through the entire range of motion. The harder you pull, the harder the Mini-Gym resists your pull. Because there is no negative phase, strength gains are not as rapid as they are with other equipment. Hydra Fitness and Eagle Performance systems combine the isotonic and isokinetic methods by automatically adjusting to the strength and speed of the individual.

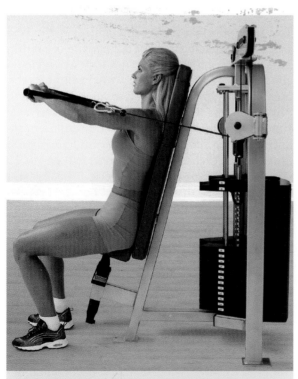

Many different types of equipment for the home and gym are available for people to customize strength and endurance training to find what works best for them.
Lifefitness

Isometric exercises are like weight-training movements in which the weight is so heavy that it cannot be moved. These exercises involve a steady muscle contraction against immovable resistance for 6 to 8 seconds such as pushing against a desk or a wall with both hands. Strength gains appear to be specific to the angle and do not transfer into increased strength throughout the full range of motion.

Calisthenics is the oldest form of weight training. Using the body as resistance, calisthenics are a safe, practical, and effective method of developing muscular strength and endurance. Because the resistance is low (body weight) and the individual must perform a high number of repetitions to bring about fatigue, calisthenics is more effective for developing muscular endurance than strength. Calisthenics is also an ideal, safe strength- and endurance-training method for preadolescent children.

Professional athletes and fitness experts prefer isotonic movements with free weights for the development of muscular strength and endurance, muscle mass, and speed. Special equipment that allows either isotonic or isokinetic movement is excellent for rehabilitating from injury, focusing on specific body areas, and improving general body development. This equipment is relatively safe, and the individual can perform movements without a spotter or partner.

Home-Fitness Equipment

The home-fitness strength equipment boom has continued into the new century. Unfortunately, a multitude of approaches and claims make it difficult for consumers to make wise choices. Rating each piece of strength-training equipment on the market today is nearly impossible, let alone keeping up with the new items that are constantly appearing. One way to increase your chances of making a sound choice is to answer each of the following questions before consulting a certified strength and conditioning coach at your college or university:

- What type of equipment is likely to help you best meet your training objectives? Do you favor isotonic workouts, isotonic and isokinetic methods combined, or machines that take full advantage of the negative phase of each exercise? If you have sufficient space and work out with others, you may want to consider free weights and some special bench and squat racks.

- How much do you want to spend? High-quality machines work more smoothly, make the workout more enjoyable, and are less likely to break down.
- How much space do you have for your workout area? You may need to choose equipment that folds up or takes up limited space.
- How safe is the equipment? You can safely use most home weight-training equipment without a spotter or partner.
- Does the item give you a complete strength-training workout? Some machines train only a few body areas, forcing exercisers to use free weights to supplement the machine.
- How much weight or resistance is available for each exercise? If you can almost move the maximum resistance provided for a given exercise, you are certain to need additional weight in the future as you progress. Some equipment items will not permit the use of additional weight, which forces you to add repetitions and possibly change your objectives. If you are primarily interested in adding muscle weight and strength, you need equipment that allows the addition of heavy weight.
- Do you like using the equipment? Before buying any item, take time to find a local fitness center, high school, or university that will allow you to complete a workout or two on the equipment. A 5-minute session in a store does not give you enough exposure to make a well-informed decision.
- What do others who possess this equipment say about the item? Ask the salesperson for names of a few people who have bought the item. Take the time to call and inquire. The information you learn may keep you from impulsively buying an inferior item.

After you have thought through these questions, you are ready to meet with an expert and make a decision. One thing is certain: You will not experience the amazing results shown in TV commercials and infomercials unless you become a dedicated user over a period of years and combine your hard work with proper nutrition and aerobic exercise.

Amount of Resistance (Weight) to Use

The weight with which you can perform a specific number of repetitions is called the RM (repetition maximum). The 9RM, then, is the amount of weight that would bring you to almost complete muscle failure on the ninth repetition—you could not perform even one additional repetition. After you decide on the range of repetitions for your training objective, your starting weight is the RM for the lower repetition (for example, with a six-to-nine cycle, your starting weight is 6RM).

Number of Repetitions to Complete

The number of consecutive times you perform each exercise is called repetitions. A high number (10 to 20) with lighter weights favors the development of endurance, whereas a low number (3 to 5) with heavier weights tends to favor strength development.

Number of Sets to Complete

One group of repetitions for a particular exercise is a set. Depending on your training objectives and the method of progression you select, three to five sets are recommended. You should perform sets consecutively for each exercise before moving on to another muscle group. To avoid excess muscle soreness and stiffness, beginners should start with one set and gradually work up to three over a period of 3 to 4 weeks.

Amount of Rest Between Sets

The time you take between each set is the **rest interval**. Muscle fibers will recover to within 50% of their capacity within 3 to 5 seconds and continue to near full recovery after about 2 minutes. In a program designed to increase strength only, the rest interval is less important and should approach 1 minute. For muscular endurance training, however, the rest interval should gradually decrease from 2 minutes to about 30 seconds over a 6- to 8-week period. Unless you slowly decrease the rest interval between repetitions or increase the number of repetitions, you will not improve muscular endurance.

Amount of Rest Between Workouts

For a total-body workout, you will receive the best results when you allow at least 48 hours of rest (alternate-day training) between workouts. With shorter rest periods, complete recovery does not occur, and you do not receive the full benefits of your workout. For split-body routines

rest interval—The amount of time taken between sets.

that emphasize the upper body one day and the lower body the next, you can train for 6 consecutive days before taking a day of rest. If too much time (4 or more days) elapses before the next workout, acquired strength and endurance gains begin to diminish.

Speed for Completing Exercises

For most training objectives, you should return the weight to the starting position (negative phase) at half the speed you used to complete the positive phase. For example, if you bench-pressed the weight overhead in 1 second, you should take 2 seconds to lower the weight. You should raise the weight slowly enough to eliminate the help of inertia in the positive phase and lower the weight under control to receive the full benefit of the negative phase. If you simply drop the weight in the negative phase of each exercise, you fail to exercise your muscles during half the workout and gain far less benefit.

Application of the Principle of Specificity

To gain strength and endurance in a particular muscle, muscle group, or movement, you must specifically train the muscle or muscles in a similar movement. To improve sprinting speed by increasing your strength and endurance, for example, you must identify the muscles involved in sprinting and choose isotonic exercises that strengthen those muscles in a movement similar to the sprinting action.

Application of the Overload Principle

Strength gains occur either by muscle fibers producing a stronger contraction or by recruitment of a higher proportion of the available fibers for the contraction. The overload principle improves strength both ways, providing you systematically and progressively increase the demands on the muscles over time and tax them beyond their accustomed levels. In other words, during each workout, your muscles must perform a higher volume of work than they did in the previous workout. You achieve this by increasing the amount of resistance (weight) on each exercise or the number of repetitions or sets.

Application of the Progressive Resistance Exercise (PRE) Principle

As training progresses and you grow stronger, you must continuously increase the amount of resistance (weight) if continued improvement is to occur. One way to apply the PRE principle is to choose your starting weight and the lower limit of repetitions for each exercise. If you are using three sets of six to nine repetitions, for example, you would perform six repetitions for each exercise on your first workout. In the second, third, and fourth workouts, you would complete seven, eight, and nine repetitions, respectively. Then you would add 5 pounds of weight to each upper-body exercise and 10 pounds to each lower-body exercise and return to performing three sets of six repetitions.

Each of the following methods has been effective in the development of muscular strength and endurance. To avoid boredom and help overcome plateaus (periods when improvement is slow or nonexistent), add variation to your program. A good approach is to alternate your program among these methods every 3 to 4 weeks.

Rest-Pause Method and the Set System

Numerous other methods of progression in weight training have been shown to be effective. The rest-pause method involves completing a single repetition at near maximal weight (1RM), resting for 1 to 2 minutes, completing a second repetition, resting again, and so on until the muscle is fatigued and cannot perform one additional repetition. The set system involves use of multiple sets (3 to 10) of about five to six repetitions for each exercise.

Burnout Method

The burnout method uses 75% of maximal weight for as many repetitions as possible. Without any rest interval, the lifter removes 10 pounds from the starting weight and performs another RM set. The lifter repeats the procedure until the muscle does not respond (burnout). Each designated muscle group goes through the same demanding process.

Supersets

Supersets involve the use of a set of exercises for one group of muscles followed immediately by a set for their antagonist. For example, one set of arm curls (biceps) is followed by a set of bench presses (triceps).

Pyramid System

The pyramid system is the most common method of increasing strength. Begin with light weights, multiple sets per exercise, and many repetitions.

Myth and Fact Sheet

Myth	Fact
1. Strength training will make you inflexible.	**1.** Strength training will actually improve your flexibility providing you go through the full range of motion on each exercise and stretch properly before and after each workout.
2. Strength training makes females unfeminine and masculine.	**2.** With three to four strength-training sessions per week, it is impossible to acquire large, bulky muscles. A program using a moderate number of repetitions and weight will improve your feminine appearance.
3. Strength training will convert your fat to muscle.	**3.** Fat (adipose) and muscles are separate tissue types. You cannot convert one to the other. When you burn more calories than you eat, fat cells shrink. Strength training causes muscle tissue to increase in size and helps your skin fit you better after weight loss.
4. Sit-ups are the best belly-flattening exercise.	**4.** Although exercises such as the abdominal curl and crunch are helpful in flattening the abdomen, decreasing your caloric intake has a greater effect. Reduced calories will shrink the fat cells in your abdominal area; the girth-control program described in this chapter will improve the muscular strength and endurance of your abdominal muscles. You must use both programs to obtain a flat abdomen.
5. If abdominal exercises do not hurt, they will not work.	**5.** You can improve your abdominal strength and endurance without pain. In fact, it is good advice to back off when a burning sensation occurs to prevent muscle soreness and injury.
6. Without steroids, it is next to impossible to add muscle mass.	**6.** You can safely add 1 to 2 pounds of muscle a month (up to a half pound per week) without steroids through weight training and sound nutrition.
7. Unlike men, women who engage in weight training progress very slowly.	**7.** The quality of muscle tissue and the ability to produce force are identical in men and women. When they use identical weight-training programs, women and men respond similarly.
8. Weight training is a good aerobic activity.	**8.** Typical weight-training programs have little or no effect on aerobic fitness. Circuit weight training involving 20- to 30-minute sessions, two to three sets, 15 to 22 repetitions, 12 different exercises, and limited rest intervals can enhance aerobic capacity by 5 to 8%, about half the effect of a conventional aerobics program.
9. Elderly men and women in their 60s, 70s, and 80s should avoid weight training.	**9.** Quite the contrary. Older individuals need weight training the most to prevent loss of muscle mass, prevent slowing of metabolism, and increase muscular strength and endurance to maintain independence and continue to do daily chores and enjoy life. Although the skeletal muscles of the elderly respond more slowly to strength training, you can add muscle mass and become stronger at any age. Without such a program you only become weaker.
10. Machines are better than free weights.	**10.** Both have advantages and disadvantages. Free weights can mimic many different sports movements and allow much more variation in exercises. Most machines involve a guided two-dimensional movement pattern that limits variation. Machines generally provide resistance at a single joint, so the exerciser develops only part of a motor skill. Unlike free weights, machines do not require the lifter to stabilize the load, a situation that is distinct from the demands of sports and other activities. On the other hand, compared with free weights, machines tend to be smoother, less dangerous, and more fun to use. Perhaps most important, using machines does not require a spotter.

After each set, increase the amount of weight and decrease the number of repetitions. One five-set routine may involve 100 (pounds) × 10 (repetitions), 110 × 8, 120 × 5, 130 × 5, and 140 × 3. Another might be 75 × 10, 125 × 8, 175 × 5, 225 × 3, and 275 × 2. The key is to increase the weight and decrease the repetitions progressively.

Double Pyramid System

In the double pyramid, you reach the top set before coming down and completing the other sets with less weight: 75 × 10, 95 × 8, 110 × 5, 140 × 3, 110 × 5, 95 × 8, 75 × 10.

Superslow Training

Superslow training involves completing each repetition at about one-third the normal speed. This method requires less weight because you cannot use the inertial effects of fast movement. Superslow training forces you to contract the muscles through their full range of motion, emphasizes the important negative phase (the return to the starting position) that you should do slowly, and reduces the chance of injury. This form of training does require slightly more discipline and time to complete a workout. If you are training to enhance sports performance, you should complete movements more rapidly on the positive phase (muscle-contracting phase). Few sports involve slow movements, and you must "train fast to be fast."

When to Expect Results

Just how fast you progress depends on your initial level of strength, your training habits, the intensity and length of your training program, and genetic factors that govern your potential for strength gains and the speed at which those gains occur. Strength gains of 8 to 50% have been reported. The fastest improvement occurs in individuals who have not engaged in weight training previously and whose programs involve large-muscle exercises, heavier weights, multiple sets, and more training sessions.

You should see significant strength gains after only 8 to 12 weeks of training. But be patient, because it will take approximately 12 months to change the general appearance of your body and add 10 to 12 pounds of muscle mass.

Signs of Overtraining

Those who notice a plateau or drop in performance over time may be experiencing the overtraining phenomenon. Overtraining is likely to occur when you train too aggressively, train too soon after being ill or injured, shorten the rest period between workouts, or simply fail to follow the guidelines presented in this chapter. The condition occurs because your body does not have adequate time to recuperate from one workout to another. Some of the signs of overtraining are extreme muscle soreness and stiffness following a workout, a gradual increase in soreness, loss of appetite, loss of weight, constipation or diarrhea, inability to complete a normal workout, and an unexplained drop in the amount of weight you can successfully lift in several exercises. If two or more of these symptoms develop, you should immediately reduce the intensity, frequency, and duration of your workouts. Short workouts with light weights twice per week for several weeks should give your body ample time to recover and allow you to resume your normal routine.

Maintenance of Strength and Endurance Gains

After you have acquired the level of muscular strength and endurance desired, one or two vigorous training sessions per week will maintain most of the improvement that has occurred.

Lifting Techniques

To avoid injury and obtain maximum benefits from each workout, observe the following techniques.

Warm-Up and Cool-Down

To warm up properly, perform 4 to 5 minutes of walking and light jogging to raise body temperature and then stretch for 6 to 8 minutes (see chapter 6). The first of three sets can serve as a light set with a high number of repetitions (15 to 20) and low weight (20RM) for most workouts. You will need additional warm-up sets if you are going to execute maximum lifts. Stronger athletes also seem to need more warm-up sets. When warming up before maximum-lift attempts, you should perform the first warm-up set with weights of 50 to 70% of the RM weight to be attempted, and the second set at 75 to 80%. If you are performing any of the Olympic lifts, you may need as many as 10 to 12 warm-up attempts before executing a maximum effort. A 4- to 5-minute stretching period at the close of your workout will help prevent muscle soreness and aid in improving your range of motion.

Full Range of Motion

For each exercise, you should move through the full range of motion without locking out the joint. For the arm curl, for example, you move the weight as close to the chest as possible on the positive phase before returning to the starting position, without locking the elbow joint. When you are lifting heavy arm or leg weights, you are much more likely to injure a joint that is fully extended at either the beginning or ending phase of the exercise.

Proper Breathing

One recommended breathing procedure is to breathe out during the working or exertion phase of the exercise and inhale during the relaxation phase. If you are taking several breaths during the execution of one repetition, you are breathing too quickly and inhaling and exhaling at the wrong time. You should also avoid the tendency to hold your breath throughout the exertion phase. When you fail to exhale, the flow of blood to your heart decreases, which in turn reduces blood flow to the brain and causes you to become dizzy and possibly to faint. Holding your breath is particularly dangerous when you are performing overhead exercises. For individuals with high blood pressure, proper breathing is essential during the completion of each repetition.

Sequence of Exercises

You should arrange exercises to prevent fatigue from limiting your lifting ability. One approach is to exercise the large-muscle groups before exercising the smaller muscles. If the smaller muscles that serve as connections between the resistance and the large-muscle groups fatigue prematurely, you will find it difficult to exhaust the large-muscle groups. For an effective workout, the abdominal muscles, used in most exercises to stabilize the rib cage, should remain relatively unfatigued until the latter phases of the session. A typical sequence that applies the concept of large to small is the following: (1) hips and lower back, (2) legs (quadriceps, hamstrings, calves), (3) torso (back, shoulders, chest), (4) arms (triceps, biceps, forearms), (5) abdominals, and (6) neck.

Form and Technique

Carefully following the specific form tips identified for each exercise in figure 7.3 is important. In addition, you can apply these general techniques to most exercises and equipment.

- Assume the basic stance by placing your feet slightly wider than shoulder-width apart with your feet parallel. Some lifters place the stronger leg back in a heel-toe alignment.
- Place your toes just under the bar in the starting phase of exercises in which the barbell is resting on the floor.
- Keep your back erect (unless it contains the muscle group being exercised) with your head up and your eyes looking straight ahead.
- Grasp the bar with your hands a shoulder-width apart using one of three grips:
  1. Overhand. Grasp the bar until your thumbs wrap around and meet your index fingers. You may place your thumbs next to your index fingers without wrapping your hand around the bar if you prefer.
  2. Underhand. Grasp the bar with your palms turned upward away from your body. Your fingers and thumbs are wrapped around the bar.
  3. Mixed grip. Combine the overhand and underhand grip, with each hand assuming one of the grips.
- Avoid leaning backward to assist your performance of a repetition.

Hints for weight-training exercises are provided in figure 7.3. These suggestions will help you prevent injury and improve the effectiveness of each exercise.

Progression

Regardless of the training method you follow, you can apply several important concepts to develop stronger and bigger muscles.

- Keep a training log. Tracking your workouts is the key to building strength and muscle. Recording the amount of weight lifted, number of sets and repetitions, and the rest interval allows you to systematically increase the load each workout. You can also multiply the amount of weight (pounds) you lift in each exercise by the number of times you lift it (repetitions). You then increase that number every workout by increasing the number of repetitions, completing more sets, or adding weight.

Bench press

Equipment: Barbell, bench rack, spotter
Movement: Using an overhand grip, slowly lower the bar to the chest, then press back to the starting position.
Hints: Bend knees at 90° and keep feet off the bench and the floor.
Muscle groups: Pectoralis major, anterior triceps, deltoid

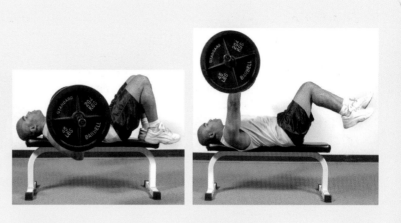

Incline bench press

Equipment: Incline bench, squat rack, spotter
Movement: Using an overhand grip, slowly raise and lower the bar to the chest (both feet flat on the floor).
Hints: Use a weight rack to support the weight above the bench. Avoid lifting the buttocks or arching the back while lifting.
Muscle groups: Anterior pectoralis major, anterior deltoid, triceps

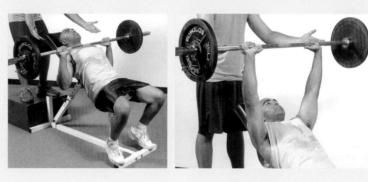

Power cleans

Equipment: Barbell
Movement: Using an overhand grip, pull the bar explosively to the highest point of your chest. Rotate hands under the bar and bend your knees. Straighten up to standing position. Bend the arms, legs, and hips to return the bar to the thighs, then slowly bend the knees and hips to lower to the floor.
Hints: Grasp the bar at shoulder width. Start with knees bent so that hips are knee-level. Keep head up and back straight.
Muscle groups: Trapezius, erector spinae, gluteus, quadriceps

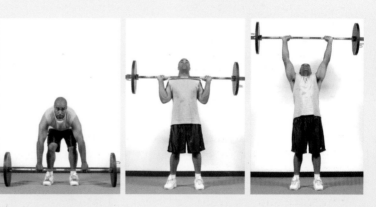

Dead lift

Equipment: Barbell
Movement: Using a mixed grip, bend knees so that hips are close to knee level. Straighten knees and hips to standing position. Bend at knees and hips to return.
Hints: Keep the head up and back flat. Grasp bar at shoulder width.
Muscle groups: Erector spinae, gluteus, quadriceps

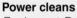
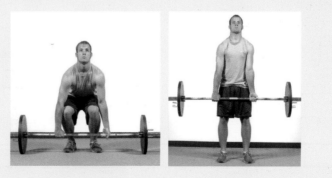

Figure 7.3 Barbell and dumbbell exercises.

(continued)

Bent arm flys

Equipment: Dumbbells
Movement: Using an underhand grip, hold a dumbbell in each hand above the shoulders with the elbows slightly bent.
Hint: Keep elbows slightly bent at all times.
Muscle group: Pectoralis major

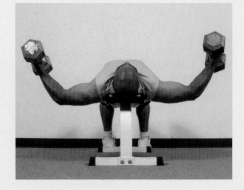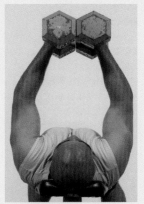

Barbell rowing

Equipment: Barbell
Movement: Using an overhand grip, hold the barbell directly below your shoulders. With elbows leading, pull the barbell to chest and hold momentarily. Then slowly return to the starting position.
Hints: Grasp bar slightly wider than shoulder width. Refrain from swinging or jerking the weights upward to the chest region.
Muscle groups: Latissimus dorsi, rhomboids, trapezius

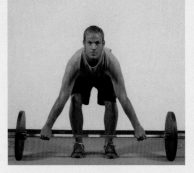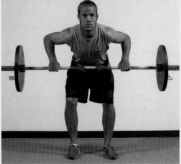

One dumbbell rowing

Equipment: Dumbbell
Movement: Using an underhand grip, kneel with one hand and one knee on exercise mat or bench. Pull the weight upward to chest.
Hint: Hold dumbbell briefly at chest before returning.
Muscle group: Latissimus dorsi

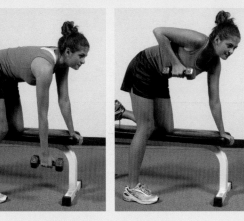

Shoulder shrug

Equipment: Barbell
Movement: Using an overhand grip, elevate both shoulders until they nearly touch the earlobes, then relax and return bar to the thighs.
Hint: Keep the extremities fully extended.
Muscle group: Trapezius

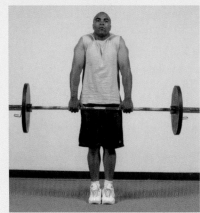

Figure 7.3 *(continued)*

Military press

Equipment: Barbell

Movement: Using an overhand grip, slowly push bar overhead from chest until both arms are fully extended.

Hints: Keep neck and back erect, and knees extended and locked. Avoid jerky movements and leaning.

Muscle groups: Deltoids, triceps

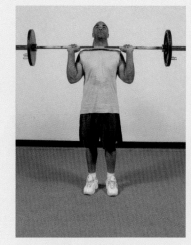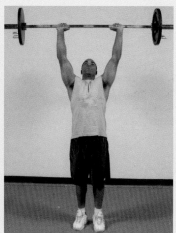

Upright rowing

Equipment: Barbell

Movement: Using an overhand grip, raise bar to the chin, and then return to thighs.

Hints: Grasp bar 15 to 20 centimeters apart. Keep elbows higher than the hands. Maintain an erect, stationary position.

Muscle group: Trapezius

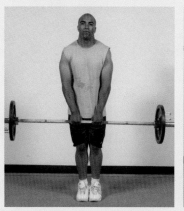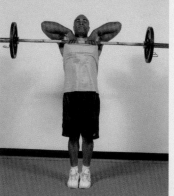

Bent-over lateral raise

Equipment: Dumbbells

Movement: Using an overhand grip, grasp dumbbell in each hand and draw arms to shoulder level. Slowly return to hanging position.

Hints: Keep knees and elbows slightly bent. Hold weights for 1-2 seconds before returning to hanging position.

Muscle groups: Posterior deltoids, latissimus dorsi, rhomboids

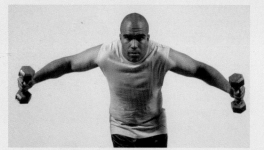

Two-arm curl

Equipment: Barbell

Movement: Using underhand grip, raise bar from thighs to chest level, and return.

Hint: Keep body erect and motionless throughout.

Muscle group: Elbow flexors

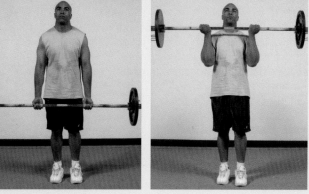

(continued)

Reverse curl

Equipment: Barbell
Movement: Using overhand grip, raise bar from thighs to chest level, and return.
Hint: Use less weight than used in two-arm curl.
Muscle groups: Upper arm flexors, hand extensors, finger extensors

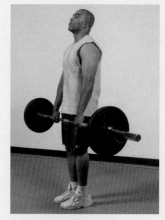 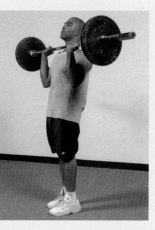

Seated dumbbell curl

Equipment: Dumbbells
Movement: Using an underhand grip, curl one or both dumbbells to the shoulder, then slowly return the weight to the sides of the body.
Hint: Keep the back straight throughout the movement.
Muscle group: Elbow flexors

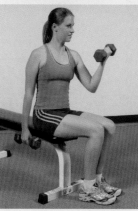

Close grip bench press

Equipment: Barbell, squat rack, spotter
Movement: Using an overhand grip, slowly lower the barbell to the chest and press back to the starting position.
Hints: Grasp center of bar (hands 2 to 4 inches apart). Bend knees at 90°; keep feet off the bench and the floor so as to avoid arching the back. Keep elbows in; extend arms fully.
Muscle groups: Triceps, anterior deltoids, pectoralis major

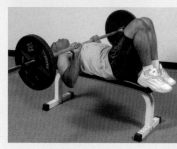 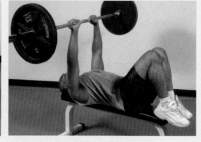

Standing or seated triceps

Equipment: Dumbbell
Movement: With both hands grasped around the inner side of one dumbbell overhead, lower the weight behind your head, then return.
Hint: Keep the elbows close together throughout the maneuver.
Muscle groups: Triceps, deltoids

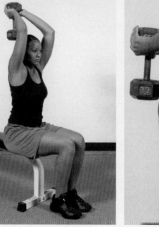 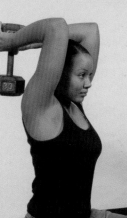

Figure 7.3   *(continued)*

Barbell wrist curl

Equipment: Barbell

Movement: Using an underhand grip, let the bar hang down toward the floor and then curl toward you.

Hints: Grasp center of bar (hands 2 to 4 inches apart). Keep forearms in steady contact with the bench while moving the weight.

Muscle group: Wrist flexors

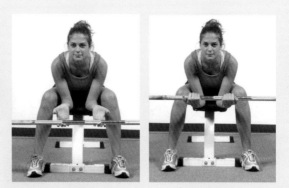

Reverse wrist curl

Equipment: Barbell

Movement: Using an overhand grip, and moving the wrists only, raise bar as high as possible, and return to the starting position.

Hints: Grasp barbell at shoulder width. Movement should only be at the wrist joint.

Muscle group: Forearm extensors

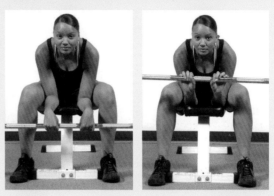

Front squat

Equipment: Barbell, squat rack, chair or bench, spotters

Movement: Using an overhand grip, flex legs to a 90° angle. Return to standing position.

Hints: Point the chin outward slightly. A chair or bench can be placed below the body (touch buttocks slightly to surface).

Muscle groups: Quadriceps, gluteals

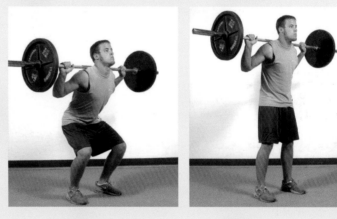

Lunge with dumbbells

Equipment: Dumbbells

Movement: Using an overhand grip, alternate stepping forward with each leg, bending the knee of the lead leg, and lowering the body until the thigh of the front leg is level to the floor. Barely touch the knee of the rear leg to the floor before returning to the starting position.

Hints: Keep your head up and upper body erect throughout the exercise. Avoid bending front knee more than 90°.

Muscle groups: Quadriceps, gluteals

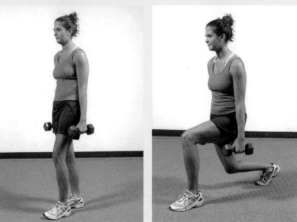

(continued)

Heel raise

Equipment: Barbell, squat rack, spotters, 2- to 3-inch board

Movement: Using an overhand grip, the body is raised upward to maximum height of the toes.

Hints: Alter the position of the toes from straight ahead to pointed in and out. Keep the body erect.

Muscle groups: Gastrocnemius, soleus

One dumbbell heel raise

Equipment: Dumbbell, 2- to 3-inch board

Movement: Using an overhand grip, shift entire body weight on the leg next to the dumbbell, and raise the foot off the floor behind. Raise the heel of the support foot upward as high as possible and hold momentarily.

Hint: A wall is useful for balance, but avoid using free hand for assistance.

Muscle groups: Gastrocnemius, soleus

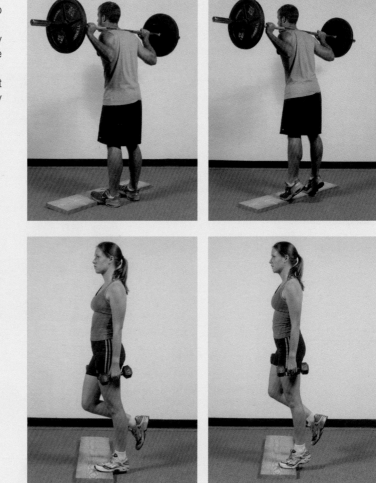

Figure 7.3   *(continued)*

Studies show that more than 70% of those who set goals and kept records stayed with their programs for a year compared with only 25% who kept no records.

- You do not have to exercise to complete muscle failure on the last repetition of each set. As muscles fatigue, they use fewer fast-twitch fibers, which have the greatest potential for size and strength gains. The solution is to use a weight that allows you to get through the final repetition. For body exercises such as a push-up, double the number of sets and decrease the repetitions by 50%. If you were doing three sets of 20 push-ups, change to six sets of 12 to 15.

- Change exercises every 4 to 6 weeks. Muscle strength and size improve faster when you periodically introduce new exercises and techniques. Switch to a completely new training approach every 8 to 12 weeks.

- Use mirrors to make certain that your form is correct.

- Avoid playing to your strengths by concentrating on those muscle groups that are already strong and large. A common imbalance, for example, is the ratio of quadriceps (front of thigh) to hamstring (back of thigh) strength.

Correcting the imbalance so that your hamstring muscles are at least 75 to 80% as strong as your quadriceps will reduce the chance of injury. You should also correct imbalances between the right and left side of the upper and lower extremities.

■ Never try to lift more weight than you can handle. Finding your new 1RM (amount of weight you can lift just one time) for each exercise should not occur more than two or three times per year. An injury associated with overlifting can set you back for months and even result in having to eliminate an important training program.

■ Be patient and stay with the program for a minimum of a year (3 to 4 workouts per week), or about 160 to 200 workouts.

Avoiding Injury

With proper supervision, injuries associated with improper lifting technique, horseplay, and using too much weight are uncommon. Observing the following precautions will reduce the danger of weight training:

■ Complete a general warm-up session that brings about perspiration before beginning your weight-training workout.

■ Perform one or two sets of shoulder and knee exercises with light weight before beginning your workout routine.

■ If you experience joint pain, do not try to train through it. Discontinue weight training and seek treatment.

■ Complete each repetition through the full range of motion with perfect form.

■ Use light weight for two or three sessions after a layoff of 2 weeks or more and when adding a new exercise.

■ Use maximal lifts sparingly—once or twice per year and only with proper supervision and spotting assistance.

■ Protect the knees at all times. Squat only to a 90-degree angle by placing a chair behind you to govern the depth of the bend. Avoid bouncing at the end of a squat.

■ Perform the Olympic lifts only with proper supervision and spotting.

■ Use a 10- to 12-minute static stretching session after each weight-training session.

■ Allow a minimum of 48 hours of rest after each workout unless you are completing upper-body exercises one day and lower-body exercises the next.

■ Secure collars and engage pins before attempting a lift.

■ Avoid holding your breath during the lift.

■ Return the barbell to the floor, rack, or starting position in a controlled manner.

■ Bend your knees when moving heavy weight from one place to another for storage.

Barbell and Dumbbell Exercises

Figure 7.3 shows specific exercises, describes the equipment needed, outlines the basic movement, gives helpful hints, and identifies the muscle groups involved in barbell and dumbbell exercises. This information will help you choose exercises that train the important muscle groups in your sport or activity. Table 7.2 includes some of the many barbell and dumbbell exercises and their variations for a basic resistance program designed to improve your strength, muscular endurance, and muscle size.

Girth Control

Almost everyone wants a flat tummy. A flat midsection is strongly associated with fitness and wellness in our society. A large belly can make people appear much older than they really are, and it also can be a sign of poor health—evidence of accumulating fat that may lead to hypertension, stroke, heart disease, adult-onset diabetes, and other ailments. Some fat around the midsection is not necessarily unhealthy. Practically everyone acquires at least a small spare tire (fat on both sides of the hips) and some abdominal fat. Becoming obsessed with this natural change is a mistake. As you reach the third and fourth decades of life, maintaining the flat midriff you had in your teens may be impossible.

Most people attempt to solve the girth-control problem by using unnatural and worthless devices such as girdles, corsets, weighted belts, rubberized workout suits, and special exercise equipment that promises a flat belly with just minutes of use daily. Although you will not find it easy, you can bring back some of the lost

TABLE 7.2—Basic and Alternative Weight-Training Programs for General Body Development

Exercises	Repetitions	Starting weight (RM)	Speed of contraction
BASIC PROGRAM			
Two-arm curl	6-10	8	Moderate
Military press	6-10	8	Moderate
Sit-up (bent knee)	25-50	30	Rapid
Rowing (upright)	6-10	8	Moderate
Bench press	6-10	8	Moderate
Squat	6-10	8	Rapid
Heel raise	15-25	20	Rapid
Deadlift (bent knee)	6-10	8	Rapid
ALTERNATIVE I			
Reverse curl	6-10	8	Moderate
Triceps press	6-10	8	Moderate
Sit-up (bent knee)	25-50	30	Rapid
Shoulder shrug	6-10	8	Moderate
Squat jump	15-25	20	Rapid
Knee flexor	6-10	8	Rapid
Knee extensor	6-10	8	Rapid
Pullover (bent arm)	6-10	8	Moderate
ALTERNATIVE II			
Wrist curl	6-10	8	Moderate
Side bender	6-10	8	Moderate
Lateral raise	6-10	8	Moderate
Straddle lift	6-10	8	Rapid
Supine leg lift	6-10	8	Rapid
Hip flexor	6-10	8	Rapid
Leg abductor	6-10	8	Rapid
Forward raise	6-10	8	Moderate

youth in your abdominal area by completing the program described in Discovery Activity 7.2: Obtaining a Flat, Healthy Abdomen at the end of this chapter.

Body Shaping (Sculpting)

Changing the shape of your body, or body sculpting, requires a 1- to 2-year commitment and the following steps and exercise programs:

- Engage in a sound, long-term caloric restriction program such as the 10-point program described in chapter 8 (page 222) to shrink fat cells in the back of the upper arms, abdomen, hips, waist, and thighs. Keep in mind that although you cannot change fatty tissue to muscle tissue, you can reduce the size of fat cells through a combination of diet and exercise.

- Continue your regular aerobic workouts three to four times weekly to maintain health, preserve cardiovascular fitness, and expend enough calories to put you in a calorie deficit of approximately 250 to 500 per day (1/2 to 1 pound of fat per week).

- Use the bodybuilding exercises described in the following section to add muscle mass and definition throughout your body and make your skin fit better in areas where you have shrunk fat cells (back of upper arms, thighs, hips, abdomen, and buttocks). A serious approach involves daily strength-training exercises, alternating from the upper body one day to the lower body the next and resting on Sunday.

- Although you cannot spot reduce (lose body fat only in areas exposed to exercise), you can concentrate on problem areas by completing multiple sets and five or six different exercises for each muscle group. Combining this approach with caloric restriction and shrinking of fat cells can result in greater definition.

- Plan to stay with the program for 2 years and remain patient for 5 to 6 months for noticeable results. You did not get in this shape in 6 months, and you cannot expect to reach your ultimate goal in the same short period.

Target Bodybuilding

Per A. Tesch (1999) used the state of the art technology of MRI (magnetic resonance imaging) to show in detail which muscles do the work in the most important arm and leg exercises performed by bodybuilders. His program trains all major muscle groups and involves 10 to 12 exercises and variations of exercises for each muscle group. These exercises and variations target each muscle within groups and all heads of the biceps (brachialas, lateral, medial); triceps (lateral, long, and medial); thigh (adductor brevis, adductor longus, adductor magnus, biceps femoris, gracilis, rectus femoris, sartorius, semitendinosus, vastus medialis, vastus lateralis, and vastus intermedius); and calf (soleus, medial gastrocnemius, lateral gastrocnemius, tibialis anterior, tibialis posterior, popliteus, extensor digitorum longus, and peroneus longus). By periodically altering specific exercises and their variations (grip position on the barbell, direction and movement of repetitions), the program targets each muscle to the fullest for complete development. Follow this procedure for each major body area.

- **Standard Program.** Single exercise (three sets of 10 to 12 repetitions) for each muscle group, two workouts weekly.

- **Intermediate Program.** Split routine, two to four exercises per muscle group (three to four sets of 10 to 12 repetitions). Various body parts are trained on alternate days, 3 to 4 days weekly.

- **Advanced Program.** Split routine, three to five exercises per muscle group (four to five sets of 10 to 12 repetitions) using a 5- to 6-day per-week regimen.

Beginning, intermediate, and advanced programs can be developed for each muscle group. For example, the thigh program trains all three major muscle groups (knee extensors, knee flexors, and the adductor muscles) using nine different exercises to increase muscle mass, develop definition, and change the contours of the body. Similar exercise prescriptions are available for the biceps and triceps, calf, and other body areas. In combination with a good aerobics program and calorie reduction, this program can change the contours of your body over a 1- to 2-year period.

Summary

Importance of Strength and Endurance Strength and endurance training provides health-related

Behavioral Change and Motivational Strategies

Several things may interfere with your strength-training progress. Here are some common barriers (roadblocks) and strategies for overcoming them and moving toward your training goals.

Roadblock	Behavioral Change Strategy
You are aware of your need to engage in strength training but just cannot seem to stay interested enough to avoid skipping workouts.	The first month of any exercise program is the most difficult. Muscle soreness, discomfort, and a body that looks the same can discourage you at this stage. Try some of these techniques to get through this critical period.

- Set a realistic goal for each exercise, such as increasing by 10 pounds the amount of weight you can move after 3 weeks.
- Measure and record the size of your upper arm, upper leg, and abdominal area. Make these notations in a journal.
- Avoid remeasuring yourself until you have added 10 pounds to most of the exercises in your program. You will meet this goal at your own pace, and when you do you will have acquired additional muscle mass.
- Use a more realistic approach to determining your progress than merely feeling various muscle groups and pinching fat to assure yourself of new firmness, more muscle, and less fat.

After 3 or 4 months of training, you seem to have leveled off or reached a plateau. Improvement is occurring so slowly that you are becoming discouraged and feel you have already improved as much as you can.	What you are experiencing happens to everyone. Initial gains in strength and endurance are always much greater than those you achieve months later. Consider some behavioral changes to help overcome this leveling off:

- Incorporate a fun day into your weekly schedule, preferably on the day you are most likely to skip. Use lighter weights, rest longer between sets and exercises, and enjoy yourself.
- Use social support by finding a partner or group of people at about your level to work out with, and encourage one another to put a strong effort in your remaining two workouts weekly.
- Incorporate a maximum lift day into your workout routine once every 12 weeks to demonstrate how you are progressing in each exercise. Use this session to reestablish your 1RM and record the results.

List other roadblocks you are experiencing that seem to be reducing the effectiveness of your strength-training program.	Now list the behavioral change strategies that can help you overcome the roadblocks you listed. If necessary, refer back to chapter 4 for behavioral change and motivational strategies.

1. _____

2. _____

3. _____

1. _____

2. _____

3. _____

benefits for people of all ages. Such training burns calories, adds muscle mass, prevents the slowing of metabolism with age, and helps control body weight and body fat throughout life. Over a period of 6 to 12 months of this training, your general physical appearance, body image, and self-concept will improve. Strength training also aids in the development of the skeletal system, improves bone-mineral content, adds muscle mass, enhances glucose metabolism, reduces coronary-disease risk factors, and helps manage lower back pain, diabetes, and geriatric fragility.

Strength and endurance also increase energy and productivity on the job and in recreational activities and reduce the incidence of sports- and work-related injuries. Finally, strength and endurance training plays a major role in the rehabilitation of soft-tissue injuries such as muscle strains, tears, and contusions.

Factors Affecting Muscular Strength and Endurance A muscle is composed of fibers and myofibrils bound together by layers of connective tissue. Fiber tissue is of three general types: slow-twitch, oxidative (aerobic) fiber; fast-twitch, oxidative, glycolytic fiber; and fast-twitch, glycolytic fiber. Strength training predominantly affects the fast-twitch fibers, whereas endurance training affects the slow-twitch fibers. Genetics and the number, size, and distribution of your fast- and slow-twitch fibers govern your strength and endurance potential. Everyone can increase muscle size, strength, and endurance with training.

Strength-Training Principles Three basic training methods are commonly used to develop strength and endurance: isotonics, isokinetics, and isometrics. In an isotonic or isokinetic contraction, the muscle shortens during the positive phase as weight is brought toward the body and lengthens in the negative phase as the weight is returned to the starting position. No muscle shortening occurs when force is applied to an immovable object (isometric contraction). Isotonic and isokinetic workouts are more beneficial to sports performance than isometric workouts are.

Altering Training Variables to Meet Specific Objectives By manipulating the number of sets, repetitions, rest intervals, and the speed of contraction, you can alter your programs to focus on strength, muscular endurance, general body development, muscle mass, speed and explosive power, or rehabilitation from injury.

Before buying home strength-training equipment, you should take time to determine your training objectives, analyze your available space and funds, try out the equipment, and consult with a strength and conditioning coach.

Lifting Techniques Sound lifting techniques with free weights or special equipment require careful warming up and cooling down with stretching, using the full range of motion on each repetition, breathing properly, using a partner or spotter, and paying attention to ideal form in each exercise.

Barbell and Dumbbell Exercises You can choose from a variety of exercises to focus on the major muscle groups of the body. One sound approach is first to identify the key muscles involved in the activity or those you want to train and then to select specific weight-training exercises that activate those muscles, preferably in a similar movement.

Girth Control To obtain a flat abdomen, you must restrict your daily calories enough to shrink the fat cells in the abdominal area and engage in a series of high-repetition abdominal exercises daily. You cannot change fatty tissue to muscle tissue, and muscle tissue will not change to fatty tissue when exercise ceases. Abdominal exercises alone will only improve the strength and endurance of your abdominal muscles; little or no change will take place in the size of your stomach unless you also restrict calories.

Body Shaping Proper use of the correct weight-training exercises and training principles can alter the way you look in a period of 1 to 2 years. Programs can add muscle and definition to all major muscle groups.

Discovery Activity 7.1

Finding Your 6RM for Each Exercise: Your First Weight-Training Workout

Name _____ **Date** _____

Instructions: Your first weight-training session focuses on mastery of the proper form for each exercise and finding the amount of weight you can lift a maximum of six times for each exercise.

- Ask an instructor to show you the proper form and technique for each exercise in the basic program in table 7.2. Use light weight and practice this form as an instructor observes your technique.

- Return to each exercise and find your 6RM. If you can bench-press 90 pounds just six times but not seven, you have a 6RM of 90 pounds. This is your starting weight for the bench press. Take your time and begin each exercise with a weight you know you can handle. If you complete six repetitions easily, rest 2 minutes, add 5 to 10 pounds, and again attempt to complete six repetitions. The first low estimate also serves as a warm-up procedure for each exercise. Continue this procedure until you find the weight that permits only six

repetitions. Record your starting weight in table 7.A. If you have a good idea of how much weight you can lift, begin with that amount. Rest 2 to 3 minutes and either add or remove weight before attempting the next set.

TABLE 7.A

Exercise	Repetitions	Starting weight
Two-arm curl	6-10	_____ (8RM)
Military press	6-10	_____ (8RM)
Rowing (upright)	6-10	_____ (8RM)
Bench press	6-10	_____ (8RM)
Squat	6-10	_____ (8RM)
Heel raise	15-25	_____ (15RM)
Deadlift (bent knee)	6-10	_____ (8RM)
Sit-ups (crunch)	25-50	_____ (25RM)*

*Hold a light weight of 5 to 11 lb with both hands behind the head.

From *Physical fitness and wellness, third edition,* by Jerrold S. Greenberg, George B. Dintiman, and Barbee Myers Oakes, 2004, Champaign, IL: Human Kinetics.

Discovery Activity 7.2
Obtaining a Flat, Healthy Abdomen

Name _____ **Date** _____

Instructions: Take a moment to measure and record the size of your waist. Now apply the pinch test or use skinfold calipers 1 inch to the right of your navel and on the left side of your hip to locate the excess fat. If you can pinch more than an inch in those areas, consider following the program described in this activity.

A girth-control program is designed to flatten your belly and improve the strength and endurance of your abdominal muscles. Two sound principles govern the program:

1. Consume fewer calories than you burn and remain in a negative caloric balance daily for a few months. Keep in mind that fat, or adipose, tissue and muscle tissue are different tissue types; you cannot transform one to the other, no matter what you do. Reducing caloric intake to produce a fat loss of 1 to 2 pounds per week (see chapter 8) will shrink the size of your fat cells in the abdominal area. Engaging in an aerobic exercise program three to four times per week will burn extra calories and allow consumption of sufficient nutrients and calories to spare protein, thus reducing the loss of lean-muscle tissue that occurs when you diet without exercise.

2. Supplement your dietary management with aerobic exercise (see chapter 5) and the six abdominal exercises described in this activity. For each exercise, work toward 50 repetitions daily. Begin with the maximum number you can perform in one set and add 2 to 5 repetitions each day until you reach 50. Complete these exercises daily and expect to train for 3 to 4 months before you notice significant results. Remember that these abdominal exercises only strengthen muscles that lie beneath the fat. Unless you reduce calories to shrink the fat cells, you will merely have firm abdominal muscles beneath the fat, with little reduction in the size of your stomach.

Lower Abdominals

- **Reverse curls.** Lie on the floor with your fingers locked behind your head and your knees bent. Contract your lower abs to curl your hips off the ground about 3 to 5 inches, bringing your knees toward your chest. Slowly return to the floor. Do not whip your legs; let the abs do the work. Remember to press your lower back into the floor throughout the exercise.

- **Knee tucks.** Lie on your back with your hands supporting your head. Tuck one knee to your chest and extend the other straight a few inches off the floor. Hold for two counts and switch legs. Some hip flexor work is involved, but keeping your low back pressed to the floor will work the lower abs isometrically.

Internal and External Obliques

- **Oblique twisters.** Lie on your back, bend your knees, and point both knees to the left. Extend your arms over your right hip. Slowly curl your shoulders and upper back off the floor to a half upright position. Reverse the curl to return to the floor. Repeat with the opposite side.

- **Twisting crunches.** Lie on your back with your knees bent and your ankles crossed and fixed. Contract your abdominals to lift your shoulders and upper back off the floor. Twist your trunk, bringing your left elbow to your right knee. Repeat to the opposite side.

(continued)

Discovery Activity 7.2 *(continued)*

Upper Abdominals

- **Crunches.** Lie on your back with your knees bent and feet flat on the floor. Your hands support your head. Look at the ceiling and contract your abs to lift your shoulders and upper back off the floor. Lift one knee and bring it in toward your elbow. Press your low back to the floor, hold briefly, and then return your leg to the floor.

- **Gravity fighters.** Start with your knees bent, feet flat, and body rounded to a position 45 degrees off the floor. Cross your arms over your chest and tuck your chin. Gradually lower your body until your shoulder blades touch the floor. Reverse the movement to the starting position.

From *Physical fitness and wellness, third edition,* by Jerrold S. Greenberg, George B. Dintiman, and Barbee Myers Oakes, 2004, Champaign, IL: Human Kinetics.

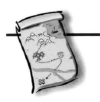

Discovery Activity 7.3

Service-Learning for Weight Training

Many communities conduct youth sports leagues—soccer leagues, basketball leagues, baseball leagues, or other organized sports leagues. Volunteers who coach and conduct these leagues, even those who are knowledgeable about the particular sport, often have limited knowledge of physical fitness. Weight training, although not traditionally a part of what is taught during these organized sport activities, can help participants become more proficient. You can offer to conduct a weight-training workshop for youth participants at the beginning of the sports season. Often, players and coaches participate in an orientation session before the season starts. This event would be a good time to introduce the availability of the weight-training workshop and to schedule sessions for the various teams or the league as a whole. Make sure to incorporate weight-training activities that are appropriate for the age group and specific to the sport in question.

From *Physical fitness and wellness, third edition,* by Jerrold S. Greenberg, George B. Dintiman, and Barbee Myers Oakes, 2004, Champaign, IL: Human Kinetics.

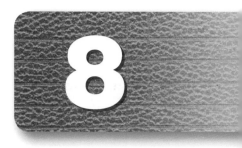

Body-Fat Loss and Weight Control

Chapter Objectives

By the end of this chapter, you should be able to

1. identify the major causes of obesity and overfatness in the United States;

2. evaluate and determine your ideal weight and percentage of body fat;

3. define overweight, overfat, and obesity;

4. describe a sound, long-term weight-loss program;

5. discuss the role of exercise in weight and fat management;

6. differentiate between anorexia nervosa and bulimia; and

7. identify the key behaviors linked to weight and fat loss and describe how to use several behavior-modification techniques to achieve your desired weight.

Susan has always been preoccupied with her weight. As far back as she can remember, she was too fat. For years she considered it purely a genetic problem. After all, her father is obese, and her mother is stocky. She thinks that perhaps the cards are stacked against her. As an adult she has tried every diet described in *Good Housekeeping* and *Redbook* or that appeared on the bestseller list. Perhaps she can't do anything about it. According to the literature, diets don't work, and she hates to exercise. Why diet for a lifetime when you need to lose only 8 to 10 pounds?

Is there any hope for women and men like Susan? This chapter provides the answers to these and other questions about weight control.

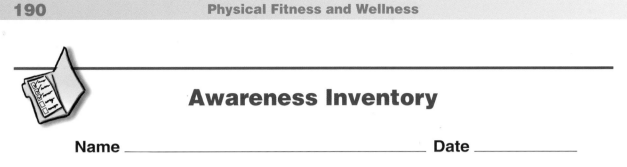

Awareness Inventory

Name _____ **Date** _____

Check the space by the letter T for the statements that you think are true and the space by the letter F for the statements that you think are false. The answers appear following the list of statements. This chapter will present information to clarify these statements for you. As you read the chapter, look for explanations for the reasons why the statements are true or false.

T___ F___ 1. The upward spiral of weight gain that has occurred in the United States for the past 20 years has now reversed for college students.

T___ F___ 2. Obesity places individuals at higher risk of developing hypertension, heart disease, gallbladder stones, and various cancers.

T___ F___ 3. Calories burned at rest (basal metabolism) account for less than 40% of the calories expended over a 24-hour period.

T___ F___ 4. Individuals are considered obese if they have more than 23% (men) or 28% (women) body fat.

T___ F___ 5. Bulimia is more common than anorexia nervosa and occurs in males and females.

T___ F___ 6. Research shows that regular exercise and calorie restriction shrink the stomach and produce a feeling of fullness with less food after 3 to 4 months.

T___ F___ 7. Strength training that increases muscle mass will also increase basal metabolism, burning more calories at rest with each pound of muscle added.

T___ F___ 8. Because snacking between meals is a major cause of weight and fat gain, the best approach for most college students is to eliminate snacking altogether.

T___ F___ 9. Skipping either breakfast or the noon meal three or four times per week is an effective approach to body weight and fat loss.

T___ F___ 10. Cellulite is recognized by the medical profession as a special form of fat that diet and exercise can completely eliminate.

Answers: 1-F, 2-T, 3-F, 4-T, 5-T, 6-T, 7-T, 8-F, 9-F, 10-F

From *Physical fitness and wellness, third edition*, by Jerrold S. Greenberg, George B. Dintiman, and Barbee Myers Oakes, 2004, Champaign, IL: Human Kinetics.

Analyze Yourself

Assessing Your Body Weight and Fat-Loss Behavior

Name _____ **Date** _____

Instructions: Indicate how often each of the following occurs in your daily activities and exercise sessions. Respond to each item with a number from 0 to 3, using the following scale:

0 = Never   **1** = Occasionally   **2** = Most of the time   **3** = Always

____ **1.** I use skinfold measures or hydrostatic (underwater) weighing as my primary method of determining whether I am overfat.

____ **2.** I avoid skipping a meal even if I only have time to consume some raw fruits or vegetables on the run.

____ **3.** I drink a minimum of six glasses of water each day.

____ **4.** I take special care to consume the correct amount of protein daily.

____ **5.** I avoid all fad diets and rarely fast or use other attempts to attain quick weight loss.

____ **6.** I avoid binge eating and never use any form of purging such as self-induced vomiting or laxatives.

____ **7.** I avoid use of weight-loss pills to depress appetite or eliminate fluid (diuretics).

____ **8.** I buy low-fat foods and request low-fat products when eating out.

____ **9.** I engage in an aerobic exercise program three to four times weekly and strength training two to three times weekly.

____ **10.** I confine my between-meal snacking to low-calorie fruits and vegetables.

Scoring: Excellent = 25-30

Good = 19-24

Poor = Below 19

Trends in Body-Fat Loss and Weight Control

During the late 19th century in the United States, human muscle power provided 33% of the energy needed to run farms, homes, and factories. Today, muscular effort contributes less than 1% of the energy. Most people in the United States work in office-bound, service-oriented jobs and use machines, computers, and pens and pencils to accomplish their tasks. The jobs we do and the types of energy needed for those jobs have changed over the past 100 years. The human body has remained the same, however, as we became victims of a technology-oriented lifestyle.

As a result, adult **obesity** in the United States has risen at an epidemic rate during the past 20 years. Although one of the national health objectives for the year 2010 is to reduce the prevalence of obesity among adults to less than 15%, studies indicate that the situation is worsening rather than improving. Table 8.1 shows this alarming trend from 1991 through 2000 by category: age, race, ethnicity, educational level, and smoking status. In every area, the percentage of obese individuals increased each year. In the year 2000, the prevalence of obesity among U.S. adults was 19.8%, a total that reflects a 61% increase since 1991. Results of the National Health and Nutrition Examination Survey (NHANES) in 1999 indicate that an estimated 61% of U.S. adults are **overweight,** defined as having a body-mass index (BMI) of 25 or more. A total of 38.8 million American adults met the classification for obesity, defined as having a body-mass index score of 30 or more. That figure represents an estimated 19.6 million men, 19.2 million women, and increases in obesity rates in nearly every subgroup of the U.S. population.

The news on the prevalence of overweight among children and adolescence is no better. Initial results of the 1999 National Health and Nutrition Examination Survey (NHANES), using measured heights and weights, reveal that approximately 13% of children ages 6 through 11 and 14% of adolescents ages 12 through 19 are overweight, representing a 2 to 3% increase in the percentages identified in data from a 1988-94 study. Data on overfatness and obesity using the percentage of body fat rather than weight charts or the BMI reveal similar findings.

The increased number of overfat children will result in significantly more overfat adults in the future. With each passing decade, the typical U.S.

> **obesity**—An excessively high amount of body fat or adipose tissue in relation to lean body mass.
>
> **overweight**—Increased body weight in relation to height when compared with some standard of acceptable or desirable weight.

adult accumulates additional excess fat and loses some lean-muscle tissue until by middle age over 50% of adult men and women in the United States are overfat or obese.

At all ages, we are growing several pounds heavier each decade. Although our average height is also increasing, most of this weight gain is fat, not muscle.

The trend must be brought under control because overweight conditions and obesity are associated with numerous disorders and early death. According to Stunkard (1993; NIH, 1998a) overweight and obese individuals (BMI of 25 and above) are at increased risk for

- high blood pressure and hypertension,
- high blood cholesterol and dyslipidemia,
- type 2 (non-insulin-dependent) diabetes,
- insulin resistance and glucose intolerance,
- hyperinsulinemia,
- coronary heart disease,
- angina pectoris,
- congestive heart failure,
- stroke,
- gallstones,
- cholescystitis and cholelithiasis,
- gout,
- osteoarthritis,
- obstructive sleep apnea and respiratory problems,
- some types of cancer (such as endometrial, breast, prostate, and colon),
- complications of pregnancy,
- poor female reproductive health (such as menstrual irregularities, infertility, irregular ovulation),
- bladder control problems (such as stress incontinence),
- uric acid nephrolithiasis, and
- psychological disorders (such as depression, eating disorders, distorted body image, and low self-esteem).

The greater the degree of obesity, the more likely and the more serious the preceding health prob-

TABLE 8.1—Prevalence of Obesity Among U.S. Adults, by Characteristics: Behavioral Risk Factor Surveillance System (1991-2001), Self-Reported Data

Characteristics	BRFSS data by year					
	1991	1995	1998	1999	2000	2001
PERCENTAGE OBESE						
Total	12.0	15.3	17.9	18.9	19.8	20.9
GENDER						
Men	11.7	15.6	17.7	19.1	20.2	21.0
Women	12.2	15.0	18.1	18.6	19.4	20.8
AGE GROUPS						
18-29	7.1	10.1	12.1	12.1	13.5	14.0
30-39	11.3	14.4	16.9	18.6	20.2	20.5
40-49	15.8	17.9	21.2	22.4	22.9	24.7
50-59	16.1	21.6	23.8	24.2	25.6	26.1
60-69	14.7	19.4	21.3	22.3	22.9	25.3
≥70	11.4	12.1	14.6	16.1	15.5	17.1
RACE, ETHNICITY						
White, non-Hispanic	11.3	14.5	16.6	17.7	18.5	19.6
Black, non-Hispanic	19.3	22.6	26.9	27.3	29.3	31.1
Hispanic	11.6	16.8	20.8	21.5	23.4	23.7
Other	7.3	9.6	11.9	12.4	12.0	15.7
EDUCATIONAL LEVEL						
Less than high school	16.5	20.1	24.1	25.3	26.1	27.4
High school degree	13.3	16.7	19.4	20.6	21.7	23.2
Some college	10.7	15.1	17.8	18.1	19.5	21.0
College or above	8.0	11.0	13.1	14.3	15.2	15.7
SMOKING STATUS						
Never smoked	12.0	15.2	17.9	19.0	19.9	20.9
Ex-smoker	14.0	17.9	20.9	21.5	22.7	23.9
Current smoker	9.9	12.3	14.8	15.7	16.3	17.8

From CDC Behavioral Risk Factor Surveillance System (BRFSS).

lems become. In addition, poor nutrition and physical inactivity account for some 300,000 premature deaths in the United States each year.

The death rate for obese men ages 15 to 69 is 50% higher than that of normal-weight persons and 30% higher than that of people classified as merely overweight. Estimates are that every 10%

increment above normal weight reduces life span by 1 year. Moreover, the quality of life declines dramatically in obese individuals.

This chapter examines the critical aspects of weight control: causes of obesity, assessment, safe weight-loss methods, the role of exercise in weight and fat management, underweight and eating disorders, and the role of behavior-modification techniques in helping young people manage body weight and fat during the late teenage and early adult years.

Causes of Obesity

According to the Centers for Disease Control (CDC), numerous factors influence overweight and obesity, including the following:

Behavior—eating too many calories while not getting enough physical activity will lead to overweight or obesity.

Environment—home, work, school, or community can provide barriers to or opportunities for an active lifestyle.

Genetics—heredity plays a large role in determining how susceptible people are to overweight and obesity. Genes also influence how the body burns calories for energy or stores fat.

The CDC also indicated that behavioral and environmental factors are the main contributors to overweight and obesity and provide the greatest opportunities for prevention and treatment.

Inactivity and overeating are clearly two major causes of obesity and overfatness. Studies show that children are spending more time watching TV, using computers, and playing video games. The proximity and availability of food and the limited time devoted to free play and exercise are producing a nation of overfat and obese youth, who will eventually become overfat and obese adults. The problem is complex. Researchers have identified many additional factors that play a role in both the prevention and treatment of obesity, such as those discussed in the following sections.

Early Eating Patterns

Most experts agree that the eating habits formed in infancy and childhood carry over into the adult years. Rats exposed to unlimited milk, for example, continue to eat more and exercise less after they are weaned than rats that receive only limited milk. In other words, rats that are overfed

before weaning become sedentary adult rats that overeat, become fat, and suffer from early cardiorespiratory disease. In contrast, rats that eat less before weaning continue to eat less, exercise more, live longer, and experience less cardiorespiratory disease. The response in humans is similar. Children who are inactive and who overeat are also more likely to continue those behaviors later in life and become overfat adults.

Environmental forces appear to influence eating patterns more than physiological forces such as hunger do. Negative eating behavior may begin in infancy. Some experts feel that bottle feeding, for example, may predispose infants to obesity. Bottle-fed babies are approximately three times more likely to be overfat than breast-fed babies are. Bottle feeding fails to provide the solace of breast feeding and tends to produce anxiety, which may provoke overeating. Breast-

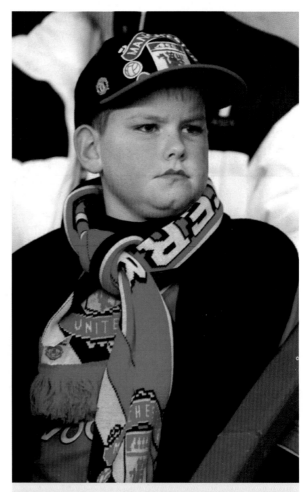

Overweight children are likely to grow into overweight adults.

Empics

fed babies also learn to stop feeding when the richest portion of the milk gives way to more watery milk. The bottle does not provide this natural mechanism, so bottle-fed babies require more calories to satisfy their hunger.

Perhaps a more important problem is feeding babies solid foods too early, which may contribute to the production of excess fat cells. Experts recommend that parents start feeding their infants solid foods at the age of 5 months rather than earlier, except for cases of very large or fast-developing babies. Following this recommendation is not easy for sleep-deprived mothers who long for the day the baby sleeps through the night without waking for a feeding.

Growing children are unlikely to be obese if they themselves decide when to stop eating at a meal. Forcing children to clean the plate is a mistake. This practice forces them to overeat. Making sweets plentiful, using them as rewards, and celebrating the fat baby compound the problem, shorten the life span, encourage premature heart disease, create undesirable eating habits, and destine the child to a life of restricted eating because of the high number of fat cells formed in early life. A lean child with a great deal of energy and vitality is healthier and more likely to be healthy later in life.

At no stage in life is excess fat desirable; however, the earlier in life a child is obese, the greater the chance that the child will eventually be of normal weight. The later in life a child is obese, the less likely it is that he or she will ever return to normal weight. An obese adolescent, for example, has approximately a 1 in 16 chance of returning to normal weight as an adult. The fatter a person is at any age, the less likely it is that he or she will ever return to normal weight. Parents should therefore start children off right and avoid overfeeding them. If children's mechanism for pushing up from the table when they are full is undermined, they are certain to need plenty of real push-ups in their adult years to control weight.

Fat Cells

Our fat cells form early in life and increase in both size and number until the end of adolescence. Calorie restriction will decrease only the size of fat cells, not the number. With a large number of fat cells formed, a return to an overfat condition is easy. This circumstance partially explains why adults who were fat babies often have difficulty keeping their weight down. These extra adipose

hypertrophy—The enlargement of existing fat cells.

hyperplasia—New fat-cell formation.

cells also affect metabolism and result in the need for fewer calories to maintain normal weight than are needed by someone who generally remains at normal weight. Unlike muscle, fat requires little energy to maintain, and additional fat weight will not increase metabolic rate.

The number of fat cells in the human body grows rapidly during three stages of development: (1) the last trimester of pregnancy (in the unborn child), (2) the first year of life, and (3) the adolescent growth spurt. Children acquire fat by an increase in the size of existing adipose cells (**hypertrophy**) and by new fat-cell formation before adulthood (**hyperplasia**). New fat cells are unlikely to form after age 21 (approximately) unless someone becomes extremely obese.

The number of fat cells present in people varies widely. A nonobese person has approximately 25 to 30 billion fat cells, whereas an extremely obese person may have as many as 260 billion. A formerly obese adult may never be cured because weight loss does not reduce the number of existing cells; it only reduces their size.

Fat is the primary energy reserve of the body. The natural distribution and amount of fat varies considerably between men and women. Some experts identify the appropriate body fatness in women as 20 to 27% compared with 12 to 15% in men. Achieving a body-fat level below the level of essential fat represents no health advantage for either sex and may be detrimental to health.

Weight and fat management is a more difficult task for women than it is for men because about 12% of fat in women is essential fat (as opposed to 4 to 7% in men), which includes an extra 5 to 9% of sex-specific fat in the breasts, pelvic region, and thighs. The childbearing role and the fact that women generally have smaller bodies requiring fewer calories also make it more difficult for a woman to lose fat and weight than for a man.

Fat accumulates in different sites on men and women. In general, men tend to have fat receptors in the abdominal area and fat inhibitors in the buttocks, hips, and upper legs. This partially explains why most men develop a beer belly and rarely accumulate fat in other areas. Women tend to have fat receptors in the hips, buttocks, and thighs and often have fat inhibitors in the abdomen. Various patterns of obesity exist in both sexes, with most obese individuals distributing fat throughout the body. Android (excessive fat in the lower body) and gynoid (excessive fat in the abdomen) obesity may occur in both men and women. Researchers have examined the so-called pear shape (fat accumulation in the hips and lower body common in women) and apple shape (fat accumulation in the abdominal area common in men). The apple shape with large fat accumulation around the midsection and chest may impose greater risk for heart disease than does the pear shape.

Because most women need significantly fewer calories to maintain their lower body weight, they find it more difficult to achieve a large negative calorie balance daily and lose weight rapidly. A 120-pound woman may need only 1,800 calories daily, for example. A 1,000-calorie deduction leaves only 800 calories to obtain adequate nourishment and energy—a nearly impossible task. A 200-pound man, however, may require as much as 3,000 calories daily to maintain weight. A 1,000-calorie daily deficit still leaves a total of 2,000 calories—enough for sufficient nourishment and energy.

We must all become more tolerant of our bodies and accept the fact that our percentage of body fat will increase slightly with age and that aging will alter the shape and appearance of our bodies regardless of our best exercise and eating efforts. Overemphasis on thinness and a youthful body is dangerous for both sexes and often leads to self-concept problems and serious eating disorders.

Genetics

The genes we inherit influence our body weight and the amount and disposition of fat. Children of overfat or obese parents, particularly the biological mother, are much more likely to develop weight problems. Twin studies also support the influence of genetics on overfatness and obesity. Heredity may link to weight and fat problems in a number of other ways, such as predisposition to consuming sweet, high-fat foods; impaired hormonal functions (insulin and cortisol); lower basal metabolic rate; differences in calories used during the metabolism of food; inability of nutrients to suppress the appetite control center; differences in the ability to store fat and burn calories during light exercise; and the tendency to develop more fat cells.

Ongoing research on the presence of a so-called fat gene and the development of drugs to control hunger permanently offer hope for overweight individuals in the future. Keep in mind, however, that environment is still critical. Genetics merely predispose individuals or provide them with the tendency to become fat—a problem that regular exercise and proper nutrition can help overcome.

Role of the Stomach

Scientists have been trying to determine why it is so much easier for most people to lose weight than it is to keep it off. New evidence suggests that it is the stomach, rather than the brain, that causes people to eat more and regain lost weight. Levels of the appetite-boosting hormone ghrelin, secreted by the stomach, rise significantly in dieters after they lose weight and drop in those who have undergone stomach-reducing procedures such as gastric bypass. Although cells in the small intestine produce small amounts of ghrelin, the stomach manufactures most of the hormone. The more weight dieters lose, the higher their level of ghrelin. Levels of ghrelin are also higher just before dieters lose weight. We have known for years that the hypothalamus gland controls food intake and that messengers from the brain activate it. Ghrelin is the first hormone from outside the brain that is known to affect the hypothalamus. Ghrelin peaks before each meal and falls afterward. Ghrelin not only boosts appetite but also acts on other tissues to slow metabolism and reduce fat burning.

Researchers feel that a drug capable of blocking the action of ghrelin would help people both lose weight and keep it off. The hormone may also provide help in gaining weight to those who have lost excessive amounts because of cancer, AIDS, anorexia nervosa, bulimia, or other conditions.

Metabolic Factors

Even small changes in metabolic rate translate into large increases in body fat and weight. A 10% decline in metabolism, for example, could result in an annual weight gain of about 15 pounds for the average individual. Aerobic exercise increases metabolic rate both during and after the exercise session. The afterburn continues for 20 minutes to several hours, depending on the duration and intensity of the workout. Coffee, tea, cocoa, colas, other caffeine-containing foods and drinks, and amphetamines and other drugs increase metabolic rate. In midafternoon, metabolism tends to slow, making this an excellent time to perform aerobic exercise that will boost metabolic rate.

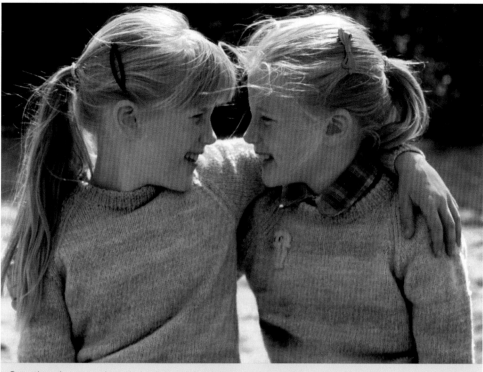

Genetics plays a major role in determining body weight and fat.

Jim Whitmer Photography

As one ages, metabolism also slows; by age 50, metabolic rate may have decreased by as much as 15 to 25% in a sedentary individual. In those who have remained active through a combination of aerobic exercise and strength training, metabolic rate slows only slightly. Loss of muscle mass is one of the leading causes of reduced metabolic rate with aging.

Viruses and Obesity

Studies show that 20 to 30% of overweight humans are infected with adenovirus-36, compared with 5% of the lean population. Mice and chickens infected with a common human virus put on much more fat than uninfected animals do. The same virus is more prevalent in overweight humans. Researcher Nikil Dhurandhar, MD, believes that the virus also increases the number of fat cells, which encourages animals and humans to store more fat. Clearly, viruses do not cause all obesity. The connection, however, is another of many health conditions, such as ulcers, that have recently been found to be caused by infections. We need more evidence before these findings can provide any practical benefits in the prevention and treatment of overweight conditions and obesity.

Environmental Factors

Although heredity plays an important role, environment is also critical. Sound exercise and eating and drinking habits can overcome the genetic tendency to be either thin or fat.

One of the clearer causes of obesity and overfatness in children is watching television. People on television programs eat about eight times per hour, and commercials generally advertise high-calorie, high-fat foods. Television watchers notice these cues and tend to eat more often and consume more high-fat, high-calorie foods. In addition, television watching is a passive activity. Almost any activity will burn more calories than watching television does. Although restricting the number of television-watching hours for all children and teenagers is a good idea, it is critical to do so for the overfat child.

Other environmental influences, such as eating and exercise habits of parents, food availability, and nutritional knowledge, may not be as important as was once believed. Experts feel that genetic influences account for about 70% of the differences in body-mass index (BMI) that occur later in life and that childhood environment has less influence than was once thought. Still, the environment has an influence on obesity. Nongenetic factors are important determinants of body fat. These factors are reversible and capable of overcoming some of the genetic factors that make us fat.

Set-Point Theory

The human body regulates its functions with tremendous precision. Body weight is one of those functions. Each individual appears to have an ideal biological weight, or set point, and will defend it against pressure to change. Those who succeed in losing or gaining weight generally return to their set-point weight in a few months or years. Within 24 hours of beginning a very low calorie diet, for example, the dieter's metabolic rate (amount of calories burned at rest) slows by 5 to 20% as a means of conserving energy, making it more difficult to lose weight. The body is convinced it is starving, and caloric conservation is a way of hanging on to the energy for a longer period. In addition, once excess fat cells are eliminated, the central nervous system receives a signal to alter feeding behavior by increasing caloric intake so that the body can maintain the set point. In other words, some experts feel that an internal thermostat regulates body fat and weight and triggers an increase in food intake when fat and weight fall too far. Overcoming the set point is difficult. Willpower and other factors that aid in tolerating the discomfort of hunger are poor defenses against a computer-like system that never quits.

Research suggests that one of the ways to take it off and keep it off may be to lower the thermostat. Yo-yo dieting (the cycle of losing and regaining weight and fat) may have the opposite effect and result in a higher setting on the thermostat, with the body then defending an even higher weight. This premise may explain why people who complete several cycles of losing and regaining 10 pounds find it nearly twice as hard to lose weight and twice as easy to gain weight on their next attempt. With each yo-yo cycle, the individual acquires extra body fat and loses some muscle mass. Regular aerobic exercise four to five times a week combined with a sound nutritional plan appears to lower the thermostat over time and allow loss of weight and maintenance of that lower weight.

set point—A theory postulating that each individual has an ideal weight (the set point) that the body will attempt to maintain against pressure to change it.

Body Composition

Many people have an ideal body image that they would someday like to achieve. For some, such an image may be unrealistic. Regardless of your motivation to change, several methods derived from research or actuarial tables may help you set realistic goals for a better-looking body.

Obesity, or the accumulation of excess fat for one's age or body type, is generally determined by hydrostatic (underwater) weighing or skinfold measures. The ideal percentage of body fat for college-age students is approximately 11 to 15% for males and 18 to 22% for females. Men who have more than 23% body fat and women who have more than 28% body fat are in the obese category. An overweight condition refers to increased body weight in relation to height and is generally determined by comparison to some standard of acceptable or desirable weights. These methods provide a less accurate indication of obesity. Being more than 20% (men) or 30% (women) above desirable weight on weight charts or having a score of 30 or above on the body-mass index (BMI) places an individual in the obese category. The BMI divides obesity into three classes: I, or moderate = 30.0-34.9; II, or severe = 35.0-39.9; and III, or very severe = 40.0 and above.

A simple method of estimating proper body weight is to use the Metropolitan Life Insurance height-weight standards shown in table 8.2. Charts of so-called ideal weight for men and women are based on data associating average weights by height and age with long life. Before 1980, figures indicated that those who weighed less than their recommended weight on the charts lived up to 20% longer than other people did. The charts, which became the national guide for determining overweight and obesity for the public, worked on the theory that the greater the weight, the greater the risk of death. The validity of such data is now being questioned because it is evident that less-than-average weights may involve health risks even greater than those associated with overweight and that the U.S. preoccupation with slimness may not be much of a health advantage.

Authorities do not dispute that people who are much heavier than average (more than 20% above ideal weight on the charts) obtain health benefits from weight reduction. Even small weight loss, for example, may aid the diabetic patient. For those in normal health who are at average or near average weight, fewer benefits are associated with losing weight. The key factor that determines what is too much or too little is body fat, not total body weight.

Determining Ideal Body Weight From Height and Weight Charts

Check your ideal weight on table 8.2. You can determine frame size by wrapping your thumb and middle finger around your opposite wrist. If the thumb and finger do not meet, you have a large frame. If they just meet or barely overlap, you have a medium frame, and if they overlap, you have a small frame. For a more accurate indicator of frame size, follow the instructions in table 8.3.

Using table 8.2 as the range for your desirable body weight, see how your actual weight compares. If you fall 20% below or above the range for your height, you are roughly classified as underweight or overweight; 30% above classifies you as obese. Keep in mind that this table provides only a rough guide to desirable weight. An individual can be considerably above a weight range and still have normal or even below-normal body fat. This circumstance is particularly common in muscular men and women. Conversely, it is possible to fall within the desired range and still have excess body fat.

Most people place far too much emphasis on height-weight charts as a measure of their desirable weight. Some experts feel that we should throw both the bathroom scale and height-weight charts into the nearest garbage can. Body weight provides no indication of what is important—not how much you weigh but how much fat your body contains and how fit you are. Height-weight

TABLE 8.2—Metropolitan Life Insurance Height and Weight Table

MEN					WOMEN				
HEIGHT		FRAME			HEIGHT		FRAME		
Feet	Inches	Small	Medium	Large	Feet	Inches	Small	Medium	Large
5	2	128-134	131-141	138-150	4	10	102-111	109-121	118-131
5	3	130-136	133-143	140-153	4	11	103-113	111-123	120-134
5	4	132-138	135-145	142-156	5	0	104-115	113-126	122-137
5	5	134-140	137-148	144-160	5	1	106-118	115-129	125-140
5	6	136-142	139-151	146-164	5	2	108-121	118-132	128-143
5	7	138-145	142-154	149-168	5	3	111-124	121-135	131-147
5	8	140-148	145-157	152-172	5	4	114-127	124-138	134-151
5	9	142-151	148-160	155-176	5	5	117-130	127-141	137-155
5	10	144-154	151-163	158-180	5	6	120-133	130-144	140-159
5	11	146-157	154-166	161-184	5	7	123-136	133-147	143-163
6	0	149-160	157-170	164-188	5	8	126-139	136-150	146-167
6	1	152-164	160-174	168-192	5	9	129-142	139-153	149-170
6	2	155-168	164-178	172-197	5	10	132-145	142-156	152-173
6	3	158-172	167-182	176-202	5	11	135-148	145-159	155-176
6	4	162-176	171-187	181-207	6	0	138-151	148-162	158-179

Weights at ages 25 to 59 are based on lowest mortality. Weight in pounds is given according to frame (in indoor clothing weighing 5 lb for men and 3 lb for women; shoes with 1" heels). For frame size standards, see table 8.3.

Reproduced, by permission, from Metropolitan Life Insurance Company, 1980, *Statistical Bulletin. Source of basic data: Society of Actuaries and Association of Life Insurance Medical Directors of America, 1979 Build Study.* This information is not intended to be a substitute for professional medical advice and should not be regarded as an endorsement or approval of any product or service.

TABLE 8.3—Approximating Frame Size

MEN		WOMEN	
Height in 1" heels	Elbow breadth	Height in 1" heels	Elbow breadth
5'2"-5'3"	2 1/2"-2 7/8"	4'10"-4'11"	2 1/4"-2 1/2"
5'4"-5'7"	2 5/8"-2 7/8"	5'0"-5'3"	2 1/4"-2 1/2"
5'8"-5'11"	2 3/4"-3"	5'4"-5'7"	2 3/8"-2 5/8"
6'0"-6'3"	2 3/4"-3 1/8"	5'8"-5'11"	2 3/8"-2 5/8"
6'4"	2 7/8"-3 1/4"	6'0"	2 1/2"-2 3/4"

Extend your arm and bend the forearm upward to a 90-degree angle. Keep your fingers straight and turn the inside of your wrist toward your body. If you have a caliper, use it to measure the space between the two prominent bones on either side of your elbow. Without a caliper, place the thumb and index finger of your other hand on these two bones. Measure the space between your fingers against a ruler or tape measure. Compare the result with the elbow measurements on this table for medium-framed men and women. Measurements lower than those listed indicate that you have a small frame. Higher measurements indicate a large frame.

Reprinted, by permission, from Metabolic Medical Center, 2003, "Approximating frame size." Avalable: http://www.metabolicmedicalcenter.com/idealweight.html#frame2 [October 13, 2003].

charts have several additional limitations: Non-Caucasians are underrepresented, age is not considered, and desirable weights are too high for young people and too low for the elderly (but correct for those in their 40s). Merely pinching certain body parts provides ample information to alert you to the need to lose body fat but not necessarily body weight.

Determining Percentile of Body Fat

A more important consideration in goal setting for a better-looking and healthier body involves not body weight but the amount of **adipose tissue** your body contains. Weight control is simply another name for fat control, and measurement of body fat is essential in setting goals for your body.

The ideal percentage of body fat is approximately 20 to 27% for females and 15 to 19% for males. Men are considered obese if they have more than 23% body fat, women if they have more than 28% body fat (see table 8.4).

Because about half of all body fat lies just beneath the skin, it is possible to pinch certain body parts, measure the thickness of two layers of skin and the connected fat, and estimate the total percentage of fat on the body.

You can measure the thickness of four skinfold sites with a caliper. Considerable practice is needed, however, before accurate measurements can be taken. Take a moment to complete Discovery Activity 8.1: Determining Your Percentage of Body Fat at the end of this chapter to develop your

TABLE 8.4—Fatness Ratings of College-Aged Men and Women

BODY FAT (PERCENTAGE)		
Rating	Men	Women
Very low fat	5-7.9	12-14.9
Low fat	8-10.9	15-17.9
Ideal fat	11-14.9	18-21.9
Above ideal fat	15-17.9	22-24.9
Overfat	18-22.9	25-27.9
High fat	≥23	≥28

skills and determine your estimated percentage of body fat.

Determining Body-Mass Index (BMI)

Body-mass index (BMI) provides a ratio between body weight and height and is quickly becoming the standard way of defining obesity for the public. Former Surgeon General C. Everett Koop proposes the use of BMI standards for physicians to identify and treat obesity. Federal guidelines suggest that people keep their BMIs under 25. The surgeon general's guidelines establish a chart for physicians to consult to determine patients' level of risk (minimal, low, moderate, high, very high, or extremely high) and suggest treatments:

- BMIs of 19 to 25 (desirable; minimal and low risk): attention to diet, increased physical activity, and lifestyle changes
- BMIs of 26 to 29 (increased health risk; moderate risk): all of the preceding and a low-calorie diet (800 to 1,200 calories daily)
- BMIs of 30 to 40 (obese; high and very high risk): all of the preceding, drug therapy, and a very low calorie diet
- BMIs over 40 (extremely obese; extremely high risk): all of the preceding and surgery

To determine your BMI, see Discovery Activity 2.1: Your Physical Fitness Profile (page 43) and figure 2.6 (page 39).

Although the CDC and the surgeon general have adopted BMI scores as the national test for obesity, some health professionals have criticized the method. A minor calculation change in the government's 1998 standard, for example, lowering BMI for overweight from 27 to 25, classified an additional 30 million Americans as overweight. The test also incorrectly classifies as many as 5 to 10% of the population as overweight or obese. Muscular athletes, such as a 6-foot, 190-pound man and a 6-foot-1, 220-pound man, are labeled overweight and obese. These heights and weights are common among athletes in various sports who may have less than 10% body fat. Although its advocates argue that the BMI test is easy to understand and calculate, it is not much better than standard height-weight charts in determining overweight and obese conditions. Technically, the BMI and height-weight charts should be used only to identify individuals who are overweight. Obesity and overfatness must be determined by hydrostatic weighing, skinfold measures, and other tests that measure percentage of body fat. The BMI test also overestimates the relationship between overweight and health when what creates the health problems is excess body fat. Experts agree that the incidence of overweight and obese children in the United States has increased to epidemic proportions, regardless of the test used, and that we should put the test argument to rest and emphasize prevention.

Several other methods are available to estimate percentage of body fat. **Electrical impedance** is a quick method. Electrodes are attached to the wrist and ankle. In less than 2 minutes, a printout provides the percentage of fat and ideal body weight. Subjects must follow certain nutritional and exercise rules for 24 hours before the test. **Hydrostatic weighing** is a reasonably accurate

adipose tissue—Fatty tissue.

electrical impedance—A quick, fairly accurate means of determining an individual's percentage of body fat that uses electrodes attached to the wrists and ankles to determine the percentage electronically.

hydrostatic weighing—A method of measuring body fat by submerging an individual in water.

method of estimating body fat. In this test the subject sits on a scale in a tank of water, exhales as completely as possible, and is then submerged for approximately 10 seconds while his or her weight is recorded. The proportions of lean body mass and fat mass are determined from calculations that involve weight underwater, weight out of water, and known densities of lean and fatty tissues.

Weight Loss Versus Fat Loss

Weight loss and the loss of body fat are not the same. Losing weight is much easier than shrinking fat cells. A typical diet producing a 10-pound weight loss that does not involve aerobic exercise and strength training may result in fat loss of only 6 or 7 pounds and a loss of 2 to 4 pounds of lean-muscle tissue. Obviously, the ideal program would produce a 10-pound loss of body fat because losing any amount of lean-muscle tissue is undesirable. Fad diets, any diet without exercise, and rapid weight loss of more than 2 to 3 pounds per week are likely to result in considerable loss of lean-muscle mass. The problem is compounded by the fact that most of the lost weight that is regained is fat, not muscle. The result is less muscle mass and a slowing of resting metabolism, which accounts for the majority of daily calories burned. For many who engage in unsound diet practices, each cycle of losing and regaining 10 pounds increases the percentage of body fat and the ratio of fat to muscle.

This chapter focuses on sound concepts and principles that safely and effectively control both body fat and body weight.

Safe Weight-Loss Procedures

Losing weight incorrectly can be dangerous. Read this section carefully and avoid beginning any fad or unfounded diet that promises miraculous results in just days or weeks. Consult your physician about a safe, effective diet and exercise plan that fits your lifestyle and current health status.

Hunger and Appetite

Hunger is generally considered physiological, an inborn instinct, whereas **appetite** is a psychological, or a learned, response. This difference helps explain why it is so common to have an appetite and eat when you are not hungry; conversely, some very thin people or those with eating disorders may experience hunger without appetite. Hunger is an active experience, whereas appetite is passive.

Satiety

The feeling of fullness or satisfaction that prompts us to stop eating is called **satiety,** one of the key regulators of eating behavior. Some experts feel that eating behavior is always in operation except when the satiety signal turns it off. Just how that happens is unknown, although a number of theories have been advanced. The **glucostatic theory** of hunger regulation suggests that blood-glucose levels and the exhaustion of liver glycogen may account for the starting and stopping of eating.

The liver stores about 75 grams of glycogen, or more than 300 energy units (calories). When liver glycogen levels fall significantly, feelings of hunger may occur. The **lipostatic theory** suggests that the number of fat-storing enzymes on the surfaces of fat cells regulates hunger in some way. The message that the cells send to the brain in this theory has not been identified. The **purinegic theory** is relatively new and untested and proposes that the circulating levels of purines, molecules found in DNA and RNA, govern hunger. Exactly where and how the brain receives these messages is also unknown. The **hypothalamus gland** appears to be important in regulating eating and satiety. Damage to this area can produce eating disorders and severe weight loss or gain.

Other factors seem to influence satiety as well. Hormones secreted by the pancreas when blood-glucose levels rise too high (insulin) or drop too low (glucagons) also affect satiety and the desire to eat. Ingesting too many simple carbohydrates at one time by eating a candy bar, for example, will rapidly elevate blood-sugar levels and produce an insulin response that eventually drops blood glucose below normal levels, a condition sometimes referred to as bonking. The faster the rate of entry of simple carbohydrates, the greater the release of insulin. Too much insulin is also responsible for driving sugar to the muscles

hunger—A physiological response of the body indicating a need for food involving unpleasant sensations.

appetite—The desire to eat; pleasant sensations aroused by thoughts of the taste and enjoyment of food.

satiety—A state in which there is no longer a desire to eat.

glucostatic theory—A theory about hunger regulation suggesting that blood-glucose levels determine whether one is hungry or satiated through the exhaustion of liver glycogen.

lipostatic theory—A theory about hunger control suggesting that the size of fat stores signals us to eat.

purinegic theory—A theory about hunger suggesting that the circulating levels of purines, molecules found in DNA and RNA, govern hunger.

hypothalamus gland—A portion of the brain that regulates body temperature and other functions; thought to be important in the regulation of food intake.

and liver for storage as glycogen, amino acids to muscles, and fat to adipose tissue for storage. Rapid changes in blood-glucose levels produced by ingesting large amounts of concentrated sugars may be part of the puzzle that affects both satiety and energy levels. Although the premise is not scientifically proven, some experts feel that the ratio of dietary carbohydrates to protein controls the relative levels of insulin to glucagon every time one eats and helps maintain satiety. A sample meal may involve carbohydrate intake that contains no more than twice the calories as the protein consumed. Such a meal may contain 20% of calories from protein and no more than 40% from complex carbohydrates (fruits, vegetables, grains). Simple carbohydrates are kept to a minimum. This approach does increase the previously recommended daily intake of protein of 12 to 15% of calories to 20% and reduces complex carbohydrate intake from 45 to 40%. Avoiding anything but small amounts of simple carbohydrates in the form of concentrated sugars and increasing protein intake slightly can help prevent extreme fluctuations in blood-glucose levels that commonly occur during the day and help control your appetite by aiding satiety.

Still other hormones, such as endorphins, the body's natural painkillers, and cortisol may affect satiety. Blood concentrations of digestive hormones such as cholecystokinin (CCK), secretin, gastrin, and others increase and combine with stomach distention to help control hunger.

Eating behavior appears to occur in response to numerous signals. The possibility also exists that an inherited, internal regulatory defect is at least partially responsible for obesity, rather than its being a purely learned behavior or genetically caused.

Obviously, we have much to learn about the causes of obesity. Experts propose many other theories. Understanding the difference between hunger and appetite and the factors suspected of controlling food intake will help you control your body weight and fat.

Controlling Appetite

From the limited information available, we know that two basic approaches to controlling appetite are somewhat effective: (1) keeping the stomach full of low-calorie food and drink and (2) raising the body's blood-sugar level. Increasing your fluid intake (particularly your water consumption) and consuming complex carbohydrates such as raw fruits and vegetables both between meals and at mealtimes will keep the stomach relatively full. New raw-grain products are also available that are equally effective. Eating small amounts of candy, such as one or two chocolate squares, 20 or 30 minutes before a meal or when you have the urge to snack, is another technique. Slow eaters (those taking 20 minutes or more) also experience elevated blood-sugar level and are less likely to overeat.

Just why appetite becomes unruly in some individuals and not others is still a mystery. The fact that Americans spend over $200 million each year on over-the-counter appetite suppressants that have little effect on permanent weight loss coupled with alarming data on the continued epidemic of obesity in the United States makes it clear that much is still to be learned.

The theory that external signals or triggers prompt overeating in the absence of hunger and are responsible for overfatness and obesity has been somewhat abandoned now that researchers are aware that these external cues govern thin people as well. Still, some experts think that weight-loss patients who have been unsuccessful should examine their reactions to the sight, smell, and thought of food to determine the influence of these external cues. University of Pennsylvania researcher Kelly Brownell lists five questions to ask yourself to determine whether external cues affect your eating behavior:

1. Do you feel like eating dessert when it looks appetizing even after eating a large meal?

2. Do you always have room in your stomach for something you like?

3. Does a buffet excite you?

4. If you drive by a bakery or fast-food outlet and smell the food, do you want to eat regardless of when you ate last?

5. Do you feel like eating when you see a picture of a delicious dessert in a magazine?

If the answer to any or all of these questions is yes, you can take a number of steps to reduce exposure to food and food cues, such as keeping high-risk foods out of the house, cutting off a small portion of a dessert and putting the rest away before sitting down to eat, placing high-risk foods out of reach and sight, and being aware that the craving to eat will disappear in seconds or minutes, making it easier to ride out the urge before reaching the supermarket or fast-food outlet.

Drugs and Weight Loss

The search continues for a safe, effective drug, free of undesirable side effects and potential for abuse, to aid in reducing body fat. Appetite-suppressant drugs (stimulants) such as Dexedrine and Benzedrine reduce appetite for only a short time, and most users quickly develop tolerance to the drugs. These drugs can also be addictive and cause nervousness, dizziness, weakness, fatigue, and insomnia. The FDA has approved two other over-the-counter appetite-suppressant ingredients. Phenylpropanolamine (PPA) hydrochloride, a chemical relative of amphetamines, is found in some cold remedies and in products such as Dexatrim and AcuTrim. Benzocaine numbs the taste buds and other sensory signals to reduce the desire for food. But both drugs seem to produce only modest weight loss at best.

Experimental medications such as naloxone and naltrexone have significantly reduced food intake in laboratory animals, but these results have not occurred with human subjects.

New drugs or agents such as phentermine that increase energy metabolism by mimicking the effects of moderate exercise in obese people and helping the body use more fat as fuel are also being tested. Fiber pills, diuretics (water pills), and a host of other diet aids with so-called magic ingredients such as spirulina, ephedrine, inositol, chromium picolinate, and ginseng are currently available. Unfortunately, not one has been shown to be an effective weight-loss aid. For example, chromium picolinate, one of the more popular ingredients, allegedly reduces fat, builds lean-muscle mass, suppresses appetite, and increases metabolism, but no evidence supports these claims.

In September 1997 the FDA requested the removal of the drugs fenfluramine, sold as Pondimin, and dexfenfluramine, sold as Redux. The popular use of the so-called fen-phen combination to shed pounds has been linked to serious heart valve problems. Dieters who have taken either of these drugs should immediately stop taking the pills and see a physician for heart monitoring and possibly a strict exam for a heart murmur.

Although new drugs continue to become available and researchers are closer to finding solutions to the prevention and treatment of obesity, no magic bullet in the form of a pill that will safely and effectively reduce your appetite and control body weight and fat is yet available. Prescription medications may aid weight loss when you work with your physician or dietitian and combine medication with diet control, modifying problem behaviors, and increasing physical activity. Using over-the-counter weight-loss drugs without the supervision of a physician should be avoided because such drugs are ineffective and unsafe.

Calorie Counting

If you are overfat according to the guidelines in this chapter, you may want to consider an exercise and diet regimen to lose body fat and weight. When you set goals for body-fat loss, you can expect to lose about .5 millimeters of body fat per week with an appropriate combination of diet and exercise. For example, if you are now classified as above-average fat, you can realistically expect to reach the average-fat category after a 10-week program.

As a first step in losing body fat, turn to Discovery Activity 8.2: Determining Your Caloric Needs at the end of the chapter to determine how many calories you need to maintain your present weight. These figures will help you decide how much to increase your daily energy expenditure and how much to reduce your daily caloric intake to meet your weight- and fat-loss goals. You can then reduce your caloric intake and increase your exercise expenditure to produce slow, safe weight and fat loss.

How Exercise Helps

Pleasing side effects that often accompany weight loss of more than 5 to 10 pounds are an enhanced self-concept and an increased energy level. Remember that the weight you choose as a target is one that, once reached, you must maintain for the rest of your life. The acceptance of a healthy lifestyle, not just weight loss per se, is what will most likely keep your thin self going in the future. Regular vigorous exercise is an essential part of this healthy, holistic lifestyle.

In 2001 the American College of Sports Medicine issued a position statement on appropriate intervention strategies for weight loss and prevention of weight regain for adults. Overall, they contend that if you expect to lose body fat and weight and then maintain that lower level, you need both to restrict your caloric intake and to engage in regular exercise. By remaining physically active, you will be able to consume more calories daily. The alternative is to remain mildly hungry most of your life. This formula for weight-loss maintenance seems simple, yet the fact that most people desire to control their weight but remain unsuccessful at maintaining body-fat losses for more than a few months addresses the complexity of the problem. Among individuals with a lower level of education, studies have shown that few were using these recommended strategies for losing and maintaining weight. The promotion of increased physical activity coupled with healthy eating habits should be a primary educational goal among high school students of all ethnicities because the 1999 National Youth Risk Behavior Survey reported that adolescents may prefer to use tobacco as a form of weight control, which adds to long-term cardiovascular risks (Lowry et al., 2002). The key to weight loss through exercise is volume, not intensity. Longer, slower walks, jogs, and exercise sessions will burn more calories than shorter workouts. Secretary of Health and Human Services Tommy Thompson is applying this concept with his staff to attack the obesity epidemic by handing out small step counters and encouraging people to take 10,000 steps daily, a figure that researchers indicate is needed to control body weight (Mulrine 2003). With the average walking step from the tip of the back toe to the tip of the front toe in normal work activity at about 18 to 20 inches (except when walking at the recommended 4 mph or 15-minute mile pace), this amounts to approximately three miles per day. This would be considered close to the minimum steps and distance one should cover to help control weight.

Numerous scientific studies have been conducted to identify perceived barriers associated with weight loss and weight-loss maintenance among high-risk populations. Results revealed that some of the perceived barriers for weight loss and weight-loss maintenance among racially and ethnically diverse women include

- lack of programs addressing the women's concerns,
- traditional ethnic cooking and eating patterns,
- cultural acceptance of a larger body type and less negative views toward overweight individuals among African American and Hispanic women,
- occupational and personal stress,
- lack of social support, and
- dietary readiness to lose weight.

One major reason for attrition from weight-loss maintenance programs is lack of motivation after termination of an organized program. We have also learned that many individuals are more likely to maintain exercise programs when they self-select the activity. Additionally, several studies show that follow-up classes that reinforce diet and exercise behavior modification are effective in maintaining long-term weight-loss outcomes (Weinsier et al., 2002; Bronner and Boyington, 2002). Many other reasons support the inclusion of both diet and exercise in a weight-loss or weight-management program.

Exercise Depresses Appetite and Improves Satiety

Regular exercise not only helps control hunger but also improves satiety by making you feel full with less food. As you continue to exercise four to five times each week and consume fewer calories, your stomach will shrink in size until only about 3 cups of food will cause you to feel full or satisfied instead of the normal four cups. By exercising regularly and avoiding meal skipping, you keep from becoming too hungry, a major cause of overeating in one sitting that eventually will increase your stomach size. Combining exercise with calorie restriction helps reduce the amount of food and calories you eat to feel satisfied because the size of your stomach will decrease. The results are loss of body weight and fat and less difficulty in maintaining your new weight.

Exercise Increases the Number of Calories You Burn at Rest

Of all the calories you expend, you burn approximately 65 to 70% while in a resting state. The number of calories you use in a resting state is

> **basal metabolism**—The number of calories burned to maintain body functions while in a resting state.

referred to as **basal metabolism.** Small changes in basal metabolism, such as those that occur following exercise, result in big changes in weight and fat loss. Both aerobic exercise and strength training will increase resting metabolism. Exercise burns calories both during the workout and for 20 minutes to several hours after exercise ceases (afterburn) by keeping your metabolic rate above the normal resting baseline. A 3-mile jog or swim, for example, doesn't expend only the 200 or 300 calories burned during the activity; it also burns an additional 25 to 40 calories per hour for the next several hours. The total benefit of a 3-mile run, then, may be as high as 400 calories.

Exercise Can Lower Your Set Point

According to the set-point theory, you possess an inborn computer-like mechanism that regulates energy balance and body weight and fat by modifying your caloric intake and expenditure. In other words, your body is programmed to be a certain weight (the set point). If you initiate a very low calorie diet in an attempt to deviate from this set point weight, your body will make metabolic changes (starvation response) to conserve energy, defend your current weight, and defeat the diet attempt. The theory may explain why some people maintain normal weight throughout life and others are unable to lose weight (because the body vigorously defends the set-point weight).

Regular aerobic exercise can adjust or reset your set-point weight to a new lower level. Physical activity produces a lower weight, less body fat, and a new energy balance. Your body now defends this lower set point, making it difficult for you to gain weight.

Exercise Burns a High Number of Calories and Increases Metabolic Rate

Although any amount of exercise is helpful, keep in mind that it is important to follow our exercise guidelines for weight loss presented in chapter 3, "Principles of Exercise." Evidence indicates that most people who exercise to lose weight do not exercise enough. According to a 1998 national survey by the Centers for Disease Control and Prevention, 62.7% of overweight Americans were exercising for the purpose of losing weight, but only 28% said they exercised 30 minutes per day, 5 days per week. The average person walked three times weekly. A program that involves aerobic activity five times weekly for a minimum of 30 minutes for each workout plus two or three weight-training sessions to add muscle mass or at least prevent loss of lean-muscle mass will be much more effective. Some studies indicate that it takes a full hour per day of moderate exercise such as brisk walking to lose weight and body fat.

Strength-training programs involving weights add muscle mass and increase metabolism permanently. Keep in mind that fat is a dormant tissue that requires few calories to maintain. Muscle tissue, on the other hand, requires considerable calories to maintain. Estimates are that every pound of additional muscle increases the metabolic rate 30 to 40 calories per 24-hour period. If you add 5 pounds of muscle over a 6-month period, your metabolic rate may increase by as much as 200 calories daily. This translates into about 6,000 calories monthly, or nearly 2 pounds of fat (2,500 calories equals 1 pound of fat). This change is obviously significant.

The best system for controlling body weight is changing your eating habits and beginning an exercise program you enjoy and are likely to continue throughout life. If you change your behavior in these two areas, you will go through life at your ideal body weight and fat. Complex forces carefully regulate body weight, but the formula for weight loss is simple. If you eat more calories than you burn through activity, a positive caloric balance will produce weight gain. If you burn up more calories than you eat, a negative caloric balance will cause weight and fat loss.

Table 5.2 (page 122) shows the number of calories used per hour in various activities. The figures do not reflect the additional effects of afterburn or the changes in metabolic rate that occur from muscle-weight gain. Walking, bicycling, swimming, dancing, jogging, and other aerobic activities are all effective means of exercise for weight loss. Some types of physical activity and sports are relaxing and enjoyable. Other activities are superior in terms of weight-loss and aerobic benefits.

When you choose a particular exercise program, consider the following:

- You are more likely to continue exercising in activities you enjoy.
- Activities that expend a moderately high number of calories per minute and allow you to continue exercise for 30 to 90 minutes are the best choices.

- Lifelong physical-recreational sports that provide heart-lung benefits are superior.
- The choice you make should allow you to start at your present fitness level and progress to higher levels later.

Exercise Brings Needed Calcium to the Bones

Because of normal aging and weight loss, bones lose calcium and other minerals and become brittle. You need adequate calcium in your diet (see chapter 10) plus weight-bearing exercise (walking, jogging, running, aerobic dance) to increase the amount of calcium that reaches the bones and thereby helps prevent osteoporosis.

Exercise Changes the Way Your Body Handles Fats

Exercise helps lower and maintain serum cholesterol (LDL) and triglycerides. HDL (high-density lipoprotein, the good cholesterol) increases, and the ratio of HDL to total cholesterol improves. High HDL counts and a high ratio of HDL to total cholesterol (1 to 4 or higher) have been associated with a lower incidence of heart attacks.

Exercise Increases Fat Loss and Decreases the Loss of Lean-Muscle Tissue

Although weight-loss programs strive to reduce body fat, most also result in the loss of lean-muscle tissue. This result is undesirable at any age because it reduces the number of calories you burn at rest, alters your appearance, and leaves you with less muscle to perform daily activities. Sound programs that combine exercise (aerobic activities and weight training) with reduced caloric intake not only prevent lean-muscle loss but also add muscle mass and increase resting metabolism. Although fat is a dormant tissue and maintained at rest with little energy expenditure, muscle tissue requires a considerable number of calories to maintain. For every pound of muscle mass you add, resting metabolic rate increases 30 to 40 calories per 24-hour period. Adding muscle weight is one of the most significant long-term ways exercise helps you lose and maintain a lower body weight and fat throughout life.

Regular Aerobic Exercise Increases Your Energy Level for Both Work and Play

The sound approaches to weight loss presented in this chapter allow you to consume enough calories to maintain an energy level that will allow you to exercise daily. Other typical low-calorie diets (fewer than 800 to 1,000 for women and 1,200 to 1,400 for men) put the body in a starvation mode of conserving calories by slowing your resting metabolic rate and robbing your energy and motivation to work out. You should consume a sufficient number of calories daily to prevent the body from adopting this starvation mode. Because you are then less likely to skip workouts, you will burn more calories, lose more fat and weight, and increase your energy level for work and play.

Exercise Will Improve Your Appearance and Self-Concept

Most people begin an exercise and weight-management program to look and feel better. An important part of the motivation to continue a lifetime approach to weight control is derived from your self-concept and how you feel about your body. Everyone has parts of their body that they are satisfied with and parts with which they are unsatisfied. Although weight and fat loss without the benefit of exercise will improve appearance in clothing, the loss of lean muscle tissue and large amounts of fatty tissue may result in a less firm body, skin that does not fit as well, and an appearance that fails to improve self-concept. The correct approach will improve your appearance by adding muscle mass and firmness, decreasing body fat, and improving the way skin fits in areas where you lost large amounts of fat deposits.

Exercise Provides a Wide Range of Health Benefits

Evidence continues to mount linking regular exercise to the prevention of various types of cancer, cardiovascular disease and stroke (lower LDL cholesterol and triglycerides; higher HDL cholesterol), osteoporosis (weight-bearing exercise such as walking, jogging, running, step aerobics, and aerobic dance brings needed dietary calcium to the bones), hypertension, and gall bladder problems (by preventing obesity). In addition, exercise contributes to an improved immune system, stress reduction, mental-emotional health, self-concept, and an improved sex life. Physically active individuals also live longer than the least physically active. Studies show that death rates increase as fitness levels decline. Another important benefit for the elderly is the evidence that weight training and flexibility training help people remain independent longer. Acts such as getting out of a chair or automobile, tying

shoes, and walking become easier as strength and flexibility improve.

Special Diets

The average diet lasts only 1 to 2 weeks for several reasons: boredom, monotony, lack of energy, fatigue, depression, complicated or expensive meal planning and buying, and failure to lose weight and fat fast enough. A sound weight-loss approach must suit your food preferences, budget, time constraints, and need for structure and social support if it is to have long-term weight-control potential by producing permanent changes in your eating and exercise habits. Unfortunately, too many people choose diet magazines, books, or ads that promise some secret, easy method of quickly and effortlessly shedding pounds and fat—sometimes without exercise and while eating as much as they want. Many of these diets do not work and are potentially dangerous. Safe, effective, long-term management of body weight and fat involves a lifelong plan of proper nutrition and regular exercise. Quick weight-loss approaches provide only a temporary fix, with over 90% of those who try any of them regaining the lost weight within 6 to 18 months. In the meantime, they may have exposed their bodies to many health hazards.

Table 8.5 analyzes some of the more popular commercial diet approaches that fall in the three categories identified by the National Research Council: do-it-yourself programs (books, programs, or self-help groups with little structure and no help from health professionals), nonclinical programs (somewhat structured with the help of health professionals), and clinical programs (highly structured with involvement from physicians, exercise therapists, and dietitians). Keep in mind that no single approach to weight and fat loss will work for everyone, and not all diets are safe for every individual. You should therefore consult your physician before beginning any approach to weight loss.

Before you initiate any type of diet, complete Discovery Activity 8.3: Ten-Point Weight-Loss Program for a Sound, Safe Diet at the end of this chapter. If your approach does not adhere to the 10-point guidelines in the activity, the diet is not safe and could have serious health consequences. If you have found an approach that worked for you in the past and you insist on dieting, adapt the plan and incorporate all 10 guidelines to protect your health.

TABLE 8.5—Commercial Approaches to Weight Management

Program	Category	Approach	Advantages	Disadvantages
Weight Watchers	Nonclinical	Low energy, group sessions	Safe, provides group support	Slow weight loss possibly discouraging
Slim Chance in a Fat World	Do-it-yourself	Low energy	Safe	Does not promote permanent weight management, no group support
Atkins Diet Revolution, Scarsdale Medical Diet	Do-it-yourself	Low carbohydrate	Rapid weight loss	May result in water loss, ketosis, and rapid weight regain; no group support
Jennie Craig	Nonclinical	Low energy, behavior modification	Safe	Expensive, does not promote behavior change
Weight to Live	Clinical and nonclinical options	Low-energy formula or food, behavior modification, exercise recommended	Safe, rapid loss, group support	Expensive
Optifast	Clinical	Low-energy formula	Rapid weight loss	Expensive, requires medical monitoring, does not promote permanent weight management
Slim Fast	Do-it-yourself	Low-energy formula	Convenient, safe	Does not promote permanent weight management, no group support
Fit or Fat	Do-it-yourself	Exercise and diet recommended	Safe	No group support

Reprinted, by permission, from L.A. Smolin and M.B. Grosvenor, 1997, Nutrition, science, and application, 210. Copyright © 1997 (Saunders College Publishing and Harcourt Brace College Publishers). Reprinted by permission of John Wiley & Sons. Inc.

Snacking

Between-meal and late-evening snacking is a leading cause of overfatness. Some people often consume over 1,000 calories between eight o'clock and midnight, or nearly one-third of a pound of fat. Yet it is unrealistic to expect people to avoid snacking altogether. In fact, planned snacking on the right foods can help you control hunger and eat less. Snacks likely to be low in calories are those that are thin and watery (tomato juice), crisp but not greasy (celery, carrots, radishes, cucumbers, broccoli, cauliflower, apples, berries, other fresh fruits and vegetables, and raw grains), and bulky (salad greens). Prepare a tray of these nutritious, low-calorie snacks and place it in the front of your refrigerator. Most snackers are compulsive and consume the first thing they see.

Characteristics of the Ideal Diet Plan

Less than 5% of dieters who lose 10 or more pounds are able to keep the weight off for a period of 12 months or more. Evidence clearly indicates that dieting does not work and does not produce lasting weight and fat loss. In addition, the type of dieting that most people resort to is dangerous and sometimes fatal. Unfortunately, the majority of people who are unhappy with their weight chase the same 10 pounds of body fat throughout life. A mere 10 pounds is responsible for the unhappiness of millions of individuals and inspires the use of unsound, unsafe practices. If those who are only slightly overfat could learn to accept their bodies, they would avoid considerable hardship and heartbreak.

The ten-point program in Discovery Activity 8.3 provides sound nutrition and exercise advice. You should follow it throughout life, including the period when you are involved in some type of diet.

Evidence suggests that the typical moderate-fat diet programs such as those advocated by the American Heart Association and Weight Watchers are the healthiest ways to keep off the pounds. Most other approaches and diets are nutritionally unsound and lack long-term data to support their effectiveness. Although most popular diets produce weight loss, only a few are capable of maintaining the new weight and body-fat levels for longer than 6 to 12 months.

The safest and most effective way to lose weight is to reduce calories and increase physical activity. Consult with your personal physician or health care professional for advice that will meet your needs. Government research can provide recommendations based on science so that people can make informed choices about appropriate weight loss. The fact is that most people who are attempting weight loss are not using the correct method to achieve or maintain positive results.

Underweight Conditions and Eating Disorders

The problems of gaining weight are just as complex as those associated with weight loss. Hunger, appetite, and satiety irregularities; psychological factors; metabolic problems—all can cause dangerous underweight. For those who need additional weight and muscle for sports or who merely want to be and appear stronger, gaining a pound is just as difficult as losing a pound is for others.

Gaining Weight

A drug-free program to gain muscle weight requires dedication to both diet and exercise. With a sound approach, individuals strive to add no more than a half pound of muscle per week. This rate of gain is about as fast as the body can add lean-muscle tissue. Faster approaches involving too many calories are almost certain to add adipose tissue.

A sound strength-training program, such as weight training, is an absolute must for muscle-weight gain (see chapter 7). Training for several hours six times weekly, alternating muscle groups each workout, may be necessary.

The nutritional support for a sound weight-gain program involves

- an increase in food (about 400 to 500 additional calories daily) that provides high calories in a small volume to keep you from getting uncomfortably full,
- a slight increase in total protein intake (14 to 15% of daily calories), and
- a slight reduction in total fat intake (18 to 20% of daily calories).

Extra calories should come from complex carbohydrates (45 to 50% of daily calories) to provide long-term energy and for **protein sparing.** Most individuals who have difficulty gaining weight do not eat enough calories to support their vigorous workout schedule. Using protein or amino acid tablets is hazardous and a waste of money. In most cases, individuals already consume more protein than they need; adding more in the form of supplements is unnecessary. Chapter 11 discusses the health implications of creatine, androstenedione, anabolic steroids, and caffeine.

Eating Disorders

The current overemphasis on flat bellies, lean thighs, firm buttocks, and slimness is at least partially responsible for aggravating two serious eating disorders that can lead to death: **anorexia nervosa** and **bulimia.** Both disorders are known only in developed nations and are most common in higher economic groups.

Anorexia Nervosa

The number of cases of anorexia nervosa is increasing and now occurs in nearly 1 of every 100 women, 95% of whom are young women. The disease is four to five times more common in identical twins than in fraternal twins, suggesting an inherited predisposition to the disease. Unfortunately, our culture encourages anorexia nervosa.

A typical case involves a young woman from a middle-class family who values appearance more than self-worth and self-actualization. Typically, family ties are strong, and the young woman is efficient, eager to please her parents, and somewhat of a perfectionist. An absentee or distant father is also common. The characteristic behavior of anorexia is obsessive and compulsive, resembling addiction. Anorexics may become obsessed with the idea that they are, or will

---

protein sparing—Consuming sufficient amounts of dietary carbohydrates and fat each day to prevent the conversion of dietary and lean-muscle protein to glucose.

anorexia nervosa—An eating disorder that involves lack or loss of appetite to the point of self-starvation and dangerous weight loss.

bulimia—An eating disorder found most often in women involving some method of purging and binge eating followed by self-induced vomiting or the use of laxatives to expel the unwanted food.

Myth and Fact Sheet

Myth	Fact
1. Overweight and obese people are always big eaters.	**1.** In both children and adults, studies show that the major cause of an overweight or obese condition is inactivity followed by overeating. The major problem for the majority of overfat people in the United States is inactivity. A regular exercise program is still the best health-insurance policy and the best approach to weight and fat loss.
2. The major part of excess weight and fat is water.	**2.** This statement is not true. Do not restrict your water intake in any way. Water is essential to the proper function of every body system. Fluid retention is common while dieting because water remains in the spaces freed by the disappearance of fat. This fluid generally remains for 2 to 3 weeks and often obscures actual weight loss. Drink water freely at all times, particularly when you are restricting your calories. The majority (about 80%) of excess weight is fat, not water.
3. There's nothing wrong with resorting to quick weight-loss diets.	**3.** You should lose weight at the rate of no more than 2 pounds weekly. Very low calorie diets that produce rapid weight loss have a number of pitfalls: (1) They are dangerous and possibly life-threatening; (2) rapid weight loss is usually followed by rapid weight gain; (3) your percentage of body fat increases each time you lose and reacquire the weight; and (4) you do not consume sufficient carbohydrates to spare protein, resulting in lean-tissue loss even from the heart muscle itself. Sufficient cardiac tissue loss to the heart might cause serious rhythm problems.
4. Special foods and exercise can eliminate cellulite.	**4.** From a medical point of view, cellulite does not exist as a particular form of fat. Fat is merely fat, although the size and appearance of fat cells vary in different body parts and in different people. The lumpy, dimplelike deposits called cellulite tend to be most visible in women and often appear on the thighs, back of the legs, and buttocks. These deposits are merely large fat cells that show through the somewhat thinner skin of women. Thicker skinned males tend not to develop this appearance unless they become extremely fat. Prevention is easier than treatment and focuses on getting proper nutrition, maintaining normal weight and fat, and avoiding rapid weight-loss attempts or yo-yo dieting.
5. Remaining fat is better than losing weight and ending up with wrinkled skin.	**5.** You are partially correct. Staying somewhat fat is better than losing and then regaining body weight rapidly. If you lose weight and fat slowly through a combination of diet and exercise and lose only 10 to 15 pounds, skin wrinkling is unlikely. Including weight training as part of your exercise routine is also helpful. As your fat cells shrink, the added muscle mass will help your skin fit you better in some areas, such as the back of the arm. If you have more than 15 pounds to lose, work with your physician on a 6- to 12-month program.
6. Sit-ups will remove fat from the abdomen.	**6.** To flatten your abdomen, you must reduce your calorie intake, exercise regularly, and perform abdominal exercises. With calorie restriction, the fat cells in the stomach will shrink, and your stomach will get smaller. Your sit-up routine (see chapter 7) will strengthen the underlying muscle tissue. Both adipose and muscle tissue need to be changed; you cannot convert fat tissue to muscle tissue, nor will muscle tissue change to fat when you become sedentary.

7. The more you perspire, the more weight you lose.

7. No permanent weight-loss benefit results from excessive sweating. Once you replenish fluids, weight will be back to normal. In fact, a 30-minute workout will burn more calories in cold weather than it will in hot, humid conditions.

8. I can't be overweight when I weigh the same now at age 40 that I did at age 19.

8. If you have remained active with regular aerobic exercise and strength training, you are probably not overweight or overfat. If you have been sedentary the past 5 years or more, it is almost certain that your ratio of lean muscle to fat tissue has changed. Although you may weigh the same, your percentage of body fat is likely to have increased and your percentage of lean-muscle mass has probably declined. Use one of the methods of determining body-fat percentages to evaluate your present state.

9. Body weight and percentage of body fat are the best indicators of health.

9. Studies continue to show what has been suspected for years: regular aerobic exercise such as walking, jogging, cycling, or swimming is good for the heart; plays a role in the prevention of numerous diseases and disorders; and reduces the risk of mortality, regardless of whether you are overweight or overfat. All exercising individuals derive health benefits from exercise, even without fat and weight loss. Although excess body fat is unhealthy, being thin is not the key; what is important is being fit. Fitness is every bit as important in evaluating one's health as body weight and fat are.

10. Laxatives help you lose weight.

10. The use of laxatives causes gastrointestinal trouble and can result in dehydration and undernourishment. Being fat is better than endangering your health. You cannot safely defecate away unwanted pounds.

11. The herb ephedra is a safe, effective weight-loss product.

11. Physicians consider ephedra so dangerous that they ban its use. The Food and Drug Administration is taking steps to ban products containing ephedra. Athletes commonly use it to aid weight loss and provide energy for training and competition. Reports have linked these herbs to more than 100 deaths and thousands of visits to the emergency room or physician's office. These herbs are extremely dangerous, and like the drug, are almost certain to be banned in the near future. Avoid using any herbs containing ephedra.

12. Weight-reducing pills are a safe approach to depressing the appetite.

12. The use of drugs and drug combinations to depress appetite is dangerous and sometimes fatal. Drug usage is an attempt to cause weight loss by increasing metabolic rate, curbing the appetite, or causing fluid loss. Amphetamines and diuretics are the two most commonly used diet pills. Amphetamines toy with the thyroid gland, cause nervousness, speed up metabolism, and require increasingly stronger dosages as tolerance develops; diuretics result in rapid fluid loss. Both are dangerous, ineffective approaches to weight loss.

13. Reducing aids such as vibrators, body wraps, rubber suits, steam baths, and massages effectively remove fat from the body.

13. Each of these popular gimmick approaches to weight loss results in little calorie burning and is ineffective. To lose weight and fat, you must engage in exercise that burns a high number of calories, such as aerobics. You then achieve a negative caloric balance and lose weight and fat.

become, fat. They may fear the transition from girlhood to womanhood that results in a more curvaceous figure, and they become determined to stave it off by controlling their weight. They carry this starvation approach to the extreme of undernourishment until total-body weight is dangerously low. Even at that extreme, anorexics may still feel fat and continue to starve themselves, sometimes literally to death.

Young female anorexics generally develop **amenorrhea.** Females must reacquire 17 to 22% body fat before the menstrual cycle resumes. Thyroid hormone secretions, adrenal secretions, growth hormones, and hormones that regulate blood pressure reach abnormal levels. The heart pumps less efficiently as cardiac muscle weakens, the chambers diminish in size, and blood pressure falls. Heart-rhythm disturbances and sudden stopping of the heart may occur because of lean-tissue loss and mineral deficiencies, producing sudden death in some patients. Other health problems include anemia, gastrointestinal problems, atrophy of the digestive tract, abnormal function of the pancreas, blood-lipid changes, dry skin, decreased core temperature, and disturbed sleep.

Early treatment is essential in preventing permanent damage. Without treatment, about 10% of anorexics die of starvation. Forced feeding may temporarily improve health, but the condition

> **amenorrhea**—Loss of at least three consecutive menstrual cycles when they are expected to occur.

can reappear unless the person receives proper psychological and medical therapy. Treatment focuses on restoring adequate nutrition, avoiding medical complications, and altering the psychological and environmental patterns that have supported or permitted the emergence of anorexia. About 5% of those in treatment eventually reach 25% of their desired weight, and 50 to 75% resume normal menstrual cycles. After treatment ends, about 66% fail to eat normally and 7% die (of which 1% commit suicide).

Bulimia

Bulimia is more common than anorexia nervosa and occurs in males as well as females. Between 10 and 20% of all college students are estimated to be bulimic. Only 5% of those students meet the criteria for anorexia nervosa, and less than 1% are actively anorexic. The typical profile of victims is similar to that of those suffering from anorexia nervosa, although bulimics tend to be slightly older and healthier, malnourished but closer to normal weight. The bulimic binge is generally not a response to hunger, and the food is not consumed for nutritional value. As the person repeats the binge-vomit cycle, medical problems

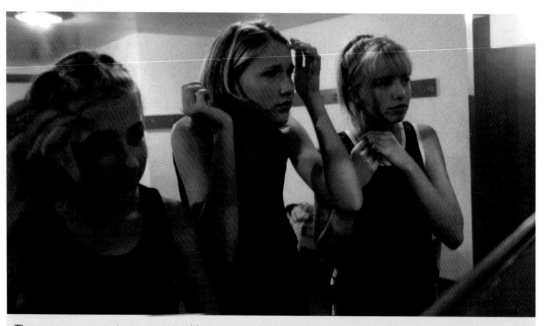

The pressure among teenagers to achieve some perceived ideal look can result in health and nutrition problems.

PhotoDisc

grow. Fluid and electrolyte imbalances may lead to abnormal heart rhythm and kidney damage. Infections of the bladder and kidneys may cause kidney failure. Vomiting results in irritation and infection of the pharynx, esophagus, and salivary glands; erosion of the teeth; and dental caries. In some cases, the esophagus or the stomach may rupture.

Bulimics are more cooperative and somewhat easier to treat than anorexic patients are because they seem to recognize that the behavior is abnormal. Most treatment programs attempt to help people gain control over their binge eating and encourage consumption of a minimum of 1,500 calories daily. Lithium and other drugs have been shown to reduce the incidence of bulimic episodes by 75 to 100%. Antidepressant medication can help most bulimics.

Table 8.6 identifies the most common symptoms of eating disorders. You may recognize some of these behaviors in a friend or colleague and be instrumental in helping him or her seek treatment. Dentists may be the first health professional to spot bulimia because self-induced vomiting brings stomach acid to the mouth and damages tooth enamel. Damage from purging generally occurs inside the upper front teeth and produces sensitivity, thinning, and chipping.

Summary

Trends in Body-Fat Loss and Weight Control
Over the past decade the percentage of obese individuals (children and adults) in the United States has steadily increased, continuing the trend of the previous decade. People of all ages are several pounds heavier than those of the previous decade were. Unfortunately, the increase comes because of additional body fat, not muscle. Unless this trend changes, the health consequences will be astronomical.

Causes of Obesity Overfatness and obesity are caused by a number of factors, with both genetics and environment playing key roles. Although inheriting the tendency to become fat is a disadvantage, environment can overcome this

TABLE 8.6—Common Symptoms of Eating Disorders

Symptoms	Anorexia nervosa*	Bulimia nervosa*	Binge-eating disorder
Excessive weight loss in relatively short time	x		
Continuation of dieting although bone-thin	x		
Dissatisfaction with appearance, belief that body is fat even though severely underweight	x		
Loss of monthly menstrual periods	x	x	
Unusual interest in food and development of strange eating habits	x	x	
Eating in secret	x	x	x
Obsession with exercise	x	x	
Serious depression	x	x	x
Bingeing—consumption of large amounts of food		x	x
Vomiting or use of drugs to stimulate vomiting, bowel movements, and urination		x	
Bingeing but no noticeable weight gain		x	
Disappearance into bathroom for long periods to induce vomiting		x	
Abuse of drugs or alcohol		x	x

*Some individuals suffer from anorexia and bulimia and have symptoms of both disorders.

From U.S. Department of Health and Human Services, NIH Publication No. 94-3477, 1994.

Behavioral Change and Motivational Strategies

Some of the more critical eating behaviors associated with weight gain that have high potential for behavioral change include drinking high-calorie drinks instead of water, consuming too much sugar, consuming too many foods high in saturated fat, binge eating, between-meal snacking, overeating at lunch and dinner, skipping breakfast or lunch, and failing to plan snacks. Important exercise behaviors that people can change include weekend leisure inactivity, long hours spent watching television, and having no regular exercise program.

You should remember that you are in complete control of your eating and exercise behavior. You have the power to alter behavior that is contributing to overfatness. Figure 8.1 includes some of the most common behavioral principles of weight loss. These suggestions should help you prepare specific motivational strategies to eliminate roadblocks.

I. Stimulus control
  A. Shopping
    1. Shop for food after eating.
    2. Shop from a list.
    3. Avoid ready-to-eat foods.
    4. Don't carry more cash than you need for items on your shopping list.
  B. Plans
    1. Plan to limit food intake.
    2. Substitute exercise for snacking.
    3. Eat meals and snacks at scheduled times.
    4. Don't accept food offered by others.
  C. Activities
    1. Store food out of sight.
    2. Eat all food in the same place.
    3. Remove food from inappropriate storage areas.
    4. Keep serving dishes off the table.
    5. Use smaller dishes and utensils.
    6. Avoid being the food server.
    7. Leave the table immediately after eating.
    8. Don't save leftovers.
  D. Holidays and parties
    1. Drink fewer alcoholic beverages.
    2. Plan eating habits before going to parties.
    3. Eat a low-calorie snack before parties.
    4. Practice polite ways to decline food.
    5. Don't be discouraged by an occasional setback.
II. Eating behavior
  A. Put your fork down between mouthfuls.
  B. Chew thoroughly before swallowing.
  C. Prepare foods one portion at a time.
  D. Leave some food on the plate.
  E. Pause in the middle of the meal.
  F. Do not read, watch TV, or do other things.
III. Reward
  A. Solicit help from family and friends.
  B. Help family and friends provide this support in the form of praise and material rewards.
  C. Use self-monitoring records as basis for rewards.
  D. Plan specific rewards for specific behaviors (behavioral contracts).
IV. Self-monitoring through diet diary
  A. Record time and place of eating.
  B. Record type and amount of food.
  C. Note who is present and how you feel.
V. Nutrition education
  A. Use diet diary to identify problem areas.
  B. Make small changes that you can continue.
  C. Learn nutritional values of foods.
  D. Decrease fat intake and increase intake of complex carbohydrates.
VI. Physical activity
  A. Routine activity
    1. Increase routine activity.
    2. Increase use of stairs.
    3. Keep a record of distance walked each day.
  B. Exercise
    1. Begin a mild exercise program.
    2. Keep a record of daily exercise.
    3. Increase the exercise gradually.
VII. Cognitive restructuring
  A. Avoid setting unreasonable goals.
  B. Think about progress, not shortcomings.
  C. Avoid imperatives like "always" and "never."
  D. Counter negative thoughts with rational restatements.
  E. Set weight goals.

Figure 8.1   Behavioral principles of weight loss

Reprinted with permission by the *American Journal of Clinical Nutrition.* © AM J Clin Nutr. American Society for Clinical Nutrition.

Roadblock	Behavioral Change Strategy
Snacking before bedtime is a major problem. You seem to get hungry after nine o'clock in the evening and often devour everything in sight.	You have identified one of the major eating habits contributing to weight and fat gain. To reduce the number of calories consumed between your evening meal and bedtime, try the following: ▪ Go to bed by 10 o'clock or earlier; the longer you stay up the more likely you are to eat and drink. ▪ Prepare a tray of fruits and vegetables for snacking and place it in the front of your refrigerator for easy access. ▪ Take a 2- or 3-mile walk several hours after your evening meal. ▪ Drink two or three glasses of water 2 hours after your evening meal.
You find that you are able to control snacking during the day but overeat at mealtime until you are stuffed and uncomfortable.	Try some of the following suggestions to reduce your intake at mealtime: ▪ Eat one or two chocolate squares or drink 3 or 4 ounces of fruit juice about 30 minutes before mealtime to raise your blood-sugar level. ▪ Drink two 8-ounce glasses of water at mealtime before you eat anything. ▪ Measure food quantities and prepare only the amount you want to eat. ▪ Eat a small amount of dessert first, followed by your salad. ▪ Take small portions and eat slowly, taking at least 30 minutes to complete the meal. ▪ Never skip breakfast or lunch and never let yourself become too hungry; being famished is the main cause of overeating at the evening meal. ▪ Take a walk or exercise an hour before mealtime.
You simply cannot seem to find time to exercise, and by the time the workday is over, you are too exhausted even to consider it.	Lack of time is the number one excuse of the sedentary individual. In most cases, even extremely busy people can work a 30-minute exercise session into their schedule. Evaluate each of the following to determine which suggestion may work for you: ▪ Walk 2 or 3 miles each day during your lunch break just before you eat. ▪ Exercise moderately about 2 hours after your evening meal just before bedtime. ▪ Consider getting up an hour earlier for a 30-minute exercise session followed by a shower. ▪ Look into muscle-toning programs that you can perform at your desk and in your vehicle.
Circle the behaviors in figure 8.1 that you feel the lack of may contribute to your weight problem or to a potential weight problem in the future.	Now prepare a list of some of the things you might do to eliminate the barriers and alter your behavior. Refer to the specific strategies discussed in this chapter, and if you need to, refer back to chapter 4 for behavioral change and motivational strategies. 1. _____ 2. _____ 3. _____

predisposition. Inactivity and overeating are still the two major behaviors associated with weight and fat gain.

The body appears to defend its biological weight, referred to as set point, by resisting attempts to lose weight. Lowering the set point requires regular aerobic exercise and reduced caloric intake for 6 to 12 months or until it is evident that the body is now defending the lower weight and fat levels.

Overeating in infancy, bottle feeding instead of breast feeding, and early consumption of solid foods before the age of 5 months may contribute to the development of excess fat cells and overeating later in life.

Fat cells increase in number only until growth ceases, at which time one becomes fat only through the enlargement of existing adipose cells. Adults who become obese may develop some new fat cells.

Small changes in metabolism result in large increases or decreases in weight over a period of 6 to 12 months. Only a small percentage of individuals with weight problems suffer from an underactive thyroid gland.

Levels of the appetite-boosting hormone ghrelin, secreted by the stomach, affect the hypothalamus gland and produce hunger, encourage eating, and increase fat storage. Researchers are searching for a drug that blocks the action of ghrelin to help people lose weight and keep it off.

The number of calories we burn at rest account for most of the calories expended in a 24-hour period. Inactivity and loss of muscle mass with aging lower one's metabolic rate and significantly contribute to excess stored fat and weight gain. Regular weight training that prevents loss of muscle tissue or adds more muscle can produce the opposite effect and increase the number of calories burned in a resting state.

Adenovirus-36 is six times more likely to be present in the body of overweight humans than in those of normal weight. Researchers feel that the virus contributes to overweight and obesity by increasing the number of fat cells and fat storage.

Body Composition   A number of methods are available to determine ideal body weight and percentage of body fat. Height-weight tables should be used only as a guide to ideal weight because they provide no indication of percentage of body fat, the key factor in determining health risks.

By measuring the thickness of two layers of skin and the underlying fat, you can secure an estimate of total-body fat and identify ideal body weight. A number of different skinfold sites can be used. Electrical impedance and underwater weighing are more accurate techniques, but those methods require special equipment.

Safe Weight-Loss Procedures   Hunger is a physiological, inborn instinct designed to control food intake, whereas appetite is a psychological, learned response. Although numerous theories have been advanced to explain how the body controls food intake, the exact signals that cue us to consume food have not been positively identified.

Calories count, and the body handles the matter with computer-like precision, storing 1 pound of fat for every 3,500 excess calories consumed.

Exercise is essential to the control of body weight and fat. Regular aerobic exercise depresses appetite, minimizes fat loss, maximizes the loss of lean-muscle tissue, burns a high number of calories, brings needed calcium to the bones, and changes the way the body handles dietary fat.

Numerous new drugs designed to curb appetite, increase metabolic rate and exercise metabolism, deaden taste buds, and increase burning of fat as energy are being tested and evaluated. The search for the magic pill that will help everyone attain ideal weight and body fat continues. Even if researchers develop such a pill, people will need to use it in combination with a lifetime of sound nutrition and fitness practices.

Special Diets   Most special diets fail, in many cases within 5 to 7 days. Approximately 90% of those who succeed in losing weight will regain it within a year.

Dieting is extremely dangerous and can prove fatal if the dieter does not observe certain nutritional guidelines. The best approach is to develop sound exercise and eating habits that one can follow throughout life.

Underweight and Eating Disorders   Gaining weight is just as difficult as losing weight. A complete program of muscle-weight gain requires sound nutritional support and an organized weight-training program that involves up to six 2-hour workouts weekly.

The number of cases of anorexia nervosa and bulimia continue to increase in the United States. As long as U.S. society places high value on slimness, this trend will continue. Both disorders are extremely difficult to treat and can produce numerous health consequences and even death.

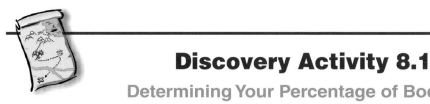

Discovery Activity 8.1

Determining Your Percentage of Body Fat

Name _____ **Date** _____

Instructions: One way to determine your percentage of body fat is to measure the thickness of four skinfolds. The procedure for measuring skinfold thickness is to grasp a fold of skin and subcutaneous (just under the skin) fat firmly with the thumb and forefinger, pulling it away and up from the underlying muscle tissue. Attach the jaws of the calipers 1 centimeter below the thumb and forefinger. All measurements should be taken on the right side of the body with the subject standing.

Working with a partner, practice taking each other's measurements in the four areas described below:

- **Triceps**—With the arm resting comfortably at the side, take a vertical fold parallel to the long axis of the arm midway between the tip of the shoulder and the tip of the elbow.
- **Biceps**—With the arm in the same position, take a vertical fold halfway between the elbow and top of the shoulder on the front of the upper arm.
- **Subscapula**—Just below the scapula (shoulder blade), take a diagonal fold across the back.
- **Suprailiac**—Just above the hipbone, take a diagonal fold following the natural line of the iliac crest.

Record the information in the following section to complete your evaluation. For example, John is a 20-year-old who weighs 185 pounds. His four skinfold measurements were 16, 12, 37, and 15. Follow his evaluation to help you understand the procedure:

_____ **1.** Sum the four skinfold measures in millimeters (16 + 12 + 37 + 15 = 80 millimeters).

_____ **2.** Find the percentage of body fat for this total from table 8.A. Moving down in the first vertical column to 80 and over to the 17 to 29 age group for males in column 2, we find that John has about 24.8% fat.

_____ **3.** Find the ideal percentage of body fat from table 8.4. John's ideal fat percentage is 14.9% or less.

_____ **4.** Figure the percentage of fat to lose to reach the ideal percentage. John has about 10% too much fat (24.8 − 14.9 = 10) and therefore needs to lose 10% of his body weight.

_____ **5.** Calculate the total pounds of fat loss needed to reach ideal weight (10% × 185 = 18.5 pounds of fat).

_____ **6.** Find the ideal weight. With 14.9% fat (high end of recommended ideal body fat for college men), John's ideal weight is 167 (185 − 18 = 167) pounds.

(continued)

Discover Activity 8.1 *(continued)*

TABLE 8.A—Fat As a Percentage of Body Weight on the Sum of Four Skinfolds, Age, and Sex

Skinfolds (mm)	PERCENTAGE OF FAT, MALES (AGE IN YR)				PERCENTAGE OF FAT, FEMALES (AGE IN YR)			
	17-29	30-39	40-49	≥50	16-29	30-39	40-49	≥50
15	4.8	—	—	—	10.5	—	—	—
20	8.1	12.2	12.2	12.6	14.1	17.0	19.8	21.4
25	10.5	14.2	15.0	15.6	16.8	19.4	22.2	24.0
30	12.9	16.2	17.7	18.6	19.5	21.8	24.5	26.6
35	14.7	17.7	19.6	20.8	21.5	23.7	26.4	28.5
40	16.4	19.2	21.4	22.9	23.4	25.5	28.2	30.3
45	17.7	20.4	23.0	24.7	25.0	26.9	29.6	31.9
50	19.0	21.5	24.6	26.5	26.5	28.2	31.0	33.4
55	20.1	22.5	25.9	27.9	27.8	29.4	32.1	34.6
60	21.2	23.5	27.1	29.2	29.1	30.6	33.2	35.7
65	22.2	24.3	28.2	30.4	30.2	31.6	34.1	36.7
70	23.1	25.1	29.3	31.6	31.2	32.5	35.0	37.7
75	24.0	25.9	30.3	32.7	32.2	33.4	35.9	38.7
80	24.8	26.6	31.2	33.8	33.1	34.3	36.7	39.6
85	25.5	27.2	32.1	34.8	34.0	35.1	37.5	40.4
90	26.2	27.8	33.0	35.8	34.8	35.8	38.3	41.2
95	26.9	28.4	33.7	36.6	35.6	36.5	39.0	41.9
100	27.6	29.0	34.4	37.4	36.4	37.2	39.7	42.6
105	28.2	29.6	35.1	38.2	37.1	37.9	40.4	43.3
110	28.8	30.1	35.8	39.0	37.8	38.6	41.0	43.9
115	29.4	30.6	36.4	39.7	38.4	39.1	41.5	44.5
120	30.0	31.1	37.0	40.4	39.0	39.6	42.0	45.1
125	30.5	31.5	37.6	41.1	39.6	40.1	42.5	45.7
130	31.0	31.9	38.2	41.8	40.2	40.6	43.0	46.2
135	31.5	32.3	38.7	42.4	40.8	41.1	43.5	46.7
140	32.0	32.7	39.2	43.0	41.3	41.6	44.0	47.2
145	32.5	33.1	39.7	43.6	41.8	42.1	44.5	47.7
150	32.9	33.5	40.2	44.1	42.3	42.6	45.0	48.2

Skinfolds (mm)	PERCENTAGE OF FAT, MALES (AGE IN YR)				PERCENTAGE OF FAT, FEMALES (AGE IN YR)			
	17-29	30-39	40-49	≥50	16-29	30-39	40-49	≥50
155	33.3	33.9	40.7	44.6	42.8	43.1	45.4	48.7
160	33.7	34.3	41.2	45.1	43.3	43.6	45.8	49.2
165	34.1	34.6	41.6	45.6	43.7	44.0	46.2	49.6
170	34.5	34.8	42.0	46.1	44.1	44.4	46.6	50.0
175	34.9	—	—	—	—	44.8	47.0	50.4
180	35.3	—	—	—	—	45.2	47.4	50.8
185	35.6	—	—	—	—	45.6	47.8	51.2
190	35.9	—	—	—	—	45.9	48.2	51.6
195	—	—	—	—	—	46.2	48.5	52.0
200	—	—	—	—	—	46.5	48.8	52.4
205	—	—	—	—	—	—	49.1	52.7
210	—	—	—	—	—	—	49.4	53.0

In two-thirds of the instances the error was ± 3.5% of body weight as fat for the women and ± 5% for the men.

Reprinted, by permission, from J.V.G.A. Dumin and J. Womersley, 1975, "Body fat assessed from total body density and its estimation from skinfold thickness," *British Journal of Nutrition* 32: 95.

From *Physical fitness and wellness, third edition*, by Jerrold S. Greenberg, George B. Dintiman, and Barbee Myers Oakes, 2004, Champaign, IL: Human Kinetics.

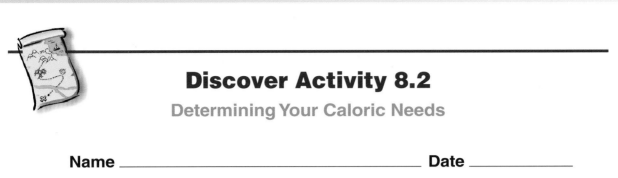

Discover Activity 8.2

Determining Your Caloric Needs

Name _____ **Date** _____

Instructions: Complete each of the following steps carefully to identify how many calories you need daily to attain and maintain your ideal weight as determined in Discovery Activity 8.1: Determining Your Percentage of Body Fat.

1. Rate your level of physical activity from the list below by honestly estimating your activity level.

Activity Pattern	Calories Needed per Pound
Very inactive (sedentary, never exercise)	13
Slightly inactive (occasional physical activity)	14
Moderately active (fairly active on the job, engage in aerobic exercise twice weekly)	15
Relatively active (almost always on the go, engage in aerobic exercise three to four times weekly)	16
Frequent strenuous activity (daily aerobic exercise for an hour or more)	17

2. Multiply your rating (calories per pound) by your weight. A sedentary 18- to 21-year-old female who weighs 130 pounds, for example, would need 1,690 calories per day (130 × 13 = 1,690). In theory, if she is consistently eating more than 1,690 calories daily, she is gaining weight.

3. Multiply your physical activity rating by your ideal weight from Discovery Activity 8.1. This figure is the number of calories you need each day to maintain your ideal weight. The ideal weight in the example in Discovery Activity 8.1 is 167 pounds. Because John is sedentary, he needs only 13 calories per pound and 2,171 calories daily to maintain that weight (167 × 13 = 2,171).

You can eventually reach your ideal weight by consuming only the number of calories necessary to maintain that weight. Some clinics in the United States use this sound approach to weight and fat loss. You are more likely to maintain weight loss that occurs slowly and safely.

From Physical fitness and wellness, third edition, by Jerrold S. Greenberg, George B. Dintiman, and Barbee Myers Oakes, 2004, Champaign, IL: Human Kinetics.

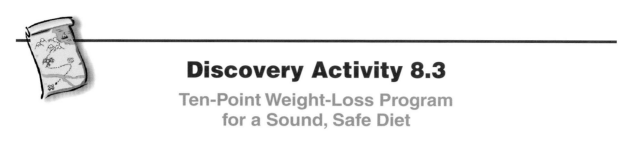

Discovery Activity 8.3

Ten-Point Weight-Loss Program
for a Sound, Safe Diet

Name _____ **Date** _____

Instructions: Although most people are aware that fad diets are an unwise choice for permanent loss of weight and fat free from the risk of illness, millions continue to try practically any new, highly publicized diet on the market. Quick weight-loss programs with some secret, easy method of rapidly shedding pounds are often too much to resist. Unfortunately, unsound dieting is dangerous and can result in permanent negative health consequences and even death.

- Before you even consider using a gimmick diet, consult your physician about your personal health concerns and ask your dietitian to evaluate the entire program.
- Compare the fad diet to the 10-point weight-loss program on page 222 by completing the following chart. Study the fad diet carefully and place a yes or no in the column to the right of each of the 10 criteria for a sound, safe diet.
- If you placed a no in the right-hand column, even in one area, the diet is suspect and possibly unsafe if used for longer than a few days. If you placed a no in the right-hand column in two or more areas, don't consider its use, even for a day.
- You can duplicate and use this form with any diet. In the column to the left, Monday through Sunday, check off each area as you meet that criterion that particular day. On most days, you should have a check in each column, regardless of the diet you are following.

(continued)

Discovery Activity 8.3 *(continued)*

Ten-Point Healthy Weight-Loss Program
Daily Check Sheet

Name _____ Date _____ Starting weight _____ % Body fat _____

Daily calories = 8 × _____ (ideal wt) = _____ Weekly weigh-in: _____

Daily requirements

M T W T F S S		Yes or no
General:		
Δ Δ Δ Δ Δ Δ Δ	1. Buy food carefully by reading labels and searching for nutritious low-calorie, low-fat, low-salt foods. Keep records of calorie, food, and fluid intake, at the time you consume it.	_____
Δ Δ Δ Δ Δ Δ Δ	2. Consume no less than 8 calories per pound and no more than 10 calories per pound of ideal weight daily for weight loss, 12 to13 for maintenance. The goal is to lose 2 to 3 pounds per week.	_____
Δ Δ Δ Δ Δ Δ Δ	3. Take one multiple vitamin/mineral daily and 1,500 milligrams of calcium for women. Do not skip meals.	_____
Δ Δ Δ Δ Δ Δ Δ	4. Consume no more than 2,000 milligrams of salt daily (midrange of 1,100 to 3,300 recommended) by eliminating table salt and reducing consumption of processed products.	_____
Fluid intake:		
Δ Δ Δ Δ Δ Δ Δ	5. Drink 12 to 15 8-ounce glasses of water for weight loss, 8 to 10 for maintenance. Consume no more than two carbonated drinks and limit alcohol to a maximum of one (women) to two (men) drinks daily.	_____
Food intake:		
Δ Δ Δ Δ Δ Δ Δ	6. Eat the proper number of servings from five food groups: (1) bread, cereal, grains, pasta; (2) vegetables; (3) fruits; (4) low-fat milk, yogurt, cheese; (5) meat, fish, poultry, dry beans, eggs, nuts. Consume 25 to 35 grams of dietary fiber.	_____
Δ Δ Δ Δ Δ Δ Δ	7. Consume adequate protein. Your ideal body weight in pounds × .36 = daily protein needs in grams. For example, 140 pounds × .36 = 50 grams of protein (4 calories per gram = 200 calories).	_____
Δ Δ Δ Δ Δ Δ Δ	8. Reduce fat consumption to 25% of total calories (saturated = 5%, monounsaturated = 10%, and polyunsaturated = 10%). Forty-five percent of your weight in pounds is the number of grams of fat you can eat daily; only 20% of these should be saturated. Reduce your intake of trans-fatty acids by limiting use of margarine (choose the softest tub margarine you can find), cookies, doughnuts, and other products made with trans fats.	_____
Δ Δ Δ Δ Δ Δ Δ	9. Snack on low-glycemic index foods (apples, cherries, kidney beans, navy beans, chick peas, lentils, dates, figs, peaches, plums, yogurt, tomato soup); avoid high glycemic index items (sucrose, maple syrup, corn syrup, honey, bagels, candy, carrots, crackers, molasses, potatoes, raisins, bread, soda, sports drinks with sugar).	_____
Exercise:		
Δ Δ Δ Δ Δ Δ Δ	10. Complete 30 minutes of aerobic exercise daily and two to three weight-training sessions weekly.	_____

Record your deficit or surplus calories for today _____

Figure 8.2   Ten-Point Healthy Weight-Loss Program

From *Physical fitness and wellness, third edition,* by Jerrold S. Greenberg, George B. Dintiman, and Barbee Myers Oakes, 2004, Champaign, IL: Human Kinetics.

Discovery Activity 8.4

Service-Learning for Weight Loss

Many American youths are overweight. This situation is so pervasive that one of the national health objectives for the year 2010 is to decrease the number of overweight youth. You can contribute to the achievement of this objective. Many schools offer various after-school programs. Some of these programs concern athletics, and others consist of tutoring or teaching computer skills. You could offer to conduct a weight-loss program for youth as part of a school's after-school program. Your program should be available to all youth interested in losing weight and should be consistent with the content of this chapter. In addition, you might consider developing written material about weight loss and nutrition to be sent home to parents or guardians so that what students learn can be incorporated into home menus. Furthermore, you could lobby the school administration to make foods consistent with weight loss available in the school cafeteria and the school's vending machines. As part of the program you develop, make sure to discuss inappropriate weight-loss techniques and eating disorders such as anorexia nervosa and bulimia with the youth participants.

Body Image

Chapter Objectives

By the end of this chapter, you should be able to

1. define body image as well as assess your own body image;
2. discuss the cultural, diet, and exercise influences on body image;
3. list several eating disorders, and discuss their causation, prevalence, and treatment; and
4. describe the relationship between body image and muscle dysmorphia, steroid use, and cosmetic surgery and makeovers.

Spring was coming and Jose was concerned. He could easily hide his "love handles" during the winter. All he had to do was wear a baggy sweater or sweatshirt, or keep his jacket on while indoors. But those strategies wouldn't hold up during spring and summer. What was Jose to do, especially when his friends expected him to go to the beach with the whole crowd?

Jose is not alone in being concerned—and sometimes embarrassed—about his body. One need only look at the popularity of diet books and cosmetic surgery and the prevalence of eating disorders. Too many of us do not accept our bodies. We have poor body images.

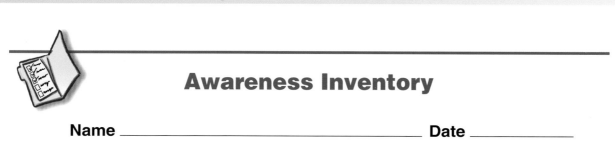

Awareness Inventory

Name _____ **Date** _____

Check the space by the letter T for the statements that you think are true and the space by the letter F for the statements that you think are false. The answers appear following the list of statements. This chapter will present information to clarify these statements for you. As you read the chapter, look for explanations for the reasons why the statements are true or false.

T ___ F ___   1. Most people are generally satisfied with their weight.

T ___ F ___   2. Women tend to be more dissatisfied with their weight than they are with other parts of their bodies, whereas men are more dissatisfied with their abdomens.

T ___ F ___   3. A significant percentage of girls don't start reading fashion magazines until they are in high school and are therefore unaffected by body images in those magazines.

T ___ F ___   4. Models in magazines and actors and actresses in films look perfect because generally they are.

T ___ F ___   5. The average American woman is 5 feet, 4 inches tall and weighs 144 pounds.

T ___ F ___   6. A study of the winners of the Miss America Pageant showed that their body shapes have remained relatively constant over the years.

T ___ F ___   7. Approximately 48 million adult Americans are on diets because these diets are successful in helping them achieve the body image they desire.

T ___ F ___   8. People who try to lose weight by exercise alone are no more successful than those who try to lose weight by dieting alone.

T ___ F ___   9. Because athletes need to be healthy to be competitive, they tend not to engage in disordered eating patterns.

T ___ F ___ 10. Muscle dysmorphia is a condition that bodybuilders may experience when they overtrain.

Answers: 1-F, 2-T, 3-F, 4-F, 5-T, 6-F, 7-F, 8-F, 9-F, 10-T

Analyze Yourself

Assessing Your Body Image

Name _____ **Date** _____

How healthy is your body image? To determine the answer to that question, circle the answer that best reflects how often you engage in the behaviors listed.

	Never	Sometimes	Often	Always
1. I dislike seeing myself in mirrors.	0	1	2	3
2. When I shop for clothing I am more aware of my weight problem and consequently I find shopping for clothes somewhat unpleasant.	0	1	2	3
3. I am ashamed to be seen in public.	0	1	2	3
4. I prefer to avoid engaging in sports or public exercise because of my appearance.	0	1	2	3
5. I feel somewhat embarrassed about my body in the presence of someone of the other sex.	0	1	2	3
6. I think my body is ugly.	0	1	2	3
7. I feel that other people must think my body is unattractive.	0	1	2	3
8. I feel that my family or friends may be embarrassed to be seen with me.	0	1	2	3
9. I find myself comparing myself with other people to see if they are heavier than I am.	0	1	2	3
10. I find it difficult to enjoy activities because I am self-conscious about my physical appearance.	0	1	2	3
11. Feeling guilty about my weight problem preoccupies most of my thinking.	0	1	2	3
12. My thoughts about my body and physical appearance are negative and self-critical.	0	1	2	3

Now, add up the number of points you have circled in each column: 0   + _____ + _____ + _____

Score interpretation

The lowest possible score is 0, which indicates a positive body image. The highest possible score is 36, which indicates an unhealthy body image. A score higher than 14 suggests a need to develop a healthier body image.

Source: Nash, J.D. 1997. *The New Maximize Your Body Potential*, Palo Alto, CA: Bull Publishing. Reprinted with permission of the publisher.

From *Physical fitness and wellness, third edition*, by Jerrold S. Greenberg, George B. Dintiman, and Barbee Myers Oakes, 2004, Champaign, IL: Human Kinetics.

Body image refers to the mental image we have of our physical appearance. Many factors influence body image, including how much we weigh, how our weight is distributed, our values about physical appearance, our concepts of good physical appearance, our ethnic and cultural background, what we see in people around us, what we hear through the media, and what we hear from others. Those with a better body image tend to be more confident and self-assured.

Body image in our society often tends to be problematic. Many people are dissatisfied with their bodies and experience the associated negative consequences. A survey conducted by Psychology Today (Garner, 1997) found that 89% of women polled wanted to lose weight and 22% of men wanted to gain weight. Some women also reported avoiding pregnancy because of a fear of what a pregnancy would do to their bodies. Table 9.1 cites percentages of 4,000 male and female respondents who reported dissatisfaction with specific parts of their bodies. Finally, recognizing the influence of the mass media on their perceptions of their bodies, 93% of women and 89% of men wanted models in magazines to represent the natural range of body shapes rather than the idealized versions they usually presented.

In another study, girls in grades 5 through 12 said they wanted to lose weight because of the pictures in magazines (Field et al., 1999). Interestingly, only 29% of the 548 girls interviewed were overweight. Even more alarming, one-third of these girls were in elementary school. Even at that age, 50% of the girls reported reading fashion magazines at least two to five times per month.

TABLE 9.1—Dissatisfaction With Body Parts

	Women	Men
Overall appearance	56%	43%
Weight	66%	52%
Height	16%	16%
Muscle tone	57%	45%
Breasts or chest	34%	38%
Abdomen	71%	63%
Hips or upper thighs	61%	29%

Reprinted with permission from *Psychology Today Magazine*, Copyright (1989 Sussex Publishers, Inc.).

body image—The mental image one has of one's body.

Those who read these magazines were three times as likely to have unrealistic body expectations.

The Elusive Perfect Body

What does the perfect body look like? To answer that question requires delineating the purposes we have in mind. Looking at successful female athletes can give us a clue. For example, the best female swimmers tend to be relatively tall and look like a capital Y from the front, with wide, flexible shoulders, long arms and hands, a narrow waist, and lightweight legs. Swimmers get by with more body fat than other athletes do because it lets them ride higher in the water. Top speed skaters, in contrast, are shorter and rather average from the waist up but tend to have heavily muscled legs with rather short thighs. Female gymnasts, on the other hand, have a lean, petite frame, small breasts, and long arms. The point is that a body that works for one purpose may be dysfunctional for another. As one observer noted, "The perfect body is one that will allow you to do things you enjoy and allow you to live life to the fullest—without compromising your health" (Barnette, 1993).

Why Models Look So Perfect

A quick glance at the covers of major fashion and sports magazines, and at their ads inside, usually depict men and women with perfect bodies. The same can often be said about actors in movies. These bodies seem almost too perfect to believe. Can these people really look like this all the time? The answer, of course, is no. To capture this perfect body image, models prepare meticulously for that millisecond when the camera's shutter captures their pose. Movie stars may spend months before shooting begins working with a personal trainer and controlling their diets to sculpt their bodies. Clothes, makeup, and lighting are carefully chosen to create the desired image. Hair styling, body makeup, and skintight outfits further enhance the image. As if that were not enough, after the photo or film is taken, editing refines the image to make it perfect. *Playboy* magazine regularly slims models' waists and thighs before publishing photos, and *Penthouse* magazine routinely augments breast size. Rumors are that when a playmate's rear end was judged to be not up to standard, a digital image of a more appealing rear end was used as a replacement.

The lesson to learn here is not to believe everything you see. Even the most beautiful and handsome models do not have perfect bodies. Consequently, for us to expect to have one is unrealistic. If we believe that a perfect body is possible and we can't acquire one, we subject ourselves to a lifetime of dissatisfaction about an important part of who we are.

These findings are not unexpected when one considers that the average American woman is 5 feet, 4 inches tall and weighs 144 pounds, whereas the average female model is 5 feet, 9 inches tall and weights 109 pounds. Furthermore, the typical fashion mannequins in stores have large breasts.

Girls grow up influenced by Barbie dolls with unrealistic body size and appearance. Add beauty pageants to the mix, and the situation becomes even more problematic. A study of the winners of the Miss America Pageant from 1922 to 1999 found that an increasing number of winners were in the range of undernutrition, as measured by body-mass index (Rubinstein and Caballero, 2000). Although pageant winners' heights increased by about 2%, their weights decreased by 12%. Boys are not immune to similar influences. They are subjected to muscular and defined bodies of Ken dolls and GI Joe action figures and see those as the body images they strive to achieve.

The result of these influences is that 85% of first-year male and female college students desire to change their body weight (Williams, 1996). Fully 40% of adult men and 55% of adult women are dissatisfied with their body weight.

Cultural Influences

Culture and ethnicity influence body image and body type. The National Health and Nutrition Examination Study (National Center For Health Statistics,1999) reported that 49% of African American and Hispanic women were overweight, as were 47% of Mexican American women. In addition, white men showed a steep increase in obesity. Other studies have found African American adolescent females to be happier with their bodies and less likely to diet than are European adolescent females.

A study of a large number of adolescent Caucasian, Latino, and African American males and females disclosed that the three ethnic groups differed significantly in their reports of body-image disturbances. A much higher percentage of Caucasian participants reported body-image concerns than did Latino or African American participants, who did not differ significantly from each other (Barry and Grilo, 2002).

The typically Western pattern of body dissatisfaction has overshadowed the traditional notions of female beauty among Asian women as well. Studies of Taiwanese college students found distorted body image and related risk factors leading to eating disorders to be common. Studies of Chinese undergraduates in Hong Kong and undergraduates in Iran found body-shape dissatisfaction among the women, even when they were not obese.

Diet

The diet business in the United States relishes these attitudes about weight and body image. After all, it is quite profitable for them. At any given time 48 million adult Americans, including 60% of adult women, are on a diet. We spend over $36 billion annually on diet products. In spite of these costs, relatively few people have long-term success controlling their weight. We have discussed weight control earlier in this book. Suffice it to say here that long-term weight control is a function of a permanent change in one's eating habits and incorporating physical activity into one's lifestyle.

Exercise

Exercise plays an important role in body image and self-esteem. One of the benefits of exercise relates to its effect on body weight. Studies have compared the ability of people to lose weight through various means. When people try to lose weight by diet alone, they are less successful than when they try to lose weight by exercise alone. The most successful strategy combines diet and exercise. In addition, with exercise as part of a weight-loss program, body-mass index improves. Exercise also helps tone muscles so that appearance is enhanced even if the scale shows no weight loss.

With these bodily changes comes greater self-esteem. Feelings of confidence and greater self-assurance accompany enhanced body image. And with greater self-esteem, one's relationships can improve, work and school productivity can increase, and general life satisfaction can be the result.

One reason that exercise can lead to weight loss is its effects on appetite. Moderate exercise decreases appetite. Recognizing this, if you are trying to lose weight, you might want to exercise before a meal. Another benefit of exercise is that it strengthens muscle tissue. Muscle tissue requires more calories to maintain itself than fat tissue does. Consequently, as lean-muscle tissue increases, the body burns more calories. As a result, resting metabolic rate, which accounts for approximately 70% of the calories we burn, increases, and greater weight loss occurs.

Of course, weight control is not magical. Controlling weight requires a permanent change in diet and adoption of a regular program of physical activity.

Issues Related to Body Image

Some people are so concerned about their body image that they develop health problems. These include eating disorders, obsessive and excessive muscular development, steroid use, and a variety of cosmetic surgeries.

Eating Disorders

Although we know that achieving a flawless body is impossible, some people are willing to pay a high cost to be attractive and try to perfect their bodies. Of course, the desire to control body weight to keep it within the recommended range is a healthy desire. To want to look attractive is also understandable. Yet some people go beyond the normal weight-control measures. Their fear of fat drives them to extreme behaviors. They may engage in binge eating (overeating) or compulsive dieting. Either of these behaviors can have dire health consequences. Although not limited to athletes, a desire to be competitive often results in eating disorders. One researcher found that among athletes, 15% of swimmers, 62% of gym-

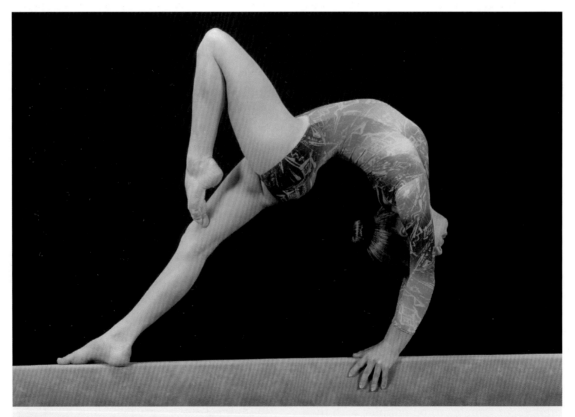

Elite athletes, particularly in sports such as gymnastics, can struggle with body image as much as other people do.
Corbis

nasts, and 32% of all varsity athletes showed disordered eating patterns (Wardlow, 1997).

Cultural beliefs and attitudes have been identified as significant contributing factors in the development of eating disorders. Rates of these disorders appear to vary among different racial and ethnic groups, and they change across time as cultures evolve. Yet emerging data on dieting disorders have indicated higher rates in some ethnic groups than previously recognized, among both American ethnic minorities and those in other countries. For example, a large-scale study of eating disorders in Iran found body dissatisfaction, a desire to be thin, and eating disorders to occur among female adolescents at rates comparable to those reported by studies in Western societies (Nobakht and Dezhkam, 2000).

Anorexia nervosa and bulimia, two eating disorders discussed here, are commonly believed to affect Caucasian women more than they do African American women at every age of comparison (Gordon et al., 2002). But a 1996 review of scientific studies on eating behaviors among American ethnic minority women found eating disturbances to be equally common among Hispanic and Caucasian females. They also found eating disturbances to be more frequent among Native American females than among Caucasian females. Like most other researchers, they reported a lower frequency among African American and Asian females (Crago, Shisslak, and Estes, 1996).

Risk factors for eating disorders are generally greater among ethnic minority females who are younger, more overweight, better educated, and more assimilated with White, middle-class values. Other studies also document an increase in eating disorders and pathological eating attitudes among ethnic minorities who report complex cultural expectations. When cultural demands are in conflict, eating disturbances often occur. For instance, a study of college women found that high pressure to assimilate was correlated with body dissatisfaction and bulimic symptoms among both African American and Hispanic women (Perez et al., 2002). Data such as these have prompted reconsideration of the view that ethnic minority populations are protected from eating disorders.

One eating disorder is anorexia nervosa, a condition in which an individual severely limits caloric intake. Anorexia nervosa is sometimes described as self-induced starvation. The diagnosis for anorexia nervosa appears in figure 9.1. Anorexia can be fatal, as it was for popular singer Karen Carpenter. Most people with anorexia are

A. Refusal to maintain body weight at or above a minimally normal weight for age and height (for example, weight loss leading to maintenance of body weight less than 85% of that expected or failure to make expected weight gain during period of growth, leading to body weight less than 85% of that expected).

B. Intense fear of gaining weight or becoming fat, even though underweight.

C. Disturbance in the way in which one's body weight or shape is experienced, undue influence of body weight or shape on self-evaluation, or denial of the seriousness of the current low body weight.

D. In postmenarcheal females, amenorrhea, that is, the absence of at least three consecutive menstrual cycles. (A woman is considered to have amenorrhea if her periods occur only following administration of hormones, for instance, estrogen.)

Specific Types

Restricting type: During the current episode of anorexia nervosa, the person has regularly engaged in binge-eating or purging behavior (that is, self-induced vomiting or the misuse of laxatives, diuretics, or enemas).

Figure 9.1 *DSM-IV:* Diagnostic criteria for anorexia nervosa.

White females under 25 years of age who have as their goal extreme thinness. They are willing to starve themselves and overexercise to reach that goal. Some males, especially models, can also be anorexic. Although the exact causes of anorexia nervosa are not known, it appears to be a result of several factors. Certainly one factor is society's emphasis on the "perfect" female body. Another factor may be an attempt to avoid dealing with issues related to intimacy and sexuality. But a major influence in the development of anorexia is the issue of control. Some people may feel that their weight is the only factor they can control in a world in which expectations of others seem difficult to fulfill.

In one study, 93% of female college athletes reported eating disorders. Fifty-one percent of women's gymnastics programs reported eating disorders among team members, a far greater percentage than in any other sport. One world-class gymnast at a well-known university admitted that her entire team would binge and vomit together after meets. Christy Henrich, another world-class gymnast, was 4 feet, 10 inches tall and weighed

muscle dysmorphia—Excessive weight training despite already having a muscular body.

steroids—Synthetic versions of the male hormone testosterone.

95 pounds at the peak of her career. Believing that she was too fat, she got her weight down to 61 pounds and eventually died of multiple organ failure at 22 years of age. Shortly before that, she had reduced her weight to 47 pounds (Dying to Win, 1994).

Another eating disorder is bulimia nervosa, in which a person periodically eats a lot of food and then purges the food through vomiting, laxatives, diuretics, and exercise. Bulimia differs from anorexia in several ways. First, the bulimic does not have thinness as a goal. Rather, he or she has an obsessive fear of becoming fat. Second, the bulimic tends to be older than the anorexic. Approximately 2% of the population is bulimic, with 95% of those being female. The diagnostic criteria for bulimia nervosa appear in figure 9.2.

A. The person engages in recurrent episodes of binge eating. An episode of binge eating is characterized by both of the following:

1. Eating, in a discrete period of time (for example, within any 2-hour period), an amount of food that is definitely larger than most people would eat during a similar period of time and under similar circumstances

2. A sense of lack of control over eating during the episode (for instance, a feeling that one cannot stop eating or control what or how much one is eating)

B. The person engages in recurrent inappropriate compensatory behavior to prevent weight gain, such as self-induced vomiting; misuse of laxatives, diuretics, enemas, or other medications; fasting; or excessive exercise.

C. The binge-eating and inappropriate compensatory behaviors both occur, on average, at least twice a week for 3 months.

D. Body shape and weight unduly influence self-evaluation.

E. The disturbance does not occur exclusively during episodes of anorexia nervosa.

Specific Types

Purging type: During the current episode of bulimia nervosa, the person has regularly engaged in self-induced vomiting or the misuse of laxatives, diuretics, or enemas.

Nonpurging type: During the current episode of bulimia nervosa, the person has used other inappropriate compensatory behaviors, such as fasting or excessive exercise but has not regularly engaged in self-induced vomiting or the misuse of laxatives, diuretics, or enemas.

Figure 9.2 *DSM-IV:* Diagnostic criteria for bulimia nervosa.

Still another eating disorder is binge-eating disorder (BED). Recurrent binge eating but not inappropriate weight-control behaviors characterize this condition. Persons with BED do not purge and, therefore, tend to be obese. The diagnostic criteria for binge-eating disorder appear in figure 9.3.

Muscle Dysmorphia

Another issue related to body image is **muscle dysmorphia.** Muscle dysmorphia refers to bodybuilders who, despite their muscular bodies and high fitness levels, consider themselves puny. In this case, weight training can become a dangerous obsession. These people are chasing the "perfect" body and have lost perspective about their actual body image. As many as 10% of male bodybuilders and 84% of female bodybuilders may suffer from "reverse anorexia." When the quest for massive size overtakes one's life, career, and relationships, self-esteem, ironically, can also suffer, and the possibility of physical injury increases. One researcher studied muscle dysmorphia in a sample of 323 female and male college students and found it common among athletes and non-athletes alike (Goodale, Watkins, and Cardinal, 2001).

Steroid Use

The use of drugs to change body size is another dangerous practice related to body image. **Steroids** are synthetic versions of the male hormone testosterone. People sometimes use steroids to achieve body mass quickly. As many as half a million Americans under the age of 18 may use steroids (National Institute on Drug Abuse, 1999), and one study found that 2.7% of high school students use steroids (Begley and Brant, 1999). About 6.5% of adolescent boys and 1.9% of girls reported using steroids without a prescription.

Steroids may have some benefits. For example, they can help female runners keep thin, use less energy during running, and hasten muscle recovery. But steroids produce side effects. Women can develop lower voices, grow more body and facial hair, develop male-pattern baldness, experience enlarged clitorises, have decreased breast size, and experience changes in or cessation of menstruation. Males may experience testicular shrinkage, impotence, infertility, baldness, prostate cancer,

---

A. The person engages in recurrent episodes of binge eating. An episode of binge eating is characterized by both of the following:

   1. Eating, in a discrete period of time (for example, within any 2-hour period), an amount of food that is definitely larger than most people would eat during a similar period under a similar circumstance.

   2. A sense of lack of control over eating during the episode (for instance, a feeling that one cannot stop eating or control what or how much one is eating).

B. The binge-eating episodes are associated with three or more of the following:

   1. Eating much more rapidly than normal.

   2. Eating until feeling uncomfortably full.

   3. Eating large amounts of food when not feeling physically hungry.

   4. Eating alone because of being embarrassed by how much one is eating.

   5. Feeling disgusted with oneself, depressed, or extremely guilty after overeating.

C. Marked distress regarding binge eating is present.

D. The binge eating occurs, on average, at least 2 days a week for 6 months.

E. The binge eating is not associated with the regular use of inappropriate compensatory behaviors (for example, purging, fasting, excessive exercise) and does not occur exclusively during the course of anorexia nervosa or bulimia nervosa.

Figure 9.3 *DSM-IV:* Proposed diagnostic criteria for binge-eating disorder.

American Psychiatric Association. *Diagnostic and Statistical Manual of Mental Disorders,* 4th ed. Washington, DC: American Psychological Association, 1994.

the development of breasts, or have difficulty or pain in urinating. Other side effects include liver malfunction, kidney disorders, increased serum cholesterol levels, a cessation of growth and bone development, aggression and violence, and bouts of depression. Furthermore, steroid use is illegal and therefore can have dire social consequences.

Cosmetic Surgery and Makeovers

In the quest for the "perfect" body, some people resort to surgery to alter body parts. One need only look at television and film stars for evidence of this trend. These public figures seek the fountain of youth in the surgeon's knife. As we observe these stars and their newfound youthful appearances and continue our quest for the perfect look, many of us are deciding we want a similar change. After all, with technologies such as liposuction, implants, and plastic surgery (cosmetic surgery) available to us, why should we not take advantage of the opportunity to be more attractive and avoid showing our age? Let's look more closely at some of these alternatives.

Liposuction

Liposuction is a technique for removing adipose (fat) tissue with a suction-pump device. A hollow suction tube attached to a special vacuum is inserted in small incisions in the skin. Liposuction is primarily used to remove fat around the abdomen, breasts, legs, face, and upper arms. It is the most popular cosmetic surgery in the United States, especially among women 30 to 49 years of age. Liposuction on a single body location can cost anywhere between $1,600 and $2,500, the cost of which is usually not covered by health insurance. Although liposuction can be helpful in removing fat in some areas, many people are surprised to learn that it results in an average loss of only 3 pounds of weight. As the procedure has grown in popularity, the number of inexperienced and incompetent practitioners offering the procedure has also grown. Even in the hands of a skilled surgeon, liposuction is not risk free. Some patients have ended up with scaring or rippling of the skin, and some need a follow-up procedure within 6 to 12 months to fix uneven results.

Breast Implants

Breast implants have been used for many years to enhance the size of the female breast. In recent years, concerns have developed that implants can

> **liposuction**—A surgical technique for removing adipose (fat) tissue with a suction-pump device.
>
> **rhinoplasty**—Surgery to alter the shape of the nose, colloquially referred to as a nose job.
>
> **tummy tuck**—A surgical procedure to remove excess skin and fat from the lower abdomen that also involves tightening the abdominal muscles.

cause systemic disease, that they can rupture or fail, and that such ruptures may produce toxicity. Although most researchers agree that implants are not the culprit described in the media, implant manufacturers have taken the easy way out and settled lawsuits from implant users. Of course, some women want their breast size reduced. In a culture that focuses extreme attention on the female breast, it is no wonder that women who believe that their breasts are too small or too large are willing to undergo these procedures to feel better about themselves. Feminists are quick to ask what males would do if society placed similar emphasis on penis size.

Cosmetic Surgery

Besides those just described, many other cosmetic surgery procedures are being performed. For the most part, White women are electing to have these surgeries. Statistically, approximately 16% of the total number of cosmetic surgeries are done on men, and only 6% on African Americans. After liposuction, the most prevalent cosmetic procedure is **rhinoplasty** (a nose job). Rhinoplasty usually takes 1 to 2 hours and costs between $2,700 and $4,700 (sometimes even more). Health insurance does not cover the procedure unless the structure of the nose impedes breathing. Potential negative outcomes include patients' dissatisfaction with the aesthetics of the new look, difficulty in breathing, or the formation of fibrous scar tissue.

Another type of cosmetic surgery is the **tummy tuck.** More extensive than liposuction, the tummy tuck removes excess skin and fat from the lower abdomen and involves tightening the abdominal muscles. The tummy tuck usually requires a hip-to-hip lower abdominal incision. This procedure usually costs between $4,700 and $6,400, and health insurance does not provide coverage.

Other forms of cosmetic surgery include face-lifts, upper and lower eyelid reduction, and chin implantation. Sometimes chemicals such

Myth and Fact Sheet

Myth	Fact
1. Most Americans are satisfied with their bodies.	1. Various studies have found Americans to be highly dissatisfied with their bodies. Women are typically more dissatisfied than men are, but both sexes want a better body image. Women tend to want to improve their weight, whereas men tend to want to improve their abdomens and have "washboard abs."
2. If you are unlucky enough to be born with a body type that you feel is unattractive, you can't really do anything to improve your body image.	2. You may not be able to do anything to improve your body (for example, you may have too large a nose), but you can do things to be more accepting of your body. You can use selective awareness by identifying parts of your body that you value and appreciating them more. Body image is the perception you have of your body, and you can perceive your body more positively if you realize that parts of it are worthy of your admiration.
3. The perfect body is one that is thin, tall, and curvy, with low body fat.	3. The perfect body doesn't exist. Different body types are best for different purposes. Body fat may be desirable for a swimmer or football player. A short body may be best for a jockey, and a thin body may be best for a gymnast. Besides, seeking the elusive perfect body may not be worth the sacrifice it requires, especially because it is unattainable anyhow.
4. Exercise may use up calories and be good for losing weight, but it increases your appetite. Therefore, the best way to lose weight is by dieting.	4. Studies have shown that the best way to lose weight is through a combination of diet and exercise. Exercise alone is a more effective weight-loss method than is dieting alone. One reason for that is that exercise decreases one's appetite.
5. Eating disorders represent a loss of control over one's eating patterns. To respond to this issue, the person needs to regain control over his or her diet.	5. Eating disorders often result from an obsession with maintaining control for people who believe they have little control over aspects of their lives other than food. Demonstrating that they are in control of their food intake by starving themselves serves their need for control.

as silicone or botox can be used. In short, just about any part of the body can be altered if one is motivated enough to do it and can afford the procedure. Many people are even changing the body to be more aesthetically appealing (in their opinion) with tattoos and body piercing. Although the most common sites for body piercing are the face or ears, people pierce their tongues, nipples, abdomen, and genitals. None of these cosmetic procedures is risk free. With piercing, for example, comes the risk of infection.

Summary

Body Image   Body image refers to the mental image we have of our bodies. Body image may be influenced by how much we weigh, how our weight is distributed, our values about our physical appearance, our concepts of a good physical appearance, our ethnic and cultural background, what we see in others around us, what we hear through the media, and what we hear from others. Many people in our society are dissatisfied with

Behavioral Change and Motivational Strategies

Many factors influence your perception of your body. Here are some barriers (roadblocks) to developing a positive body image and strategies for overcoming them.

Roadblock	Behavioral Change Strategy
You have friends who are more attractive than you are, and their good looks make you feel dissatisfied with your body.	You can engage in self-talk by identifying your positive attributes and being prepared to focus on those when you feel particularly unconfident about your body image. Remember, the parts of yourself that need improvement coexist with parts of you that are laudable. Don't neglect focusing on those parts when you feel vulnerable. You could also use the behavior change technique of placing reminder notes on your refrigerator or bathroom mirror that cite your positive attributes.
Family and friends often criticize you about your weight and appearance.	Make a list of your good qualities and read it when others try to get you down. Be sure to include the good things that other people say about you as well. Remember that many people love and respect you, despite the hurtful comments that you sometimes hear. That realization should help you focus on the reasons why you too should love and respect yourself, including your body.
You often think about your negative attributes and wind up depressed and embarrassed about your body.	Use contracting to encourage the stopping of negative thoughts. Reward yourself every time you recognize that you have been having negative thoughts and seek to decrease the number of times those thoughts crop up. Another way to use thought stopping is to wear a rubber band on your wrist. Every time you recognize that you have a negative thought related to body image, snap the rubber band. You'll soon tire of the discomfort of the snapping rubber band and decrease the number, or at least the time devoted to, those thoughts.
You have attempted to improve your body but have been unable to stick with any program. This is frustrating for you.	You appear to be at the decision, or determination, stage of the stages of change theory. What you need to do now is to plan a program tailored to your lifestyle—a program that you would enjoy participating in and that will meet the goal of improving your body. Often it is advisable to seek the help of someone with expertise in planning these programs. A private trainer, if you can afford one, is a viable option. If your financial resources are limited, your instructor or a faculty member in the physical education department might be willing to help. Don't be bashful in asking for this kind of assistance.
List roadblocks that interfere with your working on improving your body image.	Now cite behavioral change strategies that can help you overcome the roadblocks you just listed. If necessary, refer back to chapter 4 for behavioral change and motivational strategies.

1. _____

2. _____

3. _____

1. _____

2. _____

3. _____

their body images. Females are most dissatisfied with their weight, and males are most dissatisfied with their abdomens.

The Elusive Perfect Body Different body types are appropriate for different activities. A body that works for one purpose may be dysfunctional for another. No one body is the best. The most appropriate body is one that allows someone to do the things that he or she enjoys and allows that person to live life to the fullest, without compromising health.

Why Models Look So Perfect Models and actors often appear to have the perfect body, but that impression is deceiving. Movie stars and models may spend months working with a personal trainer and controlling their diets to sculpt their bodies. In addition, the clothes they wear and the lighting are carefully controlled to make the body as appealing as possible. As if that is not enough, hair styling, body makeup, and skintight outfits add to the appearance of the "perfect" body. When all of that doesn't do the trick, images are sometimes digitally altered. Breasts may be enlarged or rear ends altered with enhanced computer technology.

Cultural Influences Culture and ethnicity influence body image and body type. For example, studies have found that a higher proportion of African American, Hispanic, and Mexican women are overweight. White men show an increase in obesity in recent years. What is appealing in one culture or for one ethnic group may not be appealing in another. For example, African American adolescent females tend to be happier with their bodies and less likely to diet than are European adolescent females.

Diet At any given time, approximately 48 million adult Americans, including 60% of adult women, are on a diet. Americans spend $36 billion annually on diet products. Yet relatively few people have long-term success controlling their weight.

Exercise Exercise plays an important role in body image and self-esteem. Exercise alone is more effective in helping people lose weight than dieting alone is. The most successful weight-control strategy is a combination of diet and exercise. Exercise also helps tone muscles so that one's appearance is enhanced even if the scale shows no weight loss. One reason that exercise can lead to weight loss is its effects on appetite. Moder-

ate exercise decreases appetite. Another benefit of exercise is that it strengthens muscle tissue. Muscle tissue requires more calories to maintain itself than fat tissue does. Consequently, as lean-muscle tissue increases, more calories are burned. As a result, resting metabolic rate, which accounts for approximately 70% of the calories we burn, increases, and greater weight loss occurs.

Issues Related to Body Image Issues associated with body image include eating disorders, obsessive and excessive muscular development, steroid use, and cosmetic surgery. Among the most problematic eating disorders are anorexia nervosa (severely limiting caloric intake), bulimia nervosa (periodically binge eating and then purging), and binge-eating disorder (eating a lot of food but not engaging in inappropriate weight-control behaviors).

Another problem related to body image is muscle dysmorphia. Muscle dysmorphia refers to bodybuilders who, despite their muscular bodies and high fitness levels, consider themselves puny. For them, weight training can become a dangerous obsession. Muscle dysmorphia is common among both athletes and nonathletes.

The use of drugs to change body size is another dangerous practice related to body image. Steroids are synthetic versions of the male hormone testosterone. People sometimes use steroids to achieve body mass quickly. Women who use steroids can develop lower voices, grow more body and facial hair, develop male-pattern baldness, experience enlarged clitorises, have decreased breast size, and experience changes in or cessation of menstruation. Males may experience a cessation of growth and bone development, testicular shrinkage, increased serum cholesterol levels, infertility, decreased sexual drive, prostate cancer, kidney disorders, liver malfunction, aggression and violence, suicidal tendencies, and extreme moodiness.

In the quest for the perfect body, some people resort to surgery to alter body parts. Among the more prevalent cosmetic surgeries are liposuction (removing fat tissue with a suction-pump device), breast implants or breast reduction, rhinoplasty (nose job), tummy tucks (removing excess fat and skin from the lower abdomen), face-lifts, upper and lower eyelid reduction, and chin implantation. Some people use chemicals such as botox to alter the face, and others use body piercing to improve their body image.

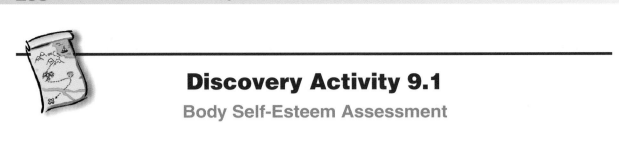

Discovery Activity 9.1
Body Self-Esteem Assessment

Name _____ **Date** _____

What do you think about your physical self? How highly do you regard your physical self? This activity will help you discover the answers to these questions. Using the scale that follows, place the number alongside each body part or body function that represents your feelings about that part of yourself.

Scale

1 = have strong feelings and wish to change

2 = do not like, but can tolerate

3 = have no particular feelings one way or the other

4 = am satisfied

5 = would not change and consider myself fortunate

Body Part or Function

_____ hair	_____ legs	_____ chest	_____ body build
_____ hands	_____ feet	_____ lips	_____ ankles
_____ nose	_____ knees	_____ teeth	_____ height
_____ wrists	_____ appetite	_____ voice	_____ eyes
_____ back	_____ fingers	_____ posture	_____ skin texture
_____ chin	_____ waist	_____ facial complexion	_____ forehead
_____ neck	_____ ears	_____ shoulder width	_____ health
_____ arms	_____ weight	_____ energy level	_____ face
_____ hips	_____ profile	_____ shape of head	

Scoring

Now add up the point values you assigned and divide the total by 35. Your score should fall between 1 and 5. If your score is below 2.5, you do not hold your body in high esteem. If your score is above 2.5, you think well of your body. In particular, look at those items to which you assigned a 1 or a 2. Those are the parts of your body or bodily functions that you think are most in need of improvement. By improving those parts or functions using safe, healthy methods or accepting who you are and what you look like, you will think better of your body.

From *Physical fitness and wellness, third edition*, by Jerrold S. Greenberg, George B. Dintiman, and Barbee Myers Oakes, 2004, Champaign, IL: Human Kinetics.

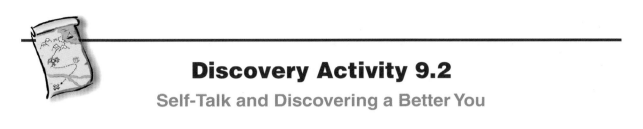

Discovery Activity 9.2

Self-Talk and Discovering a Better You

Name _____ **Date** _____

Everyone has parts of his or her body, personality, or limitations with which he or she is unsatisfied. Many people focus on those aspects of themselves and, as a result, they remain unhappy. Concurrent with parts of ourselves that we would wish to change, however, are parts of ourselves about which we are proud, happy, or satisfied. If we focused on those parts, we would achieve more satisfaction with ourselves and our lives. This way of thinking does not mean that we ignore the parts of ourselves that need improvement. Certainly, each of us should desire to grow as a person and become better. Still, to focus on the need for improvement while ignoring the many positive traits we have is dysfunctional. One way to remember that we have many positive traits is to use a technique called self-talk. You can use self-talk to convert negative thoughts to positive ones. For example, you might say to yourself, "My nose is too big," and feel sorry for yourself as a result. Using self-talk in that example, you might say to yourself, "My nose is too big, but I have very attractive blue eyes." This approach does not ignore the negative, but it adds a positive to it—a positive that is as true as the negative you might otherwise have focused on.

Identify five parts of yourself (for example, body parts, personality characteristics, physical or intellectual limitations) that you think need improvement. Alongside each part listed, write a self-talk statement that identifies a positive aspect of yourself related to the negative one you listed.

1. Negative aspect: _____

   Positive aspect: _____

2. Negative aspect: _____

   Positive aspect: _____

3. Negative aspect: _____

   Positive aspect: _____

4. Negative aspect: _____

   Positive aspect: _____

5. Negative aspect: _____

   Positive aspect: _____

Learn to work on improving the parts of yourself that require attention but do not forget the parts of yourself about which you should feel good.

From *Physical fitness and wellness, third edition,* by Jerrold S. Greenberg, George B. Dintiman, and Barbee Myers Oakes, 2004, Champaign, IL: Human Kinetics.

Discovery Activity 9.3

Service-Learning for Body Image

We have discussed the research findings that show that collegiate athletes are prone to eating disorders. You can contribute to the well-being of your college community by helping athletes on your campus recognize the implications of these disordered eating patterns, while learning more about these conditions yourself. Review the information on weight control and nutrition presented in chapter 8 and the information presented in this chapter citing which sports tend to have athletes prone to these eating patterns. Then approach the coaches of those sports and offer to conduct workshops on nutrition, weight control, and eating disorders at the beginning of the practice sessions for their competitive seasons. As part of your planning for these workshops, develop written handouts that can be distributed to the athletes so that they have a healthy eating guide to which they can refer during the season. These handouts should include the food pyramid, description of various eating disorders (for example, anorexia nervosa, bulimia nervosa), and information about other body-image issues such as dysmorphia.

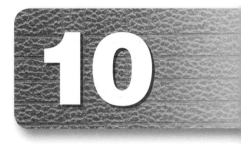

Nutrition

Chapter Objectives

By the end of this chapter, you should be able to

1. discuss the functions of the six categories of nutrients in the diet;

2. compare carbohydrates, fats, and proteins in terms of how each provides energy to the body;

3. describe a sound nutritional plan based on the recommended daily intakes (DRIs) and the USDA's food guide pyramid;

4. demonstrate the ability to read a food label;

5. discuss the role of nutrition in the prevention of disease;

6. describe the special nutritional needs of active individuals, aging individuals, and women; and

7. dispel common nutritional myths.

During Rita's freshman year, cafeteria food became unappealing. She had gained 9 pounds, had low energy, and was aware that she was eating too much fat. She also was sick several times and wondered whether any of the illnesses were related to her poor eating habits. To be honest, Rita had to admit that she simply didn't know enough about proper nutrition. Even if she discontinued the university meal plan, she would not know what to do.

This chapter focuses on Rita's concerns and presents an overview of sound nutrition to help her (and others like her) make appropriate choices in the cafeteria or prepare her own nutritional program. The discussion covers the basic food components, the energy nutrients (carbohydrates, fats, proteins), the nonenergy nutrients (vitamins, minerals, water), food density, dietary guidelines for good health and high energy, food labeling, additives, nutrition-disease relationships, cooking and cancer, nutrition and aging, and special needs of the active person.

Awareness Inventory

Name _____ **Date** _____

Check the space by the letter T for the statements that you think are true and the space by the letter F for the statements that you think are false. The answers appear following the list of statements. This chapter will present information to clarify these statements for you. As you read the chapter, look for explanations for the reasons why the statements are true or false.

T ___ F ___ 1. Saturated fat is found only in animal products such as pork, beef, and other meat products.

T ___ F ___ 2. Margarine can be consumed freely because it has no known health consequences.

T ___ F ___ 3. The primary fuel for aerobic exercise is fat.

T ___ F ___ 4. Fruits, vegetables, and grains contain no cholesterol.

T ___ F ___ 5. Trans-fatty acids form during processing when hydrogen is added to unsaturated vegetable oil to ensure consistency, prevent rancidity, and make the product more solid at room temperature.

T ___ F ___ 6. The number one cause of adult-onset type 2 diabetes is obesity.

T ___ F ___ 7. When blood-glucose levels are too high, the pancreas secretes the hormone, insulin, which removes excess glucose to storage in the liver and muscles.

T ___ F ___ 8. Glucagon is a hormone secreted by the pancreas when blood-sugar levels are too low.

T ___ F ___ 9. The fat-soluble vitamins include vitamin C and the B-complex vitamins.

T ___ F ___ 10. A large portion of the vitamins consumed in food products is absorbed, whereas only a small portion of minerals consumed is absorbed.

Answers: 1-F, 2-F, 3-T, 4-T, 5-T, 6-T, 7-T, 8-T, 9-F, 10-T

From *Physical fitness and wellness, third edition*, by Jerrold S. Greenberg, George B. Dintiman, and Barbee Myers Oakes, 2004, Champaign, IL: Human Kinetics.

Analyze Yourself

Assessing Your Dietary Behavior

Name _____ **Date** _____

Instructions: Indicate how often each of the following occurs in your daily schedule. Respond to each item with a number from 0 to 3, using the following scale:

0 = Never   **1** = Occasionally   **2** = Most of the time   **3** = Always

____ **1.** When shopping for food, I read nutrition labels before buying and select items low in fat and salt and moderate in calories.

____ **2.** I make sure I consume less than 300 milligrams of cholesterol daily.

____ **3.** I drink a minimum of six glasses of water daily, exclusive of products such as sodas, coffee, and tea.

____ **4.** I try to consume servings from the five food groups daily.

____ **5.** I limit my alcohol intake to one or two drinks daily.

____ **6.** I consume the proper amount of protein daily, even when I am restricting my caloric intake.

____ **7.** I limit my daily intake of total fat to 30% or less of my needed daily calories.

____ **8.** I consume a sufficient amount of fruits, vegetables, and grains to obtain a minimum of 25 to 35 grams of dietary fiber daily.

____ **9.** I take no more than one multiple vitamin and mineral daily.

____ **10.** As recommended on the nutrition pyramid, I consume products containing fats, oils, and sweets sparingly.

Scoring: Excellent eating habits = 25 to 30

Good eating habits; can be improved = 19 to 24

Poor eating habits; change needed = below 19

Kinds of Nutrients

Six categories of nutrients—carbohydrates, fats, and proteins (the energy nutrients); and vitamins, minerals, and water (the nonenergy nutrients)—satisfy basic body needs:

- Energy for muscle contraction
- Conduction of nerve impulses
- Growth
- Formation of new tissue and tissue repair
- Chemical regulation of metabolic functions
- Reproduction

The body's use of these nutrients for conversion into tissue, for production of energy for muscle contraction, and for maintenance of chemical machinery is called **metabolism.**

Energy Nutrients

Carbohydrates and fat provide the body with its two main sources of energy. All food has energy potential, measured in **calories.** When you see the term calorie on a food label or in reference to the number of calories the body needs or burns, it refers to kilocalories or large calories. One kilocalorie is the amount of heat required to raise the temperature of 1 kilogram of water 1° Celsius. Because the term kilocalorie is generally reserved for laboratories and technical journals, we use the term calorie throughout this chapter. The energy in one peanut, for example, can add 1° of heat to 2 gallons of water. Only carbohydrates, fats, and protein contain calories; vitamins, minerals, and water do not.

Just how much energy do these nutrients provide? Carbohydrates and protein contain 4 calories per gram, fat contains 9 calories per gram, and alcohol contains 7 calories per gram (1 gram equals about one-fifth of a level teaspoon, 100 grams equal one-half cup, 1 milligram equals .001 gram).

Recall that basal metabolism (BMR) is the minimum energy the body needs to support the ongoing activities of the cells when the body is at rest, or the work that goes on continuously without awareness. This represents the largest (60% or more) portion of your daily caloric expenditure and amounts to about 1,200 to 1,400 calories daily for an individual whose total energy expenditure is 2,000 calories. Factors such as drugs (caffeine and other stimulants), fever, growth (higher in children and pregnant women), height and weight, ingestion of a meal

(thermic effect of food), gender (males have more lean-muscle tissue), muscle mass, stress, and the thyroid hormone increase BMR. Age and reduced caloric intake (fasting, starvation, low-calorie diets) decrease BMR.

Your metabolic rate or metabolism refers to the energy you expend to maintain all physical and chemical changes occurring in the body. This includes basal metabolism, exercise metabolism (**thermic effect of exercise**), and calories expended following ingestion of food. Your total daily caloric expenditure breaks down as follows:

- Basal metabolism: 60 to 65%
- Thermic effect of exercise: 25 to 30%
- Thermic effect of food: 5 to 10%

You can determine your daily total caloric needs by completing Discovery Activity 10.1: Estimating Caloric Expenditure at the end of this chapter.

Carbohydrates

Carbohydrates are organic components of various elements that provide a continuous supply of energy in the form of glucose (sugar) to trillions of body cells. **Simple carbohydrates (monosaccharides and disaccharides)** come in concentrated form—such as refined sugar, made from cane or beet sugar, molasses, and honey—and in natural form—such as the sugars in some fruits,

---

metabolism—The sum of energy expended in carrying on the normal body processes: converting nutrients into tissue, fueling muscle contraction, and maintaining the body's chemical machinery.

calories—A large calorie, equal to 1,000 small calories; 1 calorie is the amount of heat required to raise the temperature of 1 kilogram (about 1 quart) of water 1° Celsius.

thermic effect of food—The increase in the basal metabolic rate following the ingestion of a meal; lasts 1 to 4 hours.

thermic effect of exercise—The increase in metabolism brought about by activity or muscular movement during the day.

simple carbohydrates (monosaccharides and disaccharides)—Sugars; chains of sugar molecules (one or two) found in concentrated sugar and the sugar that occurs naturally in food.

complex carbohydrates (polysaccharides)—Starch and fiber; chains of sugar molecules (three or more) found in fruits, vegetables, and grains.

adipose tissue—Fatty tissue; fat cells.

vegetables, and grains. **Complex carbohydrates (polysaccharides)** are chains of sugar molecules found in fruits, vegetables, and grains. Carbohydrates are broken down into six simple carbon-sugar molecules to permit absorption into the bloodstream. After food is eaten, blood-sugar level rises and the amount of glucose transported to the cells increases. The body converts excess sugar to glycogen and stores it for future use in the liver and muscles. Once maximum storage capacity is reached, excess sugars are converted to body fat and stored in **adipose tissue.**

Simple Versus Complex Carbohydrates

We consume simple carbohydrates (sugars) in four forms: sucrose, glucose, fructose, and lactose. Annual intake of cane and beet sugar in the United States exceeds 100 pounds per person; Americans also consume 20 to 25 pounds of syrups (glucose and fructose) each year, bringing the total intake to over 125 pounds of sugar per person per year. Consumed in these large quantities, sugar contributes directly to dental cavities, excessive weight, and body fat and indirectly to such degenerative diseases as diabetes and heart disease. As you can see from the sugar content of foods in table 10.1, a person can easily consume the equivalent of 50 teaspoons of sugar per day.

Sugar intake should be managed from infancy. Infants seem to be born with a preference for sweet foods, and it is not until early adulthood that the desire for sugar slowly decreases. You can reduce your sugar intake by reading the labels for sweeteners and sugars in products you are considering. Product labels that include the terms sucrose, glucose, dextrose, fructose, corn syrup, corn sweetener, natural sweetener, and invert sugar mean that the product contains sugar. You can further reduce your sugar intake by substituting water and unsweetened fruit juices for sodas and punches, buying fruit canned in its own unsweetened juice, cutting back on desserts, buying cereals low in sugar, reducing the amount of sugar called for in recipes, and avoiding sweet snacks. Simple sugars or so-called foodless foods contribute very little to sound nutrition and should be consumed in moderation.

We must dispel a number of popular misconceptions about the consumption of simple carbohydrates (sugars):

- "Carbohydrates are the leading cause of obesity." Excess calories and too little physical activity, not the consumption of carbohydrates,

TABLE 10.1—Sugar Content of Common Foods and Drinks

Food or drink	Size	Approximate content (teaspoons)
Beverages	12 oz	
Sodas		5-9
Sweet cider		4 1/4
Jams and jellies, candies	1 tbsp	4-6
Milk chocolate	1 1/2 oz	2 1/2
Fudge	1 oz	4 1/2
Hard candy	4 oz	20
Marshmallow	1	1 1/2
Fruits and canned juices		
Dried raisins, prunes, apricots, dates	3-5	4
Fruit juice	8 oz	2 1/2-3 1/2
Breads		
White	1 slice	1/4
Hamburger or hot dog bun	1	3
Dairy products		
Ice cream cone	Single dip	3
Sherbet	Single scoop	9
Desserts		
Pie (fruit, custard cream)	1 slice	4-13
Pudding	1/2 cup	3-5

are the biggest contributors to multiple causes of obesity.

- "Only refined sugars cause tooth decay." These sugars are the leading dietary cause of tooth decay. Sugars such as fructose in fruit and lactose in milk, and foods high in fermentable carbohydrates (bread and rice) also contribute. A more important factor is sticky foods that remain on the teeth longer and do more damage.

- "Sugar makes children hyperactive." No evidence exists to support this notion.
- "The sugar in fruit is good, and the sugar in candy is bad." Fructose (in fruit sugar) has no advantages over sucrose (in candy). Sugar is sugar and no type, including honey and brown sugar, offers a nutritional advantage over another.

Complex carbohydrates are your major source of vitamins (except vitamin B12) and minerals, an important long-term energy source and the only source of fiber. Complex carbohydrates burn efficiently, leave no toxic waste in the body, and do not tax the liver or raise blood-fat levels. Fruits, vegetables, and grains also have high **nutrition density,** providing a high percentage of our needed daily nutrients in a low number of calories. In the past 75 years, our intake of complex carbohydrates has declined by about 30% while sugar intake has increased by a similar amount. Unlike sugars, complex carbohydrates are the body's chief source of fuel. Sugar, on the other hand, provides empty calories and little long-term energy.

Complex carbohydrates should make up at least 45% of your total daily calories. You should reduce simple carbohydrates to 5 or 6% of total calories.

Soft Drinks

Sodas (junk food) now account for over 28% of our refined sugar intake, partly because of the popularity of extra-large, supersized containers such as 64-ounce big gulps. Although an occasional soda is not detrimental, habitual use is harmful. A 12-ounce soda, for example, contains 150 calories and the equivalent of 5 to 9 teaspoons of sugar. Two sodas daily can add as much as 1 pound of fat every 12 days. Even the popularity of diet sodas has failed to keep us from becoming fatter. Diet sodas, like regular sodas, crowd good foods out of the diet and contribute to poor nutrition. Sodas may also directly or indirectly increase the risk of bone fractures. Those who drink many sodas are likely to consume less milk, leafy green vegetables, and other calcium sources. Animal studies indicate that the phosphorus content of colas may lead to calcium loss and weak bones. With phosphorus plentiful in the diet, this has not been proved in humans. Many soft drinks also contain from 20 to 70 milligrams of caffeine per serving. In addition, carbonated drinks cause temporary bloating, stomach upset,

and even heartburn in some people. It is good practice to fight off the urge for a regular or diet soft drink and choose water, keeping soda intake to no more than two per day.

Energy Drinks

A new breed of concoctions containing high amounts of caffeine and sugar mixed with herbs and other substances is becoming increasingly popular among the younger generation as a pick-me-up energy drink. Although these drinks are little more than sugar and caffeine, like most existing soda pops, some experts are concerned about the already high levels of caffeine and sugar consumption and the practice of mixing energy drinks with alcohol. A few drinks also contain the drug ephedrine (a stimulant found in decongestants) that can cause deadly heart problems when combined with caffeine. The long-term effect of these drinks has some experts worried.

Fiber

As the indigestible portion of complex carbohydrates, dietary or **insoluble fiber** is a nonnutritive substance that the enzymes in the human body cannot break down. Six of the seven types of fiber are carbohydrates. Only lignin, found in fruit and vegetable skins and the woody portions of plants, is a noncarbohydrate.

Table 10.2 provides an overview of key information on fiber, including soluble and insoluble varieties, recommended daily intake, nutritional advantages of consuming adequate amounts, dangers of excess intake, and the food sources for both types. Complete Discovery Activity 10.2: Estimating Your Daily Fiber Intake at the end of this chapter to discover whether your diet contains enough fiber.

Blood-Glucose Control

The pancreas regulates blood-glucose levels. When blood-sugar levels are too high, the pancreas releases a hormone called **insulin,** which promotes the movement of glucose into certain

---

nutrition density—A measure of the nutrient value per calorie.

insoluble fiber—The indigestible portion of food after it is exposed to the body's enzymes.

insulin—A natural hormone produced in the pancreas gland that aids in the digestion of sugars and other carbohydrates; secreted when blood sugar is too high.

TABLE 10.2—All About Fiber

Characteristic	Description
Water insoluble	Cellulose, forming the cell walls of many plants, is the most abundant insoluble fiber. Cellulose and lignin (from the woody portion of plants, parts of fruit and vegetable skins, and whole grains) cannot be broken down, digested, or made to provide calories for the body.
Water soluble	Fiber types such as pectin, gums, and mucilages dissolve or swell when placed in water. Dried beans and peas (8 g per 1/2 cup), oat bran, and the flesh of fruits and vegetables are excellent sources of water-soluble fiber.
Dietary fiber	Undigested residue after the action of the body's enzymes; much more concentrated than crude fiber (1 g of crude fiber = 2-3 g of dietary fiber). Most labels that list fiber content report dietary fiber (water insoluble).
Daily needs	25-35 g. To avoid frequent bowel movements and diarrhea, increase your daily intake slowly if you are unaccustomed to adequate fiber. Add several grams daily over a period of a few weeks to give your system a chance to adjust.
Nutritional advantages of consuming adequate fiber	Insoluble fiber (dietary fiber) decreases the amount of time bacteria in food has to act on intestinal walls; collects and holds destructive bile acids and protects the intestinal wall from damage; increases stool bulk and weight and speeds the elimination of dietary carcinogens from the body; produces short-chained fatty acids as fiber ferments in the colon, which regulates the growth rate of cells lining the colon; slows absorption of food to help keep glucose and insulin levels steady; helps prevent colon cancer, rectal cancer, and diverticulitis (outpouching in the wall of the large intestine); helps eliminate constipation; maintains normal bowel movement; and helps control and maintain normal body weight and fat. Soluble fiber is associated with lower incidence of cardiovascular disease, lower blood cholesterol, and lower blood pressure. Soluble fiber may also improve blood-sugar tolerance by delaying glucose absorption and help prevent obesity by prolonging eating time and replacing calories from fat.
Dangers of excess fiber	Excess fiber binds to some trace minerals and causes excretion before the absorption of these minerals. Excessive fiber intake causes poor absorption of nutrients, interferes with the absorption of some drugs, reduces the ability to digest and absorb food by speeding up digestive time, and causes irritation of the intestinal wall. The high phosphorus content of high-fiber foods may create special problems for some individuals, such as those with kidney problems. Too much fiber blocks the absorption of some minerals, such as iron, copper, and zinc. If you now consume little fiber in your diet and are making the change to 25-35 g daily, increase your intake gradually over a period of several weeks and consume at least eight 8-ounce glasses of water daily to help your body adjust to the change.
Food sources	Complex carbohydrates (fruits, vegetables, grains) are the sole source of fiber. Both insoluble and soluble fiber are contained in some food sources, such as in the skin of fruits and vegetables (insoluble) and in the flesh of fruits and vegetables (soluble). Raw fruits and vegetables are a major source of insoluble fiber such as in dried beans and peas (8 g per 1/2 cup). Oat bran and grains are a major source of soluble fiber. Many hot and cold cereals (unprocessed bran, 100% bran, shredded wheat, oatmeal) contain 2-5 g of fiber per serving. Legumes provide about 8 g per portion (1/2 cup of garbanzo beans, kidney beans, or baked beans). Fruits provide about 2 g per serving (1 small apple, banana, orange; 2 small plums, 1 medium peach, 1/2 cup of strawberries, 10 large cherries). Vegetables also provide about 2 g per serving (broccoli, brussels sprouts, stalks of celery, small corn on the cob, lettuce, green beans, small potato, tomato), and 1 g of fiber is provided by 10 peanuts, 1/4 cup of walnuts, 2 1/2 teaspoons of peanut butter, and 1 pickle. Additional foods with fiber are breads (whole wheat, whole grain), crackers, and flours (wheat germ, wild rice, cornmeal, buckwheat, millet, rice, raisin, popcorn). Cooking does not significantly reduce the fiber content of foods.
Supplements	Two studies after 1997 found no link at all between fiber supplements and colon cancer. You should obtain your daily soluble and insoluble fiber from adequate consumption of fruits, vegetables, and grains, not from supplements.

cells, dropping blood-sugar levels. When levels are too low, the pancreas secretes a hormone called **glucagon,** which stimulates the conversion of stored liver glycogen into glucose and the conversion of noncarbohydrates into glucose to raise the blood-sugar level (see figure 10.1). The pancreas of individuals suffering from type 1 (insulin-dependent) diabetes mellitus fails to produce insulin, so it must be injected to control blood-glucose levels. The pancreas of most individuals suffering from adult-onset, type 2 (non-insulin-dependent) **diabetes mellitus** produces insulin; glucose uptake at the cellular level, however, does not occur normally, and blood-sugar levels remain high. For most of us, the pancreas does its job and, in conjunction with proper diet, maintains blood glucose at normal levels regardless of what we eat and how much we exercise.

Although use of the term is controversial, foods with a high **glycemic index** cause a rapid rise

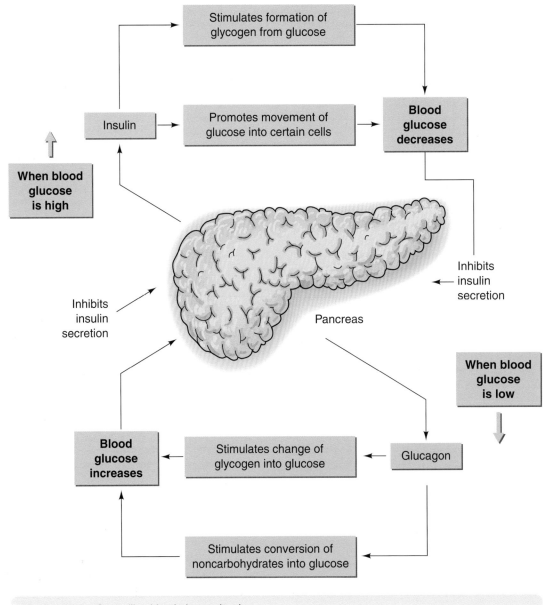

Figure 10.1 Controlling blood-glucose levels.

Reprinted from D.C. Nieman, D.E. Butterworth, and C.N. Nieman, 1992, *Nutrition, revised* 1st ed. (Dubuque, IA: Wm. C. Brown Publishers). Reproduced with permission of The McGraw-Hill Companies.

in blood-glucose levels if they are not consumed with adequate amounts of protein or foods with a low glycemic index. Foods with a high glycemic index, such as those containing large amounts of concentrated sugars, include maple syrup, table sugar, honey, molasses, bagels, raisins, white potatoes, sweet corn, and cornflakes. Foods with a low glycemic index include apples, cherries, chickpeas, lentils, dates, figs, peaches, plums, green beans, kidney beans, navy beans, red lentils, and skim milk. A rapid increase in blood-glucose levels can lead to both fatigue and hunger. (See chapter 8 for more information on controlling hunger and appetite and the role of changes in blood-glucose levels.)

Hypoglycemia

Low blood sugar (60 milligrams per deciliter or less) is called hypoglycemia. The condition is generally caused by skipping meals, eating at the wrong time, exercising longer or more strenuously than usual, or not adjusting medication properly (diabetics). Hypoglycemia is of two types: True hypoglycemia is rare and is a symptom of some severe condition such as liver problems, stomach surgery, or tumor of the pancreas rather than a disease. Reactive hypoglycemia is a common term applied to a complex set of symptoms that may or may not have anything to do with blood-sugar levels. Shortly after eating a meal, some individuals feel dizzy, unwell, or faint and ill. To diagnose hypoglycemia properly, blood samples should be taken when these symptoms are present to reveal whether they are related to blood-glucose levels (most will show normal glucose levels). Experts indicate that you should be skeptical about a diagnosis of reactive hypoglycemia and insist on testing to establish its presence. During the presence of symptoms, a blood-sugar level of 45 milligrams per deciliter (or lower) confirms the presence of significant hypoglycemia. Many patients who suspect hypoglycemia actually have blood sugars exceeding 50 milligrams, indicating that they do not suffer from this disorder. Patients meeting the 45-milligram criterion should receive further testing to rule out other problems.

Nutritional changes for hypoglycemia include eating smaller, more frequent meals; avoiding concentrated sugar; and limiting coffee and alcohol intake. A diet rich in fruits, whole grains, and vegetables is the best way to keep blood-sugar level normal. When your energy level drops between meals, eat fruits, vegetables, and grains and avoid food and drink with a high glycemic index.

glucagon—A natural hormone secreted by the pancreas that stimulates the metabolism of sugar; secreted when blood sugar is too low, a condition that causes the release of liver glycogen and its transformation into glucose.

diabetes mellitus—A disease caused by insufficient production of insulin by the endocrine portion of the pancreas; occurs in two forms: type 1 (insulin-dependent) and type 2 (non-insulin-dependent)

glycemic index—An index expressing the effects of various foods on the rate and amount of increase in blood-glucose levels.

Alcohol

For light drinkers (one or two 12-ounce beers, small glasses of wine, or average-size cocktails) who are well nourished and in good health, the occasional consumption of alcohol will have little effect on nutrition except for the additional 150 to 300 calories. Any amount of alcohol, however, slows metabolism. Consumption of larger amounts compromises your nutritional status, and a number of problems occur. These include protein deficiency; failure of intestinal cells to absorb thiamin, folate, and vitamin B12; excretion of increased quantities of magnesium, calcium, potassium, and zinc by the kidneys; dislodgement of vitamin B6, creating a deficiency that lowers the production of red blood cells; reduced capacity of the liver to activate vitamin D; and many other changes. Although proper nutrition is important for those who consume alcohol, it does not prevent changes in the excretion, absorption, and utilization of numerous nutrients.

Fats

Fat is a critical nutrient that provides a tremendous source of energy to the human body. Fat also stores and transports vitamins A, D, E, and K; carries linoleic acid (an essential fatty acid); increases the flavor and palatability of foods; provides sustained relief from hunger; and helps keep protein from being used as energy. The fatty tissue in our bodies supports organs, cushions them from injury, and aids in the prevention of heat loss. Fat is in most body tissue, with bone marrow containing 96%, liver 2.5%, and blood 0.5%. Unfortunately, too much body fat and high blood-fat levels can shorten life and increase vulnerability to numerous chronic and degenerative diseases, such as cardiorespiratory disease and cancer.

Fat in Food

The fat in food is classified as saturated, polyunsaturated, and monounsaturated. **Cholesterol** is used in the synthesis of sex hormones, vitamin D, and bile salts. Cholesterol is also associated with artery clogging and heart disease. People obtain cholesterol in two ways: The liver manufactures about 1,000 milligrams a day, and we consume 200 to 500 milligrams directly from food of animal origin (egg yolks, meat, poultry, fish, seafood, and whole-milk dairy products). Cholesterol is a **nonessential nutrient,** and the body makes all the cholesterol it needs, so there is no need to consume it in our diets.

Our dietary intake of **saturated fat** is the major culprit in raising blood cholesterol because it causes the liver to manufacture greater amounts. Dietary cholesterol intake and trans-fats also raise blood cholesterol. The average American man consumes about 337 milligrams of cholesterol a day; the average woman, 217 milligrams (table 10.3). Both genders consume an excess amount of trans-fatty acids. Healthy individuals should consume less than 300 milligrams of cholesterol daily, less than 200 milligrams if symptoms of heart disease are present. The key is to restrict your intake of saturated fat to no more than 6 ounces of lean meat, fish, and poultry per day and to use fat-free and low-fat dairy products. High-quality protein from combinations of vegetables and grains, such as rice and beans, are good substitutes for animal sources of protein and contain no cholesterol.

The average person in the United States consumes over 55 pounds of **visible fat** and over 130 pounds of **invisible fat** each year. Dietary fat contributes approximately 33 to 34% of total calories, although the recent favorable pattern of fat intake shows that more fat is being consumed from plants and less from animal sources. Because saturated-fat intake stimulates the production of cholesterol, it is important to reduce cholesterol intake to less than 300 milligrams daily and total saturated fat to less than 6 to 8% of daily calories. Both dietary saturated fat and cholesterol contribute to elevated blood-cholesterol levels.

The five kinds of foods containing the highest percentage of their calories in fat are hamburgers and meatloaf (63%); hot dogs, ham, and luncheon meats (58%); whole milk (54%); doughnuts, cakes, and cookies (54%); and beefsteak and roasts (50%). Another major source of saturated fat in our diet is the food eaten in fast-

TABLE 10.3—Cholesterol Content of Selected Foods

Food	Amount	Cholesterol (mg)
Milk, skim	1 cup	4
Mayonnaise	1 tbsp	10
Butter	1 pat	11
Lard	1 tbsp	12
Cottage cheese	1/2 cup	15
Milk, low-fat 2%	1 cup	22
Half and half	1/4 cup	23
Hot dog[a]	1	29
Ice cream, 10% fat	1/2 cup	30
Cheese, cheddar	1 oz	30
Milk, whole[a]	1 cup	34
Oysters, salmon	3 oz	40
Clams, halibut, tuna	3 oz	55
Chicken, turkey, light meat	3 oz	70
Beef[a], pork[a]	3 oz	75
Lamb, crab	3 oz	85
Shrimp, lobster	3 oz	90-110
Heart, beef	3 oz	164
Egg, yolk[a]	1	213
Liver, beef	3 oz	410
Kidney	3 oz	587
Brains	3 oz	2,637

[a]Leading contributors of cholesterol to the U.S. diet.

Reprinted from G.M. Wardlaw, P.M. Insel, and M.F. Seyler, 1994, *Contemporary nutrition: Issues and insights*, 2nd ed. (St. Louis: Mosby), 165. Reproduced with permission of The McGraw-Hill Companies.

food restaurants. Most hamburgers, hot dogs, and chicken and fish sandwiches served by major fast-food chains contain more than 50% fat and are extremely high in calories. For the percentage of calories from fat in popular fast-food selections, see appendix B.

Trans-Fatty Acids

For decades, people have used margarine rather than butter to reduce their consumption of unhealthy saturated fat. Although both products contain the same number of calories, margarine contains much less saturated fat. Research now suggests that a type of fat found in margarine may increase cholesterol levels as much as butter does. **Trans-fatty acids** form during processing when manufacturers add hydrogen to highly unsaturated vegetable oil to ensure consistency and prevent rancidity. During the process of hydrogenation, the oil creates a new chemical configuration, known as trans-fatty acids. This chemical forms in all oils that are hydrogenated, such as margarine, shortening, baked goods, commercial frying fats, and fats used by some fast-food outlets to cook french fries. In fact, any product that lists partially hydrogenated vegetable oil among its ingredients contains trans-fatty acids.

Research now suggests that high levels of trans-fatty acids not only may raise levels of bad cholesterol (LDL) almost as much as do saturated fats but also may lower levels of the good cholesterol (HDL). One study went a step further and indicated that women whose diets are high in trans-fatty acids were more likely to suffer heart disease than were women who ate little margarine and other foods high in trans-fatty acids.

According to the American Heart Association and other health organizations, the scare has been blown out of proportion, and much more research is needed. Because trans-fatty acids account for only 2 to 8% of total calories compared with 12 to 14% for saturated fat, which research clearly shows to elevate blood-cholesterol levels, individuals should continue to strive to reduce daily saturated fat intake to less than 10% of their total calories and total fat to less than 30% of their total calories. In the meantime, you would be wise to read labels carefully and reduce your intake of products that list the words "partially hydrogenated" in their ingredients. Soft tub margarine is also a wiser choice than stick margarine; the harder the margarine, the more hydrogenation was involved.

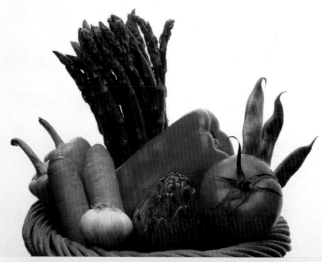

To maintain sound nutrition, choose foods lower in fat whenever possible.

PhotoDisc

cholesterol—One of the sterols, or fatlike chemical substances, manufactured in the body and consumed from foods of animal origins only; high intake is associated with elevated blood-cholesterol levels and heart disease.

nonessential nutrient—Nutrients the body can manufacture in sufficient quantities without any of that substance present in the diet.

saturated fat—Fat that contains glycerol and saturated fatty acids; found in large quantities in animal products (such as meat, milk, butter, and cheese) and in small quantities in vegetable products, with the exception of coconut oil, a highly saturated vegetable source. High intake is associated with elevated blood-cholesterol levels.

visible fat—Fat content of food that can be seen, such as the fat in butter and oils.

invisible fat—Hidden fat in food that cannot be seen, such as the fat in dairy products or egg yolks.

trans-fatty acid—A fatty acid created when hydrogen is added to an unsaturated fat.

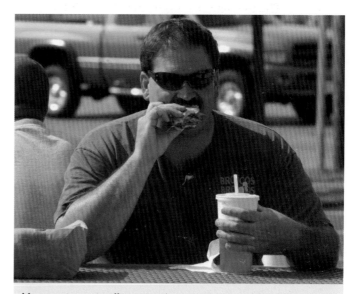

Many restaurants offer convenience and fast service, but in return they often offer foods high in calories, fat, and salt.

McDonald's Corporation recently spent huge sums of money advertising their redesigned cooking oil to reduce both saturated fat and trans-fatty acids in their fries. McDonald's small-size fries still contain 90 calories from fat, but the saturated fat calories have dropped from 20.7 to 17.0, trans-fats calories have decreased from 30 to 16, and polyunsaturated fat calories have increased from 10.8 to 29.0. The change is an improvement because saturated fat now makes up only 8.5% of total calories. Unfortunately, any amount of trans-fats is too much, and the calories and salt content are far too high, making fries, especially the large and supersized portions, a poor nutritional choice. For many people, one supersized order of fries provides about 25% of all calories and most of the salt needed in an entire day.

Polyunsaturated and **monounsaturated fats** are good substitutes for saturated fat because both contain fatty acids that are less likely to be oxidized (oxidized LDL may contribute more to plaque buildup than LDL does). You should consume about 12% of daily calories from both monounsaturated and polyunsaturated fats to replace 4 to 5% of saturated fat intake, rather than merely add 4 to 5% additional fat calories.

Artificial Fats

Artificial fats are classified into three categories based on their nutrient source: carbohydrate-based plant polysaccharides replace fat, proteins and microparticulated proteins replace fat, and fat replacers block fat absorption. The products listed below were developed to reduce caloric and fat intake by replacing the fat in food (fat substitutes) or providing the taste and feel of fat in the mouth.

- The first product to gain the approval of the Food and Drug Administration (FDA) was Simplesse® in 1990, a fat substitute available in foods such as cheese, baked goods, ice cream, frozen desserts, mayonnaise, salad dressing, yogurt, sour cream, and butter. This fat substitute is a mixture of food proteins such as egg white, whey, and milk protein that are cooked and blended into tiny round particles that trap water. This procedure causes the particles to roll over one another in the mouth and be perceived as a creamy, smooth texture much like that derived from actual fat.

- Proctor & Gamble developed Olestra after a $200 million, two-decade experiment. Olestra has the feel and flavor of real fat and is made from sugar tightly bound with fatty acids (sucrose polyester) that are nondigestible and calorie-free. It is the only artificial fat that can be used in frying. Unfortunately, Olestra is a synthetic compound of sugar and vegetable oil that tends to "scoop up" the fat-soluble vitamins A, D, E, and K, as well as nutrients such as carotenoids found in fruit and vegetables, leading to potential deficiencies in users. Olestra has also been shown to cause gastrointestinal problems such as cramps and severe diarrhea in some individuals. In November 1995 an FDA panel of experts concluded that Olestra chips were not harmful. Taste tests on potato chips, ice cream, and other products made with Olestra have also been favorable.

- Caprenin, a fat substitute designed to imitate the taste and texture of cocoa, is used in chocolate and some baked goods. Because Caprenin is poorly absorbed, it contains only 5 calories per gram instead of 9 for fat. Unfortunately, those 5 calories contain as much saturated fat as cocoa butter does.

- Salatrim is a competitor to Caprenin made from processed vegetable oils that are difficult for humans to absorb. Salatrim has a caloric profile similar to that of Caprenin (5 calories per gram) and is also high in saturated fat. The product is designed for use in baking and low-fat chocolate chips.

- Replace is manufactured from Oatrim, which is made from beta glucan (the soluble fiber in oats) and other starches, with thickeners such as guar gum. It is cholesterol-free and provides 2 grams of soluble fiber per 8-ounce serving of milk. When added to nonfat milk, the taste and texture resembles that of whole milk. The product will be used in some baked goods and processed meats.

A number of additional fat substitutes are available in dairy products, sauces, frozen desserts, salad dressings, baked goods, confections, gelatins, puddings, meat products, chewing gum, dry cake and cookie mixes, frostings and icings, condiments, and soups. The public wants the best of both worlds—the taste of fat without the calories—and will buy FDA-approved products with artificial fat if the risks are minimal. The American Heart Association's (AHA) Nutrition Committee has been looking into fat substitutes and has concluded that you should see them as just part of your healthy eating plan. Although these products have the potential to help control weight, the fact remains that obesity rates continue to rise. The debate also continues about whether the benefits of reduced calories, reduced saturated fat (in some products), and lower total fat outweigh the long-term negative side effects.

Protein

Protein, from the Greek word *proteios,* or primary, is critical to all living things. In the human body, protein is used to repair, rebuild, and replace cells; aid in growth; balance fluid, salt, and acid base; and provide needed energy when carbohydrates and fats are insufficient or unavailable. Protein is produced in the body through building blocks called **amino acids.** The body produces some of these amino acids; others are derived only from food sources. The body can manufacture **nonessential amino acids** if they are not available from the diet. The body must acquire through food sources the **essential amino acids,** 8 to 10 of which must be present in the body in the proper amount and correct proportion to the nonessential acids for normal protein metabolism to proceed. All 22 amino acids must be present simultaneously (within several hours) for the body to synthesize them into proteins that permit optimal maintenance of body growth and function.

Sources of Protein

Humans obtain protein from both animal and plant foods. In general, animal protein is superior to plant protein because it contains all the essential amino acids in the proper proportions. If one essential amino acid is missing or present in the incorrect proportion, protein construction may be blocked.

Eggs are the complete protein by which all other protein is judged. Milk, cheese, other dairy products, meat, fish, and poultry compare favorably with eggs as sources of protein. Although eggs contain about 213 milligrams of cholesterol and 5 grams of fat (60%), they are a low-calorie (75 calories) source of protein, vitamin A, riboflavin, vitamin B12, iron, zinc, phosphorus, calcium, potassium, and other nutrients. Still, you should consume no more than two to three eggs per week, and never more than one per day; eliminate or substitute other food products in recipes calling for eggs as an ingredient; and buy small eggs rather than medium, large, or extra large ones. The American Heart Association guideline of no more than 300 milligrams of cholesterol per day is difficult to follow if you start the day with an egg rather than with cold or hot cereal.

Protein containing all essential amino acids is a high-quality protein termed **complete protein.** Protein from most vegetable sources is low in some amino acids and will not support growth and development when used as the only source of protein. This is called an **incomplete protein,** or low-quality protein. Terms such as **low biological value** and **high biological value** are also used to describe the quality of protein.

To meet minimum protein needs, approximately 54 grams of protein are recommended daily for college-age males, and 46 to 48 grams for females. To determine your specific protein needs, multiply your body weight in kilograms by .8 gram. A 132-pound woman, for example, weighs 60 kilograms (132 ÷ 2.2) and needs 48 grams (60 × .8) of protein daily. Larger individuals, pregnant and lactating women, adolescents, and those who are ill may need slightly more protein. Physically active individuals generally do not require additional protein unless the weather is

polyunsaturated fat—Fat containing two or more double bonds between carbons, found in large quantities in vegetable oils, nuts, fish, and margarines.

monounsaturated fat—Fat containing one double bond between carbons, found in foods such as avocados, cashews, and peanut and olive oils.

amino acids—The basic component of most proteins.

nonessential amino acids—Amino acids that can be manufactured by the body if they cannot be acquired from food sources.

essential amino acids—Amino acids that cannot be manufactured by the body and therefore must be acquired from food sources.

complete protein—A food source that contains all essential amino acids in the correct proportions.

incomplete protein—A food source that does not contain all essential amino acids or contains several in incorrect proportions.

low biological value—A protein source such as corn and wheat that does not contain all eight essential amino acids or contains some in low proportions.

high biological value—A protein source such as meat that contains all eight essential amino acids in the correct proportions.

Myth and Fact Sheet

Myth	**Fact**
1. Margarine is a wise health choice.	**1.** Margarine and other products that contain partially hydrogenated fats produce a chemical makeup called trans-fatty acids, which have been shown to contribute to heart disease. Some new types of margarine contain no trans-fats. Canola oil margarine is a wise choice. Liquid tub or "diet" margarine also has less trans-fats. You can reduce your intake of margarine by substituting jam or jelly and avoiding baked products such as doughnuts, cookies, pies, and cakes. Unfortunately, the switch from butter to margarine decades ago was not nearly as wise a health choice as originally anticipated, and you should consume as little margarine as possible.
2. Ground beef that is lean is a good food choice.	**2.** Ground beef that is 80% lean contains 20% fat by weight, but that fat represents 70% of the total calories. That amount is far too much fat and far too many calories. Ground beef is the single most damaging food in the American diet.
3. Potato and tortilla chips should be avoided completely.	**3.** The typical brand contains 10 grams of fat, 160 calories, and 200 milligrams of sodium per ounce. Because no one eats just 1 ounce, it is important to consume such products sparingly and consider these guidelines: Choose baked potatoes rather than fried potatoes or tortilla chips; avoid fat-free chips because Olestra can cause diarrhea and will inhibit absorption of vitamins A, D, E, and K; avoid chips containing partially hydrogenated oil (trans-fats) and the high-fat chips with a lot of beta-carotene from sweet potatoes or carrots; and choose chips with 2 or 3 grams of fiber per ounce. If you are on a low-sodium diet, buy low-sodium or unsalted chips.
4. Trimming the fat removes most of the cholesterol from meats.	**4.** Cholesterol is found equally in lean meat and the fat (approximately 20 to 25 milligrams per ounce). Trimming the fat and skin is important because this saturated fat contributes more toward raising your blood cholesterol than dietary cholesterol, but you cannot cut the cholesterol out of the meat.
5. Noncalorie sweeteners are safe and help me lose weight.	**5.** These sugar substitutes do not cause tooth decay or affect blood-glucose levels and are helpful to diabetics. They appear to be safe, but their effect on obesity and overfatness is questionable. After 30 years of increased consumption of sugar substitutes, Americans of all ages have grown heavier, not lighter. Following 3 years of new studies, the once banned sweetener, Saccharin, has now been classified as safe after findings revealed that the associated laboratory-rat bladder tumors are not relevant to humans.
6. The number of food poisoning cases is rising dramatically.	**6.** Untrue. In 2002, the Centers for Disease Control and Prevention reported that the rate of E. coli fell 21%, salmonella 15%, and listeria 35%. Shigella was down 35%, campylobacter 27%, and yersina 49%. Only vibrio, a germ that shows up in raw oysters, climbed, by 83%.
7. Food products past the "sell by" date are probably spoiled.	**7.** A product past the "sell by" date may not be spoiled; one past the "use by" date is just plain dangerous. Milk may last a week or more beyond its date if stored at 45° F or below. Eggs will survive for weeks although they may be packed up to 30 days after the hen

(continued)

lays them, with the "sell by" date no more than 30 days later. Undamaged canned goods will last for years although highly acidic products (tomatoes, grapefruit, pineapple) taste better if used within 18 months. Avoid buying any product with the "use by" date expired.

8. Foods labeled as "organic" are free of pesticides.

8. A Consumers Union study found pesticide residue on 23% of organic fruits and vegetables and on nearly 75% of conventionally grown produce. One natural pesticide used by organic farmers, pryrethrum, may cause cancer, and another is linked to neurotoxic effects in rats. No produce choices on the market are free of pesticide residues, although these residues are rarely close to the limits set by the Environmental Protection Agency. Exposure to chemicals in air, water, soil, and food is believed to cause less than 1% of all cancers.

9. Imported fruits and vegetables are not safe.

9. Imported fruits and vegetables must meet the same standards as produce grown in this country.

10. "Aerobic" water sold in health stores and gyms is a wise choice.

10. "Aerobic," or oxygenated, water sells for about $2 per half liter in health food stores and gyms. Manufacturers claim that the water is infused with 5 to 10 times as much oxygen as regular water, which increases blood-oxygen levels, helps muscles, and improves performance. Studies show that none of these claims is true and that the product is a waste of money.

11. Hunger is almost nonexistent in America.

11. The Department of Agriculture reports that over 10% of Americans face hunger daily. Seventeen percent of our nation's children (over 17 million) do not have enough to eat. The report indicates that 30% of all single moms and their children went hungry or lived on the edge of hunger, as did 21% of Blacks and 20.8% of Hispanics.

12. Consuming a candy bar or nondiet cola before exercise gives me extra energy.

12. If you eat large amounts of sugar at one time, such as an entire candy bar or regular soda, the blood releases too much insulin, starting a series of complex chemical reactions. As a result, too much glucose is removed from the blood and stored in the fat cells and liver. This process can leave you with less energy than you would have had without eating the candy bar or drinking the soda. Sugar also draws fluid from other body parts into the gastrointestinal tract and may contribute to dehydration, distention of the stomach, cramps, nausea, and diarrhea. To avoid these problems, dilute concentrated fruit juices with twice the recommended water, add an equal volume of water to commercial drinks, and eat only small quantities of sugar. Sugar is absorbed faster than the muscles can use it; thus, frequent small amounts are preferable to single doses. Your blood-glucose level will reach a peak about half an hour after consumption and then decline rapidly. Eating large quantities of sugar causes more rapid decline and greater shortage of glucose for energy.

hot and profuse sweating that produces additional nitrogen loss occurs. Those living in extremely hot climates may also need slightly more protein. A minimum of 12 to 15% of the total daily calories in your diet should come from protein.

It is not difficult for most people to obtain their **dietary reference intakes (DRIs)** of protein.

Meat contains about 7 grams per ounce, milk has 8 grams per glass, and protein is plentiful in eggs and dairy products and present in small quantities in vegetables and grains. Two glasses of milk; 1 ounce of cheese; and 3 ounces of beef, chicken, or fish provide all the protein the average person needs per day.

Vegetarian Diets

More and more people in the United States are resorting to some form of vegetarianism, believing that vegetables are healthier than meats, that it is morally wrong to consume meat, or that meat is contaminated with growth-enhancing drugs.

According to polls by the Vegetarian Resource Group in Baltimore, the number of vegetarians in the United States is growing steadily. Here are some other interesting facts and statistics about vegetarians compiled by the Vegetarian Resource Group:

- Five million Americans (2.5%) eat no meat, poultry, or fish.
- Nine million (4.5%) eat no red meat.
- More than 13 million (6.7%) eat no eggs.
- Most vegetarians live in the Northeast and on the West Coast.
- Asians are more likely to be vegetarians than are members of other ethnic groups.
- The chief health benefits of a vegetarian diet are reduced risk of heart disease, diabetes, obesity, and some types of cancer.
- The chief health risks of a vegetarian diet are deficiencies in vitamin B12 and iron, which can be avoided by proper diet planning or supplements.

Vegetarians fall into four basic categories: **vegan, lactovegetarian, ovovegetarian,** and **ovolactovegetarian.** All vegetarians must plan their diets carefully to obtain their daily nutrients. Because dairy products and eggs are excellent protein sources, lacto- and ovolactovegetarians have much less difficulty than strict vegans do. Vegans must use complementary protein combinations of vegetables and grains to include proper amounts of protein in their diets. Traditional complementary protein diets include combinations of soybeans or tofu with rice (China and Indochina), peas with wheat (the Middle East), beans with corn (Central and South America), and rice with beans, black-eyed peas, or tofu (United States and the Caribbean). Other protein combinations readily available to U.S. vegans include peanut butter and whole-grain bread, whole-wheat bread, black beans, and black-bean and rice soup. These combinations of complete proteins are excellent substitutes for meat, egg, and dairy proteins.

Because fruits, vegetables, and grains contain no cholesterol, little saturated fat, and a lot of fiber, vegans tend to avoid heart disease for a decade longer than meat eaters do. Vegetarians may also be able to avoid certain kinds of diges-

tive-system cancers, but vegans are especially prone to dangerous deficiencies in iron, calcium, and vitamin B12 (available only in animal products). To combat serious nutrient shortages, vegans should follow certain daily dietary recommendations and include in their diets the following:

- Two cups of legumes daily for proper levels of calcium and iron.
- One cup of dark greens daily to meet iron requirements (for women).
- At least 1 gram of fat daily for proper absorption of vitamins.
- A supplement of fortified plant foods (like soy or nut milks or a multiple vitamin and mineral) to obtain vitamin B12.

Energy Systems

Practically all the energy your muscles use is formed by the chemical reactions of two unique pathways of energy formation: the glycolysis energy cycle and the citric acid cycle.

The majority of energy formed by glycolysis is derived from glucose, and because it is anaerobic, it can be produced quickly. The glucose used to fuel glycolysis comes from blood glucose, glycogen (the stored form of glucose), glycerol (a small fraction of stored fat molecules), and several amino acids. Most college-age people have approximately 1,400 calories of glycogen stored in the muscles and 300 stored in the liver (liver glycogen can supply glucose to muscles). Short, intense anaerobic exercises such as sprinting,

dietary reference intakes (DRIs)—The level of intake of essential nutrients considered adequate to meet the known nutritional needs of healthy persons in the United States.

vegan—Strict vegetarians who consume only fruits, vegetables, and grains.

lactovegetarian—People who eat fruits, vegetables, grains, and dairy products but avoid meat products.

ovovegetarian—people who eat fruits, vegetables, grains, and eggs but avoid meat products.

ovolactovegetarian—People who eat fruits, vegetables, grains, dairy products, and eggs but avoid meat products.

glycolysis energy cycle—The anaerobic energy pathway fueled primarily by glucose.

citric acid energy cycle—The aerobic energy pathway fueled primarily by fat, small quantities of glucose fragments, and certain amino acids.

weight training, performing pull-ups, diving, and doing push-ups are fueled by the **glycolysis energy cycle.**

The **citric acid energy cycle** uses three different types of fuel: glucose fragments produced by glycolysis, fatty acids, and certain amino acids. Fatty acids drawn from the body's fat stores are by far the largest supplier of energy in this aerobic cycle. Only in the aerobic cycle, in which oxygen is present, can fat be burned as fuel. Fat in the citric acid cycle fuels activities such as walking, jogging, running, lap swimming, aerobic dance, cycling, basketball, and soccer. These aerobic activities are ideal for weight and fat loss. Fat cannot be burned in the anaerobic cycle because oxygen is not present.

Nonenergy Nutrients

The three nonenergy nutrients are vitamins, minerals, and water.

Vitamins

Vitamins are essential in helping chemical reactions take place in the body and are required in very small amounts. Water-soluble vitamins (vitamin C and the B-complex vitamins) need to be consumed in the proper amounts over a 5- to 8-day period because they are easily dissolved in water, not stored for long periods, and are eliminated in the urine (see table 10.4). Fat-soluble vitamins (vitamins A, D, E, and K) are stored in large amounts in fatty tissues and the liver and are absorbed through the intestinal track as needed (see table 10.5).

TABLE 10.4—Summary of Information on Water-Soluble Vitamins

Name	DRI for adults[a]	Sources	Stability	Comments
Thiamin	M: 1.5 mg F: 1.1 mg	Pork, liver, organ meats, legumes, whole-grain and enriched cereals and breads, wheat germ, potatoes. Synthesized in intestinal tract.	Unstable in presence of heat, alkali, or oxygen. Heat stable in acid solution.	As part of cocarboxylase, aids in removal of CO_2 from alpha-keto acids during oxidation of carbohydrates. Essential for growth, normal appetite, digestion, and healthy nerves.
Riboflavin	M: 1.7 mg F: 1.3 mg	Milk and dairy foods, organ meats, green leafy vegetables, enriched cereals and breads, eggs.	Stable to heat, oxygen, and acid. Unstable to light (especially ultraviolet) or alkali.	Essential for growth. Plays enzymatic role in tissue respiration and acts as a transporter of hydrogen ions. Coenzyme forms flavin adenine mononucleotide (FMN) and flavin adenine dinucleotide (FAD).
Niacin (nicotinic acid and nicotinamide)	M: 19 mg NE F: 15 mg NE	Fish, liver, meat, poultry, many grains, eggs, peanuts, milk, legumes, enriched grains. Synthesized by intestinal bacteria.	Stable to heat, light oxidation, acid, and alkali.	As part of enzyme system, aids in transfer of hydrogen and acts in metabolism of carbohydrates and amino acids. Involved in glycolysis, fat synthesis, and tissue respiration.
Vitamin B6 (pyridoxine, pyridoxal, and pyridoxamine)	M: 2.0 mg F: 1.6 mg	Pork, glandular meats, cereal bran and germ, milk, egg yolk, oatmeal, and legumes. Synthesized by intestinal bacteria.	Stable to heat, light, and oxidation.	As a coenzyme, aids in the synthesis and breakdown of amino acids and in the synthesis of unsaturated fatty acids from essential fatty acids. Essential for conversion of tryptophan to niacin. Essential for normal growth.
Folate	M: 200 μg F: 180 μg	Green leafy vegetables, organ meats (liver), lean beef, wheat, eggs, fish, dry beans, lentils, cowpeas, asparagus, broccoli, collards, yeast. Synthesized in intestinal tract.	Stable to sunlight when in solution; unstable to heat in acid media.	Appears essential for biosynthesis of nucleic acids. Essential for normal maturation of red blood cells. Functions as a coenzyme: tetrahydrofolic acid.
Vitamin B12	2 μg	Liver, kidney, milk and dairy foods, meat, eggs. Vegans require supplement.	Slowly destroyed by acid, alkali, light, and oxidation.	Involved in the metabolism of single-carbon fragments. Essential for biosynthesis of nucleic acids and nucleoproteins. Role in metabolism of nervous tissue. Involved with folate metabolism. Related to growth.

(continued)

TABLE 10.4 *(continued)*

Name	DRI for adults[a]	Sources	Stability	Comments
Pantothenic acid	Level not yet determined but 4-7 mg believed safe and adequate.	Present in all plant and animal foods. Eggs, kidney, liver, salmon, and yeast are best sources. Possibly synthesized by intestinal bacteria.	Unstable to acid, alkali, heat, and certain salts.	As part of coenzyme A, functions in the synthesis and breakdown of many vital body compounds. Essential in the intermediary metabolism of carbohydrate, fat, and protein.
Biotin	Not known but 30-100 μg believed safe and adequate.	Liver, mushrooms, peanuts, yeast, milk, meat, egg yolk, most vegetables, banana, grapefruit, tomato, watermelon, and strawberries. Synthesized in intestinal tract.	Stable.	Essential component of enzymes. Involved in synthesis and break-down of fatty acids and amino acids through aiding the addition and removal of CO_2 to or from active compounds, and the removal of NH_2 from amino acids.
Vitamin C (ascorbic acid)	60 mg	Acerola (West Indian cherrylike fruit), citrus fruit, tomato, melon, peppers, greens, raw cabbage, guava, strawberries, pineapple, potato.	Unstable to heat, alkali, and oxidation, except in acids. Destroyed by storage.	Maintains intracellular cement substance with preservation of capillary integrity. Cosubstrate in hydroxylations requiring molecular oxygen. Important in immune responses, wound healing, and allergic reactions. Increases absorption of nonheme iron.

[a]M = male, F = female; NE = niacin equivalents.

Reprinted, by permission, from K.L. Mahan and M. Arlin, 1992, *Food nutrition and diet therapy* (Philadelphia: W.B. Saunders), 105-106.

TABLE 10.5—Summary of Information on Fat-Soluble Vitamins

Name	DRI for adults[a]	Sources	Stability	Comments
Vitamin A (retinol; α-, β-, γ-carotene)	M: 1,000 RE F: 800 RE	Liver, kidney, milk fat, fortified margarine, egg yolk, yellow and dark green leafy vegetables, apricots, cantaloupe, peaches.	Stable to light, heat, and usual cooking methods. Destroyed by oxidation, drying, very high temperature, and ultraviolet light.	Essential for normal growth, development, and maintenance of epithelial tissue. Essential to the integrity of night vision. Helps provide for normal bone development and influences normal tooth formation. Toxic in large quantities.
Vitamin D (calciferol)	M: 5 μg F: 5 μg	Vitamin D milk, irradiated foods, some in milk fat, liver, egg yolk, salmon, tuna fish, and sardines. Sunlight converts 7-dehydrocholesterol to cholecalciferol.	Stable to heat and oxidation.	Really a prohormone. Essential for normal growth and development; important for formation of normal bones and teeth. Influences absorption and metabolism of phosphorus and calcium. Toxic in large quantities.
Vitamin E (tocopherols and tocotrienols)	M: 10 α-TE F: 8 α-TE	Wheat germ, vegetable oils, green leafy vegetables, milk fat, egg yolk, nuts.	Stable to heat and acids. Destroyed by rancid fats, alkali, oxygen, lead, iron salts, and ultraviolet irradiation.	Is a strong antioxidant. May help prevent oxidation of unsaturated fatty acids and vitamin A in intestinal tract and body tissues. Protects red blood cells from hemolysis. Role in reproduction (in animals). Role in epithelial tissue maintenance and prostaglandin synthesis.
Vitamin K (phylloquinone and menaquinone)	M: 80 μg F: 65 μg	Liver, soybean oil, other vegetable oils, green leafy vegetables, wheat bran. Synthesized in intestinal tract.	Resistant to heat, oxygen, and moisture. Destroyed by alkali and ultraviolet light.	Aids in production of prothrombin, a compound required for normal clotting of blood. Toxic in large amounts.

[a]M = male; F = female; RE = retinol equivalents; α-TE = alphatocopherol equivalents.

Reprinted, by permission, from K.L. Mahan and M. Arlin, 1992, *Food nutrition and diet therapy* (Philadelphia: W.B. Saunders), 105.

Regardless of the claims, vitamin C does not cure or prevent the common cold. Researchers are examining large supplements of other vitamins and minerals for their disease-fighting potential and ability to assist in medical treatment. You should realize three important things about taking vitamin supplements. First, the best way to obtain adequate vitamins and minerals is from food, not from supplements. Food has the added benefit of containing fiber and water and many other chemicals. Second, most people in the United States get all the vitamins and minerals they need from their diets and do not need supplements. Third, vitamin and mineral toxicity problems occur predominantly in those who take supplements.

Minerals

Minerals are present in all living cells. They serve as key components of various hormones, enzymes, and other substances that aid in regulating chemical reactions within cells. Mineral elements play a part in the body's metabolic processes, and deficiencies can result in serious disorders. Macrominerals, such as sodium, potassium, calcium, phosphorus, magnesium, sulfur, and chlorides, are needed by the body in large amounts (more than 5 grams). Trace minerals are needed in small amounts (less than 5 grams). A minimum of 14 trace minerals must be ingested for optimum health. Iron, iodine, copper, fluoride, and zinc are the ones most important for body function. The body is composed of about 31 minerals, 24 of which are essential for sustaining life (see tables 10.6 and 10.7).

Iron

Iron is one of the body's most essential minerals. We use approximately 85% of our daily iron intake to produce new hemoglobin (the pigment of the red blood cells that transport oxygen); the remaining 15% is used for the production of new tissue or held in storage. Iron needs for college students ages 19 and over vary according to gender, with males needing 10 milligrams per day and females 15 milligrams per day. During pregnancy, the average woman needs 30 milligrams per day. After age 51 or so, both males and females need approximately 10 milligrams per day. Infants require about 6 milligrams per day for the first 6 months and 10 milligrams per day thereafter until ages 11 to 14 (growth spurt), when needs increase to 12 milligrams per day for males and 15 milligrams per day for females. Iron

deficiency results in loss of strength and endurance, rapid fatigue during exercise, shortening of the attention span, loss of visual perception, impaired learning, and numerous other physical disorders. Although the importance of sufficient dietary iron is common knowledge, many women may not get enough iron in their diets. Table 10.8 contains a variety of dietary sources of iron. In the United States iron intake has declined because of the removal of iron-containing soils from the food supply and the diminished use of iron cooking utensils. Whereas animals can ingest iron from muddy water and soil, humans must rely solely on food.

Iron deficiency anemia, a major health problem in the United States, is common in older infants, children, women of childbearing age, pregnant women, and low-income people. People must also be aware, however, that too much iron can be dangerous. Iron toxicity is rare, but a condition called iron overload occurs when the body is overwhelmed with too much iron from blood transfusions or when the body absorbs too much iron because of hereditary defects, heavy supplementation, and alcohol abuse (which increases absorption). Iron overload can cause tissue and liver damage. Rapid ingestion of large amounts of iron can also cause sudden death. Iron overdose is the second most common cause of accidental poisoning in small children. High blood-iron levels may also be related to heart disease in men.

Iron is more easily absorbed from meat, fish, and poultry (heme iron) than it is from vegetables (nonheme iron). Twice the volume of vegetable iron is absorbed when vegetables and meats are consumed during the same meal. Vitamin C also promotes iron absorption and can triple the amount of nonheme iron absorbed from foods eaten at the same meal. Table 10.9 lists dietary sources of vitamin C. The **MFP factor** enhances the absorption of nonheme iron from other foods eaten at the same meal with meat, fish, and poultry. Refer to figure 10.2 for suggestions on increasing your dietary intake of iron.

Supplementation

Some people take large doses of vitamins and minerals in the belief that these are necessary

> **MFP factor**—A factor in meat, fish, and poultry that enhances the absorption of nonheme iron present in the same foods and other foods eaten at the same time.

TABLE 10.6—Macronutrients Essential at Levels of 100 Milligrams per Day or More

Mineral	Location in body and some biological functions	DRI[a] or ESADDI[b] for adults	Food sources	Comments on likelihood of a deficiency
Calcium	99% in bones and teeth. Ionic calcium in body fluids essential for iron transport across cell membranes. Calcium is also bound to protein, citrate, or inorganic acids.	800 mg, 1,200 mg for women 19-24 yr	Milk and milk products, sardines, clams, oysters, kale, turnip greens, mustard greens, tofu.	Dietary surveys indicate that many diets do not meet recommended dietary allowances for calcium. Because bone serves as a homeostatic mechanism to maintain calcium level in blood, many essential functions are maintained, regardless of diet. Long-term dietary deficiency is probably one of the factors responsible for development of osteoporosis in later life.
Phosphorus	About 80% in inorganic portion of bones and teeth. Phosphorus is a component of every cell and of highly important metabolites, including DNA, RNA, ATP (high energy compound), and phospholipids. Important to pH regulation.	800 mg, 1,200 mg for women 19-24 yr	Cheese, egg yolk, milk, meat, fish, poultry, whole-grain cereals, legumes, nuts.	Dietary inadequacy not likely to occur if protein and calcium intake are adequate.
Magnesium	About 50% in bone. Remaining 50% is almost entirely inside body cells with only about 1% in extracellular fluid. Ionic magnesium functions as an activator of many enzymes and thus influences almost all processes.	350 mg for males, 280 mg for females	Whole-grain cereals, tofu, nuts, meat, milk, green vegetables, legumes, chocolate.	Dietary inadequacy considered unlikely, but conditioned deficiency is often seen in clinical medicine, associated with surgery, alcoholism, malabsorption, loss of body fluids, certain hormonal and renal diseases.
Sodium	30 to 45% in bone. Major cation of extracellular fluid and only a small amount is inside cell. Regulates body fluid osmolarity, pH, and body fluid volume.	500-3,000 mg	Common table salt, seafood, animal foods, milk, eggs. Abundant in most foods except fruit.	Dietary inadequacy probably never occurs, although low blood sodium requires treatment in certain clinical disorders. Sodium restriction is a necessary practice in certain cardiovascular disorders.
Chloride	Major anion of extracellular fluid, functioning in combination with sodium. Serves as a buffer, enzyme activator; component of gastric hydrochloric acid. Mostly present in extracellular fluids; less than 15% inside cells.	750-3,000 mg	Common table salt, seafood, milk, meat, eggs.	In most cases dietary intake has little significance except in the presence of vomiting, diarrhea, or profuse sweating, when a deficiency may develop.
Potassium	Major cation of intracellular fluid, with only small amounts in extracellular fluid. Functions in regulating pH and osmolarity, and cell membrane transfer. Ion is necessary for carbohydrate and protein metabolism.	2,000 mg	Fruits, milk, meat, cereals, vegetables, legumes.	Dietary inadequacy unlikely, but conditioned deficiency may be found in kidney disease, diabetic acidosis, excessive vomiting, diarrhea, or sweating. Potassium excess may be a problem in renal failure and severe acidosis.
Sulfur	Most dietary sulfur is present in sulfur-containing amino acids needed for synthesis of essential metabolites. Functions in oxidation-reduction reactions. Also functions in thiamin and biotin and as inorganic sulfur.	Need for sulfur is satisfied by essential sulfur-containing amino acids.	Protein foods such as meat, fish, poultry, eggs, milk, cheese, legumes, nuts.	Dietary intake is chiefly from sulfur-containing amino acids, and adequacy is related to protein intake.

[a]DRI = dietary reference intake.

[b]ESADDI = estimated safe and adequate daily dietary intake.

Reprinted, by permission, from K.L. Mahan and M. Arlin, 1992, *Food nutrition and diet therapy* (Philadelphia: W.B. Saunders), 137.

TABLE 10.7—Micronutrients Essential at Levels of a Few Milligrams per Day

Mineral	Location in body and some biological functions	DRI[a] or ESADDI[b] for adults	Food sources	Comments on likelihood of a deficiency
Iron	About 70% is in hemoglobin; about 26% stored in liver, spleen, and bone. Iron is a component of hemoglobin and myoglobin, important in oxygen transfer; also present in serum transferring and certain enzymes. Almost none in ionic form.	10 mg for males, 15 mg for females	Liver, meat, egg yolk, legumes, whole or enriched grains, dark green vegetables, dark molasses, shrimp, oysters.	Iron-deficiency anemia occurs in women in reproductive years and in infants and preschool children. May be associated in some cases with unusual blood loss, parasites, and malabsorption. Anemia is last effect of deficient state.
Zinc	Present in most tissues, with higher amounts in liver, voluntary muscle, and bone. Constituent of many enzymes and insulin; of importance in nucleic acid metabolism.	15 mg for males, 12 mg for females	Oysters, shellfish, herring, liver, legumes, milk, wheat bran.	Extent of dietary inadequacy in this country not known. Conditioned deficiency may be seen in systemic childhood illnesses and in patients who are nutritionally depleted or have been subjected to severe stress, such as surgery.
Copper	Found in all body tissues; larger amounts in liver, brain, heart, and kidney. Constituent of enzymes and of ceruloplasmin and erythrocuprein in blood. May be integral part of DNA or RNA molecule.	1.5-3 mg	Liver, shellfish, whole grains, cherries, legumes, kidney, poultry, oysters, chocolate, nuts.	No evidence that specific deficiencies of copper occur in humans. Menkes' disease is genetic disorder resulting in copper deficiency.
Iodine	Constituent of thyroxine and related compounds synthesized by thyroid gland. Thyroxine functions in control of reactions involving cellular energy.	150 μg of vitamin B12	Liver, kidney, oysters, clams, poultry, milk.	Primary dietary inadequacy is rare except when no animal products are consumed. Deficiency may be found in such conditions as lack of gastric intrinsic factor, gastrectomy, and malabsorption syndromes.
Selenium	Associated with fat metabolism, vitamin E, and antioxidant functions.	70 μg for males, 55 μg for females	Grains, onions, meats, milk, vegetables variable—depends on selenium content of soil.	Keshan disease is a selenium-deficient state. Deficiency has occurred in patients receiving long-term total parenteral nutrition (TPN) without selenium.
Chromium	Associated with glucose metabolism.	0.05-0.2 mg	Corn oil, clams, whole-grain cereals, meats, drinking water variable.	Deficiency found in severe malnutrition; may be factor in diabetes in the elderly and cardiovascular disease.
Tin, nickel, vanadium, silicon	Now known to be essential but DRI or ESADDI not established.			

[a]DRI = dietary reference intake

[b]ESADDI = estimated safe and adequate daily dietary intake.

Reprinted, by permission, from K.L. Mahan and M. Arlin, 1992, *Food nutrition and diet therapy* (Philadelphia: W.B. Saunders), 137-138.

to correct dietary deficiencies or prevent or cure a variety of ills. More commonly, people take the multiple-vitamin and mineral pill as an insurance policy against improper nutrition. Unfortunately, consuming too many vitamins and minerals, especially fat-soluble vitamins, which the body stores for long periods, can be toxic. The **megavitamin intake** approach may

megavitamin intake—Consuming 10 to 100 times the DRI for a particular vitamin.

hypervitaminosis—The toxic side effects that result from the consumption of excess vitamins.

result in **hypervitaminosis.** The body also has an adequate reserve storage system for key vitamins

TABLE 10.8—Dietary Sources of Iron

Food	Serving size	Iron (mg)
Beef liver	3 oz	5.3
Beef pot roast	3 oz	3.3
Chickpeas	1 cup	4.7
Chicken breast	3 oz	0.9
Chicken liver	1 each	1.7
Clams	3 oz canned	23.8
Hamburger	3 oz	2.0
Kidney beans	1 cup	3.2
Oysters	1 cup	16.6
Pinto beans	1 cup	4.5
Prune juice	1 cup	3.0
Prunes	10 med	2.1
Raisins	1 cup	3.0
Spinach	1 cup	6.4
Total (cereal)	1 cup	21.0
Tuna, canned	3 oz	2.7
Turkey, roasted	3 oz	1.7

TABLE 10.9—Dietary Sources of Vitamin C

Food	Serving size	Vitamin C (mg)
Banana	1 whole	10
Broccoli spears	1 each	141
Brussels sprouts	1 cup	100
Cabbage	1 cup	25
Cantaloupe	1/2	113
Cranberry juice	1 cup	90
Grapefruit juice	1 cup	80
Orange	1 med	70
Orange juice	1 cup	120
Potato, baked	1 each	26
Pink grapefruit	1 each	47
Snow peas	1 cup	84
Strawberries	1 cup	84
Tomatoes	1 cup	34
Tomato juice (canned)	1 cup	45
Whole milk	1 cup	2
1% milk	1 cup	2

- Eat iron-rich foods containing vitamin C to increase absorption.
- Decrease caffeinated and decaffeinated coffee intake.
- Decrease hot tea and iced tea intake.
- Eat limited amounts of beef liver.
- Use cast-iron skillets when you cook whenever possible.
- Buy only fortified or iron-enriched breakfast cereals.
- Increase intake of green, leafy vegetables.
- Eat dry iron-enriched cereals as snacks.
- Buy iron-enriched or fortified breads.
- Increase intake of legumes such as kidney beans, chickpeas, and lima beans.
- Combine animal sources of iron with vegetable sources of iron to increase absorption.
- Eat limited amounts of oysters (be careful of high dietary cholesterol intake).
- Increase intake of spinach.
- Eat limited amounts of chicken livers.

Figure 10.2 Suggestions for increasing dietary intake of iron.

and minerals to prevent health problems (see table 10.10). This reserve capacity helps prevent deficiencies when you fail to eat right for a few days or weeks, but you should not rely on it for long periods.

With few exceptions, individuals who experience toxicity problems from overdose of a specific vitamin or mineral are involved in heavy supplementation. Producing toxic reactions from food intake alone is extremely difficult. Table 10.11

TABLE 10.10—Extent of Body Reserves of Nutrients and Health Consequences of Depletion

Nutrient	Approximate time to deplete	Potential health implications
Amino acids	3-4 hr	Although you awake each morning with your amino acids depleted, no health consequences occur.
Calcium	2,500 days	Most of the body's calcium storage is in the skeletal system; drawing on this storage supply for long periods will adversely affect the bones.
Carbohydrates	12-15 hr	Short-term depletion causes no problems because the body can switch to protein and fat for energy. Long-term use of protein for energy can cause serious health problems.
Fat	25-50 days	Adipose tissue, the body's greatest reserve source of fuel, provides approximately 100,000-150,000 kcal of energy.
Iron	125 days (women), 750 days (men)	Women have a smaller reserve capacity because of monthly loss of iron in blood during menstruation.
Sodium	2-3 days	After prolonged sweating without food intake, muscle cramps, heat exhaustion, and heatstroke may occur.
Vitamin C	60-120 days	Most excess intake of this water-soluble vitamin is excreted in urine.
Vitamin A	90-360 days	Excess intake of this fat-soluble vitamin is stored in the fat cells.
Water	4-5 days	Death.

TABLE 10.11—Situations in Which Vitamin and Mineral Supplements May Be Beneficial

Situation	Supplement type
Oral contraceptive use	Folic acid, vitamin B6
Pregnancy	Iron, folic acid
Diagnosed deficiency disease (for example, anemias)	As indicated
Vegan diets	Vitamin B12, vitamin D, zinc, iron
Osteoporosis	Calcium, vitamin D, fluoride
Chronic dieting	Multivitamin and mineral
Use of drugs that interfere with the micronutrients (for example, antihypertensives and antibiotics)	As indicated by type of drug
Diseases that produce malabsorption (for example, cystic fibrosis, celiac disease)	Multivitamin and mineral or as indicated
Inadequate diets due to food allergies, alcoholism, or narrow selection of food types	Multivitamin and mineral or as indicted by type of deficiency signs

can help you decide whether you should consider supplementation.

When you extract one component of food and ingest it at very high levels in the form of a pill, you do not know whether it is helpful or harmful to the system. Phyotochemicals and antioxidants, for example, are consumed in combination with hundreds of other chemicals when obtained from food sources. This fact may explain why studies looking at the effects of supplementation on the prevention of disease have not been encouraging. Picking out a single vitamin that people normally consume with hundreds of other chemicals in food and administering it in high doses produces questionable results and is risky at best. To receive the full benefit of phytochemicals, which may help prevent cancer, you must eat the whole vegetable and fruit. Apparently, the many preventive compounds in these foods produce a synergistic effect. In other words, components in foods interact to produce a health benefit stronger than that produced by their individual effects. To aid in preventing cancer, the whole diet counts, not the individual nutrients.

Higher than normal doses of vitamins do not offer protection from various forms of cancer, cardiovascular disease, and diabetes; and very high doses of vitamins C and E may lead to health problems, including diarrhea, bleeding, and the risk of toxic reactions.

Water

The most critical food component is water. While it has no nutritional value, water is necessary for energy production, temperature control, and elimination. It is difficult to drink too much water. Although water is present in all foods, experts still recommend 6 to 8 glasses (48 to 64 ounces) of it daily in addition to your consumption of coffee, tea, and other beverages and 12 to 15 glasses (96 to 120 ounces) when you are trying to lose weight. For a more detailed discussion of daily water needs, see the section "Special Needs of the Active Individual" later in this chapter.

Food Density

You can easily determine whether a food item or meal is nutritionally dense by examining the caloric and nutrient content. A high-density food or meal provides a high percentage of key vitamins and minerals you need daily for a small percentage of your daily caloric intake. A good

cold cereal with skim milk, for example, provides about 190 calories and 20 to 30% of practically all vitamins, minerals, carbohydrates, and protein needed for the day. Because the cold-cereal breakfast contains only about 8% of a 120-pound woman's daily energy needs, the meal is considered nutritionally dense. Fruits, vegetables, and grains are examples of foods that are dense for a given nutrient or group of nutrients. Potato chips, corn chips, and cake are examples of low-density foods that supply a high percentage of daily calories and a low percentage of key nutrients.

Cold or hot cereal is an excellent way to start the day. Read the labels and choose cereals that contain no sugar, fat, or sodium and at least 2 grams of protein and 3 grams of fiber.

Dietary Guidelines for Good Health

Describing a practical plan for healthy eating is not as easy as it may sound. Complicated tables and elaborate analysis are impractical for most people. Although some record keeping is needed, a good system should allow some quick, daily spot checking without time-consuming analysis. A basic understanding of DRIs, the nutrition pyramid, and dietary recommendations for people in the United States provides such a method.

Dietary Reference Intakes (Formerly Recommended Dietary Allowances)

The recommended dietary allowances (RDAs) have been revised 10 times since they were first published in 1941. The most recent revision occurred in 1989, when the Food and Nutrition Board of the National Academy of Sciences included RDAs for protein, 11 vitamins, and 7 minerals by age groups—for men and women and for pregnant and nursing mothers. In 1995 the Food and Nutrition Board declared that a more comprehensive approach was needed to keep up with new research findings about the need for higher levels of some nutrients for disease prevention and performance; the growth in food fortification and use of dietary supplements; and findings that the RDAs did not distinguish guidelines for groups and populations from individuals. As a result, the board replaced and expanded the 1989 RDAs with dietary reference intakes (DRIs), shown in table 10.12. DRIs is a generic term used to refer to three reference values:

TABLE 10.12—Dietary Reference Intakes (DRIs)

Food and Nutrition Board, Institute of Medicine—National Academy of Sciences Dietary Reference Intakes: Recommended Intakes for Individuals

Lifestage group	Calcium (mg/d)	Phosphorus (mg/d)	Magnesium (mg/d)	Vitamin D[a,b] (μg/d)	Fluoride (mg/d)	Thiamin (mg/d)	Riboflavin (mg/d)	Niacin[c] (mg/d)	Vitamin B6 (mg/d)	Folate[d] (μg/d)	Vitamin B12 (μg/d)	Pantothenic acid (mg/d)	Biotin (μg/d)	Choline[e] (mg/d)
INFANTS														
0-6 mo.	**210***	**100***	**30***	5*	0.01*	0.2*	0.3*	2*	0.1*	65*	0.4*	1.7*	5*	125*
7-12 mo.	270*	275*	75*	5*	0.5*	0.3*	0.4*	4*	0.3*	80*	0.5*	1.8*	6*	150*
CHILDREN														
1-3 yr	500*	**460**	**80**	5*	0.7*	**0.5**	**0.5**	**6**	**0.5**	**150**	**0.9**	2*	8*	200*
4-8 yr	800*	**500**	**130**	5*	1*	**0.6**	**0.6**	**8**	**0.6**	**200**	**1.2**	3*	12*	250*
MALES														
9-13 yr	1,300*	**1,250**	**240**	5*	2*	**0.9**	**0.9**	**12**	**1.0**	**300**	**1.8**	4*	20*	375*
14-18 yr	1,300*	**1,250**	**410**	5*	3*	**1.2**	**1.3**	**16**	**1.3**	**400**	**2.4**	5*	25*	550*
19-30 yr	1,000*	**700**	**400**	5*	4*	**1.2**	**1.3**	**16**	**1.3**	**400**	**2.4**	5*	30*	550*
31-50 yr	1,000*	**700**	**420**	5*	4*	**1.2**	**1.3**	**16**	**1.3**	**400**	**2.4**	5*	30*	550*
51-70 yr	1,200*	**700**	**420**	10*	4*	**1.2**	**1.3**	**16**	**1.7**	**400**	**2.4[f]**	5*	30*	550*
>70 yr	1,200*	**700**	**420**	15*	4*	**1.2**	**1.3**	**16**	**1.7**	**400**	**2.4[f]**	5*	30*	550*
FEMALES														
9-13 yr	1,300*	**1,250**	**240**	5*	2*	**0.9**	**0.9**	**12**	**1.0**	**300**	**1.8**	4*	20*	375*
14-18 yr	1,300*	**1,250**	**360**	5*	3*	**1.0**	**1.0**	**14**	**1.2**	**400[g]**	**2.4**	5*	25*	400*
19-30 yr	1,000*	**700**	**310**	5*	3*	**1.1**	**1.1**	**14**	**1.3**	**400[g]**	**2.4**	5*	30*	425*
31-50 yr	1,000*	**700**	**320**	5*	3*	**1.1**	**1.1**	**14**	**1.3**	**400[g]**	**2.4**	5*	30*	425*
51-70 yr	1,200*	**700**	**320**	10*	3*	**1.1**	**1.1**	**14**	**1.5**	**400**	**2.4[f]**	5*	30*	425*
>70 yr	1,200*	**700**	**320**	15*	3*	**1.1**	**1.1**	**14**	**1.5**	**400**	**2.4[f]**	5*	30*	425*
PREGNANCY														
≤18 yr	1,300*	**1,250**	**400**	5*	3*	**1.4**	**1.4**	**18**	**1.9**	**600[h]**	**2.6**	6*	30*	450*
19-30 yr	1,000*	**700**	**350**	5*	3*	**1.4**	**1.4**	**18**	**1.9**	**600[h]**	**2.6**	6*	30*	450*
31-50 yr	1,000*	**700**	**360**	5*	3*	**1.4**	**1.4**	**18**	**1.9**	**600[h]**	**2.6**	6*	30*	450*
LACTATION														
≤18 yr	1,300*	**1,250**	**360**	5*	3*	**1.5**	**1.6**	**17**	**2.0**	**500**	**2.8**	7*	35*	550*
19-30 yr	1,000*	**700**	**310**	5*	3*	**1.5**	**1.6**	**17**	**2.0**	**500**	**2.8**	7*	35*	550*
31-50 yr	1,000*	**700**	**320**	5*	3*	**1.5**	**1.6**	**17**	**2.0**	**500**	**2.8**	7*	35*	550*

Note: This table presents Dietary Reference Intakes (DRIs) in bold type and Adequate Intakes (AIs) in ordinary type followed by an asterisk (*). DRIs and AIs may both be used as goals for individual intake. DRIs are set to meet the needs of almost all (97 or 98%) individuals in a group. For healthy breast-fed infants, the AI is the mean intake. The AI for other life-stage and gender groups is believed to cover needs of all individuals in the group, but lack of data or uncertainty in the data prevent being able to specify with confidence the percentage of individuals covered by this intake.

[a]As cholecalciferol. 1μg cholecalciferol = 40 IU vitamin D.

[b]In the absence of adequate exposure to sunlight.

[c]As niacin equivalents (NE). 1 mg of niacin = 60 mg of tryptophan; 0-6 months = preformed niacin (not NE).

[d]As dietary folate equivalents (DFE). 1 DFE = 1μg of food folate = 0.6μg of folic acid (from fortified food or supplement) consumed with food = 0.5μg of synthetic (supplemental) folic acid taken on an empty stomach.

[e]Although AIs have been set for choline, there are few data to assess whether a dietary supply of choline is needed at all stages of the life cycle, and it may be that the choline requirement can be met by endogenous synthesis at some of these stages.

[f]Because 10% to 30% of older people may malabsorb food-bound B12, it is advisable for those older than 50 years to meet their DRI mainly by consuming foods fortified with B12 or a supplement containing B12.

[g]In view of evidence linking folate intake with neural tube defects in the fetus, it is recommended that all women capable of becoming pregnant consume 400μg of synthetic folic acid from fortified foods and/or supplements in addition to intake of food folate from a varied diet.

[h]It is assumed that women will continue consuming 400μg of folic acid until their pregnancy is confirmed and they enter prenatal care, which ordinarily occurs after the end of the periconceptional period—the critical time for formation of the neural tube.

1. Adequate intake (AI) for a nutrient was established only when an RDA (average daily dietary intake of a nutrient that meets the requirement of 97 to 98% of healthy individuals) could not be determined. Each nutrient has either an RDA or an AI based on the intakes by a group of healthy individuals.

2. The tolerable upper intake level (UL) represents the highest intake likely to result in no risk of toxicity.

3. The estimated average requirement (EAR) is the amount needed to meet the requirement of half of all healthy individuals in a population.

The DRIs distinguish between gender and different life stages and more carefully take into consideration key factors capable of modifying the guidelines, such as bioavailability of nutrients (the degree to which ingested nutrients are absorbed and available to the body), nutrient-nutrient and nutrient-drug interactions, and intakes from food fortificants and supplements. The new title, Dietary Reference Intakes, is now the inclusive name of the new approach developed by the Food and Nutrition Board of the National Academy of Sciences.

Over the next several years, the Food and Nutrition Board DRI committees will oversee the development of reports on the use and interpretation of DRIs, upper reference levels of nutrients, and seven groups of related nutrients now in progress. Until all reports are completed, the existing RDA for a nutrient or food component not yet determined in the new DRIs will be retained. As a result, both the new DRIs and the old RDAs will need to be used until the year 2005. For now, see table 10.13 for a summary of recommendations.

Nutrition Pyramid

Although table 10.12 is extremely valuable, it does not provide a practical means of evaluating your daily nutrition unless you use computer software or elaborate record keeping. As a first step in determining whether you are meeting these dietary reference intakes, follow the food guide pyramid (see figure 10.3). This guide lists the food groups and the number of servings to consume from each group. Note that children, teenagers, and adults under age 19 should choose three servings from the milk, yogurt, and cheese group. Once you have estimated your energy needs, use the recommended servings from the food groups as shown in table 10.14.

The recommended number of servings from the five food groups provides 1,600 to 2,800 calories daily. The assumption is that if you choose a variety of foods from each group, you will meet your DRI. To determine how much of each nutrient you are eating, consult a registered dietitian or use one of the numerous inexpensive software packages that contain large databases of brand-name foods to analyze your intake.

The basic plan incorporating four food groups, originally released in 1956, was discarded in 1996 in favor of the nutrition pyramid shown in figure 10.3. The pyramid contains five food groups and emphasizes complex carbohydrates (fruits, vegetables, and grains). The small space at the top of the pyramid is not a sixth food group; rather, it singles out fats, oils, and sweets as items that people should use sparingly or not at all. Neither the meat industry nor the dairy industry is happy with the tiny spaces devoted to their products on the pyramid, although the number of servings represents the daily needs of most people in the United States. Variety, moderation, and balance, the three key elements of sound nutrition, are met by consuming the recommended number of servings from the five food groups. Recommended serving sizes are relatively small. A sandwich with two pieces of bread, for example, provides two servings of grains; one egg, 2 to 3 ounces of meat, or a small piece of fresh fruit is one serving. Those who follow the nutritional pyramid will consume less total fat, saturated fat, cholesterol, sugar, salt, and calories and more fruits, vegetables, grains, and dietary fiber. See the food composition table in appendix A for the nutritional content of common foods. People often establish poor eating habits during childhood. More than 60% of young people eat too much fat, and less than 20% eat the recommended five or more servings of fruits and vegetables each day.

Because of the alarming increases in body weight in the United States, it is anticipated that new recommendations will soon be put in effect to update the pyramid by indicating the exact size of a serving in each food group, in terms of ounces and cups, as a means of reducing the daily caloric intake of Americans by an average of 600 calories.

Dietary Guidelines for Healthy American Adults

Healthy food habits can help you reduce the risk factors for heart attack and stroke, high blood cholesterol, high blood pressure, and excess body weight. The American Heart Association Eating

TABLE 10.13—Summary of Dietary Recommendations for the American Public

Item	Current dietary intake	Recommendations
Food guide pyramid	Fifty-one percent of children and adolescents eat less than one serving of fruit a day, and 29% eat less than one serving a day of vegetables that are not fried. Nationwide average consumption of fruits and vegetables is: Never, 3.8%; 1 to 2 servings daily, 34.1%; 3 to 4 daily, 38.7%; 5 or more daily, 23.1%. Only 38% of the population are very familiar with the nutrition pyramid, 22% are somewhat familiar, and 40% are unfamiliar.	Vegetables—3 to 5 servings; fruit—2 to 4; meat, poultry, fish, dry beans, eggs, and nuts—2 to 3; milk, yogurt, and cheese—2 to 3; bread, cereal, rice, and pasta—6 to 11
Calories	Most Americans consume excess calories because supersized meals and drinks dominate the convenience store and restaurant market.	Per lb weight, active = 15-16, moderately active = 13-14, and inactive = 10-11
Carbohydrate	46% of daily calories	50%
Simple (concentrated sugars)	24-28%	5-6%
Complex fruits and vegetables	22%	45%
Protein	12-14%	12-35%
Total fat	33-34%: More than 84% of children and adolescents eat too much total fat (i.e., more than 25% of calories from fat), and more than 91% eat too much saturated fat (i.e., more than 10% of calories from saturated fat). On average, young people get 33-34% of their calories from total fat and 12-13% of their calories from saturated fat.	25-30%
Saturated fat	12-13%	5-6%
Monounsaturated fat	10-11%	12%
Polyunsaturated fat	10-11%	12%
Trans-fats		As little as possible; no safe amount determined.
Cholesterol	217 mg for women, 337 mg for men	Less than 300 mg
Salt	4,000-7,000 mg	Less than 2,400 mg (one teaspoon)
Dietary fiber	15 g	25-35 g
Fluid		
Water	4-5 glasses	6-8 glasses, 12-15 if on any type of diet
Alcohol	—	For men, no more than 2 drinks daily (2 beers, 2 glasses of wine [4 oz each], 2 shots of 100-proof vodka, bourbon, scotch); for women, 1 drink daily
Sodas	—	No more than 1-2 daily (includes diet and regular)
Coffee or tea	—	No more than 3 daily

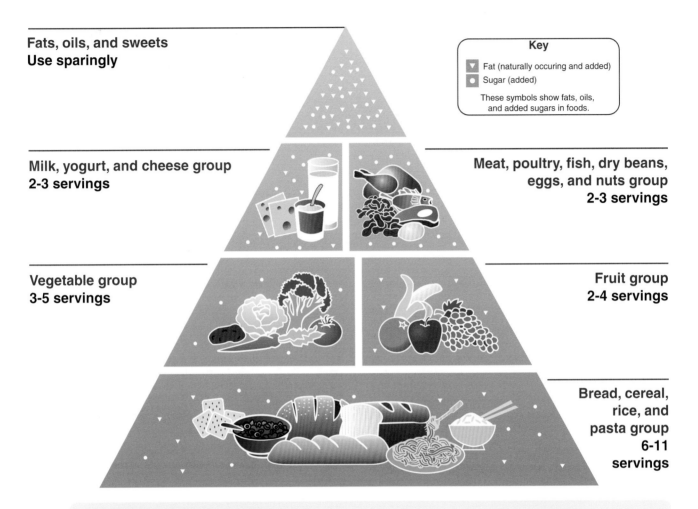

Fats, oils, and sweets
Use sparingly

Key
▽ Fat (naturally occuring and added)
○ Sugar (added)
These symbols show fats, oils,
and added sugars in foods.

Milk, yogurt, and cheese group
2-3 servings

Meat, poultry, fish, dry beans,
eggs, and nuts group
2-3 servings

Vegetable group
3-5 servings

Fruit group
2-4 servings

Bread, cereal,
rice, and
pasta group
6-11
servings

Figure 10.3 USDA food guide pyramid.

TABLE 10.14

Energy intake	1,600 kcal	2,200 kcal	2,800 kcal
Bread group	6	9	11
Vegetable group	3-4	4	5
Fruit group	2-4	3	4
Meat group	2, for a total of 5 oz	2, for a total of 6 oz	3, for a total of 7 oz
Milk, yogurt, and cheese group	2-3*	2-3*	2-3*

Older children and teens ages 9 to 18 years and adults over age 50 need 3 servings daily.

Plan for Healthy Americans, released in October 2000, is based on these dietary guidelines:

■ Eat a variety of fruits and vegetables. Choose five or more servings per day.

■ Eat a variety of grain products, including whole grains. Choose six or more servings per day.

■ Include fat-free and low-fat milk products, fish (at least two meals per week, particularly fatty fish), legumes (beans), skinless poultry, and lean meats.

■ Choose fats and oils with 2 grams or less saturated fat per tablespoon, such as liquid and tub margarine, canola oil, and olive oil.

■ Balance the number of calories you eat with the number you use each day. (To find that number, multiply the number of pounds you weigh by 14 calories. This figure is the average number of calories you use each day if you are moderately active. If you get little exercise, multiply your weight by 11 instead of 14. People who are less active burn fewer calories.)

■ Get enough physical activity to keep fit and balance the calories you burn with the calories you eat. Walk or do other activities for 60 minutes or complete 30 minutes of continuous exercise at or above your target heart rate on most or all days. To lose weight, do enough activity to use up more calories than you eat every day.

- Limit your intake of foods high in calories or low in nutrition. This category includes foods with a lot of added sugar like soft drinks and candy.

- Limit foods high in saturated fat, trans-fat, and cholesterol, such as full-fat milk products, fatty meats, tropical oils, partially hydrogenated vegetable oils, and egg yolks. Instead, choose foods low in saturated fat, trans-fat, and cholesterol from the first four points on this list. (Trans-fat comes from adding hydrogen to vegetable oil, which partially hydrogenates it. Trans-fat tends to increase blood-cholesterol levels.)

- Eat less than 6 grams of salt (sodium chloride) per day, which is about 1 1/4 teaspoons of salt, or a daily sodium intake of less than 2,400 milligrams.

- If you drink alcohol, have no more than one drink per day if you are a woman or two per day if you are a man. One drink means no more than 1/2 ounce of pure alcohol. Examples of one drink are 12 ounces of beer, 4 ounces of wine, 1 1/2 ounces of 80-proof spirits, or 1 ounce of 100-proof spirits.

Following these guidelines will help you achieve and maintain a healthy eating pattern. The benefits include healthy body weight, desirable blood-cholesterol level, and normal blood pressure. Not every meal has to meet all the guidelines, but you should apply the guidelines to your overall eating pattern over a period of several days. These guidelines may do more than improve your heart health. They may reduce your risk for other chronic health problems, including type 2 diabetes, osteoporosis (bone loss), and some forms of cancer.

To meet the dietary guidelines, the committee recommends that you choose a diet with most of the calories from grains, vegetables, and fruits, low-fat dairy products, lean meats, fish, and poultry, and fewer calories from fats and sweets. The details of these guidelines are discussed throughout this chapter.

Table 10.13 compares the current U.S. dietary intake of food and drink with the proposed dietary goals or recommendations. In most areas our current dietary intake in percentages of daily calories fails to meet the proposed goals. We have too much total fat in our total daily calories (34% instead of 25 to 30%), too much saturated fat (13% instead of 5 to 6%), too much simple carbohydrates (24% instead of 5 to 6%), too little complex carbohydrates (46% instead of 50%), and too little complex carbohydrates (22% instead of 45%). In addition, we consume too much cholesterol (more than 300 milligrams), salt (4,000 to 7,000 milligrams instead of 2,400 milligrams), and alcohol. We drink too many carbonated drinks and too much coffee and tea, we consume too many total calories, and we do not drink enough water. Obviously, taste influences our eating habits far more than our concern for health does.

Food Labeling

A law went into effect in May 1994 requiring most food products to be labeled according to strict guidelines. This label, called nutrition facts, contains information on nutrients of major concern to consumers (figure 10.4). The law requires food labels to contain the following information:

- List of ingredients, listed in descending order by weight
- Serving size
- Servings per container
- Amount per serving of total calories, calories from fat, total fat, saturated fat, cholesterol, sodium, total carbohydrate, dietary fiber, and sugars
- Protein
- Vitamin A
- Vitamin C
- Calcium
- Iron

The number of calories from the following may be listed voluntarily:

- Saturated fat
- Polyunsaturated fat
- Monounsaturated fat
- Potassium
- Soluble fiber
- Insoluble fiber
- Sugar alcohols
- Other carbohydrates

Food labels, once called the U.S. RDAs, now use daily value (DV) to help people understand how to choose foods wisely as part of a daily diet plan. The percentage of the DV supplied by

Serving size

Is your serving the same size as the one on the label? If you eat double the serving size listed, you need to double the nutrient and calorie values. If you eat one-half the serving size shown here, cut the nutrient and calorie values in half.

Calories

Are you overweight? Cut back a little on calories! Look here to see how a serving of the food adds to your daily total. A 5'4", 138-lb. active woman needs about 2200 calories each day. A 5' 10", 174 lb. active man needs about 2900. How about you?

Total carbohydrates

When you cut down on fat, you can eat more carbohydrates. Carbohydrates are in foods like bread, potatoes, fruits, and vegetables. Choose these often! They give you more nutrients than sugars like soda pop and candy.

Dietary fiber

Grandmother called it "roughage," but her advice to eat more is still up-to-date! That goes for both soluble and insoluble kinds of dietary fiber. Fruits, vegetables, whole-grain foods, beans, and peas are all good sources and can help reduce the risk of heart disease and cancer.

Protein

Most Americans get more protein than they need. Where there is animal protein, there is also fat and cholesterol. Eat small servings of lean meat, fish, and poultry. Use skim or low-fat milk, yogurt, and cheese. Try vegetable proteins like beans, grains, and cereals.

Vitamins and minerals

Your goal here is 100% of each for the day. Don't count on one food to do it all. Let a combination of foods add up to a winning score.

Nutrition Facts

Serving Size 1/2 cup (114g)
Servings Per Container 4

Amount Per Serving

Calories 90		Calories from Fat 30

	% Daily Value*
Total Fat 3g	5%
Saturated Fat 0g	0%
Cholesterol 0mg	0%
Sodium 300mg	13%
Total Carbohydrate 13g	4%
Dietary Fiber 3g	12%
Sugars 3g	
Protein 3g	

Vitamin A 80%	•	Vitamin C 60%
Calcium 4%	•	Iron 4%

*Percent Daily Values are based on a 2000 calorie diet. Your daily values may be higher or lower depending on your calorie needs.

	Calories:	2000	2500
Total Fat	Less than	65g	80g
Sat. Fat	Less than	20g	25g
Cholesterol	Less than	300mg	300mg
Sodium	Less than	2400mg	2400mg
Total Carbohydrate		300g	375g
Dietary Fiber		25g	30g

Calories per gram:
Fat 9 • Carbohydrate 4 • Protein 4

More nutrients may be listed on some labels.

Total fat

Aim low: Most people need to cut back on fat! Too much fat may contribute to heart disease and cancer. Try to limit your *calories from fat*. For a healthy heart, choose foods with a big difference between the total number of calories and the number of calories from fat.

Saturated fat

A new kind of fat? No — saturated fat is part of the total fat in food. It is listed separately because it's the key player in raising blood cholesterol and your risk of heart disease. Eat less!

Cholesterol

Too much cholesterol — a second cousin to fat — can lead to heart disease. Challenge yourself to eat less than 300 mg each day.

Sodium

You call it "salt," the label calls it "sodium." Either way, it may add up to high blood pressure in some people. So, keep your sodium intake low — 2400 to 3000 mg or less each day.*

*The AHA recommends no more than 3000 mg sodium per day for healthy adults

Daily value

Feel like you're drowning in numbers? Let the Daily Value be your guide. Daily Values are listed for people who eat 2000 or 2500 calories each day. If you eat more, your personal daily value maybe higher than what's listed on the label. If you eat less, your personal daily value maybe lower.

For fat, saturated fat, cholesterol, and sodium choose foods with a low % *Daily Value*. For total carbohydrate, dietary fiber, vitamins and minerals your daily value goal is to reach 100% of each.

g = grams (About 28 g = 1 ounce)
mg = milligrams (1000 mg = 1 g)

Key Words:

Fat free: Less than 0.61 g of fat per serving; ***Low fat***: 3 g of fat or less per serving; ***Lean***: Less than 10 g of fat, 4 g of saturated fat and 96 mg of cholesterol per serving; ***Light (Lite)***: one half less calories or no more than one half the fat of the higher-calorie, higher-fat version; or no more than one half the sodium of the higher-sodium version; ***Cholesterol free***: Less than 2 mg of cholesterol and 2 g or less of saturated fat per serving. ***To make health claims about the food must be*** *heart disease and fats*: low in fat, saturated fat and cholesterol: *blood pressure and sodium*; low in sodium; *heart disease and fruits, vegetables, and grain products*; a fruit, vegetable, or grain product low in fat, saturated fat and cholesterol, that contains at least 0.6 g soluble fiber, without fortification, per serving.

Figure 10.4 Nutrition label.

a single serving is shown for a daily diet of 2,000 and 2,500 calories. The DV may be somewhat higher or lower based on your individual calorie needs. But you can still use the percentage of DV as a frame of reference, whether you eat more or less than 2,000 calories each day. The DV is based on two sets of standards, the daily reference values (DRVs) and the dietary reference intakes (DRIs) shown in figure 10.4 and table 10.12. Consumers should read food labels to help them improve diet choices by restricting use of products high in calories, sodium, sugar, fat, saturated fat, and cholesterol and choosing high-density food (low in calories and high in the percentage of DVs for key vitamins and minerals) and high-fiber products. With only a little practice, you will be capable of making wise decisions at a glance before placing an item in the shopping cart.

Health Claims

The FDA allows food manufacturers to list health claims on food labels provided they meet certain minimum standards supporting the relationship between the product and the prevention of certain diseases. Although labels cannot state the degree of risk reduction, words such as "may" or "might" are permitted. Health claims on food labels must meet the following conditions:

- Calcium and osteoporosis—product must contain 20% or more of the DV for calcium.

- Food and cancer—product must contain no more than 3 grams of fat and be labeled a low-fat food.

- Saturated fat and cholesterol and heart disease—product must meet the definition for low saturated fat, low fat, and low cholesterol.

- Fiber-containing products such as fruits, vegetables, and grains—product must be a low-fat product and a good source of fiber, without fortification.
- Fruits, vegetables, and grains that are a good source of fiber and heart disease—product must meet the definition for low saturated fat, cholesterol, and total fat and contain at least 0.6 gram of soluble fiber, without fortification.
- Fruits and vegetables and cancer—product must contain low fat and be a good source of at least one of the following without fortification: dietary fiber, vitamin A, or vitamin C.
- Oats and heart disease—product must be low fat and contain at least 0.75 gram of soluble fiber.
- Sodium and high blood pressure—product must contain less than 40 milligrams of sodium.
- Folic acid (folate) and neural tube defects—product must be a rich source of folic acid.

How to Read a Food Label

Begin reading the label by looking at the serving size and the number of servings in the package. Labels show sizes in familiar units, such as cups or pieces, followed by the metric amount (for example, the number of grams), and are based on the amount of food people typically eat. Examine how many servings the food package contains and compare it to how much you actually eat. Serving influences all the nutrient amounts. Next, check out the total calories per serving and calories from saturated fat, total fat, cholesterol, and sodium. You should restrict high-fat, high-sodium, and high-calorie products by making certain that one serving provides only a reasonable percentage of daily value. Now check the percentage of daily value of the nutrients that are important to your health, such as vitamins A and C, calcium, and iron, to ensure that the product is a nutritious choice.

Eating enough of these nutrients can improve your health and reduce the risk of some diseases and conditions. You can also check for other important information, such as dietary fiber, protein, and carbohydrate, and learn to keep a daily mental or written record of your consumption of things you want to restrict and those you want to increase as a way of influencing meal planning that day. Finally, check the product ingredients at the bottom of the label, keeping in mind that the label lists items in descending order by weight (the ingredient that the product contains the most of is listed first; the ingredient that the product has the least of is listed last). When looking at the label, remember that

- sugar (glucose, fructose, sucrose, lactose, maple syrup) and salt (sodium chloride, monosodium glutamate, sodium potassium) may be listed in different forms;
- hydrogenated and partially hydrogenated fat indicates saturated fats and trans-fats;
- only whole grain (not enriched wheat flour) contains dietary fiber; and
- products with sugar, salt, and fats listed as the first several ingredients contain large amounts of those items and are probably unwise choices.

One of the best preventive health tips is to practice label reading at the grocery store and avoid buying certain products that can eventually result in health consequences for you and your family. To determine quickly whether the product is a good food or beverage choice, compare the percentage of daily value for calories, sodium, saturated fat, and cholesterol to the recommended percentages in table 10.13. You can do the same for healthy contents such as protein, monounsaturated and polyunsaturated fats, and dietary fiber. If a product contains 40% total fat, or 15% saturated fat, for example, it exceeds the recommended percentage of calories that you should consume daily for those fats and you should probably avoid it. On the other hand, being aware that you are consuming a product high in fat alerts you to reduce your fat intake for the rest of the day. Table 10.13 also reminds you to keep your intake of alcohol, sodas, and coffee at acceptable levels. In combination with the food guide pyramid to remind you to consume the specified number of servings from the five food groups, table 10.13 offers a built-in shopping and meal-planning guide.

Nutrition-Disease Relationships

Scientific evidence associating diet with numerous diseases has increased in the past decade. Although cause-and-effect relationships are still rather uncommon, dietary risk factors have been identified for a number of diseases and disorders (see table 10.15), and the consumption of various nutrients has been associated with the prevention of some diseases.

TABLE 10.15—Nutrition and Disease Connections

Disease or disorder	Nutrition connection	Status of research
Alzheimer's	Low levels of folic acid may increase the risk; foods rich in vitamin E and C may reduce the risk. Good nutrition over a lifetime, mainly during later life, may prevent the disease.	Some evidence
	High-fat and high-salt diets can lead to hypertension. Untreated hypertension has been linked to cognitive decline, Alzheimer's, and other forms of dementia.	Strong evidence
	High-fat and high-calorie diets double the risk of developing Alzheimer's.	Strong evidence
	Moderate alcohol intake (1-2 drinks daily for women, 1-3 for men) was associated with a reduced risk of Alzheimer's in a 6-year survey study of 5,395 people over the age of 55.	Some evidence
	Eating fish once a week reduces the risk of Alzheimer's by 60%.	Some evidence
Birth defects	American women have doubled the folic acid in their blood since the government required that flour and other grains be fortified with the vitamin in 1998. The requirement changed because of the strong link between low folic acid intake and birth defects (spinal and brain defects).	Very strong evidence
Bone strength	Longtime tea consumption may strengthen bones. Tea contains fluoride and flavenoids that include estrogen-like plant derivatives that can enhance bone strength.	Some evidence
	Vitamin A supplements can weaken the bones and increase the risk of fractures, according to a study of 465 men conducted by physicians at the University Hospital in Uppsala and reported in the January 23, 2003, *New England Journal of Medicine*. Dietary recommendations for vitamin A are 0.7 mg daily for women and 0.9 for men. Popular multivitamins contain 0.75 to 1.5 mg of vitamin A (generally listed as 2,500-5,000 international units). Men with the highest levels of vitamin A were 2 1/2 times more likely to break a hip and 65% more likely to suffer any fracture than those wit0h lower blood levels of vitamin A. Vitamin A can interfere with cells that produce new bone, stimulate cells that break down old bone, and interfere with vitamin D, which helps the body maintain normal calcium levels. Vitamin A supplements are not recommended unless specific conditions merit higher intake or deficiencies are discovered.	Good evidence
Bone loss: osteoporosis	Adequate intake of vitamin D and calcium and regular weight-bearing exercise help prevent osteoporosis.	Very strong evidence
	Of 1,100 women studied, the one-third who did not drink alcohol had three times more loss of spinal-bone mineral density than those who took 1 to 7 drinks weekly and twice as much density reduction as those who drank more than that. Similar differences were found in thighbone density.	Some evidence
Cancer (general)	Cruciferous vegetables (broccoli, cauliflower, cabbage, kale, brussels sprouts, chard, collards, mustard greens) all have compounds that boost the production of enzymes that can protect cells from cancer-causing agents. Broccoli sprouts contain up to 50 times more anticancer chemical than the mature vegetable does. Sulforaphane, found in broccoli, cauliflower, and other vegetables, prompts the body to make an enzyme that prevents tumors from forming.	Good evidence
	Phytochemicals in foods may offer front-line defense against cancer.	Good evidence
	Diets high in omega-3 fatty acids (herring, salmon, mackerel, fresh tuna, bluefish, swordfish, canned white albacore tuna) slow tumor growth.	Good evidence
	Soy foods may reduce the risk. Supplements should be avoided.	Some evidence
	All teas (green, black, and red) act as antioxidants and contain a range of beneficial chemicals that may reduce the risk of many cancers.	Strong evidence

Disease or disorder	Nutrition connection	Status of research
Cancer (general) (cont'd)	Dietary supplements have the same cancer preventive effects as a diet high in vegetables and fruits.	Very little evidence
	Beta-carotene supplements protect against cancer and heart disease.	Absolutely no evidence
	Up to 1/3 of cancers of the breast, colon, kidney, and digestive track are attributable to too much weight gain and too little exercise.	Some evidence
	American Institute for Cancer Research guidelines for cancer prevention: Choose a diet rich in a variety of plant-based foods, eat plenty of vegetables and fruits, maintain a healthy weight and be physically active, drink alcohol only in moderation if at all, select foods low in fat and salt, prepare and store foods safely, and avoid tobacco in any form.	Very strong evidence
	Coffee consumption increases the risk of some types of cancer.	Absolutely no evidence
Bladder cancer	High fluid intake (nonalcoholic drinks) is associated with a decreased risk of bladder cancer.	Some evidence
	High intake of cruciferous vegetables may reduce the risk.	Some evidence
Breast cancer	According to the American Institute for Cancer Research, high-fat, high-calorie diets increase the risk of breast cancer. Saturated-fat intake affects the progression of cancer by raising estrogen levels. Estrogen-related cancers include breast, endometrium, ovary, and prostate.	Some evidence
	Diets high in fruits and vegetables may reduce the risk.	Some evidence
	Alcohol consumption increases the risk. High folic acid intake may lower the risk in women who consume alcohol.	Some evidence
	Obesity increases the risk. An American Cancer Society study reported in the *New England Journal of Medicine* (April 23, 2003) found that 14% of cancers in men and 20% in women (90,000 deaths each year) are caused by obesity. The 16-year study of 404,576 men and 495,477 women (average age of 57) concluded that the heavier the individual, the greater the risk. Only cancer of the brain, bladder, and skin were excluded. Weighing too much is second only to smoking, which causes about 170,000 deaths annually, as a preventable cause of cancer.	Very strong evidence
	Grilling and broiling produces cancer-causing compounds (HCAs-heterocyclic amines) in red meat, poultry, and fish, which have been shown to cause tumors in animals and are suspected of increasing the risk of breast cancer in humans.	Some evidence
Colon cancer	A plant-based diet reduces the risk.	Strong evidence
	According to the American Institute for Cancer research, high-fat, high-calorie diets increase the risk of colon cancer.	Strong evidence
	Eating 2 lb of broccoli per week provides enough sulforaphane to lower colon cancer risk by half.	Good evidence
	Folic acid, calcium supplements, selenium, and vitamin E reduce the risk.	Some evidence
	High intake of red meat increases the risk of colon cancer.	Some evidence
	Obesity increases the risk.	Strong evidence

(continued)

TABLE 10.15 *(continued)*

Disease or disorder	Nutrition connection	Status of research
Colon cancer *(cont'd)*	Although a year 2000 headline reported that two studies found no connection between high fiber intake and reduced risk of colon cancer, most studies link the consumption of fruits, vegetables, and grains to the prevention of colon and other cancers. Participants in other studies altered their diets for 3-4 years and looked at whether new polyps appeared. Those who ate the most dietary fiber (over 30 grams a day) had a 20% lower risk of polyps than those who ate the least (fewer than 15 grams a day).	Strong evidence
	Regular, vigorous physical activity prevents colon cancer.	Very strong evidence
	Positive association found between colon cancer risk and diets rich in refined grains, red meat, pork, processed meat, and alcohol.	Some evidence
	Obesity increases the risk.	Strong evidence
	The unique chemical form of selenium found in broccoli reduces the risk. Dietary intake of selenium (160 μg daily) may be helpful.	Some evidence
	Fiber supplements reduce the risk.	Weak evidence
	Grilling and broiling produces cancer-causing compounds (HCAs-heterocyclic amines) in red meat, poultry, and fish, which have been shown to cause tumors in animals and are suspected of increasing the risk of colon cancer in humans.	Some evidence
Gall bladder cancer	Obesity increases the risk.	Some evidence
Gastric cancer	Flavonoids and carotenoids, found in fruits and vegetables, reduce the risk of gastric cancer.	Some evidence
Kidney cancer	Obesity increases the risk.	Some evidence
Lung cancer	According to the American Institute for Cancer research, high-fat, high-calorie diets increase the risk of lung cancer. Folate deficiency also increases the risk.	Some evidence
	Dietary selenium (160 μg daily) may reduce the risk.	Slight indication
Non-Hodgkin's lymphoma	Consuming large amounts of red meat increases the risk.	Some evidence
Oral cavity and pharynx	Excessive alcohol consumption increases the risk. Risk of upper respiratory tract cancers increases dramatically if drinkers also smoke.	Very strong evidence
Ovarian cancer	Eating lots of green, leafy vegetables is associated with reduced risk. Consumption of eggs, dairy products, and other sources of cholesterol was associated with increased risk.	Slight evidence
	No association found between caloric intake, fat, protein or dietary fiber, beta-carotene, vitamin A, and vitamin E.	Some evidence
Pancreatic cancer	According to the American Institute for Cancer Research, high-fat, high-saturated-fat, and high-cholesterol diets increase the risk of pancreatic cancer.	Suspected
	Obesity and inactivity increase the risk.	Some evidence

Disease or disorder	Nutrition connection	Status of research
Prostate cancer	Diet high in vegetables (28 or more servings weekly) and high in lycopenes (found in tomatoes, watermelon, and grapefruit) may be protective.	Some evidence
	Study of 238 men with prostate cancer and 471 who were free of the disease from Shanghai, China, cited in the *Journal of the National Cancer Institute* (October, 2002) indicates that a diet with lots of vegetables from the allium group (garlic, shallots, and onions) reduces the risk by one-half. Scallions seemed to be the most protective.	Some evidence
	Dietary selenium (160 µg daily) reduced the risk by 45-63% in one study.	Some evidence
	Two categories of vegetables (cruciferous and yellow-orange) and two individual vegetables (corn and carrots) reduce the risk.	Some evidence
	Selenium and vitamin E supplements may be protective.	Little evidence
	High consumption of dairy products increases the risk.	Conflicting evidence
	Grilling and broiling produces cancer-causing compounds (HCAs-heterocyclic amines) in red meat, poultry, and fish, which have been shown to cause tumors in animals and are suspected of increasing the risk of prostate cancer in humans.	Some evidence
Stomach cancer	Excessive alcohol intake, particularly in the form of beer, increases the risk of stomach cancer.	Some evidence
	Grilling and broiling produces cancer-causing compounds (HCAs-heterocyclic amines) in red meat, poultry, and fish, which have been shown to cause tumors in animals and are suspected of increasing the risk of stomach cancer in humans.	Some evidence
Uterine cancer	Link found between folate deficiency and uterine cancer.	Some evidence
	Obesity increases the risk.	Strong evidence
Treatment of cancer	Investigators studying how nutrition affects cancer therapy. Diets must contain sufficient calories, protein, vitamins, and minerals.	Some evidence
	Fish-oil supplements may help chemotherapy drugs work better and lessen the side effects. Safe levels for humans not yet determined.	Slight evidence
Dental cavities	High-sugar food and drink, fermentable carbohydrates, and sugared foods that remain in the mouth longer cause cavities.	Very strong evidence
	Coffee (regular, decaf, and instant) helps reduce levels of bacteria that cause tooth decay and helps keep bacteria from adhering to teeth.	Good evidence
Diabetes	Daily consumption of processed meats (hot dogs, bacon, bologna) was associated with a 50% increase in type 2 adult-onset diabetes in a study of 42,504 men aged 40-75.	Good evidence
	Failure to maintain normal weight, an overweight condition, or obesity is the main cause of type 2 diabetes. How much you eat is just as important as what you eat in controlling blood sugar.	Very strong evidence
	Regular exercise reduces insulin resistance and the body's ability to tolerate sugar and reduces the risk.	Very strong evidence
	Overweight people who consume many dairy products (more than 5 times daily) reduced the risk of insulin resistance syndrome 72%. Insulin resistant patients are at risk of developing type 2 diabetes.	Some evidence
	Weight control and regular exercise prevent adult-onset diabetes.	Very strong evidence

(continued)

TABLE 10.15 *(continued)*

Disease or disorder	Nutrition connection	Status of research
Diverticulitis	High fiber found to reduce the risk.	Strong evidence
Gallstones	Excess high-fat, high-calorie foods; very low-calorie, rapid weight-loss diets; and prolonged fasting may be contributing factors	Suspected
Heart attack	Consuming more alpha-linolenic acid (omega-3 fatty acid related to those in fish and also found in canola, flaxseed, and soybean oils, walnuts, almonds, hazel nuts, and leafy greens) reduces the risk. Even a small increase reduced coronary risk.	Strong evidence
	Consuming fish at least twice a week reduces the risk of heart disease by 30%, five times weekly by 50%.	Strong evidence
	Blood homocysteine levels, linked to a higher risk of heart disease, may be reduced with the DASH (dietary approaches to stop hypertension) diet plan.	Some evidence
	Tea (black and green) reduces the risk.	Inconclusive
	High sodium intake may increase the risk of stroke and heart attack independent of its effect on high blood pressure.	Some evidence
	Findings from the Physicians' Health Study, a long-term analysis of the habits of 22,000 doctors, indicated that men who ate a few handfuls of nuts each week (2 oz) had a 47% lower risk of sudden death due to cardiac arrest than those who ate nuts less often.	Some evidence
Heart disease	Regular exercise and limited intake of alcohol, carbohydrates, and saturated fat lower triglycerides. High triglycerides (200-400 mg/dl, borderline-high; 400-1,000 mg/dl, high), a type of fat found in foods (meats, cheeses, fish, and nuts) and manufactured in the body, are associated with ischemic heart disease independent of other risk factors.	Strong evidence
	According to the American Institute for Cancer Research, high-fat, high-saturated-fat, high-cholesterol, and high-calorie diets increase the risk of heart disease.	Strong evidence
	Garlic supplements lower blood cholesterol.	Absolutely no evidence
	Drinking modest amounts of alcohol is associated with a lower risk of coronary heart disease. Drinking higher amounts raises the risk of cancer, hypertension, stroke, birth defects, inflammation of the pancreas, damage to the brain and heart, malnutrition, osteoporosis, cirrhosis of the liver, and heart disease.	Strong evidence
	Oat bran, in combination with a low-fat, low-cholesterol, high-fiber diet significantly lowers LDL cholesterol. Other foods containing water-soluble fiber (legumes, black-eyed peas, beans, carrots, green peas, corn, prunes, sweet potatoes, zucchini, broccoli, bananas, apples, pears, and oranges) are also effective.	Strong evidence
	High blood-iron levels may contribute to heart disease.	Unknown
	Coffee consumption increases the risk.	Absolutely no evidence
Atherosclerosis	Supplementation with vitamin C may accelerate clogging of coronary arteries. People taking 500 mg of vitamin C daily for one year had a 2 1/2 times greater rate of thickening than did those who avoided supplements.	Some evidence

Disease or disorder	Nutrition connection	Status of research
Hypertension	Prevention and treatment: DASH (dietary approaches to stop hypertension) is a diet rich in calcium, magnesium, and potassium, which control blood pressure. The diet may also reduce blood homocysteine, which is linked to higher risk of heart disease. Free copies of the DASH diet are available from NHLBI Health Information Center, P.O. Box 30105, Bethesda, MD 20824-0105, 301-592-8573.	Strong evidence
	A study of 10,000 subjects from 32 countries found a correlation between low sodium intake and the incidence of hypertension.	Strong evidence
	For some individuals who are sodium sensitive, a high-sodium diet boosts blood pressure and may lead to hypertension. Lowering salt intake can be effective in controlling blood pressure in many people. You can reduce your sodium intake to less than 2,400 mg daily by reading labels; limiting intake of canned soups, sauces, cold cuts, chips, crackers, and packaged bakery goods; switching to a diet rich in fruits, grains, vegetables, and nonfat or low-fat dairy products; avoiding fast-food restaurants; reducing salt in your cooking; and avoiding the salt shaker unless food is bland.	Strong evidence
	Salt sensitivity and its effect on high blood pressure increase with age. As people grow older, they experience a decline in their ability to excrete sodium.	Strong evidence
Joint health	Gelatin dietary supplements, containing two amino acids used by the body to make collagen (component of connective tissue in joints and skin), and added vitamin C and calcium eliminate joint and bone stress.	No evidence
Liver disease	Alcohol raises the risk of liver disease.	Very strong evidence
Macular degeneration	Several studies concluded that 1-2 glasses of wine daily may prevent macular degeneration (age-related condition that can lead to partial blindness).	Some evidence
Parkinson's disease	A study of 8,004 Japanese Americans found that men who did not drink coffee were 5 times more likely to develop Parkinson's than those who drank the most (4 1/2-5 1/2 6 oz cups per day).	Some evidence

High-fat diets have been linked to cardiorespiratory disease and cancer, high sodium and alcohol intake to a small percentage of the hypertense population, and high-calorie intake and obesity to high blood pressure, diabetes, cardiorespiratory disease, and cancer. On the other hand, diets high in complex carbohydrates (fruits, vegetables, and grains) that contain vitamin A, beta-carotene, and dietary fiber have been tied to the prevention of cancer (colon, stomach, and so on), diverticulitis, and constipation, and low-fat diets have been linked to the prevention of cardiorespiratory disease and certain types of cancer.

Consumers must resist the temptation, however, to consume very large amounts of any nutrient identified as having the potential for disease prevention or treatment until researchers find supportive evidence. In early 1996 the National Cancer Institute researchers shut down a $42 million vitamin study of 18,000 smokers almost 2 years early because too many of those being given high doses of beta-carotene supplements were dying. The government declared that beta-carotene supplements do not protect people against cancer or heart disease and might increase smokers' risk of deadly tumors. Another study of 22,000 individuals receiving megadoses (10 times the average recommended daily intake) of beta-carotene for 12 years found no evidence of either harm or benefit from beta-carotene supplementation. A study of 34,000 postmenopausal women produced similar results, indicating that those who ate foods rich in vitamin E, especially nuts and seeds, had less than half the risk of death from heart disease as did women who ate minimal amounts. No benefit was found among women who took vitamin E pills (*U.S. News and World Report*, 1996).

Evidence suggests that supplementation in many areas does not adequately replace the complex mix of chemicals and high-fiber, low-fat content of foods such as fruits, vegetables, and grains. The fact that phytochemicals and antioxidants found in many foods may help prevent disease does not necessarily mean that heavy intake through supplementation will produce similar effects. Again, you should stress moderation, variation, and balance, in all aspects of your diet.

Cooking and Cancer

Grilling and broiling produces cancer-causing compounds (HCAs-heterocyclic amines) in red meat, poultry, and fish, which have been shown to cause tumors in animals and are suspected of increasing the risk of breast, colon, stomach, and prostate cancer in humans. The fat that drips onto the hot coals or stones produces another cancer-causing substance called PAHs (polycyclic aromatic hydrocarbons) that are deposited back onto food through smoke and flare-ups.

You need not stop grilling. Follow these tips recommended by the American Institute for Cancer Research (AICR) for safe grilling:

- Instead of grilling muscle meat, grill vegetables in the form of veggie burgers, pizza, tofu, or quesadillas and grill fruit as a dessert.
- Marinate meats with half a cup per pound before grilling to reduce the HCAs by as much as 92 to 99%.
- Trim fat and choose lean, well-trimmed meats with less fat to drip into the flames. Remove skin from poultry and avoid ribs, sausages, and other high-fat meats.
- Precook meats, fish, and poultry in the oven or microwave and then grill for only a short time to add flavor.
- Keep meat portions small to shorten grilling time. The AICR recommends eating no more than 3 cooked ounces (the size of a deck of cards) of red meat a day.
- Fix the drips and avoid allowing juices to drip onto the flames or coals by using tongs to turn the meat. Avoid piercing meat, cover the grill with punctured aluminum foil, avoid placing meats directly over coals, and use a bottle of water to control flare-ups.
- Flip meats frequently. Using low heat and turning often accelerates cooking, destroys bacteria, and prevents formation of HCAs.
- Remove all charred or burned portions of food before eating.

Cooking meat in vegetable oils heated at very high temperatures or in repeatedly reheated oil, a practice followed in some restaurants, increases the formation of various mutagens that can damage DNA and increase cancer risk. French fries and other deep-fried foods served in restaurants absorb some of the damaging fat they were cooked in, which is still another reason to eat these products sparingly and never reuse cooking oil.

Depending on the cooking method used, other foods also increase the risk of cancer. A chance finding in a Swedish study published April 24, 2002, showed that frying and baking at high temperatures produced high levels of acrylamide in a wide range of previously unsuspected food. Acrylamide may also occur from grilling, roasting, and barbecuing. Significant levels have not been found in raw or baked foods. Industry manufactures the chemical as a white powder to produce gels used for water treatment, for paper making, as a soil-conditioning agent, and in the construction of dam foundations, tunnels, and sewers. Because the chemical was only recently discovered in food at these levels, its effects on humans is unknown, although it is suspected of being a carcinogen.

To date, high levels have been found in home-cooked, precooked, processed, and packaged food and chips prepared from potatoes (french fries, chips, crisps, crisp breads, and cereals). Other foods are also suspected of containing high levels of acrylamide. Among the foods tested, fast-food french fries had the highest levels, with large orders containing 39 to 82 micrograms, over 300 times the EPA-recommended limit. One-ounce portions of Pringles potato crisps contained about 25 micrograms, with corn-based Fritos and Tostitos containing half that amount or less. Regular and Honey Nut Cheerios contained 6 or 7 micrograms. Table 10.16 shows the approximate amounts in other tested foods.

Possible risks to human health from acrylamide would occur from long-term exposure. Obviously, we all have been consuming products containing this chemical for decades. Clark University researcher Dale Hattis estimates that acrylamide currently causes several thousand cancers per year in Americans. Acrylamide is one of numerous substances in food that is potentially detrimental to health at high levels. Although even a balanced diet will not eliminate all risks, these initial findings provide additional evidence for Americans to reduce their consumption of greasy french fries, chips, and snack foods and return to a more healthy diet that includes a minimum

TABLE 10.16—Acrylamides in Foods

Tested food	Micrograms per serving
Water, 8 oz	EPA limit 0.12
Boiled potatoes, 4 oz	0
Old El Paso® taco shells, 3, 1.1 oz	1
Ore Ida® french fries (uncooked), 3 oz	5
Ore Ida® french fries (baked), 3 oz	28
Honey Nut Cheerios®, 1 oz	6
Cheerios®, 1 oz	7
Tostitos® tortilla chips, 1 oz	5
Fritos® corn chips, 1 oz	11
Pringles® potato crisps, 1 oz	25
Wendy's® french fries, Biggie, 5.6 oz	39
KFC® potato wedges, jumbo, 6.2 oz	52
Burger King® french fries, large, 5.7 oz	59
McDonald's® french fries, large, 6.2 oz	82

of five servings of fruits and vegetables daily to help protect against some cancers. Cooking these products at a lower temperature also decreases the presence of acrylamide.

Plastic Wraps and Bowls

The ingredients in plastic wraps, plasticizers, are suspected of contributing to cancer and other health problems. In case there is a connection, you can easily avoid problems by following these suggestions:

- All wraps are approved for microwave use by the FDA and most do not contain plasticizers. To be safe, buy only polyethylene wraps.
- Keep wraps from touching food by tenting it loosely and allowing room for steam to vent by not sealing the edge.
- Use waxed paper or paper towels instead of plastic wrap.
- Remove plastic wraps before defrosting meat in the microwave.
- Use only plastic containers labeled microwave safe.
- Never reuse frozen dinner trays.

Food Additives

Most people think that food additives, particularly chemical and artificial, are unhealthy and unnecessary. The truth is that many additives, such as preservatives and vitamins and minerals, keep food safe and healthy. Emulsifiers and flavoring agents improve texture, consistency, and appearance. Without additives, our food would spoil and be unsafe, less nutritious, and more expensive. We do not need to be concerned about most artificial ingredients in food. Manufacturers have been required to prove the safety of new additives since 1958, when the FDA set guidelines for their use. Most of the widely used and controversial additives are on the GRAS list (generally recognized as safe). The FDA continuously reevaluates the list and has banned some additives and restricted others.

Food Contamination

Although our food supply is one of the safest in the world, over 76 million become ill, 300,000 are hospitalized, and 5,000 die each year from foodborne or beverage-contaminated illnesses. Over 250 different diseases have been identified. Most are infections caused by bacteria (such as Salmonella and E. coli 0157:H7), viruses (such as calicivirus and hepatitis A), and parasites (such as Cryptosporidium and Cyclospora). Harmful toxins or chemicals account for some poisonings. The Centers for Disease Control summarized the following information in CDC Fact Book, 2000-2001 to help you reduce the incidence of foodborne disease in your household.

Raw foods of animal origin (meat and poultry, eggs, unpasteurized milk, and shellfish) are the most likely to be contaminated. Filter-feeding shellfish strain microbes from the sea and are likely to be contaminated if the seawater contains pathogens. Foods that contain products of many individual animals, such as bulk raw milk, pooled raw eggs, or ground beef, are particularly hazardous because a pathogen present in any of the animals may contaminate the whole batch. A single hamburger may contain meat from hundreds of animals. A single restaurant omelet may contain eggs from several chickens. A glass of raw milk may contain milk from hundreds of cows. A broiler chicken carcass can be exposed to the drippings and juices of many thousands of other birds that went through the same cold-water tank after slaughter.

Raw fruits and vegetables are also vulnerable. Because washing decreases but does not eliminate contamination, everyone is at risk. The use of unclean water, for example, can contaminate large amounts of produce. Fresh manure used to fertilize vegetables can also contaminate them. Alfalfa sprouts and other raw sprouts pose a particular challenge because the conditions under which they sprout are ideal for growing microbes as well as sprouts and because they are eaten without further cooking. A few bacteria present on the seeds can grow to a large number of pathogens on the sprouts. Unpasteurized fruit juice can also be contaminated if pathogens are in or on the fruit used to make it.

Although the incidence of foodborne illness is declining, the Centers for Disease Control recommends observing the following precautions to reduce your risk (*CDC Fact Book*, 2000-2001):

- Cook foods to the proper temperatures and use a thermometer to determine the internal temperature of meat. Ground beef should be cooked to an internal temperature of 160°F, poultry to 180°F, and eggs until the yolk is firm.

- Separate: Don't cross-contaminate one food with another. Wash hands, utensils, and cutting boards after they have been in contact with raw meat or poultry and before they touch another food. Place cooked meat on a clean platter rather than back on the one that held the raw meat.

- Chill: Refrigerate foods promptly. Bacteria grow quickly at room temperature.

- Clean: Wash hands and surfaces often. Wash your hands with soap and water before preparing food and avoid preparing food for others if you have a diarrheal illness. Rinse fresh fruits and vegetables in running tap water to remove visible dirt and grime. Because bacteria grow on the cut surface of fruits and vegetables, avoid contaminating these foods while slicing them on a cutting board.

- Report: Report suspected foodborne illnesses to your local health department. Calls from concerned citizens are often how outbreaks are first detected. If a public health official contacts you to find out more about an illness you had, your cooperation is important. In public health investigations, talking to healthy people can be as helpful as talking to ill people. Officials may need your cooperation even if you are not ill.

Consult your physician for any diarrheal illness that is accompanied by high fever (temperature over 101.5°F, measured orally), blood in stools, prolonged vomiting that prevents you from keeping liquids down, signs of dehydration, including a decrease in urination, a dry mouth and throat, and feeling dizzy when standing up, and diarrheal illness that lasts more than 3 days. See your physician as soon as possible. In the meantime, replace the lost fluids and electrolytes immediately and continue adequate fluid intake. Sports drinks such as Gatorade do not replace the losses correctly, so you should not use them for the treatment of diarrheal illness. Your physician may recommend solutions such as Ceralyte, Pedialyte, or Oralyte and an appropriate course of action. Because there are many different types of illnesses, your physician may prescribe various kinds of treatments. Viruses cause many diarrheal illnesses that will improve in 2 or 3 days without antibiotic therapy, which has no affect on viruses. Other treatments can help the symptoms, and careful hand washing can prevent the spread of infection to other people.

Nutrition and Aging

Scientists have been searching for decades for ways to slow the aging process. Evidence from the study of rodents and rhesus monkeys indicates that those who want to live longer and healthier lives should stop eating before they are full and reduce their caloric intake. Dietary restriction has been shown both to increase an animal's fitness and to slow the aging process. According to Richard Windruch of the University of Wisconsin in Madison, this is the only intervention that slows the rate of aging in warm-blooded animals. For example, female mice on a maximally calorie-restricted diet lived to an age of 45 months, nearly 20 months longer than mice that consumed as much as they wanted. Calorie-restricted mice and rats also maintained better cardiovascular fitness, improved glucose utilization, and had stronger immune responses—processes that falter with aging. The incidence of cancer also declined. Experts feel that calorie restriction is the most effective inhibitor of carcinogenesis known in rodents and rhesus monkeys.

Just how much were calories restricted? The mice received well-balanced meals with 65% fewer calories than their unrestricted counterparts. Some began the restricted diet at an early age, and others after they reached sexual maturity. Early restriction caused stunted bone growth and delayed sexual maturation.

To date, no long-term studies involving humans have suggested such a drastic reduction in calories. An individual who consumes 800 calories daily but needs 2,000 calories would find it quite difficult to obtain proper nutrition and energy levels. Previous studies reduced the calories of mice and rats by only 30 to 40%, which would be a much more realistic target for humans. In any case, until more evidence is available, simply follow the guidelines in this chapter, avoid overnutrition and overfatness, and exercise three or four times weekly (*Journal of NIH Research*, 1995).

Special Needs of the Active Individual

Active individuals who follow the nutritional plan in this chapter do have a few special nutritional needs. These areas and general recommendations are summarized in a joint position statement by the American College of Sports Medicine, the American Dietetic Association, and the Dietitians of Canada (2000):

- During times of high physical activity, energy and macronutrient needs, especially carbohydrate and protein intake, must be met to maintain body weight, replenish glycogen stores, and build and repair tissue.
- Fat intake should be adequate to provide the essential fatty acids and fat-soluble vitamins, and sufficient calories for weight management.
- About 20 to 25% of the energy (calories) should come from fat.
- Consuming adequate food and fluid before, during, and after exercise helps maintain blood glucose during exercise, maximize exercise performance, and improve recovery time.
- Exercising individuals and athletes should be well hydrated before exercise and drink enough fluids during and afterward to balance fluid loses.
- Consuming sports drinks containing carbohydrates and electrolytes will provide fuel for the muscles, help maintain blood glucose and the thirst mechanism, and decrease the risk of dehydration or hyponatremia (decrease in

the plasma sodium concentration caused by an excess of water relative to solute).

- Vitamin and mineral supplements are not necessary if adequate energy to maintain body weight is consumed from a variety of foods and the five food groups. Those who restrict energy intake, use severe weight-loss practices, eliminate one or more foods from their diets, or consume high-carbohydrate diets with low micronutrient density may need supplements.
- Nutritional erogenic aids should be used with caution and only after careful evaluation of the product for safety, efficacy, potency, and whether it is a banned or illegal substance.
- A qualified expert should provide nutritional advice only after reviewing an individual's health, diet, use of supplements and drugs, and energy requirements.

To help you manage your diet properly during involvement in regular exercise, a more detailed discussion of these key areas and others follows.

Eating Enough Calories

If you are neither losing nor gaining weight, you are taking in the correct number of calories daily to maintain your present weight and fat level. Weigh yourself at exactly the same time of day and under the same conditions, preferably in the morning on rising. If no weight gain or loss is occurring, you have no real need for complicated record keeping of caloric intake and expenditure, unless you wish to lose or gain weight.

You can estimate the number of calories you need from table 10.17. Multiply your body weight by the calories recommended per pound for your activity level to obtain an estimate of your needs. Your body has an infallible computer that accurately registers your caloric intake daily; the output is body-weight changes. Refer to Discovery Activity 10.1 for a more accurate indication of your energy expenditure.

Your source of calories is also an important factor in providing sufficient energy for exercise. The percentage of calories from carbohydrates, fats, and protein, shown in table 10.13, is sufficient for most exercising individuals. Increasing your complex carbohydrate (fruits, vegetables, grains) intake from 45% to 60% of total calories will increase your energy level. You should decrease total fat intake by 10% to 12%.

TABLE 10.17—Approximate Number of Calories Needed Daily per Pound of Body Weight

Age ranges	7-10	11-14	15-22	23-35	36-50	51-75
MALES						
Very active	21-22	23-24	25-27	23-24	21-22	19-20
Moderately active	16-17	18-19	20-23	18-19	16-17	11-15
Sedentary	11-12	13-14	15-18	13-14	11-12	10-11
FEMALES						
Very active	21-22	22-23	20-21	20-21	18-19	17-18
Moderately active	16-17	18-19	16-18	16-17	14-15	12-13
Sedentary	11-12	13-14	11-12	11-12	9-10	8-9

Sedentary = no physical activity beyond attending classes and desk work; moderately active = involved in a regular exercise program at least 3 times weekly; very active = involved in a regular aerobic exercise program 4-6 times weekly, expending more than 2,500 calories per week during physical activity.

Protein Sparing

Eating sufficient fruits, vegetables, and grains is critical for the exercising individual. When the body does not have adequate carbohydrates available for energy, it will convert dietary protein and lean protein mass (muscle) to glucose to supply the nervous system. When this occurs, loss of lean-muscle tissue takes place throughout the body, including major organs such as the heart. Failing to spare protein for long periods may jeopardize health. A sufficient amount of complex carbohydrates in your diet will spare protein, provide a high level of energy, and protect your health.

Carbohydrate Loading or Supercompensation

The body has an adequate supply of energy available in the form of glucose and glycogen for performing regular exercise or competing in a sport. Glucose (sugar in the blood available for energy) and glycogen (the chief storage form of carbohydrates) are available in the blood, muscles, and liver and provide sufficient energy for most anaerobic workouts.

Individuals who compete in marathons, triathlons, and other endurance contests lasting several hours need additional energy and can benefit from a technique called **carbohydrate loading,** or **supercompensation.** New evidence indicates that the depletion stage may be unnecessary. By merely increasing carbohydrate intake 3 to 4 days before an important exercise activity or competition, you will more than double your liver and muscle glycogen stores. Such an increase provides approximately 3,060 calories of energy—enough for practically any endurance event. Two large, high-carbohydrate meals (300 grams, 1,200 calories per meal) are recommended daily for 3 to 4 days.

Replacing Fluids (Water)

Water needs depend on the individual and on factors such as body weight, activity patterns, sweat loss, loss through expired air and urine, and amount of liquid consumed through other foods and drinks (see figure 10.5).

The active individual needs a minimum of 8 to 10 glasses (2 quarts or more) of water daily—much more in hot, humid weather. People can easily lose 1 to 2 liters of water per hour when exercising in extremely hot, humid weather. Drinking too much water generally poses no problem; water is rarely toxic, and the kidneys excrete it efficiently. The kidneys are also capable of conserving water when the body is deprived by excreting urine that is more highly concentrated. If the color of your urine is darker than a manila folder, you need to consume additional water (not fluid from other drinks). We remind you that the body needs plain water for heat regulation and proper functioning of systems.

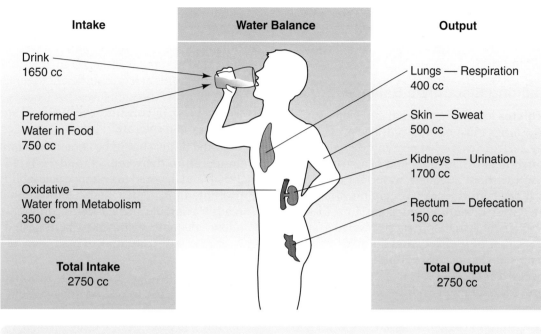

Figure 10.5   Water intake and loss.

If you exercise in hot, humid weather, thirst sensations will underestimate your needs. By the time you are thirsty, you have created a water deficit that you cannot overcome for several hours. Forced drinking (hydrating), even when no thirst sensation exists, will minimize water deficit, keep body temperature 1 to 2° lower in hot weather, result in more efficient performance, and delay fatigue. The most beneficial approach is to force down an extra glass or two of water 15 minutes before you begin to exercise. Earlier consumption may fill the bladder and make you uncomfortable during the activity.

Drink water freely before (drink generous amounts during the 24 hours before exercise and 12 to 24 ounces 15 minutes before the workout), during (drink 10 to 16 ounces every 15 minutes), and after (you need up to 150% of the water weight lost during exercise to replace losses and meet urine production obligations). A high-sodium meal after exercise also helps hydration. Water is the single most important substance in preventing heat-related illnesses and in restoring the body to normal following exercise in hot, humid weather. For the quickest absorption, drink plain water chilled to about 40°F. (For additional discussion of water and

carbohydrate loading (supercompensation)—An attempt to reduce carbohydrate intake to near zero for 2 to 3 days (depletion stage) before resorting to a high-carbohydrate diet for 3 to 4 days (loading phase) to raise glycogen stores in skeletal muscles and the liver to increase energy levels on the day of competition.

hyponatremia—Abnormally low concentrations of sodium ions in the circulating blood.

its role in preventing heat exhaustion, muscle cramps, and heatstroke, see chapter 13).

Too much water can cause problems in hot, humid weather in some individuals who perspire profusely. With the consumption of high amounts of water under these conditions, the ratio of blood sodium to water changes dramatically, producing a condition referred to as **hyponatremia**. Symptoms include nausea, fatigue, stupor, and, in extreme cases, seizures and death. It is the most common electrolyte disorder, occurring in up to 1% of patients admitted to the hospital and in 50% of patients with AIDS. Mineral deficiencies, use of diuretics, AIDS, and other diseases are also known causes. For those who sweat heavily during long exercise sessions, an electrolyte solution such as Gatorade® diluted with 50% more water may help prevent or delay the onset of this condition.

Maintaining Electrolyte Balance

Electrolytes lost through sweat and water vapor from the lungs must be replaced. The proper balance of electrolytes is what prevents dehydration, cramping, heat exhaustion, and heatstroke. Too much salt without adequate water, for example, draws fluid from the cells, precipitates nausea, and increases urination and potassium loss. A salt supplement is therefore rarely needed in spite of the weather or intensity and duration of exercise. The salt that occurs naturally in food, salt in processed food, and salt from the saltshaker will provide sufficient sodium even for active individuals.

Potassium is critical to maintaining regular heartbeat, and it plays a role in carbohydrate and protein metabolism. Profuse sweating over several days can deplete potassium stores, by as much as 3 milligrams per day. The average diet provides only 1.5 to 2.5 milligrams daily. If you sweat profusely and exercise almost daily, you may need five to eight servings of potassium-rich foods each day. Excellent sources of potassium include orange juice, skim milk, bananas, dried fruits, and potatoes. A potassium supplement is not recommended because too much potassium is as dangerous as too little.

Ionic chloride is part of hydrochloric acid and serves to maintain the strong acidity of the stomach. Loss of too much chloride upsets the acid–base balance of the body. Adding chlorine to public water provides this valuable element and makes water safe for human consumption.

For replacing fluids, electrolytes, and carbohydrates consider the following position stand on exercise and fluid replacement of the American College of Sports Medicine (1996):

- Individuals should consume a nutritionally balanced diet and drink adequate fluids during the 24-hour period before an event, especially during the period that includes the meal before exercise, to promote proper hydration before exercise or competition.
- Individuals should drink about 500 milliliters (about 17 ounces) of fluid about 2 hours before exercise to promote adequate hydration and allow time for excretion of excess ingested water.
- During exercise, athletes should start drinking early and at regular intervals in an attempt to consume fluids at a rate sufficient to replace all the water lost through sweating (that is, body weight loss), or consume the maximal amount that they can tolerate.
- Ingested fluids should be cooler than ambient temperature (between 59° and 72°F [15° and 22°C]) and flavored to enhance palatability and promote fluid replacement. Fluids should be readily available and served in containers that allow adequate volumes to be ingested with ease and with minimal interruption of exercise.
- Addition of proper amounts of carbohydrates and electrolytes to a fluid replacement solution is recommended for exercise events of duration greater than 1 hour because they do not significantly impair water delivery to the body and may enhance performance. During exercise lasting less than 1 hour, there is little evidence of physiological or physical performance differences between consuming a carbohydrate-electrolyte drink and plain water.
- During intense exercise lasting longer than 1 hour, individuals should ingest carbohydrates at a rate of 30 to 60 grams per hour to maintain oxidation of carbohydrates and delay fatigue. People can achieve this rate of carbohydrate intake without compromising fluid delivery by drinking 600 to 1,200 milliliters per hour of solutions containing 4 to 8% carbohydrates. The carbohydrates can be sugars (glucose or sucrose) or starch (e.g., maltodextrin).
- Inclusion of sodium (0.5 to 0.7 gram per serving) in the rehydration solution ingested during exercise lasting longer than 1 hour may enhance palatability, promote fluid retention, and possibly prevent hyponatremia in certain individuals who drink excessive quantities of fluid. There is little physiological basis for including sodium in an oral rehydration solution to enhance intestinal water absorption as long as sodium is sufficiently available from the previous meal.

Replacing Iron

Iron deficiency can lead to loss of strength and endurance, early fatigue during exercise, shortening of attention span, loss of visual perception, and impaired learning. Adolescent girls are more apt to be iron deficient than females are at any other age. During menstruation, female athletes of all ages should discuss the need for an iron supplement with their physicians.

Many female athletes engaging in intense chronic aerobic exercise have reported abnormal menstrual cycles. Although much research has been conducted to find the causes of this phenomenon, we still are unable to define clearly who will have abnormal menstrual cycles and why. Most women and nonendurance athletes have **eumenorrhea.** With chronic endurance exercise, however, an increased percentage of female athletes report **oligomenorrhea.** Some researchers estimate that 5 to 40% of female athletes, depending on the sport, are oligomenorrheic, as compared with 10 to 12% in the general female population. One research project reported that 45% of female track and cross-country runners who ran more than 80 miles per week experienced irregular menstrual cycles. A smaller percentage report **amenorrhea.** Only 2 to 3% of women in the general population are amenorrheic. Yet in activities such as distance running, as many as 34% of women are reportedly amenorrheic. The incidence of amenorrhea decreases to 23% of joggers and to only 4% among a nonrunning control group. Runners were defined as those running more than 30 miles per week at very high intensity. Joggers ran from 5 to 30 miles per week but all at low to moderate intensity.

As shown in numerous studies, the decrease in menstrual function is often directly related to the intensity and duration of exercise. For women engaging in very intense training in ballet dancing, figure skating, distance running, gymnastics, and cycling, irregular menstruation may be the norm rather than the exception. Some female athletes have reported the absence of menstruation for months or even years while engaging in high-intensity endurance exercise.

Sports Anemia

Researchers have found that female endurance athletes are especially prone to periods of iron deficiency. This type of anemia is often called sports anemia because of its nature. Several causes have been proposed for this transient anemia that occurs in female and other endurance athletes, particularly during the early phases

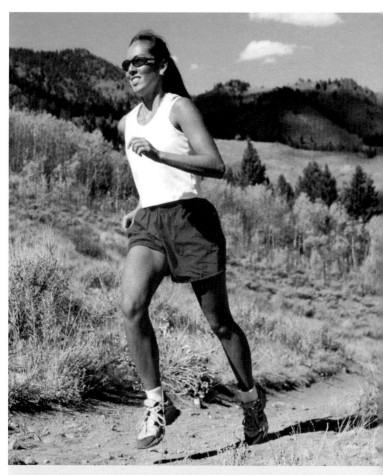

Women who seriously train in intense endurance activities often experience irregular menstruation.
PhotoDisc

electrolytes—Chemical compounds (water, sodium, potassium, chloride) in solution in the human body capable of producing electric current; important in the prevention of cramps, heat exhaustion, and heatstroke.

eumenorrhea—Regularly occurring menstrual cycles.

oligomenorrhea—Reduced, scanty, or irregular menstruation.

amenorrhea—Absence of the menstrual cycle.

hemodilution—An increase in the plasma volume (fluid portion of blood) that exceeds the increase in the total amount of hemoglobin produced, creating symptoms of anemia.

of a training program. One suspected factor is **hemodilution.** When a person begins a heavy aerobic training program, an increase occurs in both the plasma volume and the total amount of hemoglobin produced. The proportional increase in the plasma volume, however, is greater than the increase in the hemoglobin, and the hemoglobin level apparently is lower. In simpler terms, the blood is less concentrated, so the athlete has less hemoglobin for any given amount of blood. Thus, with less oxygen being delivered to the tissues with every heartbeat, the athlete appears anemic. This condition is usually transient and lasts from approximately 2 to 8 weeks during the initial training period.

Another possible cause of sports anemia is a diet inadequate in iron, especially heme iron sources. Exercisers who consume large quantities of junk food may meet the caloric requirements to maintain their body weight, in spite of strenuous training schedules. The iron-to-calorie ratio, however, may in fact be extremely low. In one report, 42% of the female distance runners studied were modified vegetarians, ingesting less than 200 grams of meat a week. This excessively low intake of such a rich source of heme iron partially explains the inability of many female athletes to meet the suggested intake of iron. We recommend that coaches regularly include an assessment of iron status as part of the medical screening for all athletes.

Any combination of these factors will likely result in the transient anemia that plagues some endurance athletes. Because women often have lower normal values of hemoglobin than men do, strenuous exercise is of some concern. Iron supplementation cannot reverse true sports anemia. Sports anemia appears to be a temporary response to exercise; thus, no treatment is required.

Osteoporosis

A crippling disease common to older people in general, and to older women in particular, is osteoporosis. With this disease, the bones become porous and fragile and break with little exertion. Last year, more than a million adults in the United States suffered bone breaks because of this degenerative disease.

Special Considerations for Women

Furthermore, at least one-third of all women age 65 or older will suffer a fracture of the spine at some point in their lives. Such fractures can be difficult to treat because the break is usually not clean. The bone literally explodes into countless fragments that cannot be reassembled. If an artificial joint-replacement operation is not possible, the person may be confined to a wheelchair for years.

Although osteoporosis is more common in women than it is in men, this crippling disease constitutes a primary health concern for most older adults. The causes of osteoporosis are multiple and somewhat confusing. Though we strongly recommend that men and women meet the recommended dietary reference intake (DRI) for daily calcium intake, it is not yet clear whether adequate calcium intakes can prevent osteoporosis or merely help slow it down.

Developing Peak Bone Mass

Peak bone mass develops up to age 24. Between the ages of 25 and 30, peak bone mass is usually maintained. After approximately age 30, however, bone loss begins to occur. Although this process cannot be reversed, the rate of bone loss can often be retarded. You should be aware that your bones are strongest and most dense in your late teenage and early adult years, because you can reduce your likelihood of developing osteoporosis right now. Once the decline in bone mineralization begins, men typically experience a lifetime bone-density loss of 20 to 30%. Women have a more accelerated bone-mineral loss, resulting in lifetime bone-density losses of 50% or more.

Risk Factors

Your predisposition to developing osteoporosis depends on both environmental and hereditary factors. The single strongest predictor is age, followed by sex. Additional risk factors include nutritional status, body weight, cigarette smoking, racial or ethnic heritage, hormonal health, physical inactivity, and alcohol consumption. The effects of many of these risk factors are additive, but we do not know the relative contribution of each risk factor. We recommend that you eliminate as many risk factors as possible.

Age

Bones lose their density as you grow older because you produce less bone-building equipment and more bone-dismantling equipment. Thus, you should try to obtain enough calcium during young adulthood so that when the bone-dismantling process begins, you have optimal bone density. If you build strong bones up to

Behavioral Change and Motivational Strategies

People in the 2000s are more educated about nutrition than previous generations have been. Unfortunately, knowledge about proper nutrition does not readily translate into sound eating behavior. The typical diet of people in the United States is too high in saturated fat, cholesterol, total fat, calories, sodium, and sugar and too low in complex carbohydrates (fruits, vegetables, grains) and water. Busy schedules, lack of money, fad diets, easy access to fast-food restaurants, youthful feelings of indestructibility, culture and religion, and many other factors help explain this trend. These problems are strongly related to present and future health, behavior, mood, and energy level. A minimum amount of effort can correct some of these problems.

Roadblock	Behavioral Change Strategy
Some people simply do not seem to like water and therefore consume less than three of the recommended six to eight glasses daily. Instead, many people consume coffee, tea, high-calorie (150 calories per 12-ounce serving) soft drinks, juices, milk, beer, and other alcoholic drinks. Avoiding water allows more room for calories and salt, sugar, and fat.	You can change your liquid consumption patterns slowly and reacquire your taste for water. For a 7-day period, try the following: ■ Place your favorite glass in the bathroom and drink one full glass of water immediately on rising in the morning and another just before bedtime. You are already drinking more water than most people do. ■ Do not pass by a water fountain without taking a drink, even if you are not thirsty. Take at least five swallows (about 3 ounces). ■ Place a cold pitcher of water in the front of your refrigerator so that it is the first thing you see. ■ Drink at least one glass of water with each meal.
Much of what we eat is processed food, which is typically high in sodium. Avoiding the problem seems impossible.	Although high sodium intake may not be as much of a health hazard as originally suspected, it is a good idea to cut back. About one-third of the salt you consume comes from processed food, one-third comes from table salt, and one-third occurs naturally in food. You can do several things: ■ Restrict your visits to fast-food restaurants to no more than one per month. ■ Avoid or use very little table salt, substituting herbs and spices such as lemon and orange. Use a salt substitute that does not contain sodium potassium. Plan to take several weeks to adjust to not adding table salt to your food. ■ Read food labels and buy products with no or low salt. ■ Avoid luncheon meats, smoked meats, hot dogs, sausages, and high-salt cheeses.
Although you are aware of the association between high total fat, high saturated fat, high-cholesterol diets and heart disease, it is simply too difficult to avoid high fat in the diet.	Reducing the amount of fat in your diet can be difficult, particularly if you eat on the run and do not have time to plan meals. Doing several specific things will reduce the percentage of calories you consume from fat daily: ■ Take time to glance at the label of every product you buy. If the label indicates higher levels of fat, consider the option not to buy. ■ If you eat ice cream, buy one of the brands that use artificial fat; the taste is excellent and the product is nearly free of fat and cholesterol. Remember to consider the potential side effects that artificial fat can induce. ■ Pack a lunch every day based on the food guide pyramid consisting of fruit, vegetables, and a low-calorie sandwich. This kind of lunch will keep you from skipping a meal or running to a fast-food restaurant during the day. ■ Reduce your intake of invisible fat by reducing your consumption of chocolate, eggs, red meat, poultry skin, and dairy products. ■ Cut the skin off raw poultry before cooking, avoid frying, and choose cooking methods that do not require use of oils.

(continued)

Behavioral Change and Motivational Strategies *(continued)*

You know what constitutes a healthy, balanced diet—one that is consistent with the food guide pyramid—but you just can't seem to adhere to that diet.

Studies have shown that health knowledge has little if any relationship to health behavior. That is, your knowing that a certain behavior is healthy doesn't mean that you will behave that way. This tendency is true with nutrition. You may know what constitutes a healthy diet, but that doesn't mean you will eat one. To encourage your adoption of healthier eating habits, try these approaches:

- Plan the meals you have at home. Write these plans on a sheet of paper the night before and place the necessary ingredients on the kitchen counter so that making those meals will be easier. In this way, you will be using chaining to control your eating behavior.
- You could combine chaining with social support by planning your meals as described but doing so with a friend. In this way, each of you will have the support of the other and both of you will be more likely to adhere to a healthy diet.
- Sometimes all that is necessary to maintain a healthy diet is seeing a reminder to do so. You could use this behavioral change technique by taping a copy of the food guide pyramid on your refrigerator or pantry to encourage you to choose healthy foods.

List some roadblocks that interfere with your following sound nutritional practices.

Now list behavioral change strategies that can help you overcome the roadblocks you just listed. If you need to, refer back to chapter 4 for behavioral change and motivational strategies.

1. _____

2. _____

3. _____

1. _____

2. _____

3. _____

---

the age of 24, your skeleton will remain stronger throughout your life. To promote maximal calcium stores in the bones, experts recommend a DRI of 1,200 milligrams per day for young adults and 1,000 milligrams per day for men and women from the age of 24 to 50. One cup of either whole or 1% milk contains approximately 300 milligrams of calcium. Thus, women need over 4 cups of milk per day to meet the DRI. One cup of plain yogurt contains approximately 415 milligrams of calcium. Thus, only 3 cups of yogurt will meet the DRI.

Sex and Hormones

Both men and women lose bone density as they grow older, but women tend to lose much greater amounts than men do and are therefore more susceptible to bone breakage. After menopause, women are especially susceptible to developing osteoporosis because the ovaries decrease their estrogen output. But premenopausal women whose ovaries are removed are also at high risk because their bodies do not produce estrogen. Research has shown that young women who are long-distance runners for years are prone to athletic amenorrhea. Many of these women can have a period only following estrogen administration. If they fail to obtain estrogen-replacement therapy, these young women become highly susceptible to osteoporosis.

Obviously, men do not usually produce large amounts of the estrogen hormone. Thus, lack of estrogen cannot explain the increased incidence of osteoporosis in older men. Researchers have found that men tend to suffer more fractures when their testes have been removed or when the testes begin to lose their functional capability, as often occurs as a part of the aging process.

Both female and male sex hormones probably contribute significantly to osteoporosis.

Evidence Supporting Risk Factors

Strong evidence suggests that obesity, African ancestry, estrogen use, and high peak bone mass are related to decreased susceptibility to osteoporosis. Factors such as being of northern European descent, older age, surgical removal of ovaries before menopause, and extensive bed rest also increase susceptibility to osteoporosis (see table 10.18). Moderate evidence suggests that heavy exercisers (with the exception of underweight amenorrheic females) have a lower incidence of osteoporosis, whereas smokers and heavy drinkers are at greater risk. More research is needed to ascertain the effect of factors such as Asian ancestry, number of live births, diabetes mellitus, and caffeine consumption.

Prevention of Osteoporosis

As the previous discussion suggests, several factors are related to the delay or prevention of osteoporosis, especially exercise and calcium nutrition. The idea is to reach menopause with as much bone mass as possible through a drug-free lifestyle, sound nutrition, and regular aerobic exercise. A new nonhormonal drug, Fosamax®, has been shown not only to slow the pace at which bone mineral is lost but also to increase the replenishment phase, resulting in a net gain in bone mass. Evidence suggests that the use of Fosamax® increases bone mass by an average of 10% and significantly cuts the number and severity of bone fractures in postmenopausal women. Your physician can help you determine whether you are a good candidate for the drug in light of some of the side effects reported by some users.

Exercise

As we mentioned earlier in this textbook, much research has been conducted on the effect of exercise on the development of bone density. You may have been told since you were a child that exercising is good for you because it helps you develop stronger bones. Well, that is true, and it is important that you understand why. When you engage in activities that stress the bones, they demand that the bones strengthen their structure. We know that when muscles work, they pull on the bones and signal the bones that more tissue must be developed. Simultaneously, the hormones that promote increases in bone mineralization also promote the making of new muscle tissue.

Athletes who participated in weight-bearing exercises have exhibited as much as a 40% increase in bone mineralization when compared to a sedentary control group. Bone density increases through weight-bearing activities such as jogging, walking, aerobics, stair-stepping exercise, stair climbing, dancing, calisthenics, and even swimming. This wide range of activities makes it obvious that you can increase bone density by participating in aerobic and anaerobic exercises. To reduce bone loss after reaching peak

TABLE 10.18—Risk Factors for Osteoporosis

Factors that increase risk:	Factors that decrease risk:
Northern European ancestry	African ancestry
Female (gender)	High dietary calcium intake
Low dietary calcium intake	High peak bone mass by age 24
Older age	Heavy chronic exercise history
Postmenopausal status for women	Obesity
Surgical removal of ovaries before menopause	Estrogen use
Surgical removal of testes	
Extensive bed rest	
Increased alcohol consumption	
Cigarette smoking	
Underweight	

bone mass, however, you should engage in aerobic activity for at least 30 minutes at least three times per week.

Racial and Ethnic Heritage

African Americans tend to have bones that are 10% denser than the bones of White people. African American males tend to have the greatest average peak bone mass and to develop osteoporosis less frequently than individuals of any other race and sex group. African American females tend to have higher average peak bone mass than their White counterparts do and consequently have lower incidence of osteoporosis. For example, hip fractures occur three times more often in White females age 80 or older than in African American females age 80 or older. In the United States, other ethnic groups have lower bone density than do White people of northern European descent, yet they do not necessarily have higher rates of osteoporosis. The implication is that although race and ethnic heritage are important predictors, lifestyle factors are also important in determining susceptibility to osteoporosis.

Underweight and Physical Inactivity

Osteoporosis occurs much more frequently in women who are underweight, even among African American women. Thus, although obesity is linked strongly to all types of cardiorespiratory diseases, osteoporosis is linked equally strongly to women who are too stringent in maintaining their body weight.

For years, researchers have known that when you are confined to bed rest, your bones lose density, just as the muscles atrophy. The strong relationship between muscle strength and bone density is important because if you want to maintain strong bones, you need to engage in weight-bearing activities.

Cigarette Smoking

Smokers have a higher incidence of fractures than nonsmokers do. One reason for this may be that smokers tend to weigh less than nonsmokers do. Also, women who smoke tend to experience menopause at an earlier age than nonsmokers do.

Alcohol Consumption

Alcoholics have less bone density than nonalcoholics do. Men who are alcoholics tend to have more bone fractures than nonalcoholic males do. The possible link may be that alcohol causes the body to lose more fluid, and so more calcium is lost in the urine. Thus, calcium leaches out of the bones to maintain the blood level of calcium. In addition, alcoholics tend to have poor nutritional habits and typically avoid foods known to be rich sources of calcium. Alcohol also tends to affect the ovaries of women, upsetting the normal hormonal balance necessary to maintain healthy levels of calcium in the bones.

Finally, we recommend that you concentrate on meeting the DRI for calcium each day. Regardless of your rate of absorption or bone loss, meeting the DRI is your best protective measure from a dietary perspective. Unfortunately, most girls and adult women fail to meet the DRI for calcium during their bone-building years. Such girls are at a disadvantage because they will begin their adult lives with lower bone mass and will be more prone to osteoporosis in later years.

Figure 10.6 gives suggestions for increasing the intake of calcium in your diet. If you have problems drinking milk or eating dairy products, you can see that several kinds of meat, fruits and vegetables, and grains are excellent sources of calcium. Strive to meet the DRI for this all-important mineral each day and add quality to your life as you grow older.

Summary

Basic Food Components Six categories of nutrients satisfy the basic body needs: the energy nutrients, comprising carbohydrates, fats, proteins; and the nonenergy nutrients, comprising vitamins, minerals, water.

Carbohydrates and fats provide the main sources of energy (calories) to perform work. Simple carbohydrates found in concentrated sugar provide empty calories to the diet and little nutrition in terms of key vitamins and minerals.

Soft drinks and so-called energy drinks provide little more than unnecessary calories and caffeine, contribute to weight gain, and detract from a healthy diet.

Complex carbohydrates (fruits, vegetables, grains) are our only source of fiber and a major supplier of long-term energy. Complex carbohydrates are nutritionally dense foods, providing a high percentage of our daily needs in vitamins

- Drink low-fat milk with meals or as a snack.
- Drink orange juice that has added calcium.
- Eat canned sardines or canned fish prepared with their bones.
- Use milk instead of water when you prepare creamed soups.
- Add grated cheese to salads, tacos, spaghetti, and lasagna.
- Increase intake of broccoli and turnip greens.
- Add powdered nonfat milk to soups, casseroles, sauces, and beverages such as cocoa.
- Eat low-fat yogurt as a snack.
- Postmenopausal women should drink 3 to 5 cups of milk daily.
- Drink buttermilk with meals or as a snack.
- Make dairy products a part of your meals, especially low-fat and nonfat cheeses.
- Eat cheese as a snack or add a slice to your sandwiches.
- Drink cocoa occasionally instead of drinking hot tea or coffee.
- Teenagers should drink 4 or more cups of milk daily.
- Use low-fat or nonfat yogurt to make a low-calorie salad dressing.
- Choose calcium-rich desserts, such as ice cream, custard, or pudding.
- Pregnant and lactating women should drink 3 or 4 cups of milk daily.
- Increase intake of tofu (bean curd).
- Drink fluoridated water.
- Eat fortified breakfast cereals with skim milk.

Figure 10.6 Suggestions for increasing dietary intake of calcium.

and minerals in relatively few calories. Both insoluble (dietary) and soluble fibers provide important health benefits.

Dietary fat is a critical nutrient and a source of high energy for the human body. Fat is classified as saturated, polyunsaturated, or monounsaturated. Cholesterol, a type of fat, is found in animal sources and is manufactured by the human liver. Trans-fatty acids form when vegetable oils low in saturated fat are hydrogenated to make them more solid at room temperature. These fatty acids, present in margarine and all foods with the phrase "partially hydrogenated" on their labels, have been shown to raise bad LDL cholesterol and lower good HDL cholesterol as well as contribute to the incidence of heart disease.

Several artificial fats or fat substitutes are currently on the market, and others are being tested for safety and side effects. These products may eventually replace the fat in many of our high-fat foods and provide the same taste without the calories and health consequences.

Protein can be obtained from both animal and plant foods. In the human body, protein is used for the repair, rebuilding, and replacement of cells; growth; fluid, salt, and acid–base balance; and energy in the absence of sufficient dietary carbohydrates and fat. Protein from meat, eggs, and dairy products is termed complete because it contains all the essential amino acids in the correct proportion. The correct combinations of various vegetables and grains also compose complete protein sources. With proper planning, vegetarians can easily obtain sufficient protein in their diets without consuming meat, eggs, or dairy products.

Vitamins help chemical reactions take place in the body and are needed only in small amounts. A balanced diet provides most people with their daily need for vitamins and minerals.

Minerals are present in all living cells and serve as components of hormones, enzymes, and other substances aiding chemical reactions in cells. The body needs macrominerals in large amounts, whereas it needs only small quantities of 14 trace minerals for optimum health. You can obtain your daily mineral needs through a balanced diet.

Although it has no nutritional value, water is necessary for energy production, temperature control, and elimination. You should consume a minimum of six to eight glasses of water daily, exclusive of all other beverages.

Food Density   A food is nutritionally dense if it contains a low percentage of daily caloric needs and a high percentage of key nutrients such as protein, vitamins, and minerals. Complex carbohydrates are the most nutritionally dense foods; foods high in fat are the least dense.

Dietary Guidelines for Good Health   You can be assured of sound nutrition by planning your diet around the nutrition pyramid. The recommended servings from each of five key food groups and limited use of the sixth group (fats, oils, and sweets) will provide you with excellent nutrition. The pyramid offers a less complicated approach to sound nutrition for the layperson than do DRI tables and complicated calculations.

Dietary recommendations have also been made in terms of percentage of total calories to guide your intake of carbohydrates, protein, fat, and alcohol. Specific guidelines in grams or milligrams are also available for fiber, salt, and cholesterol.

Nutrition and Disease   The evidence associating nutritional practices with various diseases and disorders and linking sound nutrition to the prevention of some of these diseases continues to mount. Diets high in complex carbohydrates and low in fat, cholesterol, sodium, and calories offer the greatest benefits.

Nutrition and Aging   Laboratory studies with rhesus monkeys and rodents have uncovered a favorable effect of undernutrition on the aging process. Laboratory animals whose caloric intake was reduced by 30 to 60% but that were given a balanced diet lived nearly 50% longer, maintained their fitness levels and the functioning of their immune systems, and showed remarkable resistance to cancer.

Special Needs of the Active Individual   Physically active individuals who follow the nutritional guidelines presented in this chapter have only a few special needs. They must consume sufficient calories to support activity levels and prevent weight and muscle loss, consume adequate carbohydrates and fat to prevent loss of lean-muscle mass, increase water intake dramatically, maintain electrolyte balance, and take care to obtain sufficient dietary iron. Female athletes who experience decreased iron absorption and increased iron loss through the menstrual cycle are more susceptible to both iron deficiency and sports anemia.

Special Considerations for Women: Osteoporosis   Women are more susceptible than men are to certain conditions, including osteoporosis, iron-deficiency anemia, and sports anemia. All such conditions can have a debilitating effect on exercise capacity.

Osteoporosis is more commonly known as adult bone loss. Many postmenopausal women are plagued with this disease. Peak bone mass develops up to age 24. After age 30, bone loss begins to occur, regardless of how dense the bones are. Risk factors such as being female, growing older, being amenorrheic, being of northern European ancestry, being underweight, smoking cigarettes, drinking alcohol, and leading a sedentary lifestyle make individuals more prone to developing osteoporosis.

People should strive to maintain the DRI for calcium, especially in the bone-building years. Women should ingest 1,300 milligrams per day up to age 24, and men and women past age 24 should ingest 1,000 milligrams per day. Weight-bearing activities increase bone density. Thus, maintaining a lifetime physical activity program is crucial to retarding and preventing this disease.

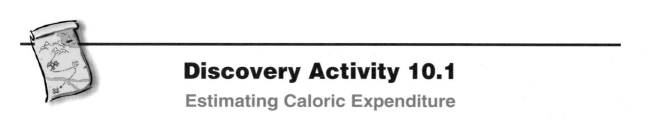

Discovery Activity 10.1

Estimating Caloric Expenditure

Name _____ **Date** _____

Instructions: The energy needs of your body depend on three factors: (1) body size, (2) age, and (3) the type and amount of your daily physical activity. Your basal metabolic rate (BMR) and caloric expenditure in normal daily activities combine to represent your required energy needs. Complete these steps to estimate your total caloric expenditure. Locate your height on scale 1 and your weight on scale 2 in figure 10.7. Using a straight edge, connect the appropriate points on scales 1 and 2. The intersection of this line with scale 3 is your body surface area.

Scale 1 Height in. / cm	Scale 3 Surface area m^1	Scale 2 Weight lb / kg
8"	2.9	340 — 160
6'6" — 200	2.8	320 — 150
4"	2.7	300 — 140
4" — 190	2.6	280 — 130
2"	2.5	260 — 120
6'0"	2.4	240 — 110
10" — 180	2.3	
8"	2.2	220 — 100
5'6" — 170	2.1	— 95
— 165	2.0	200 — 90
4" — 160	1.9	190 — 85
2" — 155	1.8	180 — 80
5'0" — 150	1.7	170 — 75
10" — 145	1.6	160 — 70
8" — 140	1.5	150 — 65
4'6"	1.4	140 — 60
— 135		130 — 55
4" — 130	1.3	120 — 50
2"	1.2	110 — 45
— 125		100 — 45
4'0"	1.1	95 — 40
— 120		90 — 35
10" — 115	1.0	85 — 35
8" — 110		75 — 30
	0.9	70 —
3'6" — 105		65 — 30
4"	0.8	60 — 25
— 100		55 — 25
		50 —

Figure 10.7 Body surface area.

Identifying BMR

Locate your BMR according to the values in table 10.A.

TABLE 10.A—Basal Metabolic Rate by Age and Gender

Age	Men	Women	Age	Men	Women
10	47.7	44.9	13	44.5	40.5
11	46.5	43.5	14	43.8	39.2
12	45.3	42.0	15	42.9	38.3

(continued)

Discovery Activity 10.1 *(continued)*

TABLE 10.A *(continued)*

Age	Men	Women	Age	Men	Women
16	42.0	37.2	32	37.2	34.9
17	41.5	36.4	33	37.1	34.9
18	40.8	35.8	34	37.0	34.9
19	40.5	35.4	35	36.9	34.8
20	39.9	35.3	36	36.8	34.7
21	39.5	35.2	37	36.7	34.6
22	39.2	35.2	38	36.7	34.5
23	39.0	35.2	39	36.6	34.4
24	38.7	35.1	40-44	36.4	34.1
25	38.4	35.1	45-49	36.2	33.8
26	38.2	35.0	50-54	35.8	33.1
27	38.0	35.0	55-59	35.1	32.8
28	37.8	35.0	60-64	34.5	32.0
29	37.7	35.0	65-69	33.5	31.6
30	37.6	35.0	70-74	32.8	31.1
31	37.4	35.0	≥75	31.8	

Determining Activity

To your BMR you must add the caloric cost for your daily activities. Calculating your precise daily energy needs every day would be impractical, but you can arrive at a close estimate. Select the figure from the following list that best describes your activity level:

40% Sedentary activities—limited to walking and sitting

50% Semisedentary activities—standing, walking, and recreational activities

60% Laborer or limited physical exercise

70% Heavy worker—regular participation in sports and other physical activities

80% Engaged in intercollegiate sports or in a vigorous daily physical fitness program

Calculating Total Energy Expenditure

Enter the values indicated and perform the necessary calculations.

1. Body surface area (from figure 10.7) _____

2. BMR factor (from table 10.A) × _____

3. BMR per hour at rest (step 1 × step 2) = _____

4. Number of hours in a day (24) × _____

5. BMR per day at rest (step 3 × step 4) = _____

6. Activity level (enter .40, .50, .60, .70, or .80) × _____

7. Activity calories (step 5 × step 6) = _____

8. BMR per day at rest (enter number from step 5) + _____

Total energy expenditure (total calories per 24 hours) = _____

From *Physical fitness and wellness, third edition*, by Jerrold S. Greenberg, George B. Dintiman, and Barbee Myers Oakes, 2004, Champaign, IL: Human Kinetics.

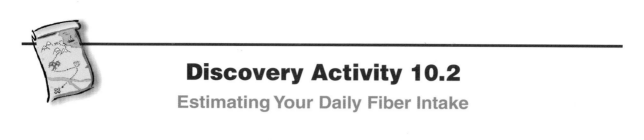

Discovery Activity 10.2

Estimating Your Daily Fiber Intake

Name _____ **Date** _____

Instructions: Record in the space provided all the fiber-containing foods you eat for a period of 3 days. Remember that you must keep records only of the amount and portion size of all fruits, vegetables, and grains eaten.

To help you estimate the grams of fiber in each food item consumed, see table 10.2. Now record in the last column the number of grams of dietary fiber you consume in each food daily. Divide the total grams by three to determine your average daily intake.

Record of Daily Fiber Intake

Day	Food item	Size or amount	Grams of fiber
1	Fruits:_____	_____	_____
	Vegetables:_____	_____	_____
	Grains:_____	_____	_____
2	Fruits:_____	_____	_____
	Vegetables:_____	_____	_____
	Grains:_____	_____	_____
3	Fruits:_____	_____	_____
	Vegetables:_____	_____	_____
	Grains:_____	_____	_____

Total grams of dietary fiber in 3 days _____

Average grams per day _____

Recommended daily intake = 35 grams

Additional daily fiber needed _____

Are you consuming at least 35 grams of dietary fiber daily? ___ Yes ___ No

From *Physical fitness and wellness, third edition*, by Jerrold S. Greenberg, George B. Dintiman, and Barbee Myers Oakes, 2004, Champaign, IL: Human Kinetics.

Discovery Activity 10.3

Service-Learning for Nutrition

Many people are familiar with the food guide pyramid distributed by the federal government to encourage Americans to eat healthy, balanced diets. The foods cited in the food guide pyramid, however, may not be appealing to all ethnic or cultural groups. Although not nearly as well known as the original food guide pyramid, adaptations that account for cultural or ethnic preferences are available. For example, there is a food pyramid for vegetarians[1], a food guide pyramid with a Mexican flavor[2], a Puerto Rican food guide pyramid[3], an east African eating guide for good health[4], a Native American food guide[5], a southeast Asian food guide[6], and food guide pyramids for other populations as well (for example, Jewish and Chinese[7]).

Select and teach an ethnic or cultural minority population how to eat in a healthy way, consistent with a food guide pyramid specific to that group's eating habits and preferences. You could conduct this workshop in a community center, a school, or a social hall used by this population for meetings and social gatherings. Local supermarkets may allow you to post flyers announcing the availability, date, and place of the workshop. The supermarket may also be willing to provide sample foods for distribution and demonstration during the workshop. Make sure to leave the participants with a handout that includes the food guide pyramid appropriate to the specific population. In that way, participants will more easily be able to develop eating patterns in their homes consistent with recommendations for healthy, balanced diets.

[1]Prouix, Lawrence G. "Feeding the Vegetarian Child," *Washington Post,* June 20, 1997, p. 20.

[2]University of California Agricultural and Natural Resources, 800-994-8849.

[3]Hispanic Health Council, University of Connecticut, Department of Nutrition With the COOP Extension, and the Connecticut State Department of Social Services.

[4]Washington State Department of Health Warehouse Materials Management, 360-664-9046.

[5]Ibid.

[6]Ibid.

[7]Penn State Nutrition Center, Multicultural Pyramid Packet, 4 Henderson Building, University Park, PA 16802, 814-865-6323.

Chemicals and Fitness

Chapter Objectives

By the end of this chapter, you should be able to

1. differentiate between drug use, misuse, and abuse and give examples of each;

2. describe the prevalence of alcohol on college campuses and make suggestions for drinking responsibly;

3. cite methods taken by colleges to control alcohol use on their campuses;

4. describe the prevalence of tobacco use and its effects on the body;

5. describe strategies to quit smoking or make smoking less harmful;

6. list and discuss the dangers of elicit drugs used by college students;

7. discuss the effects and dangers of Rohypnol and the prevention of date rape; and

8. list the drugs used to enhance athletic performance or physical appearance and discuss their safety and effectiveness.

The Thomas and Lopez families both experienced a difficult year. Glen Thomas was diagnosed with angina (pain in the chest caused by constricted coronary arteries) and started taking nitroglycerin pills periodically. His wife, Barbara, contracted a sinus infection in February, and her doctor prescribed antibiotics. In May her gynecologist recommended she begin regular doses of estrogen to replace her body's decreased production of estrogen caused by menopause. Their son, Clark, was diagnosed with attention-deficit/hyperactivity disorder, and his pediatrician put him on the drug Ritalin.

The Lopezes were no more fortunate. Felipe decided that he needed assistance to stop smoking, and his doctor encouraged him to wear a nicotine patch. Flore Lopez was diagnosed with high blood pressure and instructed to take hypertension medication daily. And Melinda, the Lopezes' teenage daughter, was found to be anemic and began taking an iron supplement each day.

More than ever before, drugs—prescription and nonprescription—are available to treat medical and psychological conditions, thereby improving the quality of our lives. Without these drugs, the Thomases and the Lopezes would not feel as well each day and would probably live shorter lives or have their activities limited.

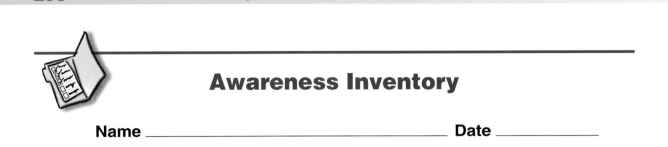

Awareness Inventory

Name _____ **Date** _____

Check the space by the letter T for the statements that you think are true and the space by the letter F for the statements that you think are false. The answers appear following the list of statements. This chapter will present information to clarify these statements for you. As you read the chapter, look for explanations for the reasons why the statements are true or false.

T ___ **F** ___   1. The inappropriate use of a legal drug is referred to as drug abuse.

T ___ **F** ___   2. Using an illegal or legal drug for purposes other than for what it was intended is referred to as drug misuse.

T ___ **F** ___   3. With a blood alcohol level (BAL) of .08 and above, an individual is declared legally intoxicated in most states.

T ___ **F** ___   4. A male weighing 150 pounds who consumes two beers or two glasses of wine within 1 hour will have a blood alcohol high enough to be declared legally drunk in most states.

T ___ **F** ___   5. Young adults aged 18 to 22 enrolled full-time in college in 2001 were less likely to report current cigarette use than were their peers not enrolled full-time.

T ___ **F** ___   6. Moderate drinkers have lower risk of heart disease than nondrinkers do.

T ___ **F** ___   7. Smokeless tobacco users are about 50 times more likely to develop oral cancer than nonusers are.

T ___ **F** ___   8. The use of anabolic steroids to acquire muscle mass, improve appearance, and enhance sports performance is safe and effective as long as a 7-day drug-free period occurs for every 3 weeks of use.

T ___ **F** ___   9. Androstenedione is banned by the NCAA, the International Olympic Committee, and the National Football League.

T ___ **F** ___ 10. Amphetamines are drugs that stimulate the central nervous system.

Answers: 1-F, 2-F, 3-T, 4-F, 5-T, 6-T, 7-T, 8-F, 9-T, 10-T

From Physical fitness and wellness, third edition, by Jerrold S. Greenberg, George B. Dintiman, and Barbee Myers Oakes, 2004, Champaign, IL: Human Kinetics.

Analyze Yourself

Assessing Your Drug Use Behavior

Name _____ **Date** _____

Instructions: Indicate how often each of the following occurs in your daily activities and parties. Respond to each item with a number from 0 to 3, using the following scale:

0 = Never   **1** = Occasionally   **2** = Most of the time   **3** = Always

____ **1.** I avoid binge drinking and the consumption of more than five drinks on the same occasion.

____ **2.** I monitor my intake of alcohol at parties and avoid consuming more than one drink per hour.

____ **3.** I avoid driving a vehicle after consuming alcohol, even if I had only one drink.

____ **4.** I refuse to ride in a vehicle with a driver who has been drinking and make sure that there is a designated, nondrinking driver when attending parties away from home.

____ **5.** I avoid all use of anabolic steroids.

____ **6.** I will not use, experiment with, or even try an illicit drug such as cocaine, heroin, Ecstasy, or marijuana.

____ **7.** I read the label on all medication (over-the-counter and prescription) and follow the directions carefully.

____ **8.** I avoid the use of over-the-counter or prescription tranquilizers and sedatives unless a physician prescribes them for me.

____ **9.** I avoid the use of any type of growth hormone or supplementation with an amino acid (arginine, ornithine, and glycine) that is promoted as a way to boost the body's synthesis of testosterone.

____ **10.** I avoid use of unproven, potentially unsafe sports supplements such as creatine, androstenedione, and growth hormones.

Scoring: Excellent = 25 to 30

Good = 19 to 24

Poor = below 19

From *Physical fitness and wellness, third edition,* by Jerrold S. Greenberg, George B. Dintiman, and Barbee Myers Oakes, 2004, Champaign, IL: Human Kinetics.

You, too, are a drug user; we all are. In fact, the United States is a drug-taking society. And in many respects it is fortunate that we are. Think about the important drugs we use:

- Vaccines that provide protection from diseases that can wipe out whole societies
- Antibiotics that control previously fatal bacterial diseases
- Oral contraceptives that help some people plan families and that have a profound, though controversial, effect on our society
- Tranquilizers and antidepressants that allow people with mental illness to function

For all the good that has come from drugs, many people believe that U.S. society has become too reliant on medication and mood-altering substances. Too often, the remedy for anxiety is a tranquilizer, the response to a headache is an aspirin or some other painkiller, the answer to a problem is alcohol, and the driving force of a social occasion is an illegal drug.

Drug Use, Misuse, and Abuse

You will soon see that differentiating between drug use, misuse, and abuse is not as easy as it first appears. Start this section by listing the last 10 times you can remember taking a drug.

Drug Use

Your list probably includes an occasion when you were ill and took either a drug prescribed by your physician or one available over the counter. Perhaps you had a strained muscle from exercising and took aspirin or ibuprofen to control the inflammation and pain. If you used the drug properly, it probably helped you overcome your malady. The drug might have been so important to your health that if you had not used it, your condition might have worsened. For example, if you contract pneumonia and do not take the antibiotic prescribed for you, you might die. That act is **drug use**—that is, taking drugs as they are recommended to be used and for the purposes for which they were recommended.

Drug Misuse

Unfortunately, some people ruin a good thing. They take too many aspirin tablets in too short a time or ingest ibuprofen without drinking enough fluids. The result could be intestinal problems such as bleeding stomach caused by damage to

stomach tissue. Inappropriate use of a legal drug is **drug misuse.**

Drug Abuse

Use of an illegal drug or use of a legal drug for purposes other than for what it was intended is **drug abuse.** Common abused drugs include marijuana, cocaine, heroin, anabolic steroids, and amphetamines. People often take these drugs for the euphoria they produce rather than for any medical or physiological reason. Legal drugs that people sometimes abuse include Demerol (meperidine), Dilaudid (hydromorphine), and Darvon (propoxyphene). These drugs are prescription pain relievers that are sometimes sold illicitly for their narcotic effects.

Drugs That Are Difficult to Categorize

Although the differentiation between drug use, misuse, and abuse may at first appear clear, a number of drugs and drug usages are difficult to categorize. For example, how would you classify tobacco products? They are legal but cause the body harm. What about alcoholic beverages? In this case, the amount of drug used (the dosage) might dictate its categorization. And in which category would you place over-the-counter diet remedies? They, too, can be taken in excessive amounts or in place of changes in eating and exercise habits.

Space dictates that we limit our discussion of drugs and fitness and the effects of drugs on health and wellness. Consequently, we have chosen to discuss only the more prevalent drugs or those with direct application to physical fitness.

Alcohol

Studies indicate that alcohol use in 2001 increased with age for youths, from 2.6% at age 12 to a peak of 67.5% for persons 21 years old. The use of alcohol also remained steady among older age groups. For people aged 21 to 25 and those aged 26 to 34, the rates of current alcohol use in 2001 were 64.3 and 59.9%, respectively. Use was slightly lower for persons in their 40s.

The highest prevalence of both **binge drinking** and **heavy drinking** in 2001 occurred among adults 18 to 25 (38.7%), with the peak rate at age 21 (48.2%). Binge and heavy-use rates for college students were 42.5 and 18.2%. More males (22.0%) than females (15.9%) reported binge drinking in 2001. Heavy alcohol use was reported by 13.6% of those aged 18 to 25 and by 17.8% of persons aged 21 (*NHSDA,* 2001). Young adults aged 18 to 22 enrolled full time in college were more likely than their peers not enrolled full-time (this category includes part-time college students and persons not enrolled in college) to report all three levels of drinking in 2001. Past-month alcohol use was reported by 63.1% of full-time college students compared with 53.3% of their counterparts who were not enrolled full-time.

Drinking also starts much earlier than age 18. More than one-fourth of high school seniors report weekly use of alcohol (PRIDE, 1996). The situation is probably similar to what occurs on college campuses throughout the United States (see figure 11.1). Alcohol is the drug of choice on college campuses and leads to many accidents, fights, suspensions and expulsions from school, injuries, and even death. All this occurs despite the fact that the legal drinking age is 21.

People drink for many reasons: to relax, to be sociable, to have something to do with their hands during social occasions, and to decrease inhibitions and become less shy. When people limit their drinking to, say, a single **drink,** alcohol-related problems usually do not occur. When they ingest too much alcohol in too short a time,

drug use—The proper use of a drug.

drug misuse—The inappropriate use of a legal drug.

drug abuse—The use of an illegal drug or the use of a legal drug for purposes other than those it was intended for.

binge drinking—Five or more drinks on the same occasion at least once in the 30 days before survey (includes heavy use).

heavy drinking—Five or more drinks on the same occasion on at least 5 different days in the past 30 days.

The U.S. Department of Health and Human Services reports these statistics pertaining to college students and alcohol:

- Of the current student population in the United States, between 2 and 3% will eventually die from alcohol-related causes, about the same number that will earn advanced degrees, master's and doctorate degrees combined.

- For the more than 12 million college students in the United States, the annual consumption of alcoholic beverages totals over 430 million gallons. To visualize this, imagine an Olympic-sized swimming pool filled with beer, wine, and distilled spirits. In a single year, the student body of each college in the country drinks the contents of one pool.

- Over half of all college students participate in drinking games that involve the consumption of extremely large quantities of alcohol. In these games, students consume an average of 6 to 10 drinks in a short time.

- Approximately 35% of college newspaper advertising revenue comes from alcohol advertisements.

- Fraternity members drink more frequently and more heavily than other college students do.

- Depending on the particular study, between 53 and 84% of college students get drunk at least once a year. Between 26 and 48% get drunk once a month.

- College administrators believe that alcohol is a factor in 34% of all academic problems and in 25% of dropouts.

- Almost half of college athletes who drink admit that their use of alcohol has had a harmful or slightly harmful effect on their athletic performance.

Figure 11.1 Facts and figures on college students and alcohol.

From U.S. Department of Health and Human Services, 1991, *Prevention resource guide: College youth,* Pub. no. (ADM) 91-1803 (Washington, DC: U.S. Department of Health and Human Services).

take alcohol with other drugs or medications, or combine it with events requiring coordination and speedy reflexes (such as driving a vehicle), however, serious consequences can result.

Effects of Alcohol

Alcohol affects the body in many different ways. Alcohol causes blood vessels in the head to dilate, which can lead to headaches. It also increases heart rate and blood pressure while at the same time constricting (narrowing) the blood vessels supplying the heart. And when the liver is subjected to excessive doses of alcohol over time, it, too, can be damaged. **Cirrhosis** of the liver is a condition to which alcoholics are prone; it is irreversible and sometimes leads to death. Malnutrition, cancer (of the liver, esophagus, nasopharynx, and larynx), endocrine and reproductive problems, neurological disorders, and mental illness are but a few other potential effects of alcohol abuse.

Numerous studies have found a link between moderate drinking (one to two drinks per day) with protection from heart disease. The most well-established effect of alcohol is an increase in HDL, or good, cholesterol. Regular physical activity and weight loss also raise HDL choles-

terol. Alcohol or substances such as resveratrol (res-VAIR-ah-trol) found in alcoholic beverages are also thought to reduce the risk of heart attack or stroke by preventing platelets in the blood from sticking together and reducing clot formation, in an effect similar to that produced by aspirin. In spite of this evidence, the American Heart Association does not recommend drinking wine or any other form of alcohol to gain these potential benefits.

Alcohol and Pregnancy

In spite of strong public education efforts on its dangers, 12.9% of women aged 15 to 44 who were pregnant used alcohol in 2000 and 2001, and 4.6% were binge drinkers. Obviously, pregnant women shouldn't drink alcohol in any form. Alcohol can cause serious harm to the baby, including causing birth defects.

a drink—One can or bottle of beer, glass of wine or a wine cooler, shot of liquor, or mixed drink with liquor in it.

cirrhosis—A scarring of cells of the liver associated with excessive use of alcohol.

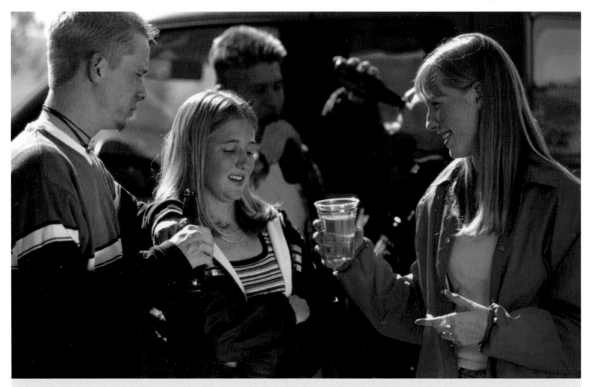

Alcohol is the most frequently used drug by both high school and college students, and troublesome acts are too often a consequence.

Getty Images

How to Take Control of Your Drinking

As you can see in Table 11.1, alcohol can significantly impair your physical functioning. To be physically fit, remain healthy, and possess a high level of wellness requires either abstaining from ingesting alcohol or drinking responsibly. That means limiting the amount of alcohol ingested to no more than one drink containing no more than 0.6 fluid ounce of alcohol per hour (the amount your liver can metabolize in an hour), drinking only when it is appropriate and never when you are driving, and refraining from drinking when you need good judgment.

Yet saying no to alcohol is often easier said than done. Imagine that your friends drink alcohol every time you socialize. They either go to a bar near campus, bring in beer and sit around and drink, or attend a party where alcohol is available. If you do not drink, they will think you are strange. You fear that they might not want anything more to do with you. What can you do?

You can adopt any of the following strategies:

- Take one drink and nurse it for a long time to limit the amount of alcohol you ingest.
- Tell your fiends you are taking medication that prohibits you from drinking.

- Invite someone to join you who also does not want to drink. With company, you will find it easier to withstand peer-group pressure.
- Practice refusal skills in which you assertively tell your friends that you prefer not to drink. By not being judgmental, you can be assertive without turning them off. For example, you might say, "You can drink if you like, but I would prefer not to." You might have to say this several times for your friends to believe that you mean it, but once they do, they will usually accept your decision.

If you do decide to drink, however, follow these guidelines:

- Drink in moderation.
- Never drink on an empty stomach. Food in your stomach will slow down the absorption of the alcohol.
- Never drink when you are taking medication.
- Never ingest alcohol in combination with other drugs.
- Drink slowly.
- Dilute your drinks with water or a mixer.
- Do not drink and eat salty or spicy foods at the same time. The salts and spices will make you thirsty, and you will drink more.

TABLE 11.1—Blood-Alcohol Level (BAL) Effects and Metabolism*

BAL	Effects and symptoms	Approximate hr to metabolize
<0.03	Little observable effect.	2-3
0.03-0.05	Changes in mood and behavior, gregarious.	4-5
0.05-0.10	Legally drunk in most states (.08), unsteady walking or standing, impaired vision and loss of motor coordination; 3-4 drinks within 1 hr will produce a BAL of 0.08 to 0.10 in the average male and a higher value in females.	6-9
0.10-0.15	Driving is extremely dangerous as vision and judgment become more impaired; uncoordinated; pleasant euphoria.	10-19
0.15-0.30	Severe intoxication; slurred speech, loss of alertness and coordination; staggering walk; aggressive, obnoxious behavior; possibly followed by depression, lethargy, and sleep.	20-24
0.30-0.40	Severe intoxication; difficulty remaining conscious.	25-35
0.40-0.50	Severe intoxication; stupor, unconsciousness, coma, and death may occur.	36 or more

*Because the effect of alcohol on the human body and the rate of metabolism are altered by the rate of consumption, type of beverage (beer and wine contain substances that slow absorption; carbonation speeds absorption), gender (women metabolize alcohol slower than men do), body weight (more body mass and blood dilute the effect), tolerance (cellular adaptation to alcohol varies), presence or absence of food and other drugs (illegal, prescription, over-the-counter) in the stomach, and other factors, the preceding information provides only a general indication of the body's immediate response to alcohol consumption.

Too many people have a problem with alcohol. To determine whether you have a problem with alcohol, complete Discovery Activity 11.1: Signs of Alcoholism at the end of this chapter.

Alcohol on College Campuses

A number of strategies have been developed in response to the problem created by alcohol on college campuses. These include, but are not limited to, the following:

- Some universities have offered dry bars, that is, bars that only serve nonalcoholic beverages. Here students can gather and meet as they do at bars that serve alcohol but with neither the pressure nor the opportunity to ingest alcohol. An example is the University of Maryland's Dry Dock.

- Some universities have offered hangover-free Friday night gatherings that include music and dancing.

- A national organization has formed to educate students about how to drink responsibly, how to prevent friends who have been drinking from experiencing problems (such as driving drunk), and how to control their own drinking. This organization, funded by the alcohol industry, is called BACCHUS (Boost Alcohol Consciousness Concerning the Health of University Students) and is now present on many campuses across the United States.

- College theater groups have presented skits educating students regarding responsible use of alcohol. An example is the Wellesley College's Alcohol Information Theater (Project WAIT).

- Sporting and other events on campuses that once boasted of having kegs of beer are refraining from the alcohol connection. An example is George Washington University, which used to have a "Miller's Rocks the Block" party with free beer, T-shirts, and hats. Now, although the beer distributors are still present on the George Washington campus, they no longer provide beer; instead, they sponsor a superdance for muscular dystrophy.

- On many campuses, college administrators have prohibited beer kegs at parties and require that food and soft drinks be served where beer is available. Roanoke College in Virginia instituted such a policy .

- Universities such as William and Mary College, the University of Virginia, James Madison University, and Louisiana State University have instituted dry fraternity and sorority rushes.

- At the University of Maryland, campus-area alcohol retailers have begun a program entitled SUDS (Students Understanding Drinking Sensibly). They distribute SUDS T-shirts and buttons, train local bartenders, and arrange for local police officers to have breathalyzers available for those drinkers who voluntarily choose to have their blood-alcohol levels tested.

What is your campus doing to respond to both the pressure to drink and the problems resulting from the consumption of alcohol? If you decide to become proactive, you can obtain assistance from the organizations listed in figure 11.2.

Tobacco

Another prevalent drug is tobacco and its products, including cigarettes, cigars, pipes, and chewing tobacco. The U.S. government estimates that tobacco use is responsible for one of every six deaths in the United States and is the most preventable cause of death and disease in our society. Tobacco use is the major risk factor for heart and blood diseases; chronic bronchitis and emphysema; cancers of the lung, larynx, pharynx, oral cavity, esophagus, pancreas, and bladder; and other problems such as respiratory infections and stomach ulcers. Cigarette smoking accounts for approximately 440,000 deaths each year, including 21% of coronary-disease deaths, 87% of lung-cancer deaths, and 30% of all cancer deaths. Smokers of more than two packs of cigarettes a day are 15 to 25 times more likely to die of lung cancer than are people who never smoked (U.S. Department of Health and Human Services, 2002).

Smoking Rates

An estimated 66.5 million Americans reported current use (past-month use) of a tobacco product in 2001, a prevalence rate of 29.5% for the population aged 12 or older. Among that same population, 56.3 million (24.9% of the total population aged 12 or older) smoked cigarettes, 12.1 million (5.4%) smoked cigars, 7.3 million (3.2%) used smokeless tobacco, and 2.3 million (1.0%) smoked tobacco in pipes. Between 2000 and 2001, the percentage reporting past-month cigar smoking increased from 4.8 to 5.4%, which was similar to the rate reported in 1999 (5.5%). No other significant changes occurred in the rates of current use of other tobacco products.

Between 1999 and 2001, the rate of cigarette use among males aged 12 to 17 decreased from

Al-Anon Family Groups, Inc.
World Service Office
1600 Corporate Landing Parkway
Virginia Beach, VA 23454-5617
888-425-2666

Alcohol Policies Project Center for Science in the Public Interest
1875 Connecticut Avenue NW, #300
Washington, DC 20009
202-332-9110

Alcoholics Anonymous (AA)
World Service, Inc.
468 Park Avenue South
New York, NY 10016
212-686-1100

American College Health Association
15879 Crabbs Branch Way
Rockville, MD 20855
301-963-1100

American Council on Education
1 Dupont Circle
Washington, DC 20036
202-466-5030

Campuses Without Drugs, Inc.
National Office
2530 Holly Drive
Pittsburgh, PA 15235
412-731-8019

Coalition of (Campus) Drug and Alcohol Educators
250 Arapahoe, Suite 301
Boulder, CO 80302
303-443-5696

Commission on Alcohol and Other Drugs of the American College Personnel Association
Central Michigan University
Mt. Pleasant, MI 48859
517-774-3381

Health Promotion Resources
509 University Avenue
St. Paul, MN 55103
1-800-782-1878

Integrated Substance Abuse Consultants (INSAC)
P.O. Box 7505
Arlington, VA 22205
703-237-3840

Nar Anon Hotline
800-780-3951

National Association of Student Personnel Administrators
1 Dupont Circle, Suite 330
Washington, DC 20036
202-293-9161

Marin Institute for the Prevention of Alcohol and Other Drug Problems
24 Belvedere Street
San Rafael, CA 94901
415-456-5692

National Interfraternity Conference
3901 West 86th Street
Suite 390
Indianapolis, IN 46268
317-872-1112

National Organization of Student Assistance Programs and Professionals (NOSAPP)
250 Arapahoe, Suite 301
Boulder, CO 80302
800-972-4636

Network of Colleges and Universities Committed to the Elimination of Drug and Alcohol Abuse
Office of Educational Research and Improvement
U.S. Department of Education
555 New Jersey Avenue SW
Washington, DC 20208-5644
202-357-6265

Peterson's Drug and Alcohol Programs and Policies
Dept. 9377
P.O. Box 2123
Princeton, NJ 08543
800-338-3282

Figure 11.2 Alcohol-related groups, organizations, and programs for college students.

14.8 to 12.4%, with a similar pattern among females between 1999 and 2001 (15.0% in 1999 to 13.6% in 2001). Cigarette-smoking rates increased steadily with age up to age 21, from 1.7% at age 12 to 43.5% at age 21. After age 21, rates generally declined, reaching 18.3% for persons aged 60 to 64 years and 9.1% for persons aged 65 or older. By age group, the prevalence of cigarette use was 13.0% among 12- to 17-year-olds, 39.1% among young adults aged 18 to 25 years, and 24.2% among adults aged 26 or older.

Young adults aged 18 to 22 enrolled full-time in college in 2001 were less likely to report current cigarette use than were their peers not enrolled full-time. Past-month cigarette use was reported by 32.9% of full-time college students compared with 44.6% of their peers who were not enrolled full-time.

Perhaps the best statistical news is that the number of new daily smokers aged 12 to 17 is declining, from 1,100,000 in 1997 to 747,000 in 2000, representing a reduction in the number of youths who begin smoking on a daily basis from 3,000 per day to 2,000 per day. This trend is bad news for cigarette manufacturers in the future and good news for the health of those who do not begin the habit.

Smokeless Tobacco

Smokeless tobacco includes primarily moist or dry snuff and chewing tobacco. An estimated 6.8 million Americans (3.3%) use smokeless tobacco (Substance Abuse and Mental Health Services Administration, 2001). The rate of smokeless tobacco use is significantly higher among men (6.2%) than it is among women (0.6%). Over 90% of smokeless tobacco users are men. Smokeless tobacco users are susceptible to oral cancer, with long-term snuff users being 50 times more likely to develop oral cancer than nonusers are. Adolescent males make up the great majority of new users of smokeless tobacco. They may see their favorite athletes (usually baseball players) chew tobacco and emulate that behavior.

Effects of Tobacco on the Body

Tobacco affects the body in many ways. The nicotine in tobacco stimulates the central nervous system and therefore increases the heart rate. Tobacco use also constricts blood vessels, increases blood pressure, destroys air sacs in the lungs, and increases the production of hydrochloric acid in the stomach. The result is shortness of breath; upset stomach; cold and clammy fingers and toes; the development of heart disease, hypertension, stroke, emphysema, and digestive disorders; and lung and other cancers.

Why People Use Tobacco Products

Before reading further, complete Discovery Activity 11.2: Why Do You Smoke? at the end of this chapter. If you are not a smoker, complete the activity by guessing how most smokers would respond to the statements presented.

The purpose of tobacco advertising is to sell tobacco products—and advertisers do a good job of it, as the statistics just presented suggest. As we strive to be desirable, envied, cool, and admired, tobacco sellers encourage us to emulate the people depicted in the tobacco product ads. They are handsome and pretty, smiling and obviously happy, and appear wealthy enough to have fine furniture and expensive clothing.

People use tobacco products for other reasons as well. Tobacco provides something to do with the hands. Best friends or parents may smoke, so people may copy their behavior. Tobacco use is antiauthority (schools and workplaces disallow it and parents often object) and is therefore considered cool. It relieves boredom and is psychologically relaxing for some people, in spite of being a central nervous system stimulant. Tobacco substitutes for food and can be used to control weight.

How to Quit

Researchers have found that the best way to quit smoking is simply to quit. That might sound simplistic, but what usually happens is that smokers try to quit when they are not really committed to doing so. Eventually, they reach the point at which they are well motivated and in their next attempt are successful. For that reason it is difficult to cite any one program as better than another. The key ingredient in any program is the motivation and seriousness of the smoker wishing to quit.

Imagine you smoke cigarettes and cannot seem to quit. They relax you after dinner and give you something to do with your hands during social occasions. You have tried to quit many times without success. Do not give up. You can employ several strategies that can be effective.

You can write a contract using the form in figure 4.1 on page 91, with the goal of progressively decreasing the number of cigarettes you smoke over several weeks until you quit altogether. A friend or relative can witness the contract and check on your progress at predetermined intervals.

You can also use chaining. With this approach you want to increase the number of links in the chain leading to smoking. For example, you can take your pack of cigarettes and place it in a sweat sock. Then wrap the sock with masking tape and place it in a locked drawer as far from where you usually smoke as possible (perhaps upstairs if you tend to smoke downstairs). Next, take the key to the drawer and place it in the other sock, wrap it with masking tape, and deposit it in a drawer far away from the drawer in which the pack of cigarettes is located. Now, to smoke, you have to go through several inconveniences. Compare this to simply reaching into your pocket or pocketbook and lighting up almost without thinking.

Here are some other suggestions that can help motivated smokers stop smoking or at least lessen the harm they expose themselves to:

- Smoke only one cigarette per hour and eventually taper down.
- Smoke exactly half as many cigarettes each week as you did the week before.
- Inhale with less vigor, avoiding deep inhalation.
- Smoke each cigarette only halfway.
- Remove the cigarette from your mouth between puffs.
- Smoke slowly.
- Smoke brands with low tar and nicotine content.
- Place unlighted cigarettes in your mouth when you have the urge to smoke.
- Switch to a brand you dislike.
- Put something else in your mouth when you want a cigarette (for example, chewing gum, fruit, hard candy).
- Exercise regularly so that you do not smoke out of boredom.
- Develop the sense of wanting to do well by your body.
- Spend time in places where smoking is prohibited.
- Brush your teeth directly after every meal.
- Alter your behavior pattern. For example, avoid friends who smoke for several weeks after quitting and substitute another activity for smoking after dinner.
- Remind yourself frequently why you quit smoking.
- Use the other behavioral change techniques discussed in chapter 4 to quit smoking.

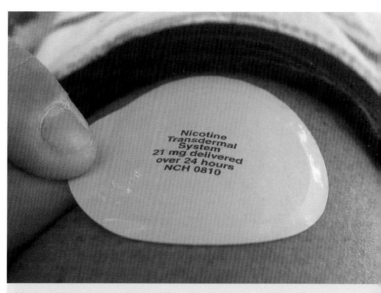

Many methods are available to smokers who truly want to quit, ranging from the nicotine patch, to nicotine gum, to a host of smoking cessation programs.

Ecstasy MDMA (methylenedioxymethamphetamine)—An illicit drug that stimulates the central nervous system and alters mood.

Ecstasy

The use of Ecstasy (MDMA) has increased from 1.3 million new users in 1999 to 1.9 million in 2000. Ecstasy has become a popular drug on college campuses throughout the United States and is often used in combination with alcohol. **Ecstasy MDMA (methylenedioxymethamphetamine)** belongs to a family of drugs called entactogens, which literally means touching within. Before being declared illegal in 1985, MDMA was used by psychiatrists as a therapeutic tool. MDMA is a mood elevator that produces a relaxed, euphoric state about 30 minutes after the user takes a 100- to 125-milligram tablet, reaching peak effect in 60 to 90 minutes. The drug is said to enhance sensations, feelings of empathy, emotional warmth, and self-acceptance and to produce loss of inhibitions, excitedness, euphoria, talkativeness, and a rush of energy. The effects subside in 3 to 5 hours.

Although Ecstasy is not physically addictive, compulsive use develops in many individuals and continued use reduces the effect. Like most drugs purchased on the street, Ecstasy varies widely in strength and contains other drugs. Possession of Ecstasy is illegal, and a conviction can result in a lengthy prison sentence. Some of the possible side effects include increased heart rate and blood pressure, sweating, dehydration, overheating, depressed appetite, dizziness, and lack of coordination. Long-term effects may include depression, brain and liver damage, and death.

Rohypnol

Rohypnol, the "date rape" drug (rophy, ruffles, roofies, ruffies, ruf up, rib, roach 2, R2, R2-do-U, roche, rope, ropies, circles, Circes, forget it, Mexican Valium) is a prescription sedative. The generic name for Rohypnol is flunitrazepam. This drug is not manufactured or approved for use in North America, but it can be found as a street drug in pill form (small white pill with a split-pill line on one side and the word "ROCHE" with numbers 1 or 2 in a circle stamped on the other) in 0.5-, 1-, and 2-milligram tablets. The drug is tasteless, colorless, and odorless and can be crushed and added to any drink, including water, without detection. Because of its use as a date-rape drug, the manufacturer has now altered the formula of Rohypnol so that it changes color when it comes in contact with liquid.

Rohypnol produces a sedative effect, amnesia, muscle relaxation, and a slowing of psychomotor responses. Sedation occurs 20 to 30 minutes after administration and lasts for several hours, longer when mixed with alcohol. Blood and urine samples reveal its presence 24 to 48 hours after ingestion. Effects include disinhibition and amnesia, excitability or aggressive behavior, decreased blood pressure, memory impairment, drowsiness, visual disturbances, semiconsciousness, dizziness, confusion, stomach disturbances, and urinary retention.

Rohypnol quickly gained acceptance in the United States in the early 1990s and is now one of the "in" drugs on high school and college campuses. "Roofies" are often combined with alcohol, marijuana, or cocaine to produce a rapid dramatic high. Even without alcohol or other drugs, users become intoxicated, slur speech, and lose coordination. The drug has been added to punch and other drinks at fraternity parties and college social gatherings to lower inhibitions and facilitate potential sexual conquest. Besides the dangers of unwanted and unprotected sex, the drug presents the risk of respiratory depression, aspiration, and even death. The amnesia-producing effect of the drug, which may prevent some users

> **Rohypnol**—A powerful sedative sold illegally on the street in the form of a pill that has been implicated in many cases of date rape.
>
> **anabolic steroids**—Drugs that are derivatives of the male sex hormone testosterone; sometimes used illegally by those desiring to increase body size, speed, or strength.

from remembering whether they took the drug or were given it by others, complicates investigation of sex-related offenses.

Keep in mind that anyone who is intoxicated from alcohol or other drugs cannot legally consent to sex and that having sex with such a person is legally rape, punishable by 20 years in prison.

Drug Taking to Enhance Athletic Performance

Athletes are competitive by nature. They try hard to beat others in their sports or, when competing against themselves, strive to do better than they have ever done before. It stands to reason that they would want whatever edge they can get. The desire to perform at their best has led some athletes to a search for drugs that can enhance performance. Among these drugs are anabolic steroids, caffeine, amphetamines, and cocaine.

Anabolic Steroids

So you want to be strong? So you want to run faster than you ever thought you could? Well, forget about all the work of weight training or exercise that makes you perspire. Try steroids. In today's quick-weight-loss, quick-fitness, quick-everything society, why not engage in quick bulking up? As we will soon see, the reason not to is simple: **Anabolic steroids** are quite dangerous.

Anabolic steroids made the news when Olympic world-record holder Ben Johnson was disqualified from receiving a gold medal for winning the 100-meter sprint at the 1988 Olympic Games. When he was routinely tested just after the race, Johnson tested positive for a steroid. The death of former professional football player Lyle Alzado of cancer, which was attributed to his use of anabolic steroids in an attempt to gain strength, also fueled publicity about these drugs.

Anabolic steroids are derivatives of the male sex hormone testosterone. They are prescribed

Myth and Fact Sheet

Myth	Fact
1. Alcohol consumption in the United States is declining.	**1.** According to the 2001 NHSDA study, the rate of alcohol use and the number of drinkers actually increased between 2000 and 2001. Almost half of all Americans age 12 or older, 48.3% or 109 million persons, were current drinkers in the 2001 survey. This estimate was roughly 5.0 million higher than the corresponding figure in 2000, when 46.6% of those age 12 or older reported current alcohol use. No significant changes were found in heavy or binge drinking.
2. Because of stricter laws and education, fewer people are driving their vehicles when drinking.	**2.** The rate of driving under the influence of alcohol increased from 10.0% in 2000 to 11.1% in 2001. Among young adults aged 18 to 25, 22.8% drove under the influence of alcohol.
3. It is safe to combine alcohol and aspirin.	**3.** The U.S. Food and Drug Administration warns that people who take aspirin regularly should not drink alcohol. Heart-disease patients should avoid combining alcohol and aspirin if their doctors prescribed aspirin for a heart condition.
4. Alcohol is really the only drug to be concerned about on college campuses.	**4.** The increased use of Ecstasy is also a major concern. Lately, college students have been combining Ecstasy with Viagra and alcohol in search of an all-night, psychedelic, love-making potion, a practice that experts indicate is extremely dangerous.
5. Date rape is easy to avoid if college students take precautions.	**5.** Precautions do reduce the risk; however, the use of the tasteless date-rape drug, Rohypnol, makes practically everyone vulnerable at parties and mixers involving large numbers of people. Students need to go to such outings in groups and come home safely the same way, with a designated nondrinking driver.
6. Androstenedione and growth hormones must be safe because athletes at all levels of competition use them.	**6.** Both drugs are dangerous and capable of producing serious, permanent side effects and even death. You can add muscle mass and improve performance without resorting to the use of unproven dangerous drugs.
7. Beer will not get you as drunk as hard liquor will.	**7.** The alcohol is what is responsible for inebriation. You can ingest just as much alcohol from beer as you can from other sources.
8. Drinking alcohol is relaxing.	**8.** A small amount of alcohol initially acts as a stimulant. Larger amounts depress the central nervous system. The feeling of relaxation, however, arises because the brain is deadened. The price paid is that other bodily functions are depressed as well, such as the ability to think clearly or perform coordinated actions. The result can be accidents or poor decisions that lead to injury or ill health.
9. The use of marijuana, cocaine, and similar drugs is the major drug problem on college campuses.	**9.** Alcohol is both the most prevalent and frequently abused drug on college campuses. Alcohol intoxication can lead to vandalism, fights, and other behaviors resulting in suspension or expulsion from school, not to mention the legal consequences.
10. Being physically fit and possessing a high level of wellness means never using drugs.	**10.** We all use drugs. We take prescribed antibiotics, we buy over-the-counter cold remedies, and we ingest aspirin or ibuprofen when our muscles ache. The key is to use safe drugs safely, in the way they were intended to be used.

as treatment for anemia and growth problems and as an aid in recovery from surgery. A black market has developed, however, and steroids are illegally used to increase body weight and muscle mass, gain power, and increase strength.

Steroids can be taken in pill form or injected directly into the bloodstream. Steroid users may take more than one steroid at a time, a practice called stacking, believing that the effect will be hastened or enhanced.

Steroid users place themselves at risk for liver cancer, high blood pressure, heart disease, and sterility. In men, steroid use can lead to atrophied testicles, prostate cancer, and breast growth. In women, it can result in menstrual irregularities, deepening of the voice, decreased breast size, baldness, and facial hair growth. In both men and women, anabolic steroid use can lead to clogging of the arteries, eating compulsions, increased aggressiveness, and hostility.

The *Physician's Desk Reference* (p. 2122) states that "anabolic steroids have not been shown to enhance athletic ability." The American College of Sports Medicine (ACSM) states that although steroids can increase body weight and muscular strength, they do not increase aerobic power or the capacity for exercise. The ACSM goes on to say that anabolic steroid use is contrary to the rules and ethical principles of athletic competition, and they deplore its use by athletes. Yet almost 5% of high school seniors, not to mention other students and athletes, use anabolic steroids illegally.

Suppose that in the gym where you work out many men and women your age look fantastic. The men are chiseled. Their muscles are round and hard, and they do not have an ounce of fat on them—or so it seems. The women are curved to perfection. They have muscles in all the right places and are round where they should be round. But you learn that they take steroids. Without the drugs, you are told, they would not look so good. You would love to look like they do and are tempted to try these drugs. How can you overcome this temptation?

You can always use selective awareness. Instead of focusing on how good you could look if you took steroids, concentrate on their potential effect on your liver, your sexual organs (atrophied or shrunken testicles if you are a male and menstrual irregularities if you are a female), and the threat they pose to your life. Imagine yourself as a perfectly chiseled corpse.

You could also use covert modeling. After watching someone weight train who looks good and does not take steroids, close your eyes and imagine that you are doing just what you observed the other person doing. Smell the smells, hear the noise, see the sights, and so forth. Make it vivid. Refer back to chapter 4 for other ways to take charge of your behavior.

Androstenedione

Androstenedione is a so-called hormone precursor that is said to increase blood levels of testosterone and increase muscle mass, strength, power, and speed. The drug was made popular by Mark McGwire during his famous 1998 record-setting home run performance in major league baseball. Athletes generally consume 50 to 200 milligrams of androstenedione daily. Many manufacturers suggest that users consume the supplement about an hour before exercise and cycle its use (3 to 4 weeks on followed by 1 week off).

Studies are underway to test the effectiveness and safety of androstenedione, although the real dangers of long-term use will not be determined for some time. According to a June 1999 study (King et al., 1999) in the *Journal of the American Medical Association (JAMA)*, androstenedione does not increase testosterone in the blood or enhance muscle as previously believed and can be dangerous. The *JAMA* study, conducted at Iowa State University in Ames, looked at 30 healthy men ages 19 to 29 with normal testosterone levels. Twenty of the men performed 8 weeks of whole-body resistance training. During that period, 10 of the men were given 300 milligrams of androstenedione a day, and the others were given a placebo. Researchers found no difference between the muscle strength or testosterone levels in the blood of those who took androstenedione and those who took the placebo. Men who took androstenedione did have raised blood levels of estrogens, the female hormones. Higher estrogen levels in men can increase the risk of heart and pancreas problems, breast development, breast cancer, pancreatic cancer, and heart disease. Other potential risks include those associated with use of other androgenic-anabolic steroids, such as kidney and liver damage, acne, premature baldness, gynecomastia (excessive development of the male mammary glands), an enlarged prostate, testicular atrophy, reduced HDL cholesterol, reduced sperm production, and heightened aggression. For females, effects could include a disrupted menstrual cycle, a deepened voice, hirsutism (increased facial hair growth), an enlarged clitoris, acne, masculinization, kidney damage, and liver damage. To date, no studies have indicated that androstenedione has any erogenic or anabolic effects in normal human subjects.

Although permitted by Major League Baseball, androstenedione is banned by the NCAA, the International Olympic Committee, and the National Football League. Major League Baseball, the National Basketball Association, and the National Hockey League are expected to follow suit.

Steroids always have side effects that may not appear for months or years, and the hormone testosterone is carefully regulated. Since the 1994 Dietary Supplement Health Education Act was passed in 1994, substances that create testosterone in the human body are not classified as drugs and can be sold over the counter (OTC drugs). As a result, products such as androstenedione are available to the consumer in spite of the potentially dangerous side effects that may occur in the future.

Creatine

Creatine (phosphocreatine or PCr) is a compound that initially resupplies muscle ATP during short, intense bursts of activity such as a 100-meter sprint, after repeated anaerobic efforts such as short sprints in basketball, soccer, rugby, football, and tennis, and following weight-training workouts. Creatine is a phosphorylated form that is manufactured in the body from amino acids (glycine and arginine) and consumed in red meat and other foods. Studies have indicated that supplementation in the form of 5 grams four times per day improved performance in some of these activities but not in others. Creatine supplementation is a legal nutritional practice similar to the widely accepted technique of carbohydrate loading for distance running and athletic events lasting 1 hour or longer. "Creatine loading" through supplementation seems to expedite resynthesis of phosphocreatine and allow subsequent exercise sessions or competition to be completed faster and with more power. Studies indicate that as many as 13% of college students use creatine supplements. Coaches and trainers also stock products such as Creatine Fuel, Growth Fuel, PhosphaGems, Pro Stuff, Hy-Gear, and Pinnacle for use by their athletes. Creatine supplementation for a month or two during training has been reported to improve sprint performance (5 to 8%) and promote gains in strength (5 to 15%) and lean body mass (1 to 3%). More research is needed on individual differences in the response to creatine, periodic or cyclical use of creatine, side effects, and long-term effects on endurance.

Because muscles can only store a certain amount of creatine, supplementation is not helpful to those who have no room for more. More evidence is needed to support the value of supplementation in gaining muscle mass. Studies reveal a number of side effects including muscle cramping, diarrhea and gastrointestinal pain, renal dysfunction, and dehydration. The FDA (Food and Drug Administration) has logged 32 complaints including cardiac arrhythmia (irregular heartbeat), cardiomyopathy (disease of the heart muscle with unknown cause), deep venous thrombosis (clot within a vein), rhabdomyolysis (an acute, potentially fatal disease that entails destruction of skeletal muscle), and death, with no conclusions to date linking these reports to creatine supplementation. Because long-term effects are unknown, the American College of Sports Medicine discourages the use of creatine, especially among teenagers. The Tampa Bay Buccaneers of the NFL have also taken a strong stand indicating that although some individuals will increase muscular size and strength with proper training and nutrition faster than non-supplemented individuals will, the side effects are too risky.

Growth Hormones

Growth hormone is produced in the pituitary gland and promotes synthesis of protein, mobilizes fatty acids from fat stores, and controls skeletal growth. Some athletes use growth hormone injections to increase muscle mass and strength.

androstenedione—A hormone precursor used to add muscle mass and strength by increasing blood levels of testosterone.

creatine (phosphocreatine or PCr)—A type nutritional supplement that users claim resupplies muscle ATP during short, intense bursts of activity such as a 100-meter sprint and other anaerobic activities by increasing muscle strength and power.

The use of growth hormone can produce serious side effects, including abnormal growth of the skin, tongue, bones of the jaw, fingers, and toes; growth of the heart and other internal organs; and death. Supplementation with amino acids arginine, ornithine, and glycine to increase growth hormone has been shown to produce only a modest increase that is of little physiological consequence.

Caffeine

Caffeine is a stimulant drug that appears in coffee, tea, chocolate, and soft drinks. Caffeine can activate the brain, thereby decreasing drowsiness and fatigue. Caffeine also increases heart and breathing rates. In addition, caffeine serves as a stimulant for skeletal muscles and enables the body to use fatty acids for energy. The result is an increase in physical work output. For those reasons caffeine has been suggested as an aid to physical fitness and athletic activities.

Caffeine consumption as an adjunct to physical activity, however, is not recommended because caffeine can have serious side effects. Depending on the dosage, caffeine can result in irregular heartbeat; hyperactivity; headaches; insomnia; an increase in low-density lipoprotein (LDL), which is associated with coronary heart disease; and low birth weight when consumed by pregnant women.

Amphetamines

Amphetamines are drugs that stimulate the central nervous system. They result in increased heart rate, blood pressure, breathing rate, and blood sugar and in high arousal levels. This psychological-arousal effect, along with the physiological-arousal effects, disguises muscle fatigue so that greater work output can occur.

People should not use amphetamines to increase work output for several reasons. First, no evidence supports the notion that their use enhances athletic performance. In fact, amphetamines may interfere with athletic performance by increasing hyperactivity when more controlled physical responses are needed. Second, amphetamine users often become dependent on these drugs and resort to taking barbiturates to come down from an amphetamine high. This yo-yo drugging effect can be dangerous. Barbiturates are extremely addictive, and withdrawing from them without medical supervision can be deadly.

caffeine—A stimulant drug present in coffee, tea, and colas and other soft drinks that have not been decaffeinated.

amphetamines—Drugs that stimulate the central nervous system, increasing heart rate, blood pressure, and other body processes.

cocaine—A drug that stimulates the central nervous system and can cause tremors, rapid heartbeat, and harmful psychological effects.

Cocaine

Cocaine is another drug that people take to improve physical performance or for "recreational" reasons. Cocaine can be snorted through the nose, smoked as crack, or injected. Like amphetamines, cocaine can increase work output by the nature of its stimulating effect on the central nervous system. It also produces a euphoria that disguises fatigue.

Cocaine, however, is not only illegal but also can result in dire health consequences. It can cause tremors and rapid heartbeat, raise blood pressure dangerously high to the point of threatening stroke, lower the effectiveness of the immune system, and decrease appetite, resulting in malnutrition. In addition, cocaine can cause acute anxiety, confusion, and depression. In a few cases, cocaine psychosis has occurred in heavy users, leading to delusions and violence.

Summary

Drug Use, Misuse, and Abuse Using drugs as they are recommended to be used and for the purposes for which they were recommended is drug use. Using a legal drug inappropriately is drug misuse. Using an illegal drug or using a legal drug for purposes other than those for which it was intended is drug abuse.

Alcohol Alcohol is the most prevalent drug on college campuses. Estimates are that between 2 and 3% of the current college student body will eventually die from alcohol-related causes. Between 53 and 84% of college students get drunk at least once a year, and between 26 and 48% get drunk once a month.

Alcohol dilates blood vessels in the head, causing headaches; narrows the blood vessels supplying the heart; damages cells in the liver; often leads to malnutrition, endocrine, and reproductive

Behavioral Change and Motivational Strategies

Many things can interfere with your desire to avoid the misuse or abuse of drugs. Here are some of those barriers (roadblocks) and strategies for overcoming them.

Roadblock	Behavioral Change Strategy
When you attend parties or hang out with your friends, they try to get you to use drugs.	Use assertiveness skills to refuse the use of drugs. To make an assertive response, first describe the situation ("When I am asked to use drugs . . ."), your feelings about the situation ("I feel as though I am being disrespected"), what you would prefer ("I would rather people respect my decision not to use drugs"), and the results if the preferred action is taken and the results if it is not taken ("If my decision not to use drugs is respected, I hang out, but if I continue to get pressure to use drugs, I will find other friends to spend time with").
You have a difficult time saying no. You live with a roommate who smokes cigarettes.	Contracting can help with this issue. Explain to your roommate that you want to avoid the effects of breathing in exhaled smoke. You are concerned about the health effects of breathing in secondhand smoke and would appreciate it if smoking occurred only outside the room or apartment. Then draw up a contract to make sure that happens. The contract should be specific regarding the behavior in question (smoking), the agreed-upon remedy (smoking only outside the room or apartment), the rewards for adhering to the action specified in the contract, and the punishment for not adhering to that action. Rewards might include doing the dishes 4 days a week while your roommate does them only 3 days a week. Punishment might be seeking other roommates and places to live.
The friends that you weight train with use anabolic steroids to achieve that "cut" look. You are tempted to do the same but are concerned about the health effects.	You can use the parts of the health belief model (chapter 4, page 94) to influence your behavior. Write down how susceptible you would be to a severe condition if you use anabolic steroids. Then list the benefits of not using anabolic steroids. Next, list the barriers to your not using steroids (for example, your friends will make fun of you) and the responses you can make to overcome those barriers. Last, place cues to action on your refrigerator, that is, notes that cite both the dangers of anabolic steroid use and the benefits of not using them.
List other roadblocks you might encounter that could influence your use of chemicals to enhance fitness.	Now cite behavioral change strategies that can help you overcome these roadblocks. If you need to, refer to chapter 4 for behavioral change and motivational strategies.

1. _____

2. _____

3. _____

1. _____

2. _____

3. _____

system problems; and can cause cancer in several body sites.

Drinking responsibly means not becoming inebriated by limiting the amount of alcohol ingested to no more than one average-sized drink (0.6 fluid ounce) an hour, drinking only when appropriate, never drinking and driving, and refraining from drinking when you need good judgment. To control drinking, drink in moderation, never drink on an empty stomach, never drink when taking medication, never ingest alcohol in combination with other drugs, drink slowly, dilute drinks, and do not eat salty or spicy foods when drinking.

Tobacco Tobacco use is the most preventable cause of death in the United States. It is the major risk factor for heart and blood disease; chronic bronchitis and emphysema; cancers of the lung, larynx, pharynx, oral cavity, esophagus, pancreas, and bladder; and other problems such as respiratory infections and stomach ulcers.

Tobacco use constricts blood vessels, increases blood pressure, destroys air sacs in the lungs, and increases the production of hydrochloric acid in the stomach. The results are shortness of breath; upset stomach; cold and clammy fingers and toes; the development of heart disease, hypertension, stroke, emphysema, and digestive disorders; and lung and other cancers.

To quit or cut down on smoking, smoke only one cigarette an hour, smoke only half the cigarette, inhale less, smoke slowly, smoke brands you dislike, place unlighted cigarettes in your mouth when you get the urge, exercise regularly as a diversion, and spend time in places where smoking is prohibited.

Ecstasy
Ecstasy (MDMA) has become a popular drug on college campuses throughout the United States. Although the drug is not physically addictive, compulsive use develops in many individuals. The drug produces serious side effects, including increased heart rate and blood pressure, sweating, dehydration, overheating, depressed appetite, dizziness, and lack of coordination. Long-term effects may include depression, brain and liver damage, and death.

Rohypnol
Rohypnol, the date-rape drug, is a prescription sedative that is tasteless, colorless, and odorless. It produces a sedative effect in 20 to 30 minutes,

amnesia, muscle relaxation, and a slowing of psychomotor responses. The drug has been added to punch and other drinks at fraternity parties and college social gatherings to lower inhibitions and facilitate potential sexual conquest. Dangers include unwanted and unprotected sex, respiratory depression, aspiration, and even death. To avoid date rape, individuals need to consume alcohol responsibly, guard their drinks at all times, travel to and from parties in groups, and take other precautions to protect themselves from unwanted consumption of the drug.

Drug Taking to Enhance Athletic Performance
Among the drugs taken in an attempt to improve athletic performance are anabolic steroids, caffeine, amphetamines, and cocaine. All these drugs present a serious threat to health.

Anabolic steroids place the user at increased risk for liver cancer, high blood pressure, heart disease, and sterility. In men, use of anabolic steroids can lead to atrophied testicles, prostate cancer, and breast growth. In women, use can result in menstrual irregularities, deepening of the voice, decreased breast size, baldness, and facial hair growth. In both men and women, anabolic steroid use can lead to clogging of the arteries, eating compulsions, increased aggressiveness, and hostility.

Caffeine is a stimulant that increases heart and breathing rates, enables skeletal muscles to use fatty acids for energy more efficiently, and decreases fatigue and drowsiness. Caffeine, however, can have serious side effects depending on the amount ingested. Using caffeine can result in irregular heartbeat; hyperactivity; headaches; insomnia; an increase in LDL, which is associated with coronary disease; and low birth weight when pregnant women consume it.

Amphetamines and cocaine are also stimulants. They can create feelings of psychological and physiological arousal. But people can become dependent on these drugs, and they can cause serious cardiac problems that can result in death.

Although the use of androstenedione, creatine, and growth hormone in the form of supplementation to enhance muscle size, strength, and power is legal, their use is not recommended because the immediate side effects are too risky and the long-term side affects are numerous and serious, some of which may cause death.

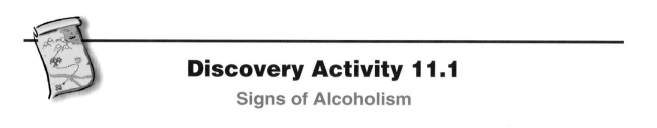

Discovery Activity 11.1
Signs of Alcoholism

Name _____ **Date** _____

Instructions: Answer each of the questions below. Then read the interpretation section to find out what your score indicates about you and symptoms of alcoholism.

Yes   No

___   ___   **1.** Do you ever drink too heavily when you are disappointed, under pressure, or have had a quarrel with someone?

___   ___   **2.** Have you ever been unable to remember part of the previous evening even though your friends say you did not pass out?

___   ___   **3.** Has a family member or close friend ever expressed concern or complained about your drinking?

___   ___   **4.** Do you often want to continue drinking after your friends say they have had enough?

___   ___   **5.** When you are sober, do you sometimes regret things you did or said while you were drinking?

___   ___   **6.** Are you having financial, work, school, or family problems because of your drinking?

___   ___   **7.** Has a physician ever advised you to cut down on drinking?

___   ___   **8.** Do you eat very little or irregularly at times when you are drinking?

___   ___   **9.** Have you recently noticed that you cannot drink as much as you used to?

___   ___   **10.** Have any of your blood relatives ever had a problem with alcohol?

Interpretation:

Any yes answer indicates that you may be at greater-than-average risk for alcoholism. More than one yes may indicate the presence of an alcohol-related problem or alcoholism and the need for consultation with an alcoholism professional. To find out more, contact the National Council on Alcoholism and Drug Dependence in your area.

Source: These questions have been excerpted from *What Are the Signs of Alcoholism?* The NCAAD Self Test, published by the National Council on Alcoholism and Drug Dependence, Inc. For a copy of this brochure, send 50 cents to NCAAD, 12 West 21st St., New York, NY 10010.

From *Physical fitness and wellness, third edition,* by Jerrold S. Greenberg, George B. Dintiman, and Barbee Myers Oakes, 2004, Champaign, IL: Human Kinetics.

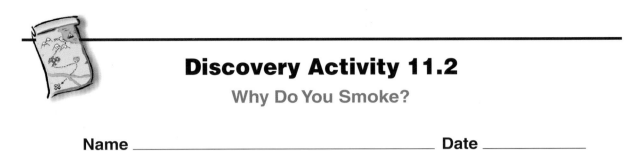

Discovery Activity 11.2

Why Do You Smoke?

Name _____ **Date** _____

Instructions: Here are some statements made by people to describe what they get out of smoking cigarettes. If you are a smoker, how often do you feel this way when smoking cigarettes? If you are not a smoker, how often do you think smokers feel this way when they smoke? Perhaps responding to these questions, even if you do not smoke cigarettes, will help you better understand why other people smoke. Circle one number for each statement. Answer all statements.

	Always	Frequently	Occasionally	Seldom	Never
A. I smoke cigarettes to keep myself from slowing down.	5	4	3	2	1
B. Handling a cigarette is part of the enjoyment of smoking it.	5	4	3	2	1
C. Smoking cigarettes is pleasant and relaxing.	5	4	3	2	1
D. I light up a cigarette when I feel angry about something.	5	4	3	2	1
E. When I run out of cigarettes, I find it almost unbearable until I can get them.	5	4	3	2	1
F. I smoke cigarettes automatically without even being aware of it.	5	4	3	2	1
G. I smoke cigarettes to stimulate myself, to perk myself up.	5	4	3	2	1
H. Part of the enjoyment of smoking a cigarette comes from the steps I take to light it up.	5	4	3	2	1
I. I find cigarettes pleasurable.	5	4	3	2	1
J. When I feel uncomfortable or upset about something, I light up a cigarette.	5	4	3	2	1
K. I am very much aware of it when I am not smoking a cigarette.	5	4	3	2	1
L. I light a cigarette without realizing I still have one burning in the ashtray.	5	4	3	2	1
M. I smoke cigarettes to give myself a lift.	5	4	3	2	1
N. When I smoke a cigarette, part of the enjoyment is watching the smoke as I exhale it.	5	4	3	2	1
O. I want a cigarette most when I am comfortable and relaxed.	5	4	3	2	1
P. When I feel blue or want to take my mind off cares and worries, I smoke cigarettes.	5	4	3	2	1
Q. I get a gnawing hunger for a cigarette when I haven't smoked for a while.	5	4	3	2	1
R. I've found a cigarette in my mouth and didn't remember putting it there.	5	4	3	2	1

Scoring

1. Enter the numbers you have circled in the test questions in the spaces below, putting the number you have circled for question A over line A, for question B over line B, and so on.

2. Add the three scores on each line to obtain your totals. For example, the sum of your scores over lines A, G, and M gives your score on stimulation; the sum of lines B, H, and N gives your score on handling, and so on. Scores can vary from 3 to 15. Any score of 11 or above is high; any score of 7 or below is low.

Scores			**Totals**	**Comment**
_____ + _____ + _____ = A G M			_____ Stimulation	A score of 11 or above suggests that you are stimulated by the cigarette to get going and keep going. To stop smoking, try a brisk walk or exercise when the smoking urge is present.
_____ + _____ + _____ = B H N			_____ Handling	A score of 11 or above suggests satisfaction from handling the cigarette. Substituting a pencil or paper clip or doodling may aid in breaking the habit.
_____ + _____ + _____ = C I O			_____ Pleasurable relaxation	A score of 11 or above suggests that you receive pleasure from smoking. Substitution of other pleasant habits (eating, social activities, exercise) may aid in eliminating smoking.
_____ + _____ + _____ = D J P			_____ Crutch: tension reduction	A score of 11 or above suggests that you use cigarettes to handle moments of stress or discomfort. Substitution of social activities, eating, or handling other objects may aid in stopping.
_____ + _____ + _____ = E K Q			_____ Craving: psychological addictions	A score of 11 or above suggests an almost continuous psychological craving for a cigarette. Cold turkey may be your best method of breaking the smoking habit.
_____ + _____ + _____ = F L R			_____ Habit	A score of 11 or above suggests that you smoke out of mere habit and may acquire little satisfaction from the process. Gradually reducing the number of cigarettes smoked may be effective in helping you stop.

Source: National Clearinghouse for Smoking and Health (USPHS).

From *Physical fitness and wellness, third edition,* by Jerrold S. Greenberg, George B. Dintiman, and Barbee Myers Oakes, 2004, Champaign, IL: Human Kinetics.

Discovery Activity 11.3

Service-Learning for Preventing Alcohol Abuse

Alcohol abuse is the most prevalent drug problem on college campuses. Irresponsible drinking can lead to accidents and aggressive behavior resulting in fights and injuries. It can also lead to disastrous health effects. On the campus of one of your authors, a student who drank excessively one night was found dead on his fraternity's porch the following morning. He might have had fun that night, but, sadly, he paid dearly for his decision to drink excessively. His friends and family continue to feel sorrow to this day.

You can have an effect on the use of alcohol on your campus. As mentioned earlier in this chapter, universities and colleges have organized alcohol-free events so that students who prefer not to drink can party safely. Conduct an inventory of such events on your campus. For alcohol-free events that do exist, interview students who have attended, or who are attending, to determine how sponsors of these activities can better organize or advertise them to attract more students. If not enough of these alcohol-free events exist on your campus, develop such events using the examples of what other colleges have done, described earlier in this chapter, and your own creativity. Write a report about what you find to be effective and leave your report for student organizers who can take your place after you graduate.

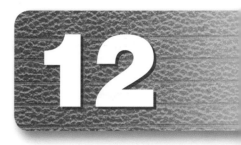

Stress Management and Physical Fitness

Chapter Objectives

By the end of this chapter, you should be able to

1. define stress, stressor, and stress reactivity;
2. list sources of stress and differentiate between distress and eustress;
3. describe the bodily changes that occur when a person experiences stress;
4. manage stress by using coping mechanisms at various levels of the stress response;
5. use time-management techniques to free up time for regular exercise; and
6. describe the role of exercise in the management of stress.

Emilio's wife died last year, and he grieved long and hard for her. He felt that her death was unfair (she was such a kind person), and a sense of helplessness crept over him. Loneliness became part of his days, and tears became the companions of his late evening hours. Some of his friends were not surprised at Emilio's own death just a year after his wife's. They officially called it a heart attack, but his friends know he died of a broken heart.

You probably know someone like Emilio—a person who died or became ill from severe stress but seemingly had few physical troubles. That is what stress can do. In this chapter you will learn how stress can change your body to make you susceptible to illness and disease or other negative influences. Contrary to what some people might tell you, it is not all in your mind. You will learn how you can prevent those negative consequences from occurring, including the role of exercise in that process.

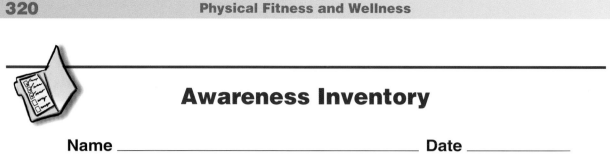

Awareness Inventory

Name _____ **Date** _____

Check the space by the letter T for the statements that you think are true and by the space for the letter F for the statements that you think are false. The answers appear following the list of statements. This chapter will present information to clarify these statements for you. As you read the chapter, look for explanations for the reasons why the statements are true or false.

T ___ **F** ___   1. Stress is defined as the reaction to a stressful occurrence.

T ___ **F** ___   2. A stressor leads to a stress reaction that increases heart rate, muscle tension, and blood pressure.

T ___ **F** ___   3. Stress reaction is the same as the fight-or-flight response.

T ___ **F** ___   4. Psychosomatic illnesses are predominantly in one's mind, with no physical manifestation.

T ___ **F** ___   5. Exercise is an effective stress-management technique, but its use is limited to relieving stress by-products (muscle tension, increased heart rate).

T ___ **F** ___   6. Stress can lead to athletic injuries, as well as contribute to traffic accidents.

T ___ **F** ___   7. Eustress is to be avoided, and meditation is one method of achieving that goal.

T ___ **F** ___   8. Autogenic training is a method of preventing stress that involves the contraction and then relaxation of various muscles in the body.

T ___ **F** ___   9. Type A behavior pattern is associated with the development of coronary heart disease predominantly because of feelings of hurriedness and polyphasic behavior.

T ___ **F** ___ 10. Adopting time-management techniques will result in saving time.

Answers: 1-F, 2-F, 3-T, 4-F, 5-F, 6-T, 7-F, 8-F, 9-F, 10-F

From Physical fitness and wellness, third edition, by Jerrold S. Greenberg, George B. Dintiman, and Barbee Myers Oakes, 2004, Champaign, IL: Human Kinetics.

Analyze Yourself

Assessing Your Physical Stress Symptoms

Name _____ **Date** _____

Instructions: Indicate how often each of the following effects happens to you either when you are experiencing stress or following exposure to a significant stressor. Respond to each item with a number from 0 to 5, using the scale that follows:

0 = never   **1** = once or   **2** = every few   **3** = every   **4** = once or   **5** = daily
            twice a year   months   few weeks   more each week

1. Cardiovascular symptoms

___ Heart pounding

___ Cold, sweaty hands

___ Heart racing or beating erratically

___ Headaches (throbbing pain)

_____ *Subtotal*

2. Respiratory symptoms

___ Rapid, erratic, or shallow breathing

___ Asthma attack

___ Shortness of breath

___ Difficulty in speaking because of poor breathing control

_____ *Subtotal*

3. Gastrointestinal symptoms

___ Upset stomach, nausea, or vomiting

___ Diarrhea

___ Constipation

___ Sharp abdominal pains

_____ *Subtotal*

4. Muscular symptoms

___ Headaches (steady pain)

___ Muscle tremors or hands shaking

___ Back or shoulder pains

___ Arthritis

_____ *Subtotal*

5. Skin symptoms

___ Acne

___ Perspiration

___ Dandruff

___ Excessive dryness of skin or hair

_____ *Subtotal*

6. Immunity symptoms

___ Allergy flare-up

___ Influenza

___ Common cold

___ Skin rash

_____ *Subtotal*

7. Metabolic symptoms

___ Increased appetite

___ Thoughts racing or difficulty sleeping

___ Increased craving for tobacco or sweets

___ Feelings of anxiety or nervousness

_____ *Subtotal*

_____ **Overall Symptomatic Total**
(add all seven subtotals)

(continued)

Analyze Yourself *(continued)*

What Does Your Score Mean?

0-35   Moderate physical stress symptoms

A score in this range indicates a low level of physical stress manifestation, hence minimal overall probability of encounter with psychosomatic disease in the near future.

36-75   Average physical stress symptoms

Most people experience physical stress symptoms within this range. This level is representative of an increased predisposition to psychosomatic disease but not an immediate threat to physical health.

76-140   Excessive physical stress symptoms

If your score falls in this range, you are experiencing a serious number and frequency of stress symptoms. You may be heading toward one or more psychosomatic diseases sometime in the future and should take deliberate action to reduce your level of stress.

Adapted, by permission, from R.J. Allen and D. Hyde, 1980, *Investigations in stress control* (Minneapolis, MN: Burgess Publishing), 101-105.

Optimal mental health (emotional and cognitive functioning) is an important factor for maintaining physical function in individuals across cultures. Yet regardless of race, ethnicity, or gender, depression and other stress-related disorders occur more often today than they did in recent years. Depressive disorders represent a major public health problem because of their high prevalence in individuals of all ages and their psychosocial effect. Most research studies, such as the National Black Women's Health Project (Scarinci et al., 2002), show that being female, having poor self-rated physical health, experiencing chronic diseases, having low socioeconomic status, being less-educated, being unmarried, and being dissatisfied with the level of social support are significant predictors of individuals with high depressive symptoms. For example, the LIDO Study (Herrman et al., 2002) surveyed symptoms of depression among nearly 20,000 individuals aged 18 to 75 years living in six countries and found that depressed persons had an overall worse health status, poorer functional status, lower quality of life, and higher use of health services in every country participating in the study.

Stress-related disorders are also common in adolescents and continue to increase among college students (Chabrol et al., 2002; Iwata and Buka, 2002). Several studies, such as the National Longitudinal Study of Adolescent Health (Rush-

ton et al., 2002) validate the increased presence of depressive symptoms and other stress-related disorders among high school adolescents, with higher incidences among ethnic minority youth. As in adults, depression in youths is more common among females than among males. Adolescent obesity is frequently associated with depression and is a strong predictor of adult obesity as well (Goodman and Whitaker, 2002; Rugulies, 2002). Recognizing that ethnic minority women tend to be more overweight and frequently display higher levels of depression than nonminority women, women of color seem to be a particularly important target group for future study (Faith et al., 2002; Leppamaki et al., 2002; Penninx et al., 2002). Overall, the association between stress-related disorders and physical functioning is often complicated because many life stresses combine to affect depression and anxiety; and, in many cases, factors that increase risk differ for men and women of varying ethnicities (Fleck et al., 2002; Myers et al., 2002; Strawbridge et al., 2002). Nonetheless, you should realize that as you learn methods to manage stress in your life, you are more likely to enjoy a healthier lifestyle as you grow older.

Stress-Related Concepts

Even the experts do not agree on the definition of **stress.** Some define it as the stimulus that causes a physical reaction (such as being afraid to take a test), whereas others view it as the reaction itself (for example, increases in blood pressure, heart rate, and perspiration). For our purposes in this text, we define stress as a combination of the cause (**stressor**) and the physical reaction (**stress reactivity**). The significance of these definitions is not merely academic. Stressors have the potential to result in stress reactivity but may not necessarily do so.

Common Stressors

Stressors can be biological (toxins, heat, cold), sociological (unemployment), philosophical (deciding on a purpose in life), or psychological (threats to self-esteem, depression). Each has the potential to result in a stress reaction.

We all encounter stressors in our daily lives. You may have stressors associated with school (getting good grades, taking exams, having teachers think well of you), with work (too much to do in a given amount of time, not really understanding what is expected of you, fear of a company reorganization), with family (still being treated as a child when you are an adult, arguing often, lack of trust), or with your social life (making friends, telephoning for dates). Even scheduling exercise into your already busy day may be a stressor.

Stress Reactivity

When a stressor leads to a stress response, several changes occur in the body. The heart beats faster, muscles tense, breathing becomes rapid and shallow, perspiration appears under the arms and on the forehead, and blood pressure increases. These and other changes prepare the body to respond to the threat (stressor) by either fighting it off or running away. For that reason, stress reactivity is sometimes called the **fight-or-flight response.** Although many people consider the fight-or-flight response harmful, it is negative only if it is inappropriate to fight or run away—that is, when it is inappropriate to do something physical. For instance, if you are required to present a speech in front of your class, you cannot run from the assignment (you will fail the class if you do so) and you cannot strike out at the instructor or your classmates. It is in these situations, when you do not or cannot use your body's preparedness to do something physical, that the stress reaction is unhealthy. Your blood pressure remains elevated, more cholesterol roams about your blood, your heart works harder than normal, and your muscles remain tense. Those reactions, in turn,

stress—The combination of a stressor and stress reactivity.

stressor—A stimulus that has the potential to elicit stress reactivity.

stress reactivity—The physical reaction to a stressor that results in increased muscle tension, heart rate, blood pressure, and so forth.

fight-or-flight response—A physiological reaction to a threatening stressor; another name for stress reactivity.

psychosomatic—Illnesses or diseases that either become worse or develop in the first place because of body changes resulting from an interpretation of thoughts.

can lead to various illnesses, such as coronary heart disease, stroke, and hypertension. At this point, pay attention to your body, particularly your muscle tension. If you think you can drop your shoulders, then your muscles are unnecessarily raising them. If you can relax your forearm muscles, you are unnecessarily tensing them. This wasted muscle tension—wasted because you are not preparing to do anything physical—is the result of stress and can cause tension headaches, backaches, or neck and shoulder pain.

Psychosomatic Disease

When built-up stress products (for example, increased heart rate and blood pressure) are chronic, go unabated, or occur frequently, they can cause illness and disease. These conditions are called **psychosomatic,** from the Greek words psyche (the mind) and soma (the body). The term does not mean that these conditions are all in the mind; instead, it means that a mind-body connection is causing the illness. An example is the effect of stress on allergies. Stress results in fewer white blood cells in the immunological system, which in turn can lead to an allergic reaction (teary eyes, stuffy nose, itchy throat). The reaction occurs because the white blood cells are what fight off allergens (the substances to which people are allergic); fewer of them will increase susceptibility to an allergic reaction.

A Model of Stress

Stress can be better understood by considering the model depicted in figure 12.1. The model begins with a life situation perceived as distressing. Once it is perceived that way, emotional arousal (anxiety, nervousness, anger) occurs that

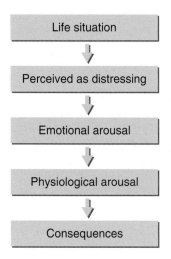

Figure 12.1 A model of stress.

in turn results in physiological arousal (increased heart rate, blood pressure, perspiration). That response can lead to negative consequences such as psychosomatic illness, low grades at school, or arguments with family and friends.

Now let us see how the model operates in a stressful situation. Imagine that you are a college senior and that to graduate this semester all you need to do is pass a physical fitness class. Imagine further that you fail this class (life situation). You might say to yourself, "This is terrible. I will not be able to start work. I must be a real dummy. What will all my friends and relatives think?" In other words, you view the situation as distressing (perceived as distressing). That perception can result in fear and insecurity about the future, anger at the physical fitness instructor, or worry about how you will obtain your degree (emotional arousal). These emotions can lead to increased heart rate, muscle tension, and the other components of the stress response (physiological arousal). As a result, you can develop a tension headache or an upset stomach (consequence).

The situation evolves as though a road winds its way through the towns of Life Situation, Perceived As Stressful, Emotional Arousal, Physiological Arousal, and Consequences. And as with any road, a roadblock can be set up that interferes with travel. Remember, a stressor only has the potential to lead to stress. A roadblock can prevent that stressor from proceeding to the next town. The essence of stress management is setting up roadblocks on the stress model to interfere with travel to the next level.

Using the example of failing a physical fitness class again, imagine that your reaction was, "It's not good that I failed this course, but I still have

my health and people who love me. They'll help me get through this." In this case, you do not perceive the life situation as distressing. Consider this change in perception a roadblock preventing emotional arousal. Without emotional arousal, physiological arousal will not occur and no negative consequences will arise. In fact, positive consequences may even develop. Maybe failing the course will cause you to study extra hard the next time, with the result that you learn much more about physical fitness and become more fit than you would have otherwise. In that instance, you experience not distress but **eustress,** stress that results in personal growth and positive outcomes.

Exercise's Unique Contribution to Stress Management

Studies confirm the positive effects of physical activity on depression and related stress disorders among individuals of all ages. Exercise contributes to self-esteem, being more positive toward others, feeling more alert and able, and having decreased feelings of depression and anxiety (Greenberg, 2002).

Exercise As a Roadblock

Exercise is a unique stress-management intervention because you can plug it in at many levels on the stress model. You achieve a life-situation intervention when you give up stressful habits (for example, cigarette smoking) because they interfere with your exercising. When you make friends through participating in a training program, you may also be using exercise as a life-situation intervention because you may be remedying loneliness and social isolation.

Exercise can be a perception intervention as well. The brain produces neurotransmitters (endorphins) during exercise, and their euphoric, analgesic effect serves to relax the brain and the rest of the body. That relaxed state helps us perceive stressors as less stressful.

Exercise is also an emotional-arousal intervention. During exercise, we focus on what we are doing, not on our problems and stressors. Engaging in physical activity can therefore be relaxing. Furthermore, numerous research studies have found that exercise enhances well-being. It reduces feelings of depression and anxiety while increasing the sense of physical competence. The result is greater self-esteem. Exercise can use up the built-up stress by-products and the body's preparedness to do something physical. Consequently, it can also be a physiological-arousal intervention.

Because we can plug it into all the levels of the stress model, exercise is particularly useful as a means of managing stress. Be careful, however, to exercise in ways recommended in this book rather than in inappropriate ways. Although exercise is an excellent stress-management coping mechanism, done incorrectly it can result in injury or discomfort. In that case, exercise will be a stressor rather than a stress reliever. And if exercise in itself is not your cup of tea but you participate anyway because you know it is good for you, you can still make it pleasant. Exercise with a friend. Listen to music while you are exercising. Engage in physical activity out of doors in a pleasant setting, listening to the birds chirping and the wind rustling through the leaves. These and other accommodations can make your exercise more pleasing and therefore make you more likely to maintain your program.

Stress and Athletic Injuries

A good deal of research demonstrates the relationship between stress and subsequent athletic injuries. One explanation for this relationship is the stress-injury model developed by Anderson and Williams (1988). According to this model, when people place themselves in stressful situations (for example, an important competition or tournament), three factors may contribute to a stress response: (1) a history of stressors (previous stressful events, past injuries, daily hassles), (2) personality characteristics (trait anxiety, external locus of control), and (3) coping resources (support of others, communication skills). Someone with a history of stressors, a personality that often interprets situations as anxiety provoking, and few resources with which to cope with these perceptions is likely to elicit a stress response. Such individuals—those with high stress—experience increased muscle tension, narrowed fields of vision, and increased distractibility. These variables cause stressful people to be prone to athletic injury. Imagine trying to move out of the way of a baseball traveling toward you at a high speed if you are distracted or if your field of vision is narrowed. Or imagine trying to avoid muscle strains, sprains, or other musculoskeletal injuries when fatigue or lack of flexibility results from the muscle tension associated with stress. The model addresses more than just sports injuries. Traffic accidents can occur when a driver is distressed and therefore not as alert or able to react as quickly to a vehicle running a red light.

Recognizing the relationship between stress and injury, some athletic programs have begun teaching their athletes stress-management techniques, with the result that fewer injuries occur. If you are interested in reading more about the stress-injury model and the research supporting its validity, see the 1996 article by Jean M. Williams in the *International Journal of Stress Management* titled "Stress, Coping Resources, and Injury Risk" (vol. 3, no. 4, pp. 209-221).

Managing Stress

To manage stress, you need to set up roadblocks at each level of the stress model.

Life-Situation Level

At the life-situation level you can make a list of all your stressors, routine ones that occur regularly and unusual ones that are often unanticipated. Then go through the list trying to eliminate as many of them as you can. For example, if you jog every day but find jogging stressful, try a different aerobic exercise or vary exercises from day to day. If you commute on a crowded highway and often become distressed about the traffic and construction slowdowns, try taking a different route. If you often argue with a friend and the associated stress interferes with your work, see the friend less often or not at all. By habit, you probably tolerate many stressors that you can eliminate and thereby decrease the stress in your life.

Perception Level

You can perceive or interpret as less distressing some of the stressors that you cannot eliminate. One way to do that is through **selective awareness.** Every situation embraces some good and some bad. Choosing to focus on the good while not denying the bad will result in a more satisfying and less distressing life. For example, rather than focus on the displeasure of standing in line

eustress—Stress that results in personal growth or development so that the person experiencing it is better for having been stressed.

selective awareness—A means of managing stress by consciously focusing on the positive aspects of a situation or person.

at the checkout counter, you can choose to focus on the pleasure of being able to do nothing during a hectic day.

Consider the story about a female college student who writes her parents that she is in the hospital after having fallen out of her third-floor dormitory window. Luckily, she landed in some shrubs and was only temporarily paralyzed on her right side (that explains why her handwriting is so unclear). In the hospital, she meets a janitor and falls in love with him, and now they are planning to elope. The reason for eloping is that he is of a different religion, culture, and ethnic background, and she suspects that her family might object to the marriage. She is confident, though, that the marriage will work because her lover learned from his first marriage not to abuse his spouse, and the jail term he served reinforced that lesson. She goes on to say in the letter, "Mom and Dad, I am not really in a hospital, have not fallen out of any window, and have not met someone with whom I am planning to elope. But I did fail chemistry and wanted you to be able to put that in its proper perspective." Now that is selective awareness.

Emotional-Arousal Level

An excellent way to control your emotional responses to stress is to engage regularly in some form of relaxation. This section describes some of the more effective ways of relaxing.

No research can help us identify which relaxation technique is best for you. The only way to determine that is to try several and evaluate their ability to make you feel relaxed. To help you do that, we have provided a relaxation technique rating scale (figure 12.2). Use it after you try each of the relaxation techniques.

To determine which relaxation technique is most effective for you, try each one presented in this chapter and evaluate it by answering these questions, using the following scale:

1 = very true
2 = somewhat true
3 = I'm not sure
4 = somewhat untrue
5 = very untrue

1. _____ It felt good.
2. _____ The technique was easy to fit into my schedule.
3. _____ It made me feel relaxed.
4. _____ I handled my daily chores better than I usually do.
5. _____ The technique was easy to learn.
6. _____ I was able to shut out my surroundings while I was practicing this technique.
7. _____ I did not feel tired after practicing this technique.
8. _____ My fingers and toes felt warmer after trying this relaxation technique.
9. _____ Any stress symptoms I had (headache, tense muscles, anxiety) before doing this relaxation technique disappeared by the time I was done.
10. _____ Each time I concluded this technique, my pulse rate was much lower than it was when I began.

Now sum the values you responded with for a total score. Compare the scores of all the relaxation techniques you try. The lower the score, the more appropriate a particular relaxation technique is for you.

Figure 12.2 Relaxation technique rating scale.

From *Physical fitness and wellness, third edition*, by Jerrold S. Greenberg, George B. Dintiman, and Barbee Myers Oakes, 2004, Champaign, IL: Human Kinetics.

Progressive Relaxation

With **progressive relaxation,** you tense a muscle group for 10 seconds, all the while paying attention to the sensations that are created. Then you relax those muscles, paying attention to that sensation. The idea is to learn what muscular tension feels like so that you will be able to recognize it when you are experiencing it and be familiar with muscular relaxation so that when you are tense you can relax those muscles. The technique is called progressive because you progress from one muscle group to another throughout the body.

Autogenic Training

Autogenic training involves imagining that your arms and legs are heavy, warm, and tingly. When you are able to imagine that, you are increasing blood flow to those areas. This precipitates the relaxation response. After your body is relaxed, think of soothing images (a day at the beach, a park full of trees and a green lawn, a calm lake on a sunny day) to relax your mind.

Body Scanning

Even when you are tense, some part of your body is relaxed, perhaps your thigh or your chest or your hand. The relaxation technique called **body scanning** requires you to search for a relaxed body part and transport that feeling to the tenser parts of your body. You can do that by imagining the relaxed part as a fiery, hot ball that you roll to the tenser parts of your body. As with all relaxation techniques, the more you practice, the more effective you will become.

Biofeedback

This technique involves using an instrument to mirror what is going on in the body and reporting the results back to the individual. Biofeedback instrumentation can measure and convey to the person numerous physiological parameters: tem-

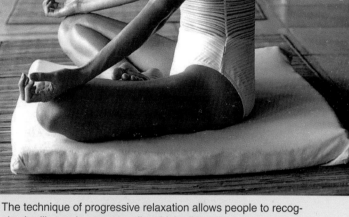

The technique of progressive relaxation allows people to recognize bodily tension more easily, which allows them to relax their muscles consciously as a response.
Digitalvision

---

progressive relaxation—A relaxation technique in which you contract, then relax, muscle groups throughout the body.

autogenic training—A relaxation technique in which you imagine that your arms and legs are heavy, warm, and tingly.

body scanning—A relaxation technique in which you identify a part of your body that feels relaxed and transport that feeling to another part of your body.

---

perature, blood pressure, heart rate, perspiration, breathing rate, muscle tension, brain waves, and many others. One interesting aspect of biofeedback is that individuals can control responses previously thought to be involuntary once the measure has been reported back to them. With biofeedback training, people can increase or decrease the physiological parameters enumerated in this paragraph. Because the body and the mind are connected, changes in either can effect changes in the other. Consequently, when a person learns to decrease heart rate and muscle tension, for example, the psychological states of anxiety and nervousness may also decrease.

Physiological-Arousal Level

At the point of physiological arousal, your body is already prepared to do something physical.

Managing stress at this level requires you to engage in some physical activity, which can range from the obvious to the obscure. Running around the block as fast as you can will use the stress by-products and do wonders for your disposition. Dribbling a basketball up and down the court mimicking fast breaks, serving 30 tennis balls as hard as you can, bicycling as fast as you can, or swimming several laps at breakneck speed can also relieve stress. Still, you need not engage in formal sports activities to relieve stress at this level in the model. You can simply punch your mattress or pillow as hard and as long as you can. You will not hurt them or yourself, but you will feel better.

Types A and B Behavior Patterns and the Exerciser

Researchers have discovered that the **type A behavior pattern** is related to the subsequent development of coronary heart disease. Type A people are aggressive and competitive, never seem

type A behavior pattern—A constellation of behaviors that makes individuals susceptible to coronary heart disease.

type B behavior pattern—A combination of behaviors that seem to protect people from contracting coronary heart disease, such as lack of hostility, anger, and aggression; cooperativeness; and the ability to focus on one task at a time.

to have enough time, do two or more things at once (this is called being polyphasic), are impatient, and become angry easily. In contrast, the **type B behavior pattern** seems to protect against the development of coronary heart disease. Type B people exhibit no free-floating hostility, always seem to have enough time to get things done and do not fret if they don't, are more cooperative than competitive, and are concerned with quality rather than quantity (they focus not on how fast they run but on the enjoyment they receive from running).

Subsequent research has clarified the relationship between type A behavior and coronary heart

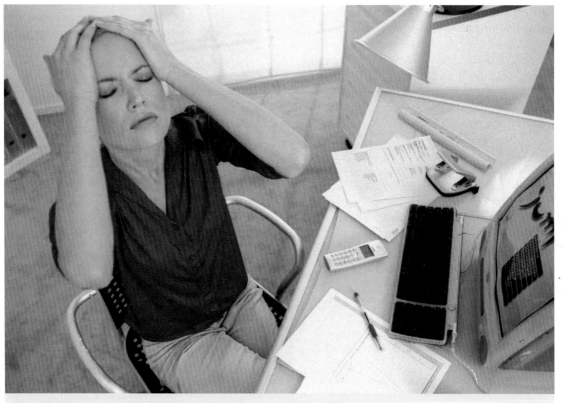

A demanding, fast-paced job can cause a great deal of stress if you let it.

Kristiane Vey/Jump

disease. Apparently, hostility is the trait of major concern. People who tend to become angry easily are more apt to develop coronary heart disease than are others.

Our friend Jorge, mentioned at the beginning of chapter 4, characterizes the type A exerciser. If you remember, on a sunny, windless day, Jorge was playing tennis when he hit one too many errant backhands. Losing control, he threw his racket over the fence, over several trees, and into the creek alongside the court. As the racket floated downstream, Jorge was at a loss about what to berate more severely, his tennis skills or his temper. This aggressiveness and hostility are classic characteristics of type A behavior.

Type A exercisers are aggressive (they may smack their golf clubs into the ground when they hit a shot off target), hostile (they may accuse their opponents of cheating), competitive (they may not be able to bear losing), and numbers oriented (they evaluate themselves on how many matches they won rather than whether they played well or enjoyed participating). If you see yourself as a type A, think about making a change. Use the behavioral change techniques and strategies presented in chapter 4 to become more like type B people. You may be healthier, and you will probably be happier.

Time Management: Freeing Up Time to Exercise

To manage stress, you need to set aside time. To exercise regularly, you also need to set aside time. Because stress can sap your attention, energy, and time, it can interfere with your exercise regimen. After all, stress can be a threat to your physical self and your self-concept. Who can blame you for postponing or canceling exercise to manage that threat? But you can organize your time better so that you have plenty of time for exercising, managing stress, and doing the myriad other things you need, and choose, to do.

To be serous about using time-management strategies, you need to realize several things:

- Time is one of your most precious possessions.
- Time spent is gone forever.
- You cannot save time. Time moves continually, and you use it, one way or another. If you waste time, you cannot go to a bank and withdraw

the time you previously saved to replace the time you wasted.

- To come to terms with your mortality is to realize that your time is limited. None of us will live forever, and none of us will be able to do everything we would like to do.

You can invest time to free up (not to save) more time than you originally invested. Then you will have sufficient time to use the stress-management techniques presented in this chapter and plenty of time to participate in a regular exercise program. The techniques we will now describe will help you do that. As you read the following suggestions for better managing your limited time, try to make direct application of these techniques to your situation. Most of these techniques you will want to incorporate into your lifestyle; others you will decide are not worth the effort or the time.

Assessing How You Spend Time

As a first step, analyze how you spend your time now. To do this, divide your day into 15-minute segments as shown in figure 12.3. Record what you are doing every 15 minutes. Review this time diary and total the time spent on each activity throughout the day. For example, you might find that you spent 5 hours attending class, 2 hours socializing, 3 hours eating meals, 2 hours watching television, 1 hour doing homework, 1 hour shopping, 2 hours listening to music, 6 hours sleeping, and 2 hours on the telephone, as shown in the example in table 12.1. Evaluate the use of time shown in table 12.1 and note in the adjustment column that the adjustments would free up 3 1/2 hours a day, which would leave plenty of time to exercise. A good way to make the changes you desire is to draw up a contract with yourself that includes a reward for being successful. Refer to chapter 4 for the most effective way to develop such a contract.

Prioritizing

One important technique for managing time is to prioritize your activities. Not all of them are of equal importance. You need to focus on the activities of major importance to you and devote time to other activities only after you have completed the major ones. One of the activities for which you should prioritize your time is exercise.

To prioritize your activities, develop A, B, and C lists. On the A list (see figure 12.4a), place

Time	Activity	Time	Activity	Time	Activity
12:00 a.m. _____		8:00 a.m. _____		4:00 p.m. _____	
12:15 a.m. _____		8:15 a.m. _____		4:15 p.m. _____	
12:30 a.m. _____		8:30 a.m. _____		4:30 p.m. _____	
12:45 a.m. _____		8:45 a.m. _____		4:45 p.m. _____	
1:00 a.m. _____		9:00 a.m. _____		5:00 p.m. _____	
1:15 a.m. _____		9:15 a.m. _____		5:15 p.m. _____	
1:30 a.m. _____		9:30 a.m. _____		5:30 p.m. _____	
1:45 a.m. _____		9:45 a.m. _____		5:45 p.m. _____	
2:00 a.m. _____		10:00 a.m. _____		6:00 p.m. _____	
2:15 a.m. _____		10:15 a.m. _____		6:15 p.m. _____	
2:30 a.m. _____		10:30 a.m. _____		6:30 p.m. _____	
2:45 a.m. _____		10:45 a.m. _____		6:45 p.m. _____	
3:00 a.m. _____		11:00 a.m. _____		7:00 p.m. _____	
3:15 a.m. _____		11:15 a.m. _____		7:15 p.m. _____	
3:30 a.m. _____		11:30 a.m. _____		7:30 p.m. _____	
3:45 a.m. _____		11:45 a.m. _____		7:45 p.m. _____	
4:00 a.m. _____		12:00 p.m. _____		8:00 p.m. _____	
4:15 a.m. _____		12:15 p.m. _____		8:15 p.m. _____	
4:30 a.m. _____		12:30 p.m. _____		8:30 p.m. _____	
4:45 a.m. _____		12:45 p.m. _____		8:45 p.m. _____	
5:00 a.m. _____		1:00 p.m. _____		9:00 p.m. _____	
5:15 a.m. _____		1:15 p.m. _____		9:15 p.m. _____	
5:30 a.m. _____		1:30 p.m. _____		9:30 p.m. _____	
5:45 a.m. _____		1:45 p.m. _____		9:45 p.m. _____	
6:00 a.m. _____		2:00 p.m. _____		10:00 p.m. _____	
6:15 a.m. _____		2:15 p.m. _____		10:15 p.m. _____	
6:30 a.m. _____		2:30 p.m. _____		10:30 p.m. _____	
6:45 a.m. _____		2:45 p.m. _____		10:45 p.m. _____	
7:00 a.m. _____		3:00 p.m. _____		11:00 p.m. _____	
7:15 a.m. _____		3:15 p.m. _____		11:15 p.m. _____	
7:30 a.m. _____		3:30 p.m. _____		11:30 p.m. _____	
7:45 a.m. _____		3:45 p.m. _____		11:45 p.m. _____	

Figure 12.3 Daily activity record.

From *Physical Fitness and Wellness, third edition,* by Jerrold S. Greenberg, George B. Dintiman, and Barbee Myers Oakes, 2004. Champaign, IL: Human Kinetics.

those activities that you must get done, those that are so important that not doing them would be extremely undesirable. For example, if a term

TABLE 12.1—Summary of Daily Activities

Activity needed	Total time spent on activity (hr)	Adjustment
Attending class	5	None
Socializing	2	1/2 hr less
Eating meals	3	1 hr less
Watching television	2	1 hr less
Doing homework	1	1 hr more
Shopping	1	None
Listening to music	2	1 hr less
Sleeping	6	None
Talking on telephone	2	1 hr less

paper is due tomorrow and you have not typed it yet, that task goes on your A list.

On the B list (see figure 12.4b) are the activities you would like to do today and need to accomplish. If you do not get them done today, however, it would not be too terrible. For example, if you have not spoken to a close friend and have been meaning to telephone, you might put that on your B list. Your intent is to call today, but if you don't get around to it, you can call tomorrow or the next day.

On the C list (see figure 12.4c) are those activities you would like to do if you get all the A-list and B-list activities done. But if you never accomplish the C-list activities, that is no problem. For example, if a department store has a sale and you would like to go browse, put that on your C list. If you do all of the As and Bs, you can go browse.

In addition, make a list of things not to do (see figure 12.4d). For example, if you tend to waste your time watching television, you might want to include that on your not-to-do list. In that way, you will have a reminder not to watch television today. Place other time wasters on this list as well.

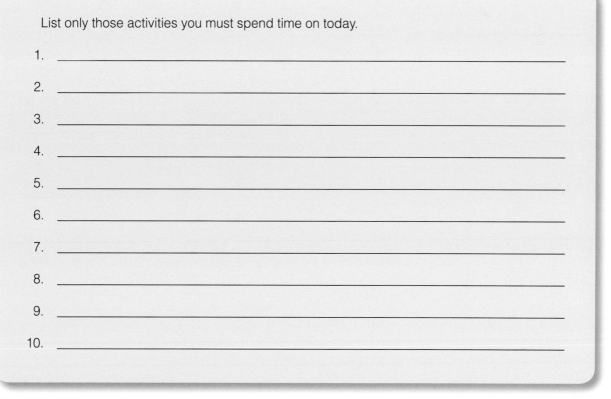

List only those activities you must spend time on today.

1. _____
2. _____
3. _____
4. _____
5. _____
6. _____
7. _____
8. _____
9. _____
10. _____

Figure 12.4a List of activities for today.

From *Physical fitness and wellness, third edition*, by Jerrold S. Greenberg, George B. Dintiman, and Barbee Myers Oakes, 2004, Champaign, IL: Human Kinetics.

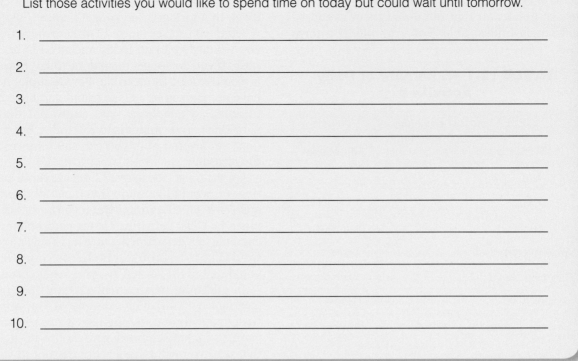

List those activities you would like to spend time on today but could wait until tomorrow.

1. _____

2. _____

3. _____

4. _____

5. _____

6. _____

7. _____

8. _____

9. _____

10. _____

Figure 12.4b List of activities for today.

From *Physical fitness and wellness, third edition,* by Jerrold S. Greenberg, George B. Dintiman, and Barbee Myers Oakes, 2004, Champaign, IL: Human Kinetics.

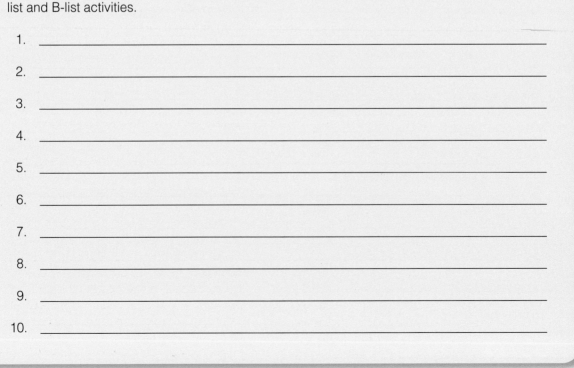

List those activities you will devote time to today only if and after you have completed all A-list and B-list activities.

1. _____

2. _____

3. _____

4. _____

5. _____

6. _____

7. _____

8. _____

9. _____

10. _____

Figure 12.4c List of activities for today.

From *Physical fitness and wellness, third edition,* by Jerrold S. Greenberg, George B. Dintiman, and Barbee Myers Oakes, 2004, Champaign, IL: Human Kinetics.

List those activities you will avoid spending time on today.

1. _____
2. _____
3. _____
4. _____
5. _____
6. _____
7. _____
8. _____
9. _____
10. _____

Figure 12.4d Not-to-do list of activities for today.

From *Physical fitness and wellness, third edition,* by Jerrold S. Greenberg, George B. Dintiman, and Barbee Myers Oakes, 2004, Champaign, IL: Human Kinetics.

Other Ways to Free Up Time for Exercise

You can use many other time-management strategies to make time for exercise.

- **Say No**—Because of guilt, concern for what others might think, or a real desire to engage in an activity, we often have a hard time saying no. Creating A, B, and C lists and prioritizing your activities will help you identify how much time remains for other activities and make saying no easier.

- **Delegate to Others**—When possible, persuade others to do things that need to be done but that do not need your personal attention. Conversely, avoid taking on chores that others try to delegate to you. This plan does not mean that you use other people to do work you should be doing or that you do not help others when they ask. What it means is that you should be more discriminating regarding delegation of activities. In other words, don't hesitate to seek help when you are short on time or overloaded. And help others when they really need it and when you have time available to do so.

- **Give Tasks the Once-Over**—Many of us will open our mail, read through it, and set it aside to act on later. This method is a waste of time. If we pick it up later, we have to familiarize ourselves with it again. As much as possible, look things over only once.

- **Use the Circular File**—How many times do you receive mail that you can easily identify from its envelope as junk mail yet still take time to open it and read the junk inside? You would be better off bypassing the opening and reading part and going directly to the throwing-out part. That procedure would free up time for more important activities, such as exercise.

- **Limit Interruptions**—Throughout the day, you will be interrupted. Recognizing this, you should schedule in time for interruptions. That is, don't make your schedule so tight that interruptions will throw you into a tizzy. On the other hand, try to keep these interruptions to a minimum. You can accomplish this in several ways. You can accept phone calls only during certain hours. You can arrange to have someone take messages so that you can call back later, or you can use an answering machine.

Do the same with visitors. You can ask anyone who visits to return at a more convenient time. If you are serious about making better use of your time, you will adopt some of these means of limiting interruptions.

■ **Recognize the Need to Invest Time**—The bottom line of time management is that you need to invest time initially to free it up later. We often hear people say, "I don't have time to organize myself the way you suggest. That would put me further in the hole." This belief is an interesting paradox. If you are so pressed for time that you believe you do not even have sufficient time to get yourself organized, that in itself tells you that you are in need of applying time-management strategies. The investment in time devoted to organizing yourself will pay dividends by allowing you to achieve more of what is important to you. After all, what is more important than your health and wellness? And what better way is there to achieve health and wellness than freeing up time for regular exercise?

Summary

Stress-Related Concepts Stress can be defined as a combination of the cause (stressor) and the physical reaction (stress reactivity). A stressor has the potential to result in stress reactivity, but it does not necessarily do so. Whether it does depends on how the stressor is perceived or interpreted. Stressors can take a variety of forms: biological (toxins, heat, cold), sociological (unemployment), philosophical (deciding on a purpose in life), or psychological (threats to self-esteem, depression).

When a stressor leads to a stress response, several changes occur in the body. The heart beats faster, muscles tense, breathing becomes rapid and shallow, perspiration appears under the arms and on the forehead, and blood pressure increases. These and other changes make up the fight-or-flight response.

When built-up stress products (for example, increased heart rate and blood pressure) are chronic, go unabated, or occur frequently, they can cause illness and disease. These conditions are called psychosomatic, meaning that they stem from a mind-body interaction that causes the illness or makes an existing disease worse.

A Model of Stress A model that can help us understand stress and its effects begins with a life situation occurring that is perceived as distressing. Once the situation is perceived that way, emotional arousal occurs (anxiety, nervousness, anger), which in turn results in physiological arousal (increased heart rate, blood pressure, muscle tension, perspiration). Negative consequences such as psychosomatic illness, low grades at school, or arguments with family and friends can follow. The essence of stress management is to set up roadblocks on the stress model to interfere with travel to the next level.

Myth and Fact Sheet

Myth	Fact
1. Stressful events of necessity cause stress and a stress reaction.	1. Stressful events only have the potential to cause a stress reaction. They need not do so if you interpret them as nonstressful.
2. You cannot really do anything about stress—it is simply a normal part of life.	2. You can manage stress in many ways so that it does not make you ill or interfere with the satisfaction you derive from life.
3. Exercise is stressful because of the toll it takes physically.	3. Exercise is an excellent way of managing stress because it relates to every level of the stress model.
4. You should try to eliminate all stress from your life.	4. There is an optimal level of stress that results in joy and stimulation and encourages your best performance. Therefore, you need some stress to make life worth living.

Behavioral Change and Motivational Strategies

Many things can interfere with your ability to manage stress. Here are some barriers (roadblocks) and strategies for overcoming them.

Roadblock

You may have a lot to do with little time to get it all done. Term papers are due, midterm or final exams are approaching, you are invited to a party, you are expected to attend a dinner celebrating your sister's birthday, your team is scheduled for an intramural game, and your professor is holding a study session.

You are not accomplishing your fitness objectives, and because of that you feel distressed. You are not running as fast as you would like to run, nor are you lifting the amount of weight you would like to lift, doing the number of repetitions you would like to do, losing the amount of weight you would like to lose, or participating in aerobic dance classes.

You try to relax but cannot. Your thoughts seem to run nonstop. Your body becomes fidgety. You are anxious to move on to do something that needs doing. Finding the time to engage in a relaxation technique is impossible. You are simply too busy.

List roadblocks interfering with your ability to manage stress.

1. _____

2. _____

3. _____

Behavioral Change Strategy

When lumped together, responsibilities often appear overwhelming. Use the behavioral change strategy of divide and conquer. Buy a large calendar and schedule the activities of the semester by writing on the calendar when you will perform them, when you will do library research for term papers, when you will begin studying for exams, and when you will read which chapters in which textbooks. Do not forget to include nonacademic activities as well. For example, write on the calendar the schedule of your intramural team and times of parties or dinners to attend. You will soon realize that you have plenty of time. You simply need to be organized. That realization will go a long way in relieving unnecessary stress.

Use the goal-setting strategies outlined in chapter 4. Set realistic fitness goals, give yourself enough time to achieve them, and make your workout fun. If you are distressed because your goals seem elusive, perhaps they are. Maybe they are too difficult to achieve, at least in the time you have allotted. If you are injuring yourself regularly, perhaps your fitness program is too difficult or too intense. Use gradual programming and tailoring to devise a program specific to you and your current level of fitness.

Use material reinforcement to encourage the regular practice of relaxation. Whenever you set aside time to relax, reward yourself with something tangible. You might put aside a certain amount of money or buy a healthy snack. Another behavioral change technique that could help is boasting. Be proud of taking time to relax and share that feeling of pride with friends. Doing so will make you feel good and be more likely to engage in that relaxation technique again.

You will also need to assess your relaxation method periodically. Use table 12.1 to help you perform this assessment. You will find that some relaxation techniques are more effective for you than others are, so you will learn which ones to use regularly.

Cite behavioral change strategies that can help you overcome the roadblocks you just listed. If you need to, refer back to chapter 4 for behavioral change and motivational strategies.

1. _____

2. _____

3. _____

The goal, however, is not to eliminate all stress. Certainly, some stress (distress) is harmful. On the other hand, some stress is useful because it encourages peak performance, or eustress.

Exercise's Unique Contribution to Stress Management Exercise is a unique stress-management intervention because you can plug it in at many levels on the stress model. A life-situation intervention occurs when you give up stressful habits because they interfere with exercising. You perform a perception intervention when your brain produces neurotransmitters during exercise that make you feel relaxed. When you focus on the physical activity and ignore problems and stressors, you have achieved an emotional-arousal intervention. And you carry out a physiological-arousal intervention when you use the built-up stress by-products by doing something physical.

Managing Stress Managing stress involves interventions at each of the levels of the stress model. At the life-situation level, you can assess routine stressors and eliminate them. At the perception level, you can use selective awareness. At the emotional-arousal level, you can do progressive relaxation, autogenic training, body scanning, biofeedback training, and medita-

tion. At the physiological level, you can exercise regularly.

Types A and B Behavior Patterns and the Exerciser People who are aggressive and competitive, never seem to have enough time, do two or more things at once, are impatient, and become angered easily exhibit type A behavior patterns. Type As are prone to coronary heart disease, with the most harmful characteristic being free-floating hostility. Type B people—those who exhibit no free-floating hostility, always seem to have enough time to get things done, are more cooperative than competitive, and are concerned with quality rather than quantity—seem to be protected from developing coronary heart disease.

Time Management: Freeing Up Time to Exercise You cannot save time, but you can free up time by being more organized. Some effective time-management strategies include assessing how you spend time so that you can make sensible adjustments, prioritizing your activities, learning to say no so that you do not take on too many responsibilities, delegating tasks to others, looking things over only once, avoiding spending time on junk mail, and limiting interruptions. Time invested in applying time-management strategies will pay off by freeing up time for important activities such as regular exercise.

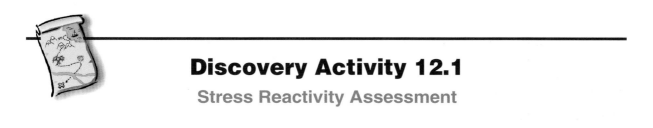

Discovery Activity 12.1

Stress Reactivity Assessment

Name _____ **Date** _____

How does your body respond to a stressful event? This assessment will help you discover that information. While seated in a comfortable position, determine how fast your heart beats at rest using one of these methods. (Use a watch that has a second hand.)

1. Place the first two fingers (pointer and middle finger) of one hand on the underside of your other wrist, on the thumb side. Feel for your pulse and count the number of pulses for 30 seconds.

2. Place the first two fingers of one hand on your lower neck, just above the collarbone; move your fingers toward your shoulder until you find your pulse. Count the pulse for 30 seconds.

3. Place the first two fingers of one hand in front of your ear; move your fingers until you find a pulse. Count the pulse for 30 seconds.

Multiply your 30-second pulse count by two to determine how many times your heart beats each minute while you are at rest. Now close your eyes and think of either someone you really dislike or some situation you experienced that really frightened you. If you are recalling a person, think of how that person looks and smells and what he or she does to incur your dislike. Really feel the dislike, do not just think about it. If you recall a frightening situation, try to place yourself back in that situation. Sense the fright, be scared, vividly recall the situation in all its detail. Think of the person or situation for 1 minute and then count your pulse rate for 30 seconds, as you did earlier. Multiply the rate by two and compare your first total with the second.

Most people find that their heart rates increase when they are experiencing stressful memories. This increase occurs despite lack of any physical activity; the very thoughts increase heart rate. This experiment demonstrates two things: the nature of stressors and the nature of stress reactivity.

Source: Jerrold S. Greenberg, *Comprehensive Stress Management,* 7th ed. New York: McGraw-Hill, 2002, p. 10.

From *Physical fitness and wellness, third edition,* by Jerrold S. Greenberg, George B. Dintiman, and Barbee Myers Oakes, 2004, Champaign, IL: Human Kinetics.

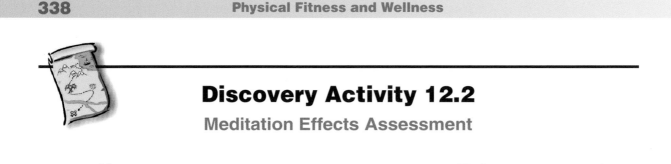

Discovery Activity 12.2
Meditation Effects Assessment

Name _____ **Date** _____

Learning how to meditate is easy. Just close your eyes and repeat the word "calm" or "one" or some other relaxing word in your mind every time you exhale. Make sure not to eat anything or ingest a stimulant beforehand. Stimulants such as caffeine or nicotine will interfere with your ability to relax. Do this for 20 minutes but recognize that no one can stay focused on a word for that long. As soon as you realize that your mind has wandered, just return to repeating the relaxing word as you did before.

To measure whether meditation has a relaxing effect on you, follow these instructions:

1. Using one of the techniques presented in Discovery Activity 12.1, determine your resting pulse rate per minute. Place that number in the space marked "Pulse rate before meditating."

2. After determining how fast your heart beats at rest, meditate for 20 minutes. Be sure not to set an alarm clock because your heart rate will speed up when it goes off. Merely look at your watch when you think 20 minutes has passed.

3. After meditating, determine your pulse rate per minute again. Place that number in the space marked "Pulse rate after meditating."

Pulse rate before meditating _____

Pulse rate after meditating _____

Difference in pulse rate _____

Most people experience a reduced heart rate after meditating (or engaging in any other relaxation technique). That finding should not be unexpected because we know that one of the effects of relaxation is to slow down the heart.

From *Physical fitness and wellness, third edition,* by Jerrold S. Greenberg, George B. Dintiman, and Barbee Myers Oakes, 2004, Champaign, IL: Human Kinetics.

Discovery Activity 12.3

Service-Learning for Stress Management and Physical Fitness

Too many of us live hectic, busy lives with little time for relaxation. Our studies, jobs, social activities, and family lives seem to compete with each other, leaving few moments for fun and enjoyment, or for physical activity. But what you have learned in this chapter can go a long way to alleviate this situation for you and others in your community. One of your authors teaches a stress-management course in which students are required to apply what they learn by teaching information and stress-management techniques to people off-campus in a service-learning assignment. Students have worked with cancer patients, school children, nursery school staff, residents and staff at nursing homes, volunteer firefighters, and others. When students teach stress-management skills to groups in the community, they learn more about the topic themselves because they want to appear knowledgeable, and therefore they study the material more thoroughly. Of course, the groups with whom they work also benefit by learning how to manage the stress they experience.

What community groups can you help to manage stress better? Perhaps you could volunteer to teach stress management at local churches, synagogues, or mosques. You might teach these skills to children in local schools or to senior citizens in local assisted-living facilities. Your campus may have an office devoted to connecting those who want to volunteer with agencies seeking volunteers. Volunteering in this way will help you learn more about this chapter's content and, at the same time, enhance the lives of people in your community.

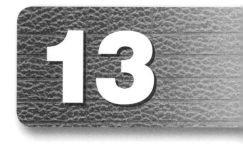

Prevention and Care of Exercise Injuries

Chapter Objectives

By the end of this chapter, you should be able to

1. design an 11-point injury-prevention plan for someone who is about to begin a new exercise program;

2. describe the body's response to soft-tissue injury and the three stages of healing;

3. discuss the correct use of cold, heat, and massage in the emergency treatment of exercise injuries;

4. demonstrate the correct technique of RICE therapy in the treatment of an ankle sprain and other soft-tissue injuries;

5. describe the proper use of common over-the-counter and prescription drugs for the treatment of soft-tissue injuries; and

6. describe the proper emergency treatment for at least 25 common exercise injuries.

Most of Lee's friends exercise regularly. Some jog, cycle, and swim; others engage in aerobic exercise classes or play sports such as tennis, racquetball, basketball, soccer, and touch football. At one time or other, it seems as if every one of them has experienced an injury of some sort. Sprained ankles, torn Achilles tendons, sore knees and backs, and inflamed shoulders and elbows are just a few of the complaints Lee hears. Lee feels good most of the time, although her weight is creeping upward and she is generally tired by late afternoon. If it were not for the risk of injury, Lee would join her friends in an aerobic activity she enjoys.

This chapter presents a program designed to keep Lee injury free while she receives the full benefits of an exercise program of her choice. Although there are no guarantees, the information in this chapter can significantly reduce Lee's risk of injury.

Entering into a fitness program involves a slight risk of injury or illness during the first month or so. Later, a key benefit of improved conditioning is the reduction in the incidence and severity of serious injuries related to exercising, jogging, and performing daily activities. The danger of injury increases considerably, however, when you fail to follow simple rules of training. For the weekend athlete, exercise can even be fatal. This chapter is designed to help you avoid common hazards and make exercise a safe, enjoyable experience. The chapter includes 11 steps for injury prevention for your body; discusses how tissue responds to injury; describes the proper use of cold, heat, and massage; provides basic treatment procedures for common injuries and illnesses; and discusses the special injury-proofing problems of women.

Awareness Inventory

Name _____ Date _____

Check the space by the letter T for the statements that you think are true and the space by the letter F for the statements that you think are false. The answers appear following the list of statements. This chapter will present information to clarify these statements for you. As you read the chapter, look for explanations for the reasons why the statements are true or false.

T ___ F ___ 1. Fibrous bands or folds that support organs, hold bones together, or attach to the bones they act on are called tendons.

T ___ F ___ 2. Soft-tissue injuries involve injury to tissue other than bones.

T ___ F ___ 3. Sudden death on the field is rare in high school athletics and involves only 1 in 200,000 participants.

T ___ F ___ 4. Immediately after sustaining an ankle sprain or pulled muscle, you should apply heat to the injured area .

T ___ F ___ 5. To stop a nosebleed, squeeze the nose between the thumb and forefinger just below the hard portion for 5 to10 minutes while seated with the head tilted forward, and avoid lying down.

T ___ F ___ 6. For most soft-tissue injuries, it is safe and effective to use RICE (rest, ice, compression, elevation) therapy.

T ___ F ___ 7. A hard blow to the right place, such as a relaxed midsection, that hampers breathing ("knocks the wind out of you") creates a dangerous situation.

T ___ F ___ 8. If the symptoms of heatstroke are present, cool the body to 102°F with ice packs and cold water, give cool drinks if the patient is conscious, and seek immediate medical attention.

T ___ F ___ 9. The strength of scar tissue that forms following an injury increases for 3 months to a year.

T ___ F ___ 10. People who have any form of a heart murmur should avoid exercise.

Answers: 1-F, 2-T, 3-T, 4-F, 5-T, 6-T, 7-F, 8-T, 9-T, 10-F

From *Physical fitness and wellness*, third edition, by Jerrold S. Greenberg, George B. Dintiman, and Barbee Myers Oakes, 2004, Champaign, IL: Human Kinetics.

Analyze Yourself

Assessing Your Injury-Prevention Behavior

Name _____ **Date** _____

Instructions: Indicate how often each of the following occurs in your daily activities and exercise sessions. Respond to each item with a number from 0 to 3, using the following scale:

0 = Never   **1** = Occasionally   **2** = Most of the time   **3** = Always

____ **1.** I avoid using rubberized suits on hot days to increase weight loss.

____ **2.** To avoid muscle cramps on hot, humid days, I drink sufficient amounts of water and may use electrolyte solutions such as Gatorade.

____ **3.** I take extra time to warm up on cold days.

____ **4.** I drink water freely before, during, and after exercise.

____ **5.** After a soft-tissue injury, such as an ankle sprain, pulled muscle, or contusion, I apply cold immediately and continue with ice therapy for 1 to 3 days.

____ **6.** I apply ice to the injured area for no more than 15 to 20 minutes each session.

____ **7.** I avoid jogging or running on hard surfaces as much as possible.

____ **8.** If a blister breaks, I trim off all loose skin and apply an antibiotic salve.

____ **9.** If any injury to the head produces dizziness or temporary unconsciousness, play is stopped, ice is applied, and medical attention is sought.

____ **10.** If I suffer a minor cut, I immediately clean it with soap and water or peroxide to remove all dirt and foreign matter.

Scoring: Excellent = 25-30

Good = 19-24

Poor = Below 19

From *Physical fitness and wellness, third edition,* by Jerrold S. Greenberg, George B. Dintiman, and Barbee Myers Oakes, 2004, Champaign, IL: Human Kinetics.

Protecting Your Body From Injury and Illness

Common sense and the application of some basic conditioning concepts can eliminate the majority of risks in most exercise programs. The 11-point injury-prevention program that follows will help minimize your risk of injury and initiate a sound, safe fitness program.

Analyze Your Medical History Before You Begin

If you are over 40 years of age, have been inactive for more than 2 years regardless of age, or are in a high-risk group (obese, hypertense, diabetic, high blood lipids), a thorough physical examination is recommended. A qualified fitness instructor can check your heart rate and blood pressure during exercise on a stationary bicycle to secure valuable information about how you will respond to an exercise program. Although the chances of a serious problem are slight for young people, they are better safe than sorry.

Competitive athletes, on the other hand, may need special attention. Although sudden death is rare (1 in 200,000 high school athletes dies while on the practice or playing field or in the arena), the occasional tragedy that occurs always receives considerable media attention. One study of 134 competitive athletes who underwent medical screening and died of cardiovascular disorders revealed that only 4 had aroused any suspicion of possible heart problems and only 1 had been diagnosed with cardiovascular disease.

To reduce the incidence of sudden cardiac arrest among high school, university, and professional athletes, the American Heart Association has made the following recommendations:

- Make preparticipation cardiovascular screening, including a physical examination and a complete and careful personal and family history, mandatory for all athletes. A detailed medical history of the immediate family may detect clues to some fatal inherited disorders that may not show up on routine physical exams.
- Conduct this screening before the athlete's initial engagement in sports and repeat it every 2 years.
- Require that a licensed physician or appropriately trained health care worker perform all screening.

- Listen to the hearts of athletes while they are both standing and lying down to identify heart murmurs and other problems.
- Include blood-pressure measurements in each physical exam.
- Develop a national standard for preparticipation medical evaluations including cardiovascular screening.

Unfortunately, eliminating all potentially fatal heart conditions is nearly impossible in spite of rigorous screening. If you suspect an inherited disorder or abnormality, ask your physician to secure a careful medical history from family members.

Improve Your General Conditioning Level

You need to be extra careful in the first month of a new exercise program when you are particularly vulnerable to muscle, joint, **ligament,** tendon, **cartilage,** and other soft-tissue injuries. Injuries of all types are more likely to occur when you are generally fatigued because the blood supply to muscles is reduced, muscle fibers are somewhat devitalized and easily torn, and joint stability and muscle groups are weakened. A state of general fatigue is common during the early stages of an exercise program. Strengthening the injury-prone areas such as the ankles, wrists, knees, shoulders, lower back, and neck (see chapter 7) before beginning a new program will help reduce the incidence of fatigue-related injuries.

Warm Up Properly Before Each Workout

At the beginning of every exercise session, you want to raise your body temperature 1 to 2°F to prepare muscles, ligaments, and tendons for vigorous movement. A fast walk, a slow jog, or a mild form of exercise specific to your workout activity for 4 to 5 minutes to elevate core temperature, followed by several minutes of stretching, will help prevent muscle pulls, strains, sprains, and lower-back discomfort and reduce muscle soreness that may occur 8 to 24 hours later (see chapter 6).

ligament—Fibrous bands that hold bones together.

cartilage—A fibrous connective tissue between the surfaces of movable and immovable joints.

Cool Down at the End of Each Exercise Session

The cool-down is a key phase of the fitness workout that exercisers should enjoy rather than avoid. Experienced joggers or runners, for example, complete the final 1/2 to 1 mile at a slow, easy pace rather than with a kick or sprint. The final 3 to 5 minutes of any workout should include some stretching as the body cools and slowly returns to a near resting state (see chapter 3). The cooldown will reduce the incidence of injury during this fatigued state of your workout and decrease muscle soreness the next day.

Progress Slowly

Adding only small increments to your workout each exercise session is wise. Too much, too soon is a common cause of muscular injuries. Plan your program over a 3- to 6-month period to maximize enjoyment and minimize pain and the risk of injury.

Runners are a group that typically add extra mileage too soon, which increases the type and seriousness of injuries that may occur. The novice runner who completes 5-20 miles weekly at a 9-12 minute mile pace is prone to shin splints, runner's knee, low back pain, and muscle soreness. Runners who cover 20-40 miles weekly may also develop stress fractures and Achilles tendonitis. The long-distance runner (40-70 miles at a 7-8 minute mile pace) and the elite marathon runner (up to 200 miles weekly at a 5-7 minute pace) develop more serious tendon pulls, stress fractures, and leg and back muscle strains. Several factors can compound the problem: running surface (a soft, level surface is preferred); running up and down curbs, which increases shock to the legs, feet, and back; sloping or banked roads, which force the foot on the higher part of the slope to twist inward excessively; overstressing tendons and ligaments; or running uphill (strains the Achilles tendon and lower-back muscles) and downhill (increases the force to the heel). Complete Discovery Activity 13.1: Evaluating Your Potential for Foot and Leg Injuries at the end of this chapter.

In your workout you should also avoid increasing your heart rate to more than 60% of your maximum during the first 2 to 4 weeks. After this acclimation period, you can train at higher heart rates more safely.

Alternate Light- and Heavy-Workout Days

Many people make the mistake of trying to exercise hard every day. The body then does not have adequate time to repair or rebuild, and exercisers may not attain the full benefit of each workout. In addition, injuries, boredom, and peaking early are much more likely to occur. Alternating light- and heavy-workout days each week reduces the chance of an exercise-related injury.

Avoid the Weekend Athlete Approach to Fitness

One sure way to guarantee numerous injuries and illnesses is to exercise vigorously only on weekends. The older weekend athlete is particularly susceptible to heart attack, and individuals of all ages increase their chances of soft-tissue injuries to muscles, tendons, and ligaments.

Early in the spring of each year and during the first major snowfall of winter, approximately 25 to 50 men die of heart attacks. The early spring victims are generally middle-aged men who recently bought an expensive pair of running shoes and decided to get in shape in just one workout. The 5-mile run they usually attempt is often the first exercise they have performed in the past year. Similarly, the snow shoveling that follows the first major snowfall is the first exposure to exercise since the previous winter. For these individuals, who may already be at risk for disease, the result is often fatal. A few months of walking as a means of preconditioning can probably prevent these deaths.

Death occasionally occurs following unaccustomed exertion in cold weather even though an autopsy reveals no signs of a heart attack. Although the condition is rare, it is a possibility when men and women try to do it all in one weekend workout. Cold air constricts the blood vessels of the skin and increases blood pressure slightly. Vigorous exercise dramatically increases blood pressure, heart rate, and the oxygen needs of the heart. Without proper warm-up and with the presence of hidden signs of heart disease, a heart attack may occur.

If you can exercise only on the weekend, avoid long bouts in hot or cold weather and abstain from strenuous exercise (jogging, running, racquetball, handball, tennis, basketball, soccer, rugby, and so on) unless you take frequent breaks. Consider supplementing your weekend routine with one other workout during the week. After a month, try increasing to two workouts during the week in addition to one on weekends. If you choose an aerobic activity and progress slowly for several months, you can minimize the risk of serious illness or injury. With three workouts weekly, you have the foundation for a good conditioning program.

Pay Close Attention to Your Body Signals

You should not ignore pain and other distress signals during exercise. Although some breathing discomfort and breathlessness is common, and minor pain may be present in joints or muscles, severe, persistent, and particularly sharp pain is a warning sign to stop exercising. Also, stop exercising immediately if you notice any abnormal heart action (pulse irregularity, fluttering, palpitations in the chest or throat, rapid heart beats); pain or pressure in the chest, teeth, jaw, neck, or arms; dizziness; lightheadedness; cold sweat; or confusion.

Paying attention to your body can also help you detect the early onset of heat-related injuries that commonly occur in hot, humid weather during an exercise session. Early awareness and treatment can prevent heat exhaustion and heatstroke and the potentially serious health consequences of these conditions. If you experience any of the symptoms described in table 13.1, stop exercising immediately, begin the suggested treatment, and seek medical attention. A careful look at your diet, including fluid intake (water, juice, electrolyte drinks), may help explain why a specific heat-related problem tends to reoccur and lead to elimination of the problem in the future.

Exercise may be inadvisable for some individuals afflicted with certain medical conditions. Study table 13.2 to identify the adjustments that you should make when you are ill, injured, or suffering from a medical condition that requires modifications. When you are obviously ill or not up to par, avoid exercise, rest a few days, and return to a lower level or an easier workout.

After each workout, let your body analyze the severity of your exercise session. The workout was probably too light if you did not sweat, and it was likely too heavy if you were still breathless 10 minutes after you stopped exercising, if your pulse rate was above 120 beats per minute 5 minutes after stopping, if you felt fatigue for more than 24 hours, if nausea or vomiting occurred, or if sleep was interrupted. To remedy these symptoms in

TABLE 13.1—Heat Injuries: Causes, Clinical Findings, and Treatment

Heat injuries	Causes	Clinical findings	Treatment
Heat syncope	Excessive vasodilation, pooling of blood in the skin	Fainting, weaknesses, fatigue	Place on back in cool environment; give cool fluids.
Heat cramps	Excessive loss of electrolytes in sweat, inadequate salt intake	Cramps	Rest in cool environment; ingest salt drinks; salt foods daily; get medical treatment in severe cases.
Salt-depletion heat exhaustion	Excessive loss of electrolytes in sweat, inadequate salt intake	Nausea, fatigue, fainting, cramps	Rest in cool environment; replace fluids and salt by mouth; get medical treatment in severe cases.
Water-depletion heat exhaustion	Excessive loss of sweat, inadequate fluid intake	Fatigue, nausea, cool pale skin, active sweating, rectal temperature lower than 104°F	Rest in cool environment; drink cool fluids; cool body with water; get medical treatment if serious.
Anhidrotic heat exhaustion	Same as water-depletion heat exhaustion	Nausea, sweating stopped, dry skin, rectal temperature lower than 104°F	Same as water-depletion heat exhaustion.
Heatstroke	Excessive body temperature	Headache, disorientation, unconsciousness, rectal temperature greater than 105.8°F	Cool body immediately to 102°F (38.9°C) with ice packs, cold water; give cool drinks with glucose if conscious; get medical help immediately.

TABLE 13.2—Disqualifying Conditions for Sports Participation

Conditions	Collision[a]	Contact[b]	Noncontact[c]	Others[d]
GENERAL HEALTH				
Acute infections Respiratory, genitourinary, infectious mononucleosis, hepatitis, active rheumatic fever, active tuberculosis	x	x	x	x
Obvious physical immaturity in comparison with other competitors	x	x		
Hemorrhagic disease Hemophilia, purpura, and other serious bleeding tendencies	x	x	x	
Diabetes, inadequately controlled	x	x	x	x
Diabetes, controlled	e	e	e	e
Jaundice	x	x	x	x
EYES				
Absence or loss of function of one eye	x	x		
RESPIRATORY				
Tuberculosis (active or symptomatic)	x	x	x	x
Severe pulmonary insufficiency	x	x	x	x
CARDIOVASCULAR				
Mitral stenosis, aortic stenosis, aortic insufficiency, coarctation of aorta, cyanotic heart disease, recent carditis of any etiology	x	x	x	x
Hypertension on organic basis	x	x	x	x
Previous heart surgery for congenital or acquired heart disease	f	f	f	f
Liver, enlarged	x	x		
SKIN				
Boils, impetigo, and herpes simplex gladiatorum	x	x		
Spleen, enlarged	x	x		
HERNIA				
Inguinal or femoral hernia	x	x	x	
MUSCULOSKELETAL				
Symptomatic abnormalities or inflammations	x	x	x	x
Functional inadequacy of the musculoskeletal system, congenital or acquired, incompatible with the contact or skill demands of the sport	x	x	x	

(continued)

TABLE 13.2 (continued)

Conditions	Collision[a]	Contact[b]	Noncontact[c]	Others[d]
NEUROLOGICAL				
History of symptoms of serious head trauma or repeated concussions	x			
Controlled convulsive disorder	g	g	g	g
Convulsive disorder not moderately well controlled by medication	x			
Previous surgery on head	x	x		
RENAL				
Absence of one kidney	x	x		
Renal disease	x	x	x	x
GENITALIA				
Absence of one testicle	h	h	h	h
Undescended testicle	h	h	h	h

[a]Football, rugby, hockey, lacrosse, and so forth.

[b]Baseball, soccer, basketball, wrestling, and so forth.

[c]Cross country, track, tennis, crew, swimming, and so forth.

[d]Bowling, golf, archery, field events, and so forth.

[e]No exclusions.

[f]Each patient should be judged on an individual basis in conjunction with his or her cardiologist and surgeon.

[g]Each patient should be judged on an individual basis. All things being equal, it is probably better to encourage a young boy or girl to participate in a noncontact sport rather than a contact sport. However, if a patient has a desire to play a contact sport and this is deemed a major ameliorating factor in his or her adjustment to school, associates, and the seizure disorder, serious consideration should be given to letting him or her participate if the seizures are moderately well controlled or the patient is under good medical management.

[h]The committee approves the concept of contact sports participation for youths with only one testicle or with one or both testicles undescended, except in specific instances such as an inguinal canal undescended testicle or testicles, following appropriate medical evaluation to rule out unusual injury risk. The athlete, parents, and school authorities should be fully informed that participation in contact sports with only one testicle carries a slight injury risk to the remaining healthy testicle. Fertility may be adversely affected after an injury. But the chances of an injury to a descended testicle are rare, and the injury risk can be further substantially minimized with an athletic supporter and protective device.

Reprinted from D. Amheim, 1989, *Modern principles of athletic training* (St. Louis: Times Mirror/Mosby College Publishing), 51-52. Reproduced with permission of The McGraw-Hill Companies.

the future, exercise less vigorously and lengthen your cool-down period.

Master the Proper Form in Your Activity

For all activities, correct form improves efficiency and reduces the risk of injury. Proper running form, for example, is important to most fitness programs. Joggers should avoid running on the toes, which produces soreness in the calf muscles. The heel should strike the ground first before rolling the weight along the bottom of the foot to the toes for the pushoff. A number of running-form problems can produce mild muscle or joint strain.

Participants in racket sports are susceptible to numerous form-related injuries (elbow, shoulder, and wrist inflammation and lower-back problems) from faulty stroke mechanics such as elbow-leg ground strokes, bent-elbow hits, muscles not firm at impact, and so on. A few professional lessons in your sport can help to reduce the risk of these types of injuries.

Dress Properly for the Weather

Weather extremes can also cause health problems during exercise. Consider the suggestions in figure 13.1 to reduce the risk of overheating on hot, humid days or overexposure on cold days. Becoming familiar with the early symptoms and

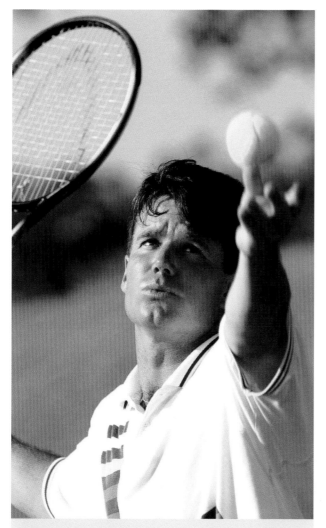

Mastering the proper form improves efficiency and reduces risk of injury. Tennis players are especially susceptible to elbow, shoulder, wrist, and lower-back problems.

Eyewire

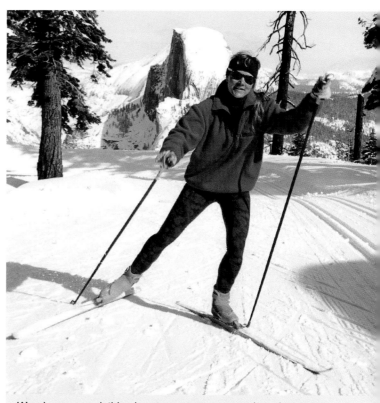

Wearing proper clothing in extreme temperatures is an important safety consideration for active people.

PhotoDisc

hypothermia—Subnormal body temperature.

frostbite—Destruction of tissue by freezing.

emergency treatment for heat- and cold-related injuries such as heat exhaustion, heatstroke, **hypothermia,** and **frostbite** is also helpful.

If you are a runner, plan your jogging course to avoid being too far out on either a hot or cold day should symptoms of heat exhaustion or over-exposure to cold occur. For example, if in cold weather you run with the wind behind you on the way out, on the way back, when you are likely to be sweating much more, you will be running into a headwind with wet clothes, which will draw heat away from your body.

Weather extremes can be dangerous. Heatstroke (when core temperature may rise to 105 or 106°F) symptoms are difficult to reverse unless immediate, rapid cooling takes place. On the other hand, a 1°F drop in core temperature will produce pain. Should body temperature drop to 94°F, shivering ceases and rigidity sets in; at 75°F, death usually occurs from heart failure.

Wearing properly fitted shoes, using appropriate equipment, avoiding gimmicky exercise devices, and using acceptable equipment for contact sports are important for injury prevention. These matters need special attention. A high-quality shoe is your best protection against injury to the feet, ankles, knees, hips, and lower back.

Use the Recommended Protective Equipment for Your Activity

The use of protective gear can reduce your risk of a serious injury in many activities. Eyeglasses for handball, racquetball, and squash; headgear for bicycling, in-line skating, ice skating, lacrosse, and football; proper wrist, knee, and elbow padding for roller skating, ice skating, and rugby—all prevent broken bones, concussions, and other serious injuries.

Hot, humid weather

- Listen to weather reports and avoid vigorous exercise if the temperature is above 90°F and the humidity is above 70%. Do your light workout on hot days.
- Avoid adding to normal salt intake. Do not use salt tablets. Increase consumption of fruits and vegetables.
- Avoid lengthy warm-up periods.
- Wear light-colored, porous, loose clothing to promote evaporation. Remove special equipment, such as football gear, every hour for 15 minutes.
- Avoid wearing a hat (except for an open visor with brim) because considerable heat loss occurs through the head.
- Never use rubberized suits that hold the sweat in and increase fluid, salt, and potassium loss.
- Remember that wet clothing increases salt and sweat loss, so change clothes when possible.
- Slowly increase the length of your workout by 5 to 10 minutes daily for 9 days to acclimate to the heat.
- Drink cold water (40°F) before (10 to 20 ounces 15 minutes before exercise), during, and after exercise. Hydrate before the workout with two or three glasses of water.

Cold weather

- Listen to weather reports and note the temperature and windchill factor. Unless the equivalent temperature is in the area of little danger, avoid exercising outside.
- Eat well during cold months; the body needs more calories in cold weather.
- Warm up carefully until sweating is evident.
- Use two or three layers of clothing rather than one heavy warm-up suit.
- Protect the head (warm hat), ears, fingers, toes, nose, and genitals. A hat should cover the ears and face. Fur-lined supporters for men can prevent frostbite to sensitive parts.
- Never use rubberized, airtight suits that keep the sweat in. When the body cools, the sweat starts to freeze.
- Keep clothing dry and change out of wet items as soon as possible.
- Slowly increase the length of your workout by 5 to 10 minutes daily for 9 days to acclimate to the cold.
- Drink cold water freely before, during, and after exercise. Let thirst be your guide.

Figure 13.1   Preventive techniques on hot and cold days for heat- and cold-related injuries.

In-line skating is an example of a relatively new activity in which the use of proper protective equipment greatly reduces injury. The number of people enjoying this form of exercise has increased dramatically in recent years, with over 22.5 million people now participating. Unfortunately, the number of related injuries serious enough to require emergency care has increased tremendously. Most skating injuries involve the wrist (32%), lower leg (13%), elbow (9%), and knee (13%). Only 7% of those injured are fully outfitted with helmet, wrist guards, elbow pads, and kneepads.

Tissue Response to Injury

The healing process is unique to each individual and to different types of tissue. Age, nutrition, and the proper use of treatment techniques also affect the way tissue responds to the injury and the healing process. An understanding of how **soft tissue** responds (heals) to **acute** and **chronic** injuries will help you understand emergency treatment techniques and reinforce the correct use of heat, cold, and massage as treatment modalities.

Healing of musculoskeletal injuries incurred through sports or exercise occurs in three phases.

These three phases have been designated as inflammation, proliferation, and remodeling.

Inflammation

This phase (the first 3 or 4 days after an injury) occurs as the body reacts initially to an injury with redness, heat, swelling, pain, and loss of function or movement. During this period, pressure on nerve endings, or **ischemia,** may produce considerable pain. Some tissue death also takes place from the initial trauma or the lack of oxygen following the trauma. Acute inflammation is actually a protective mechanism designed to keep the problem local and remove some of the injurious agents so that healing and repair can begin. Almost immediately after the injury occurs, blood flow to that area decreases for a period from several seconds to as long as 10 minutes, and coagulation begins to seal the broken blood vessels. Numerous other vascular and cellular events occur to prepare the site for the next phase.

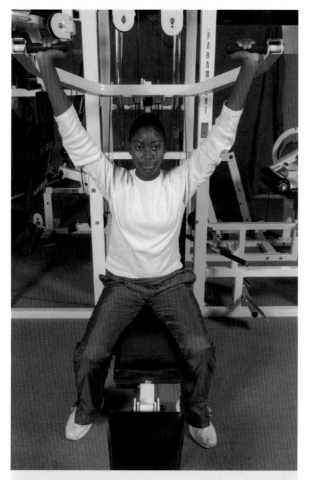

Strength training can help reduce the incidence of work- and exercise-related injuries.

Proliferation

For a period of from 2 or 3 days after the injury to about 21 days after the injury, healing begins when cellular debris, erythrocytes, and the fibrin clot are being removed. Although some scar tissue will form following soft-tissue injuries, a desirable goal is to treat the injury properly to produce as little of such tissue as possible because scar tissue is less viable than normal tissue. Primary healing occurs with little scar-tissue formation in injuries in which the edges are held closely together. With a gaping lesion and large tissue loss, considerable scar tissue forms during the healing process to replace lost tissue and bridge the gap.

Remodeling

In this phase, which overlaps the proliferation phase, scar tissue continues to increase and become stronger for 3 to 6 weeks following an injury. The strength of scar tissue increases for 3 months to a year. The complete remodeling of ligamentous tissue generally requires a year.

General Treatment Modalities

Numerous single treatments and the combined use of two or more modalities are effective in treating soft-tissue injuries.

Cryotherapy

The application of cold, or **cryotherapy,** to the skin for 20 minutes or less at a minimum temperature of 50°F causes the constriction of vessels and reduces the flow of blood to the injured area. When cold is applied for longer than 20 minutes, an intermittent period of **vasodilation** occurs for 4 to 6 minutes. Vasodilation prevents tissue damage from too much exposure to cold. At this point, cold is no longer effective. Cold also reduces muscle spasms, swelling, and pain; slows

soft tissue—Tissue other than bone.

acute—Disease or pain characterized by sudden onset and a short, severe course.

chronic—Disease or pain of slow onset and long duration.

ischemia—A condition of localized diminished blood supply.

cryotherapy—The use of cold in the treatment of injury and disease.

vasodilation—Increase or opening of the blood vessels.

metabolic rate; and increases **collagen** inelasticity and joint stiffness.

Cold applications should be used immediately after an injury and continued for several days until swelling subsides. Cold can be applied intermittently for 20 minutes every 1 1/2 waking hours in combination with compression, elevation, and rest (see information about RICE later in this chapter). The longer the cold is applied, the deeper the cooling. Ice massage can be used on a small body area by freezing water in a foam cup to form a cylinder of ice. After removing 1 or 2 inches of the foam at the top of the cup, the cup portion can serve as a handle and the ice can be rubbed over the skin in overlapping circles for 5 to 10 minutes to produce cold, burning, aching, and numbness in the area. Ice packs can be made by placing flaked or crushed ice in a wet towel or self-sealing plastic bag. Only in ice massage should ice come in direct contact with the skin.

Thermotherapy

In general, proper **thermotherapy** to an injured area raises skin temperature and increases the amount of blood flow to the area. Heat can relieve joint stiffness, pain, muscle spasms, and increase the extensibility of collagen tissues. A treatment session should never exceed 30 minutes. Additional cautions in the use of heat include the following:

- Never apply heat immediately over an area of acute inflammation.
- Never use heat over an area of decreased sensation or reduced arterial circulation.
- Never apply heat over an area of recent or potential bleeding, or over an infected area.
- Never use heat over an area of known malignancy.
- Never apply heat over an area where liniments or heat rubs have recently been applied.
- Never apply heat directly to the eyes or genitals or to the abdomen of a pregnant woman.

Heat can be safely applied by using moist heat and commercial packs as well as whirlpool and paraffin baths. You can use moist heat at home by soaking a towel in hot water and allowing it to drain for several seconds before applying it to an injured area that is already covered by four to six layers of toweling. The moist towel should not come in direct contact with the skin.

Thermotherapy using ultrasound or diathermy should be performed only by a physician, physical therapist, or licensed athletic trainer.

Massage

The use of massage to manipulate soft tissue is a helpful adjunct to heat and cold. Stroking, kneading, friction, percussion, and rapid shaking are some of the more common techniques used to increase heat, improve blood flow to the injured area, remove metabolites such as lactic acid, overcome edema, improve circulation and the venous return of blood to the heart, and aid relaxation.

Prevention and Emergency Treatment of Common Exercise Injuries and Illnesses

Additional common injuries, illnesses, and problems associated with exercise are discussed in appendix D, which serves as a guide for diagnosis, prevention, emergency treatment, and determination of the need for a physician. If in doubt, consult a physician immediately or transport the injured person to a hospital emergency room.

RICE

Emergency home treatment for most muscle, ligament, and tendon strains as well as sprains, suspected fractures, bruises, and joint inflammations involves four simple actions that make up the RICE approach.

Rest. To prevent additional damage to injured tissue, stop exercising and immobilize the injured area immediately. If the lower extremities are affected, use crutches to move about.

Ice. To decrease blood flow to the injured area and decrease swelling, apply ice (crushed in a towel or ice pack) directly to the skin immediately for 15 to 20 minutes. Use cold applications intermittently for 1 to 72 hours.

Compression. To limit swelling and decrease likelihood of hemorrhage and hematoma formation, wrap a towel or bandage firmly around the ice and injured area. An elastic wrap soaked in water and frozen in a refrigerator will apply both compression and cold.

Elevation. To help drain excess fluid through gravity, improve the venous return of blood to the heart, and reduce internal bleeding and swelling, raise the injured limb above heart level.

collagen—The connective tissue portion of the true skin and other organs.

thermotherapy—The application of heat.

Myth and Fact Sheet

Myth	Fact
1. With injuries to most body parts, you should apply heat.	**1.** Injuries to soft tissue should be treated with RICE therapy, which requires ice, not heat. Heat should be avoided for 2 to 3 days until swelling begins to subside. Early use of heat in any form increases swelling, delays healing, and can cause serious tissue changes that may require surgery to correct.
2. You should apply ice directly to your skin for 1 hour.	**2.** Ice should be applied for no more than 20 minutes. Longer periods can bring about tissue damage. Ice should not contact the skin unless ice massage is being used.
3. If you have a heart murmur, you should not exercise.	**3.** A heart murmur is an abnormal sound caused by turbulent blood flow. The difficulty may be an impaired valve that fails to close completely or narrowed valve orifices that slow the flow of blood. These conditions place a greater-than-normal load on the heart. Heart walls may increase in size, and tension increases inside the walls. The heart is less efficient and, in a sense, has to regurgitate blood twice. In what is termed a functional murmur, no structural defect is evident to account for the abnormal sounds. Although you can generally exercise safely with functional murmurs, you should consult your physician before starting an exercise program.
4. If you have the wind knocked out of you, you are in danger of dying.	**4.** The temporary inability to breathe following a blow to a relaxed midsection will slowly subside until natural breathing resumes. Meanwhile, you will gasp for breath; possibly suffer dizziness, nausea, and weakness; or even collapse. A hard blow to the solar plexus increases intra-abdominal pressure, causes pain, and interferes with the diaphragmatic cycle reflex because of nerve paralysis or muscle spasm. Breathing is only temporarily affected by a blow that momentarily paralyzes the nerve control of the diaphragm. For relief, loosen clothing at the neck and waist, apply ice to the abdomen, and breathe slowly through the nose.
5. A popping or snapping sound in your knee is a sign of serious trouble.	**5.** The sound generally comes from a tendon flipping over bony fulcrums and may be quite natural in some athletes who simply never noticed the sound before. "Joint mice," or the presence of some loose cartilage or other tissue, may also produce a clicking sound as the knee flexes and extends. Bone, tendon, ligament, or cartilage damage may not be indicated unless other symptoms are present, such as inflammation, swelling, fluid, and knee locking.
6. The concept of no pain, no gain should be followed when recovering from an injury.	**6.** Observing this practice can cause harm. You should train at a frequency, duration, and intensity that produces no pain or compensation. Favoring a sore area may eventually injure other body parts and slow your recovery. Workouts during recovery should be shorter and involve more rest between repetitions and workouts.
7. You can safely return to activity almost immediately after arthroscopic knee surgery.	**7.** In general, you should rest and rehabilitate for a minimum of 3 to 4 weeks before you return to activity after repairing minor damage to cartilage. Recovery after repair of an injury to knee ligaments such as the anterior or posterior cruciates may require as long as 6 to 12 months. Only then should you return to participation in a contact sport. Predicting recovery time is difficult because each case and each person is different. Follow the advice and rehabilitation program recommended by your orthopedic surgeon. Returning too soon could result in reinjury and a return to the operating room.

Home treatment should begin as soon as possible. The procedure should be the following: (1) Evaluate the injured area; (2) apply ice for 20 minutes; (3) compress the ice firmly against the injury; (4) replace the ice pack with a compress wrap and pad; (5) rest the injured area; (6) reapply ice within 1 to 1 1/2 hours; (7) remove the wrap and elevate the area before you go to bed; and (8) begin ice therapy immediately on rising in the morning. On the 4th or 5th day, discontinue cold treatments and begin to apply moist heat or dry heat or use a whirlpool twice daily for 15 to 20 minutes. Depending on the severity of the injury and amount of swelling and pain, you can resume mild exercise in 4 or 5 days. Another acronym to remind you of the proper procedure in treating minor injuries is PRICE; the P is a reminder to see a physician.

Considerable misinformation is available concerning proper home emergency treatment. Unfortunately, incorrect treatment can worsen the injury or produce serious side effects that may require surgery later.

Shock

Many injuries, such as fractures, concussions, profuse bleeding, heart attack, back and neck damage, and severe joint trauma, can produce shock. Shock is one of the body's strongest natural reactions to disease and injury. It slows blood flow, which acts as a natural tourniquet and reduces pain with serious injury. All three types of shock can kill: traumatic (injury or loss of blood), septic (infection induced), and cardiogenic (from a heart attack). Shock is much easier to prevent than it is to treat. You should assume that shock is present with the above injuries and illnesses, splint broken bones, handle the victim with care, stop the bleeding, and keep the victim warm at all times.

Use of Medication in the Treatment of Exercise-Related Injuries

Numerous prescription and nonprescription (over-the-counter) drugs are available to combat infection, treat fungi, control pain and bleeding, and reduce inflammation. You should consult your physician, however, before using any medication. Update your home medicine cabinet to make certain that you are stocking the basics for common illnesses and injuries. Take a moment to analyze your home pharmacy by completing

counterirritants—Medication, heat, cold, electricity, and so forth used to eliminate pain and inflammation.

Discovery Activity 13.2: Evaluating Your Home Medicine Cabinet at the end of this chapter. Then compare your findings to the recommended home pharmacy shown in table 13.3.

You can often prevent infection by including at least one antiseptic and one wound protectant in your home medicine kit. Your physician may also prescribe an antibiotic—either a topical dressing or a systemic medication.

You can control pain through the skin by applying a topical anesthetic to inhibit pain sensations through quick evaporation and cooling or by counterirritating the skin so that you are no longer aware of the pain. Liniments, analgesic balms, heat, and cold are examples of **counterirritants.**

Counterirritants trick the brain into ignoring soreness. Pain signals reach the brain along two types of nerve fibers—myelinated fibers, which are covered by a fatty material called myelin, and C fibers, which do not have the fatty covering. The C fibers transmit dull, aching types of pain and soreness, whereas the myelinated fibers transmit sharper pain. The brain can process only so many pain signals at once. When both types of nerve fibers are activated simultaneously, the myelinated fibers override the C fibers and you perceive only the sharper pain and sensations of heat, cold, and pressure, not the dull ache.

Some central nervous system drugs such as acetaminophen (Tylenol®) and aspirin reduce pain by acting on the nerves that carry the pain impulse to the brain.

One of several drugs can reduce inflammation to soft tissue. Aspirin is effective for conditions such as tendonitis, bursitis, chondromalacia, and tendosynovitis. Some enzymes can help treat swollen joints, reduce inflammation, edema, pain, swelling, and redness. NSAIDs (nonsteroidal-anti-inflammatory drugs) are also effective in eliminating inflammation. A physician's prescription and guidance are needed, however, because side effects may occur and long-term use can be dangerous.

Nutrition and Healing

Individuals who do not eat correctly and have poor nutritional status do not heal as rapidly as they might otherwise. Although the Dietary Reference Intakes (DRIs) (see chapter 10) for protein

TABLE 13.3—Your Home Pharmacy

Medical concern	Medication
Allergy	**Antihistamines**
Cold and coughs	Cold tablets, cough drops
Constipation	**Milk of magnesia**
Diarrhea	Antidiarrheal, paregoric
Eye irritations	Eye drops
Exercise injury problems (inflammation)	**Aspirin**, NSAID medication; see your physician.
Exercise injury problems (pain)	**Acetaminophen, aspirin**, use of heat and cold
Pain and fever (children)	Children's aspirin, acetaminophen, liquid acetaminophen, aspirin, rectal suppositories
Fungus	**Antifungal preparations**
Sunburn (preventive)	**Sunblock**
Sprains	**Elastic bandages**
Stomach upset	Antacid (nonabsorbable)
Wounds (general)	**Adhesive tape bandages, sodium bicarbonate (soaking agent)**
Wounds (antiseptics)	**Ethyl alcohol (60-90%)**, isopropyl alcohol
Wounds (protectant)	Topical antibiotics

Note: Items in bold print are basic requirements; other preparations are also useful and should be considered.

and some vitamins and minerals increase during periods of recovery from illness and injury, a sufficient safety margin exists in the DRI to promote normal healing and recovery, provided you are consuming adequate fluids and calories.

Summary

Protecting Your Body From Injury and Illness Many exercise-related injuries are preventable. You can significantly reduce your risk of injury and illness by using a preconditioning period before beginning your exercise program, warming up and cooling down properly, analyzing your medical history, progressing slowly in the early stages of your program, monitoring body signals, dressing properly for the activity, and mastering proper form.

Tissue Response to Injury The healing process is unique to each individual. Factors such as age, nutrition, treatment, and type and severity of the injury play a major role. In the inflammatory stage immediately following an injury, the body attempts to keep things localized to prevent further damage and aid the healing process that will occur over the next 5 or 6 weeks. Complete regeneration and repair, however, may require up to a year.

General Treatment Modalities The immediate and continued use of cold applications over the first several days after a soft-tissue injury should be followed by heat therapy during the proliferative and remodeling stages of healing. Numerous techniques to apply heat and cold can be safely used.

Prevention and Emergency Treatment of Common Exercise Injuries and Illnesses Proper home emergency treatment for a soft-tissue injury to an extremity requires the use of RICE. Certain symptoms suggest the need for immediate care by a physician. If you are in doubt, go to an emergency room or see a physician as soon as possible.

Some injuries involving fractures, concussions, bleeding, heart attack, and severe joint trauma can produce shock. Because shock is considerably easier to prevent than it is to treat, precautions

Behavioral Change and Motivational Strategies

Many things can interfere with the use of practices known to prevent injuries or to help recuperation from exercise-related injuries. Here are some of these barriers (roadblocks) and strategies for overcoming them.

Roadblock	Behavioral Change Strategy
You are in a rush to get through your exercise program and don't have time to stretch.	Either allow more time for exercising so that you have time for stretching or plan on working out for a shorter time. Self-talk can help here. Remind yourself that if you don't stretch, you increase your chances of injury. If injury occurs, you might not be able to work out for a few weeks or longer. Think of the fitness you might lose and the weight you might gain if that occurs.
You injure yourself and know that you should apply the RICE principle (rest, ice, compression, and elevation). Yet you have to get back to work and have dinner plans that evening. You decide that you'll take care of your injury tomorrow.	This situation offers a classic example of how you might use social support to manage behavior. You might telephone your coworkers and notify them of your injury. The concern you likely will receive from them and their advice to take care of the injury will go a long way toward alleviating any guilt about not returning quickly to work. Selective awareness—that is, choosing to focus on one thing rather than another—can also help. In this case, you can focus on the need to recover and not create a long-term inconvenience for your coworkers, rather than on the need to avoid inconveniencing them in the short term. Not caring for yourself right away may cause the injury to worsen and extend considerably your absence from work.
Summer is quickly approaching. You want to increase the amount of weight you lift so that you can sculpt your body and appear irresistible in a bathing suit. You know that increasing the amount of weight you lift might subject you to injury, but time is short so you decide to go for it anyhow.	In this case, you need to use chaining. That is, you should slowly increase the weight consistent with recommendations in chapter 7. If you do not, you might look great on the surgery table (a torn muscle or ruptured tendon) but not on the beach. Self-monitoring could also help. You could maintain a journal of the amount of weight you lift and, in a healthy manner, increase the weight gradually. Joining a group with whom to weight train might enable you to take better control of your training routine and make it safer. The influence of others can be supportive.
List other roadblocks you are experiencing that seem to place you at risk of exercise-related injury.	Now list the behavioral change strategies that can help you overcome these roadblocks. If necessary, refer back to chapter 4 for information about behavioral change and motivational strategies.
1. _____	1. _____
2. _____	2. _____
3. _____	3. _____

should be taken with all patients when dealing with these types of injuries.

Use of Medication in the Treatment of Exercise-Related Injuries The home medicine cabinet should contain the basic items necessary for the emergency treatment of common exercise injuries. Over-the-counter medications to treat inflammations, fungi, pain, fever, wounds, and basic problems such as allergies, colds, consti-pation, diarrhea, and eye irritations should be readily available.

Nutrition and Healing Sound nutrition is impor-tant during recovery from both injury and illness. Nutritional needs increase somewhat during the recovery period, so it is important to continue to eat well, avoid skipping meals, drink plenty of water and other fluids, and consider the use of a multiple vitamin and mineral supplement.

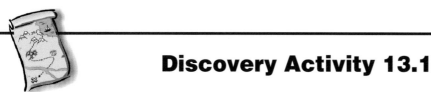

Discovery Activity 13.1

Evaluating Your Potential for Foot and Leg Injuries

Name _____ **Date** _____

Instructions: Injuries to the feet and legs are common in most sports and activities. If you continue the same activity long enough, overuse injuries are almost certain to occur. Certain aspects in the makeup of the lower extremities may require some adjustment to prevent injury. To evaluate your potential for lower-extremity injury, examine yourself carefully in the following areas:

1. Length of both legs below the ankle: Stand erect, with your ankles together, and ask a helper to measure the distance from the floor to a spot marked with a magic marker at the bony protrusion of your ankle.
2. Length of both legs above the ankle: Sit in a chair with your feet on the floor, heels together, and toes pointed. If a carpenter's level placed on both knees is uneven, your problem is above the ankle.
3. Morton's toe: Stand erect without shoes or socks and determine whether your second toe is longer than your big toe.
4. Excessive pronation: Examine your running or athletic shoes for excessive wear on the outside back of the shoe heel.

Results

1. Does the length of your legs differ by more than 1/16 inch?

2. Is the problem below the ankle or from the ankle to the knee?

3. Is your second toe longer than your big toe?

4. Are your shoes wearing evenly?

5. Are you experiencing pain in your lower back, hip, knees, ankles, or feet during or following exercise?

If you answered yes to any of the questions, consult an orthopedic physician for advice about how to prevent a future injury.

Discovery Activity 13.2
Evaluating Your Home Medicine Cabinet

Name _____ **Date** _____

Instructions: You should analyze your home medicine cabinet at least once a year and discard outdated prescriptions and other medicine. Replace used items, discard unnecessary items, place dangerous medicine out of the reach of children, and buy needed products. Because you are beginning a new exercise program, you may need some new items so that you can treat common injuries. Complete the three steps below to evaluate and update your home medicine cabinet.

1. Prepare a list of all items in your home medicine cabinet and complete the form that follows.

Item	Date	Purpose	Effectiveness
_____	_____	_____	_____
_____	_____	_____	_____
_____	_____	_____	_____
_____	_____	_____	_____
_____	_____	_____	_____
_____	_____	_____	_____
_____	_____	_____	_____
_____	_____	_____	_____
_____	_____	_____	_____

2. List all unneeded and outdated items that you can discard.

_____   _____
_____   _____
_____   _____
_____   _____
_____   _____

3. Study table 13.3 to make certain that your cabinet contains the bare necessities for treatment of common exercise injuries and ailments. List the items you are missing and may want to consider buying.

_____   _____
_____   _____
_____   _____
_____   _____
_____   _____

From *Physical fitness and wellness, third edition*, by Jerrold S. Greenberg, George B. Dintiman, and Barbee Myers Oakes, 2004, Champaign, IL: Human Kinetics.

Discovery Activity 13.3

Service-Learning for Prevention and Care of Exercise Injuries

If your college is like most, intramural sports leagues are popular. Depending on the season, teams may be competing in football, basketball, soccer, tennis, or volleyball leagues. Unfortunately, many injuries occur during intramural league games. You can help fellow students by conducting a workshop on prevention and care of athletic injuries during the intramural league orientation session. You should emphasize things participants can do to prevent injuries from occurring in the first place. Recognizing, however, that preventing all possible injuries is impossible, you should include information on the care of various athletic injuries. If possible, work with the intramural department on campus to require attendance by all participants as a prerequisite for eligibility in the league. Leave participants with handouts describing how to prevent and care for some of the more common exercise injuries and include addresses and Web sites where they can obtain valid information about other specific injuries. Once successful in educating other students on campus about prevention and care of exercise injuries, you might consider offering to conduct similar workshops for interscholastic or intramural programs at local high schools.

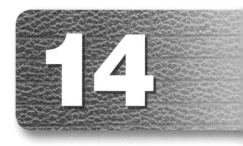

Preventing Premature Heart Disease, Cancer, and Other Diseases

Chapter Objectives

By the end of this chapter, you should be able to

1. cite the prevalence and describe the causes of heart disease;
2. cite the prevalence and describe the causes of cancer;
3. describe how to prevent or postpone the development of heart disease;
4. describe how to prevent cancer;
5. discuss the role of physical fitness in preventing heart disease, cancer, and other diseases;
6. describe several sexually transmitted infections, including signs and symptoms, effects on health, and treatment options; and

7. discuss the role of exercise in other diseases such as diabetes, obesity, hypertension, and kidney disease.

When Frank was young, he assumed he was invulnerable. He knew intellectually that he would someday die; sooner or later, everyone does. But that was not a reality Frank had internalized. In fact, he acted as though he was impervious to the effects of his health decisions. He smoked cigarettes; rarely exercised; took on too much work, thereby stressing himself out; ate poorly by often choosing fatty meals at fast-food restaurants; and spent prolonged periods lounging in the sun.

Frank eventually paid the price for his health-related choices. By the time he reached his 50th year, he had a cough diagnosed as lung cancer and had blocked arteries that threatened a heart attack. Although he had yet to develop skin cancer, his doctor warned him that cancer was possible unless he altered his exposure to the sun's harsh rays. Contributing to his heart condition was the amount of stress to which he subjected himself, the cigarettes he smoked, and his lack of regular exercise. Contributing to the threat of his developing cancer elsewhere than in the lungs was his ingestion of foods high in fat. Frank's early years may have been carefree, but his later adult life was fraught with discomfort and fear. He realized that he would not live as long as he might have.

Unfortunately, Frank's situation, extreme though it may sound, is not unusual. Too many people have experienced the death of a loved one from either heart disease, cancer, or some other disease. If you have not experienced any of these illnesses yourself, you certainly know others who have—parents, grandparents, relatives, friends. Heart disease and cancer alone account for 54% of all deaths that occur in the United States each year (National Center for Health Statistics, 2000). Throw in stroke, which is also a developmental disease associated with an unhealthy lifestyle, and you have accounted for almost 61% of the deaths that occur in this country every year.

In this chapter we will define heart disease, cancer, and other serious and potentially fatal diseases and conditions and discuss what causes them. More important, we will describe how to prevent their occurrence or at least how to delay their arrival. Much of that latter discussion pertains to lifestyle decisions that include physical fitness and wellness considerations.

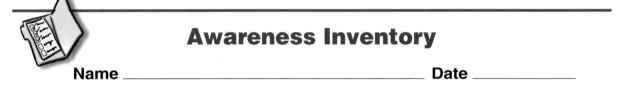

Awareness Inventory

Name _____ **Date** _____

Check the space by the letter T for the statements that you think are true and the space by the letter F for the statements that you think are false. The answers appear following the list of statements. This chapter will present information to clarify these statements for you. As you read the chapter, look for explanations for the reasons why the statements are true or false.

T ___ **F** ___ 1. The heart receives blood filled with waste products that it pumps into the lungs for elimination through breathing.

T ___ **F** ___ 2. Arrythmia is a condition in which the coronary arteries are occluded (clogged).

T ___ **F** ___ 3. Erratic beating of the heart is called atherosclerosis.

T ___ **F** ___ 4. High-density lipoproteins (HDL) are unhealthy and the result of eating a diet too high in fats.

T ___ **F** ___ 5. If coronary heart disease runs in your family, you cannot do much to avoid getting it.

T ___ **F** ___ 6. Cigarette smoking causes about 75% of all lung cancers.

T ___ **F** ___ 7. Carcinogens are medications prescribed for people who develop cancer.

T ___ **F** ___ 8. For most Americans who do not use tobacco, dietary choices and physical activity are the most modifiable determinants of cancer.

T ___ **F** ___ 9. Syphilis is the most prevalent sexually transmitted infection.

T ___ **F** ___ 10. Women usually have more difficulty than men do in determining whether they have a sexually transmitted infection.

Answers: 1-T, 2-F, 3-F, 4-F, 5-F, 6-T, 7-F, 8-T, 9-F, 10-T

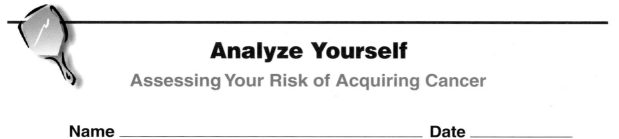

Analyze Yourself

Assessing Your Risk of Acquiring Cancer

Name _____ **Date** _____

Select the response that best describes you for each item and record the point value for each response you selected in the space provided. Total your points for each section separately.

Lung Cancer

1. _____ Sex
    a. male (2)
    b. female (1)

2. _____ Age
    a. 39 or younger (1)
    b. 40 to 49 (2)
    c. 50 to 59 (5)
    d. 60 or older (7)

3. _____ Status
    a. Smoker (8)
    b. Nonsmoker (1)

4. _____ Type of smoking
    a. cigarettes or little cigars (10)
    b. pipe or cigar but not cigarettes (3)
    c. ex-cigarette smoker (2)
    d. nonsmoker (1)

5. _____ Number of cigarettes smoked per day
    a. 0 (1)
    b. less than one-half pack per day (5)
    c. one-half to one pack (9)
    d. one to two packs (15)
    e. more than two packs (20)

6. _____ Type of cigarettes
    a. high tar and nicotine, more than 20 milligrams of tar and 1.3 milligrams of nicotine (10)
    b. medium tar and nicotine, 16 to 19 milligrams of tar and 1.1 to 1.2 milligrams of nicotine (9)
    c. low tar and nicotine, 15 milligrams of tar or less and 1.0 milligram of nicotine or less (7)
    d. nonsmoker (1)

7. _____ Duration of smoking
    a. never smoked (1)
    b. ex-smoker (3)
    c. up to 15 years (5)
    d. 15 to 25 years (10)
    e. more than 25 years (20)

8. _____ Type of industrial work
    a. mining (3)
    b. asbestos (7)
    c. uranium and radioactive products (5)
    d. never worked in an industrial field (0)

_____ *Lung total*

Colon-Rectal Cancer

1. _____ Age
    a. 39 or younger (10)
    b. 40 to 59 (20)
    c. 60 or older (50)

2. _____ Has anyone in your immediate family ever had
    a. colon cancer (20)
    b. one or more polyps of the colon (10)
    c. neither (1)

3. _____ Have you ever had
    a. colon cancer (100)
    b. one or more polyps of the colon (40)
    c. ulcerative colitis (20)
    d. cancer of the breast or uterus (10)
    e. none (1)

4. _____ Bleeding from the rectum (other than obvious hemorrhoids or piles)
    a. yes (75)
    b. no (1)

_____ *Colon-rectal total*

Skin Cancer

1. _____ Frequent work or play in the sun
    a. yes (10)
    b. no (1)

2. _____ Work in mines, around coal tars, or around radioactivity
    a. yes (10)
    b. no (1)

3. _____ Complexion—fair or light skin
    a. yes (10)
    b. no (1)

_____ *Skin total*

(continued)

Analyze Yourself *(continued)*

Breast Cancer (women only)

1. _____ Age group
   a. 20 to 34 (10)
   b. 35 to 49 (40)
   c. 50 and older (90)

2. _____ Race/ethnicity
   a. Asian (5)
   b. African American (20)
   c. White (25)
   d. Mexican American (10)

3. _____ Family history
   a. mother, sister, aunt, or grandmother
      with breast cancer (30)
   b. none (10)

4. _____ Your history
   a. previous lumps or cysts (25)
   b. no breast disease (10)
   c. previous breast cancer (100)

5. _____ Maternity
   a. first pregnancy before 25 (10)
   b. first pregnancy after 25 (15)
   c. no pregnancies (20)

_____ *Breast total*

Cervical Cancer[a] (women only)

1. _____ Age group
   a. younger than 25 (10)
   b. 25 to 39 (20)
   c. 40 to 54 (30)
   d. 55 and older (30)

2. _____ Race/ethnicity
   a. Asian (10)
   b. Puerto Rican (20)
   c. African American (20)
   d. White (10)
   e. Mexican American (20)

3. _____ Number of pregnancies
   a. 0 (10)
   b. 1 to 3 (20)
   c. 4 or more (30)

4. _____ Viral infections
   a. herpes and other viral infections or
      ulcer formations on the vagina (10)
   b. never (1)

5. _____ Age at first intercourse
   a. younger than 15 (40)
   b. 15 to 19 (30)

   c. 20 to 24 (20)
   d. 25 or older (10)
   e. never (5)

6. _____ Bleeding between periods or
      after intercourse
   a. yes (40)
   b. no (1)

_____ *Cervical total*

[a]Lower portion of uterus. These questions do not apply to women who
have had total hysterectomies.

Endometrial Cancer[b] (women only)

1. _____ Age group
   a. 39 or younger (5)
   b. 40 to 49 (20)
   c. 50 and older (60)

2. _____ Race/ethnicity
   a. Asian (10)
   b. African American (10)
   c. White (20)
   d. Mexican American (10)

3. _____ Births
   a. None (15)
   b. 1 to 4 (7)
   c. 5 or more (5)

4. _____ Weight
   a. 50 or more pounds overweight (50)
   b. 20 to 49 pounds overweight (15)
   c. underweight for height (10)
   d. normal (10)

5. _____ Diabetes
   a. yes (3)
   b. no (1)

6. _____ Estrogen hormone intake
   a. yes, regularly (15)
   b. yes, occasionally (12)
   c. none (10)

7. _____ Abnormal uterine bleeding
   a. yes (40)
   b. no (1)

8. _____ Hypertension
   a. yes (3)
   b. no (1)

_____ *Endometrial total*

[b]Body of uterus. These questions do not apply to women who have had
total hysterectomies.

Analyze Yourself (continued)

Analysis of Results

Lung

1. Men have a higher risk of lung cancer than women do given the same type, amount, and duration of smoking. Because more women are smoking cigarettes for a longer duration than they did previously, their incidence of lung and upper respiratory tract (mouth, tongue, and larynx) cancer is increasing.

2. The occurrence of lung and upper respiratory tract cancer increases with age.

3 Cigarette smokers have up to 20 times or even greater risk than nonsmokers do, but the rates for ex-smokers who have not smoked for 10 years approach those of nonsmokers.

4. Pipe and cigar smokers are at higher risk for lung cancer than nonsmokers are. Cigarette smokers are at much higher risk than nonsmokers or pipe and cigar smokers are. All forms of tobacco use, including chewing, markedly increase the user's risk of developing cancer of the mouth.

5. Male smokers of less than one-half pack per day have lung cancer rates 5 times higher than those of nonsmokers. Male smokers of one to two packs per day have lung cancer rates 15 times higher than those of nonsmokers. Smokers of more than two packs per day are 20 times more likely to develop lung cancer than nonsmokers are.

6. Smokers of low tar and low nicotine cigarettes have slightly lower lung cancer rates.

7. The frequency of lung and upper respiratory tract cancer increases with the duration of smoking.

8. Exposure to materials used in these industries has been demonstrated to be associated with lung cancer. Smokers who work in these industries may have greatly increased risks. Exposure to materials in other industries may also carry a higher risk.

Lung total:

24 or less   You have low risk for lung cancer.
25 to 49   You may be a light smoker and would have a good chance of kicking the habit.
50 to 74   As a moderate smoker your risks of lung and upper respiratory tract cancer are increased. If you stop smoking now, these risks will decrease.
75 or more   As a heavy cigarette smoker your chances of getting lung and upper respiratory tract cancer are greatly increased. Your best bet is to stop smoking now—for the health of it. See your doctor if you have a nagging cough, hoarseness, persistent pain, or a sore in the mouth or throat.

Colon-Rectal

1. Colon cancer occurs more frequently after the age of 50.

2. Colon cancer is more common in families with a previous history of this disease.

3. Polyps and bowel diseases are associated with colon cancer.

4. Rectal bleeding may be a sign of colorectal cancer.

Colon total:

29 or less   You are at low risk for colon-rectal cancer.
30 to 69   This is a moderate-risk category. Testing by your physician may be indicated.
70 or more   This is a high-risk category. You should see your physician for the following tests: digital rectal exam, guaiac slide test, and proctoscopic exam.

Skin

1. Excessive ultraviolet light causes cancer of the skin. Protect yourself with sunscreen medication.

2. These materials can cause cancer of the skin.

3. People with light complexion need more protection than others do.

Skin total:

Numerical risks for skin cancer are difficult to state. For instance, a person with a dark complexion can work longer in the sun and be less likely to develop cancer than a light-complected person can. Furthermore, a person wearing a long-sleeve shirt and wide-brimmed hat may work in the sun and be less at risk than a person who wears a bathing suit for only a short period. The risk goes up greatly with age.

The key here is whether you answer yes to any question. If so, you need to protect your skin from the sun and any toxic materials. Changes in moles, warts, or skin sores are important, and your doctor should see them.

Breast

Breast total:

100 or less   Low-risk women should practice monthly breast self-examination and have a doctor examine their breasts as part of a cancer-related checkup.
100 to 199   Moderate-risk women should practice monthly breast self-examination and have a doctor examine their breasts as part of a cancer-related checkup. Your doctor may advise periodic breast x rays.
200 or more   High-risk women should practice monthly breast self-examination and have a doctor examine their breasts as part of a cancer-related checkup. See your doctor for the recommended (frequency of breast physical examinations or x ray) examinations related to you.

(continued)

Analyze Yourself *(continued)*

Cervical

1. The highest occurrence is in the 40 and over age group. The numbers represent the relative rates of cancer for different age groups. A 45-year-old woman has a risk three times higher than a 20-year-old does.

2. Puerto Ricans, Blacks, and Mexican Americans have higher rates of cervical cancer.

3. Women who have delivered more children have higher rates of occurrence.

4. Viral infections of the cervix and vagina are associated with cervical cancer.

5. Women with earlier intercourse and with a greater number of sexual partners are at higher risk.

6. Irregular bleeding may be a sign of uterine cancer.

Cervical total:

40 to 69 This is a low-risk group. Ask your doctor for a Pap test. You will be advised how often you should be tested after your first test.

70 to 99 In this moderate-risk group, more frequent Pap tests may be required.

100 or more You are in a high-risk group and should have a Pap test (and pelvic exam) as advised by your doctor.

Endometrial

1. Endometrial cancer occurs in those in older age groups. The numbers by the age groups represent relative rates of endometrial cancer at different ages. A 50-year-old woman has a risk 12 times greater than a 35-year-old woman does.

2. Caucasians have a higher occurrence.

3. The fewer children one has delivered, the greater the risk of endometrial cancer.

4. Overweight women are at greater risk.

5. Cancer of the endometrium is associated with diabetes.

6. Cancer of the endometrium may be associated with prolonged continuous estrogen hormone intake. This circumstance occurs in only a small number of women. You should consult your physician before starting or stopping any estrogen medication.

7. Women who do not have cyclic regular menstrual periods are at greater risk.

8. Cancer of the endometrium is associated with high blood pressure.

Endometrial total:

45 to 59 You are at very low risk for developing endometrial cancer.

60 to 99 Your risks are slightly higher. Report any abnormal bleeding immediately to your doctor. Tissue sampling at menopause is recommended.

100 or more Your risks are much greater. See your doctor for tests as appropriate.

Source Unknown

From *Physical fitness and wellness, third edition,* by Jerrold S. Greenberg, George B. Dintiman, and Barbee Myers Oakes, 2004, Champaign, IL: Human Kinetics.

Heart Disease

One of the authors of this book recently moved into a new house and has experienced an extremely frustrating situation. Every few weeks the faucets have to be dismantled to clean out debris. The builder says that this is normal in a new house—that lead and material from inside the pipes accumulate and clog the faucets.

The situation with the faucets is analogous to what happens in the body's fluid system, which includes the heart, the blood, and the blood vessels. As the faucets carry water to where it is needed, so the blood vessels carry blood to where it is needed. As the pumping station somewhere in town pumps the water, so the heart pumps the blood. And as pipes can become clogged with debris, so too can blood vessels.

How the Heart Functions

The main function of the heart is to pump blood containing oxygen and nutrients to various parts of the body. The heart also receives blood filled with waste products (such as carbon dioxide) that it pumps into the lungs for elimination through breathing. If blood vessels become obstructed or rupture, thereby interfering with the passage of oxygenated blood, the part of the body deprived of blood can die. And if the heart's blood supply itself is blocked, it too can die. That is what happens when a heart attack occurs. Because the arteries supplying the heart are called the coronary arteries, any problem with them is called either **coronary heart disease (CHD)** or coronary artery disease.

Cardiovascular Heart Disease (CVD)

Cardiovascular disease (CVD), generally referred to as heart disease, is the leading cause of death and disability among adults in America today. In 1998 nearly 1 million people died from heart disease, accounting for 41% of all U.S. deaths. Estimates are that nearly 60 million Americans have one or more types of CVD. Recent studies show that heart disease imposed a high economic burden. In 2001 the economic cost of heart disease was $298 billion. In addition, the annual medical costs incurred by individuals with heart disease were generally more than twice the costs for people without CVD. Therefore, decreasing the economic burden of heart disease is of immense public health significance (Wang et al., 2002).

Some people are born with heart disease. They may be missing a heart chamber or have one that is malformed, have a valve between the chambers of the heart that does not open or close adequately, or have a weak heart that is unable to pump with enough power to expel sufficient amounts of blood throughout the body. Others may have blood vessels that do not work normally because they are malformed. Still others may have heart disease because they have had rheumatic fever (which affects the heart valves), or they may experience an irregular heartbeat known as an arrhythmia.

coronary heart disease (CHD)—A condition in which the heart is supplied with insufficient blood due to clogging of coronary arteries

occluded—Clogged arteries that no longer allow the normal amount of blood to pass through them.

plaque—A collection of blood fats and other substances that combine to clog blood vessels.

atherosclerosis—A condition in which plaque has formed and blocks the passage of blood through a blood vessel.

Coronary Heart Disease (CHD)

The most prevalent form of heart disease is CHD. The coronary arteries can become obstructed, or **occluded,** when blood fats and other substances collect on their inside walls, thereby narrowing the opening through which blood can flow (see figure 14.1). This collection of blood fats and other substances can also break loose and travel through the arteries until they catch somewhere and block the flow of blood at that point. That blockage is called a thrombosis. The clogging material is called **plaque,** and the condition is known as **atherosclerosis.** Plaque consists of fatty substances, cholesterol, cellular waste products,

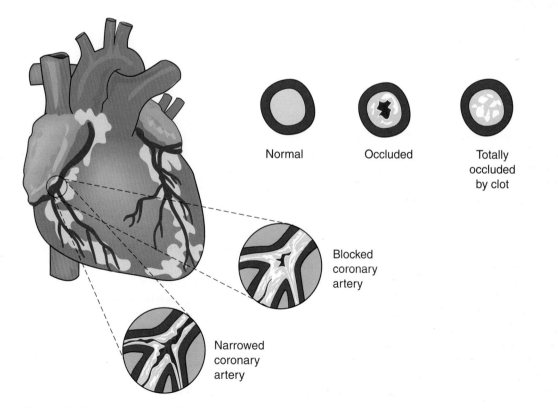

Normal

Occluded

Totally occluded by clot

Blocked coronary artery

Narrowed coronary artery

Figure 14.1 Coronary artery blockage.

calcium, and the clotting material fibrin. If blood flow is restricted, a person can become fatigued easily and may feel **angina pectoris** when active. If the coronary arteries are so narrowed or blocked that little if any blood can pass through, the part of the heart deprived of oxygenated blood can die. If that part is important or involves a large enough section of the heart, the person to whom this happens can die.

An estimated 7 million Americans suffer from CHD, the number one killer of both men and women in the United States annually. Each year, more than 500,000 Americans die of heart attacks caused by CHD. African American men and women, as well as people of other ethnic minority groups, are increasingly recognized as being at greater risk for CHD. In 2000 the National Center for Health Statistics reported an overall age-adjusted death rate per 100,000 persons for diseases of the heart among African American men of 407. The corresponding figure was 338 for Caucasian men, 219 for Native American men, 213 for Hispanic men, and 198 for Asian American men. In comparison, the heart-disease death rate for African American women was 292. The corresponding figure was 220 for Caucasian women, 146 for Hispanic women, 138 for Native American women, and 121 for Asian American women. Although the overall mortality rates for women are less than they are for men in each racial category, heart disease has also emerged as the number one cause of death among women. Based on several scientific studies, rates of heart disease and its risk factors appear to be increasing in Native American populations, but these changes have received little documentation (Sewell et al., 2002). These data validate the necessity of deepening our understanding of the underlying factors that place special groups at risk to guide us in designing interventions that explicitly address their needs.

Fat and Cholesterol

Lipoproteins consist of **triglycerides,** a blood protein (to make the fat soluble in the portion of the blood that is water), and cholesterol. Although some people are suspicious of the role of triglycerides in causing CHD, researchers have found no clear-cut association between the two. The real culprit in CHD is the cholesterol found in the foods we eat and the cholesterol manufactured by the liver. When we eat foods high in saturated fats, the liver is stimulated to manufacture cholesterol. Add that to the cholesterol in the foods of animal origin that we eat, and the amount in our blood can be excessive. The recommended daily consumption of cholesterol is 300 milligrams, but the average person in the United States consumes 1.5 to 3 times that amount. The recommended amount of saturated fat to be consumed daily is 10% of total calories. The average person in the United States consumes over three times that amount. No wonder heart disease is the leading cause of death in the United States.

Low-Density and High-Density Lipoproteins (LDLs and HDLs)

Of the several different kinds of lipoproteins, **low-density lipoproteins (LDLs)** and **high-density lipoproteins (HDLs)** have the most significance for CHD. LDLs are produced in the liver and released into the bloodstream, where they carry cholesterol to cells throughout the body. Cholesterol helps form cell membranes and the covering that protects nerve fibers; aids in the formation of vitamin D and the sex hormones androgen, estrogen, and progesterone; and helps produce bile salts that aid in digestion of fats. When LDLs carry more cholesterol than the body requires, however, they can build up on the artery walls.

HDLs are also produced by the liver and released into the bloodstream. Although they also carry cholesterol, HDLs pick up unused cholesterol and return it to the liver, where it is used to produce bile salts. In addition, it is thought that HDLs provide a protective layer to help prevent buildup of substances on artery walls.

When LDL is elevated and HDL is too sparse, arteries will likely become clogged and CHD will be promoted. HDL (the good cholesterol) levels should exceed 35 for adult men and 45 for adult women, and LDL (the bad cholesterol) levels should remain below 165. A total cholesterol-to-HDL ratio of 5 to 1 (20% of total cholesterol being of the HDL variety) begins to provide some protection from CHD. Physical activity can increase HDL levels in the bloodstream, which is one reason that exercise is recommended as a way of preventing CHD.

Other Risk Factors for Heart Disease

You already know that the foods we eat and the cholesterol our bodies produce can cause our blood vessels to become clogged. Several other conditions can cause clogged coronary arteries and the development of heart disease.

Hypertension

Hypertension is systolic blood pressure in excess of 140 millimeters Hg or diastolic blood pressure

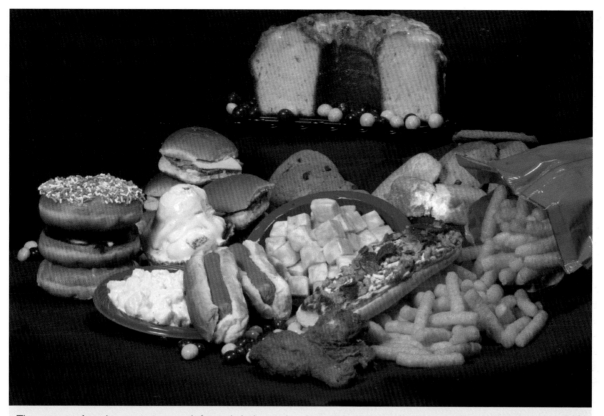

The average American eats too much fat and cholesterol, substances that contribute to both heart disease and cancer.

in excess of 90 millimeters Hg. **Systolic blood pressure** refers to the force of the blood against the arterial blood-vessel walls when the left ventricle contracts and blood is pumped out of the heart. **Diastolic blood pressure** represents the force of the blood against the arterial walls when the heart is relaxed. High blood pressure forces the heart to work harder than normal and places the arteries under stain. Eventually, hypertension contributes to heart attacks, strokes, and atherosclerosis. In 90% of high-blood-pressure essential hypertension cases, the causes are unknown. In the remaining 10%, a kidney abnormality, a tumor of the adrenal gland, or a congenital defect of the aorta (the main artery leading out of the heart) is the cause. Regular physical activity and a healthier diet are often recommended for people whose blood pressure is too high. In some cases, medication is needed to reduce blood pressure to healthier levels.

Obesity or Overweight

Excess weight places added strain on the heart and increases blood pressure and blood cholesterol. For those reasons, people who gain more than 20 pounds from what they weighed at age 18 double their risk of experiencing a heart attack.

angina pectoris—Chest pain caused by restricted blood flow to the heart.

lipoproteins—A substance consisting of lipids and proteins that travels through the blood system transporting triglycerides and cholesterol.

triglyceride—A blood protein in lipoproteins that makes fat soluble in the portion of the blood that is water.

low-density lipoproteins (LDLs)—Fatty particles in the blood that carry cholesterol to cells throughout the body.

high-density lipoproteins (HDLs)—Fatty particles in the blood that pick up unused cholesterol and transport it for processing and elimination from the body.

hypertension—High blood pressure, usually greater than 140 systolic blood pressure or greater than 90 diastolic blood pressure.

systolic blood pressure—The force of the blood against the arterial blood-vessel walls when the left ventricle contracts and blood is pumped out of the heart.

diastolic blood pressure—The force of the blood against the arterial walls when the heart is relaxed.

In addition, obesity is linked to diabetes and is usually associated with lack of physical activity, thereby further increasing the risk of heart attack.

Stress

Excessive stress also increases a person's chances of contracting heart disease because stress results in an increase in cholesterol in the blood, an increase in heart rate, higher blood pressure, and other effects detrimental to normal heart functioning. Stress results in the release of hormones called catecholamines, which prepare the body to respond physically (the fight-or-flight response). The heart beats faster, blood pressure increases, and blood-glucose and cholesterol levels increase. If stress occurs often, these detrimental effects become chronic and can lead to CHD. See chapter 12 for a more detailed description of the role of stress in the development of CHD.

Two researchers (Friedman and Rosenman, 1974) have even found a coronary-prone personality type. They call it the type A behavior pattern, characterized by being focused on time (hurried and time pressured), competitive, aggressive, hostile, and polyphasic (doing two or more things at a time). The opposite pattern, type B behavior, seems to protect people from developing CHD (see chapter 12). Recent research indicates that hostility is the major ingredient in the type A behavior pattern. That is, people who are easily angered and who are often hostile are the most susceptible to CHD. Stress also frequently interferes with people engaging in regular exercise. They become so concerned with managing the source of the stress—whether that be their classes, jobs, finances, or home lives—that they allow too little time, if any, for physical activity.

Sedentary Lifestyle

We have just discussed the effect of stress on physical activity. In addition, a sedentary lifestyle does not allow for the production of sufficient HDLs, does not strengthen the heart muscle, and cannot help control mild hypertension. To make matters worse, inactivity is associated with overweight and obesity, two other risk factors for CHD. Moreover, inactivity deprives people of an outlet for the release of built-up stress by-products (for example, cholesterol).

Smoking Tobacco

Research has linked smoking with various diseases such as cancer, emphysema, and heart disease. When a person smokes, the blood vessels constrict, thereby causing increased blood pressure. In addition, the heart speeds up in response to nicotine, a central nervous system stimulant. Furthermore, cigarettes contain substances that can damage the inside walls of the arteries. Once the walls have been damaged, cholesterol and other substances can more readily adhere to them and accumulate in the arteries. All this, coupled with the replacement of oxygen in the bloodstream by carbon dioxide from cigarette smoke, means that the heart is working too hard and that heart disease is more likely.

Family History

Not all risk factors are amenable to change. Heredity, for example, is not. Some people are born with a predisposition to heart disease. But that predisposition only means that a person has the potential to develop CHD—lifestyle will influence whether and when that happens. Some people prefer to use a family history of heart disease as an excuse of behaving in ways that are unhealthy for the heart. That choice is unfortunate because they might be able to delay or even prevent CHD if they change their behavior.

How to Prevent Coronary Heart Disease (CHD)

People can manage many of the risk factors for CHD. People can control hypertension by some combination of diet, exercise, and medication. Diet and exercise can control excess weight or obesity. A change in lifestyle and some form of regular relaxation can allow people to manage stress. Participation in an exercise program will remedy a sedentary lifestyle. People can stop smoking by joining a smoking-cessation program or by quitting cold turkey. Periodic medical screenings can be useful in analyzing blood lipids and evaluating heart function. The good news is that you have a great deal of influence over whether you develop CHD. If you are serious about preventing CHD, you can do so.

Role of Physical Activity

Physical activity is one of the most important components of a CHD-prevention program. Exercise is related either directly or indirectly to many of the risk factors. Physical activity exercises the heart muscle, encourages the production of HDLs, and aids in the control and prevention of mild hypertension. It enhances cardiorespiratory endurance and increases stroke volume of the heart (the amount of blood pumped out of the

Myth and Fact Sheet

Myth	Fact
1. If CHD runs in your family, you cannot do much to prevent getting it.	**1.** CHD is related to a number of factors, of which heredity is but one. Other risk factors include smoking, lack of exercise, fatty diets, obesity, and high blood pressure. You can do much to eliminate or diminish the effects of these risk factors.
2. All cholesterol is bad.	**2.** The cholesterol that accumulates on the walls of the arteries, LDL, is bad for you. HDLs, however, help to carry blood fats out of the body and therefore are helpful.
3. You can recognize whether your blood pressure is high, but you can do little to lower it.	**3.** High blood pressure occurs without any noticeable symptoms, but with a healthier diet and regular physical activity, you can lower blood pressure, even without medication.
4. Everything causes cancer.	**4.** This statement is simply not true. Although cancer can result from toxins, carcinogens in cigarette smoke, chemicals, and viruses, saying that everything causes cancer is merely an excuse for ignoring specific causes.
5. Cancer affects all groups of people to the same extent.	**5.** African American men and women have a higher cancer death rate than do White men and women. And White men and women contract skin cancer to a much greater extent than do African American men and women.

heart with each contraction). Exercise is also an excellent stress-management technique because it uses the stress by-products that prepare the body to respond physically to a stressor. And physical activity can help you maintain desirable weight and proper amount of lean-body mass.

These effects are direct and obvious, but physical activity offers less direct and less obvious CHD-related benefits as well. Engaging in regular exercise will tone your body, provide you with confidence in your ability to perform physically, and make you feel better about yourself. In short, exercise will improve your self-esteem. You will have less stress, produce fewer catecholamines, and therefore do less damage to your heart.

Physical activity also encourages smoking cessation. Smoking is incompatible with aerobic activity because carbon monoxide replaces oxygen in the bloodstream. Furthermore, doing one good thing for your health, such as becoming physically fit, encourages other healthy lifestyle adjustments.

For these and other reasons, an effective CHD-prevention program includes a physical activity component. The influential American Heart Association (AHA) recognizes the importance of physical activity in preventing CHD. In 1992 the

Committee on Exercise and Cardiac Rehabilitation of the Council on Clinical Cardiology of the AHA published a position paper titled Statement on Exercise: Benefits and Recommendations for Physical Activity Programs for All Americans. That AHA statement serves as a good summary of the role physical activity can play in preventing and treating CHD. In it, the AHA states the following:

> Exercise helps control blood abnormalities, diabetes, and obesity. . . . Inactivity is a risk factor for the development of coronary artery disease. . . . There is also evidence that physical activity probably alleviates symptoms of mild and moderate depression and provides an alternative to alcoholism and drug abuse.

The AHA goes on to suggest specific activities that are most beneficial:

> Activities such as walking, hiking, stair-climbing, aerobic exercise, calisthenics, jogging, running, bicycling, rowing, and swimming and sports such as tennis, racquetball, soccer, basketball, and touch football are especially beneficial when performed regularly. Brisk walking is also an excellent choice. . . . The evidence also supports the notion that even low-intensity activities performed daily can have

some long-term health benefits and lower the risk of cardiovascular disease. Such activities include walking for pleasure, gardening, yard work, housework, dancing, and prescribed home exercise.

Cancer

Cancer is a disease involving abnormal cell growth. Cells grow wildly, divide rapidly, and assume irregular shapes. Tumors develop and invade nearby normal tissue. These abnormal cells can spread to other parts of the body through the bloodstream and lymphatic system in a process called **metastasis.** The result can be disability or death (see tables 14.1 and 14.2).

Cancer is the second-leading cause of death in the United States. Lung cancer is by far the leading cause of death from cancer in both men and women, but that need not be the case. If everyone who now smokes cigarettes would

quit, the incidence of lung cancer would decline dramatically.

A comparison of cancer rates among racial and ethnic groups reveals that African Americans are more likely to develop and die from cancer than are people from any other minority group. From 1992 to 1998, the average incidence rate per 100,000 individuals for all cancer sites was 445 among African Americans, 401 for Caucasians, 283 for Asian Americans, 270 for Hispanics, and 203 for Native Americans. Furthermore, the mortality rate for all cancers combined is about 33% higher in African Americans than it is in their White counterparts (American Cancer Society, 2002). Although these rates are disproportionately high, the incidence and mortality rates from all cancers combined decreased more among African American men than they did in other ethnic minority groups between 1992 and 1998. This decline is partially due to an emerging body of research that has resulted in a growing understanding of the underlying factors affecting the risk of cancer mortality.

Cancer is more than one disease. Some cancers are caused by chemicals, others by environmental pollutants, some by radiation from the sun,

TABLE 14.1—Estimated Cancer Incidence in the United States, by Site and Gender

MALES		FEMALES	
New cases	Type	New cases	Type
11,000	Liver	12,700	Kidney
13,300	Stomach	13,000	Uterus, cervix
14,700	Pancreas	13,200	Leukemia
17,600	Leukemia	15,000	Bladder
18,900	Oral	15,600	Pancreas
19,100	Kidney	18,400	Rectum
22,600	Rectum	23,300	Ovary
30,100	Melanoma of skin	23,500	Melanoma of skin
31,900	Lymphoma	29,000	Lymphoma
41,500	Bladder	39,300	Uterus, body
50,000	Colon	57,300	Colon
90,200	Lung and bronchus	79,200	Lung
189,000	Prostate	203,500	Breast

TABLE 14.2—Estimated Cancer Deaths in the United States, by Site and Gender

MALES		FEMALES	
Deaths	Type	Deaths	Type
7,200	Brain	5,200	Liver
7,200	Kidney	5,200	Stomach
7,200	Stomach	5,300	Multiple myeloma
8,600	Bladder	5,900	Brain
8,900	Liver	6,600	Uterus, body
9,600	Esophagus	9,600	Leukemia
12,100	Leukemia	12,300	Lymphoma
13,500	Lymphoma	13,900	Ovary
14,500	Pancreas	15,200	Pancreas
23,100	Colon	25,000	Colon
30,200	Prostate	39,600	Breast
89,200	Lung	65,700	Lung

and still others by viruses. As we have already discussed, cancers also occur in different parts of the body. Even the treatment for different cancers varies. In some cases, surgery is necessary to remove the cancerous tissue. Sometimes, radiation or chemotherapy is required. Often, a combination of these three treatments is used.

Causes of Cancer

Cancer develops from a number of causes. By far the leading cause of cancer is the use of tobacco. About 75% of all lung cancer cases are thought to be caused by smoking cigarettes. Smoking a pipe or cigar or chewing tobacco can cause cancer of the mouth and its parts. The use of tobacco products is associated with cancer of the larynx, pharynx, esophagus, pancreas, and bladder.

High-fat diets are associated with cancer of the colon, rectum, prostate, stomach, and breast. Conversely, diets low in fat but high in fruits and vegetables seem to offer protection against certain cancers.

Repeated exposure to the sun is a cause of skin cancer. Radiation from the sun is the culprit here. Particularly vulnerable are people with fair skin who burn easily.

Excessive use of alcohol exposes one to the risk of oral cancer and cancers of the larynx, throat, esophagus, and liver, especially when accompanied by the use of smokeless tobacco.

Other causes of cancers include occupational hazards, such as exposure to toxins, chemicals, or other **carcinogens,** viruses, obesity, environmental pollutants (such as those contained in automobile exhaust), and hereditary and genetic factors.

Breast cancer, the most common cancer among women, is attributed to genetic susceptibility in only 5 to 10% of the cases. Hence, most cases of this disease are probably related to potentially modifiable lifestyle or environmental factors such as dietary folate intake, alcohol consumption, and physical inactivity. Defining exactly which factors affect the risk of breast or any other type of cancer is difficult because many differences exist in the prevalence, onset, causes, and mortality rates among ethnic minority and Caucasian individuals. For example, African American women have an earlier age of breast cancer onset and higher mortality rates than Caucasian women do, a circumstance not entirely explained by socioeconomic factors (Sauter et al., 2002). Mexican-descent women also have a

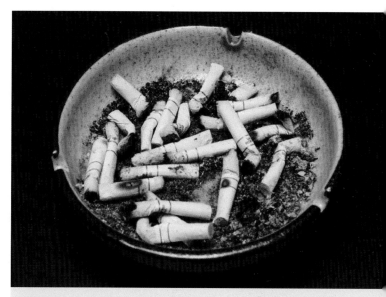

Cigarette smoking is a major reason for the high incidence of lung cancer in the United States.

PhotoDisc

> **metastasis**—The process in which cancerous cells from one part of the body travel to other parts of the body.
>
> **carcinogens**—Agents (toxins, chemicals, and so forth) that can cause cancer.

particularly high risk of late-stage breast cancer diagnosis, but they are also the least likely of the major U.S. Hispanic subgroups to undergo breast cancer screening (Wenten et al., 2002; Borrayo and Jenkins, 2001). In contrast, we also know that the incidence of breast cancer in Arab women is low compared with the rate in Western populations in other countries (Aghassi-Ippen et al., 2002).

Cancer Prevention

Although not all cancers can be prevented, in excess of 80% probably can be. If people gave up smoking, ate diets consisting of less fat and more vegetables and fruits, limited the amount of alcohol they ingested, and protected themselves from exposure to the sun, the decrease in the incidence of cancer would be significant. Here are some things you can do to decrease your chances of contracting cancer or, if you do contract it, to detect it early:

- Abstain from using tobacco in any form, including the smokeless variety.

- Eliminate or reduce your consumption of alcohol; drink only in moderation.
- Avoid contact with known carcinogens whenever possible.
- Decrease your exposure to the sun, avoid sunbathing for long periods, and use sunscreen with the appropriate sun protection factor (SPF) for your skin type any time you plan to be in the sun.

- Follow a dietary plan that increases your consumption of vitamins A and C, cruciferous vegetables (for example, cauliflower and broccoli), and fiber. Reduce your consumption of artificial sweeteners, heat-charred food, nitrite-cured or smoked foods, fats, and calories.
- Maintain recommended body weight and fat.
- Obtain cancer screenings as recommended (see table 14.3) to identify early signs of cancer.

TABLE 14.3—Summary of American Cancer Society Recommendations for Early Detection of Cancer in Asymptomatic People

Site	Recommendation
Breast	Women age 40 and older should have an annual mammogram, an annual clinical breast examination (CBE) by a health care professional, and should perform monthly breast self-examination (BSE). Ideally, the CBE should occur before the scheduled mammogram. Women ages 20 to 39 should have a CBE by a health care professional every 3 years and should perform BSE monthly.
Colon and rectum	Beginning at age 50, men and women should follow one of the following examination schedules: • A fecal occult blood test (FOBT) every year. • A flexible sigmoidoscopy (FSIG) every 5 years. • Annual fecal occult blood test and flexible sigmoidoscopy every 5 years. Combined testing is preferred over either annual FOBT or FSIG every 5 years, alone. People who are at moderate or high risk for colorectal cancer should talk with a doctor about a different testing schedule. • A double-contrast barium enema every 5 to 10 years. • A colonoscopy every 10 years.
Prostate	The PSA test and the digital rectal examination should be offered annually, beginning at age 50, to men who have a life expectancy of at least 10 more years. Men at high risk (African American men and men with a strong family history of one or more first-degree relatives diagnosed with prostate cancer at an early age) should begin testing at age 45. Patients should have information about what is known and what is uncertain about the benefits and limitations of early detection and treatment of prostate cancer so that they can make an informed decision.
Uterus	Cervix: All women who are or have been sexually active or who are 18 and older should have an annual Pap test and pelvic examination. After three or more consecutive satisfactory examinations with normal findings, the Pap test may be performed less frequently. Women should discuss the matter with their physicians. Endometrium: The American Cancer Society recommends that all women should be informed about the risks and symptoms of endometrial cancer and be encouraged to report any unexpected bleeding or spotting to their physicians. Annual screening for endometrial cancer with endometrial biopsy beginning at age 35 should be offered to women with or at risk for hereditary nonpolyposis colon cancer (HNPCC).
Cancer-related checkup	A cancer-related checkup is recommended every 3 years for people aged 20 to 39 years and every year for people age 40 and older. This exam should include health counseling and, depending on a person's age, might include examinations for cancers of the thyroid, oral cavity, skin, lymph nodes, testes, and ovaries, as well as for some nonmalignant diseases.

ACS guidelines for early cancer detection are assessed annually to identify whether new scientific evidence warrants reevaluation of current recommendations. If new evidence is sufficiently compelling to consider a change or clarification in a current guideline or the development of a new guideline, a formal procedure is initiated. Guidelines are formally evaluated every 5 years regardless of whether or not new evidence suggests a change in the existing recommendation. This procedure involves nine steps, and these "guidelines for guideline development" were formally established to provide a specific methodology for science and expert judgment to form the underpinnings of specific statements and recommendations from the ACS. These procedures constitute a deliberate process to ensure that all ACS recommendations have the same methodological and evidence-based process at their core. This process also employs a system for rating strength and consistency of evidence similar to the one employed by the Agency for Health Care Research and Quality (AHCRQ) and U.S. Preventive Services Task Force (USPSTF).

- Learn how to do breast (females) and testicular (males) self-examinations and do them regularly.
- Check for changes in your skin that might indicate skin cancer.
- Report any family history of cancer to your doctor and have that history noted on your medical records.

Table 14.4 summarizes the things you can do to prevent developing cancer.

Physical Activity and Cancer Prevention

Physical activity has been found to help prevent the onset of cancer. The exact reason for this is unclear, although researchers have proposed several theories. For example, some researchers attribute the decreased incidence of cancer among people who are physically active to their being leaner. Excess fat is associated with cancer of the colon, prostate, endometrium, and breast. Whether physical activity has a direct effect on cancer or an indirect effect by reducing body fat is unknown.

The National Cancer Institute also reports that men who exert the energy equivalent of walking 10 or more miles per week have half the risk of developing colon cancer of less active men. One theory explaining this finding is that exercise increases the rate of transit of food through the digestive tract. If carcinogens are present in the fecal stream, the faster they proceed through it, the less likely it is that they will attach them-

TABLE 14.4—Ways to Prevent Cancer

Recommendation	Notes
Do not smoke.	Cigarette smoking is responsible for 75% of all lung cancer cases. Smoking accounts for about 30% of all cancer deaths. Those who smoke two or more packs of cigarettes a day have lung cancer mortality rates 15 to 25 times greater than nonsmokers do.
Limit exposure to sunlight.	Almost all of the more than 600,000 cases of nonmelanoma skin cancer diagnosed each year in the United States are sun related. Recent epidemiological evidence shows that sun exposure is a major factor in the development of melanoma and that the incidence increases for those living near the equator.
Limit ingestion of alcohol.	Oral cancer and cancers of the larynx, throat, esophagus, and liver occur more frequently among heavy drinkers of alcohol.
Avoid smokeless tobacco.	Use of chewing tobacco or snuff increases risk of cancer of the mouth, larynx, throat, and esophagus and is highly habit forming.
Consult with physician regarding estrogen treatment.	For mature women, estrogen treatment to control menopausal symptoms increases risk of endometrial cancer and heart disease. Use of estrogen by menopausal women needs careful discussion between the woman and her physician.
Limit exposure to radiation.	Excessive exposure to ionizing radiation can increase cancer risk. Most medical and dental x rays are adjusted to deliver the lowest dose possible without sacrificing image quality. Excessive radon exposure in homes may increase risk of lung cancer, especially in cigarette smokers. If levels are found to be too high, remedial actions should be taken.
Limit exposure to occupational hazards.	Exposure to several different industrial agents (nickel, chromate, asbestos, vinyl chloride, and so forth) increases risk of various cancers. Risk from asbestos increases significantly when combined with cigarette smoking.
Eat well	Risk of colon, breast, and uterine cancers increases in obese people. High-fat diets may contribute to the development of cancers of the breast, colon, and prostate. High-fiber foods may help reduce risk of colon cancer. A varied diet containing plenty of vegetables and fruits rich in vitamins A and C may reduce risk for a wide range of cancers. Salt-cured, smoked, and nitrite-cured foods have been linked to esophageal and stomach cancer. Heavy use of alcohol, especially when accompanied by cigarette smoking or chewing tobacco, increases risk of cancers of the mouth, larynx, throat, esophagus, and liver.

selves to mucosa lining the tract and develop into cancer.

Mounting evidence shows that women who exercise regularly are less prone to develop cancer of the breast or of the reproductive system. The Black Women's Health Study (Adams-Campbell et al., 2001) suggests that strenuous physical activity in early adulthood is associated with a reduced risk of breast cancer among 64,524 African American women. Other studies have shown a similar protective effect of leisure-time physical activity among Hispanic and Caucasian women. One theory relates a lower rate of these cancers and exercise to the amount of body fat. The body needs fat to make estrogen. This theory hypothesizes that excess fat increases the risk of these cancers because it leads to the production of too much estrogen.

These findings pertain to moderate amounts of exercise and do not mean that intense exercise is also protective of cancer. Some researchers believe that intense exercise is detrimental because it suppresses the immune system, causing the body to be less able to ward off carcinogens. The discovery by researchers that prostate cancer is more common among male athletes lends credence to this theory.

The American Cancer Society reports that for "the majority of Americans who do not use tobacco, dietary choices and physical activity are the most important modifiable determinants of cancer risk" (American Cancer Society, 2002). As a result, ACS recommends the adoption of a physically active lifestyle to prevent cancer, among its other benefits. Adults are encouraged to engage in at least moderate activity for 30 minutes or more 5 or more days a week, and children and adolescents should engage in at least 60 minutes per day of moderate to vigorous physical activity at least 5 days a week. ACS further suggests that public, private, and community organizations work to create social and physical environments that encourage physical activity behaviors.

Early Detection and Diagnosis of Cancer

Despite the fact that cancer incidence and mortality rates are often highest among ethnic minorities, studies show that a disproportionate number of African American men and Hispanic women do not participate in prevention efforts that promote early screening and detection, particularly with respect to breast and prostate cancer. Studies also show that African American women are more likely to be diagnosed at a more advanced stage of breast cancer than are Caucasian women.

Many cancers are curable if they are detected early. For example, both breast and testicular cancer detected in their earliest stages are well over 90% curable. The later the cancer is detected, the less positive is the prognosis. For that reason, detecting cancer early is critical. Obtaining regular medical checkups is one way of assuring that cancers are found in their earliest stages. Table 14.3 lists recommended medical screenings. Performing regular self-examinations is another method of early detection. Two of the most frequently recommended self-examinations are of the breast for women and of the testicles for men.

Detecting Breast Cancer

The American Cancer Society stresses the early detection of breast cancer through the triad approach: mammography, clinical breast exams, and breast self-exams.

Mammography Mammography is especially valuable as an early detection tool because it can identify breast abnormalities that may be cancer at an early stage before physical symptoms develop.

Clinical Breast Exams Women between the ages of 20 and 39 should have a clinical breast exam every 3 years, and women ages 40 and older should have a breast exam by a health professional every year before their scheduled mammogram.

Breast Self-Exams Breast self-exam (BSE) allows a woman to become familiar with her own breasts and able to let her health care provider know whether she detects any changes. Women ages 20 and older should perform a BSE every month.

Detecting Testicular Cancer

Because men were not performing testicular self-examinations often enough or well enough, the American Cancer Society no longer recommends that men do them. Instead, they recommend that men obtain annual screenings from a physician.

Breast Self-Examination

If you regularly examine your breasts, you will probably notice any changes. The best time for breast self-examination (BSE) is about a week after your period ends, when your breasts are not tender or swollen. If you are not having regular periods, do BSE on the same day every month.

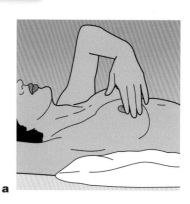

a

- Lie down with a pillow under your right shoulder and place your right arm behind your head (see figure 14.2a). Use the finger pads of the three middle fingers on your left hand to feel for lumps in the right breast. Press firmly enough to know how your breast feels. A firm ridge in the lower curve of each breast is normal.

- Move around the breast in an up and down line, a circular pattern, or a wedge pattern (figure 14.2b). Be sure to do it the same way every time, check the entire breast area, and remember how your breasts feel from month to month.

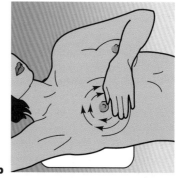

b

- Repeat the exam on your left breast, using the finger pads of the right hand. (Move the pillow to under your left shoulder.)

- Repeat the examination of both breasts while standing, with one arm behind your head (figure 14.2c). The upright position makes it easier to check the upper and outer part of the breasts (toward your armpit).

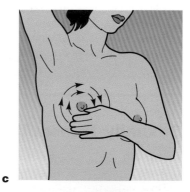

c

- For added safety you can check your breasts for any dimpling of the skin, changes in the nipple, redness, or swelling while standing in front of a mirror right after your BSE each month (figure 14.2d).

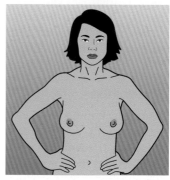

d

- If you find any changes, see your doctor.

Figure 14.2 Breast self-examination.

Testicular Self-Examination

Follow the instructions in the diagram carefully and examine your testes immediately after your next hot bath or shower. Heat causes the testicles to descend and the scrotal skin to relax, making it easier to find unusual lumps.

- Examine each testicle by placing the index and middle fingers of both hands on the underside of the testicle and the thumbs on the top. Gently roll the testicle between your thumb and fingers, feeling for small lumps (see figures 14.3, a and b).

- Changes or anything abnormal will appear at the front or side of your testicle. Did you find any unusual lumps? Are there any unusual signs of any kind? Are there any markings or lumps at any site?

- Keep in mind that not all lumps are signs of testicular cancer. Unusual lumps at any location, however, should be checked by a physician. Early detection greatly increases your chances of attaining a complete cure. Repeat the examination every month and record your findings.

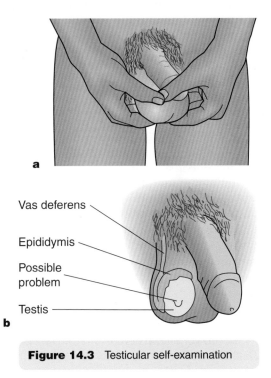

Figure 14.3   Testicular self-examination

Reprinted by permission of the American Cancer Society, Inc.

Sexually Transmitted Infections

Certain diseases can interfere with sexual activities. These used to be called venereal diseases (VD), named for Venus, the Roman goddess of love. Today, they are known less euphemistically as **sexually transmitted infections (STIs).** Although more than 20 organisms are linked to STIs, we discuss only the most prevalent STIs.

Gonorrhea

Popularly known as the "clap," the "drip," and many equally descriptive names, **gonorrhea** is caused by the Neisseria gonorrhoeae bacterium. Gonorrhea is increasing in incidence—more than 350,000 cases are reported in the United States each year, with the actual incidence estimated to be four times that amount—and is one of the most prevalent communicable diseases. The 2010 national health objective is to decrease new cases of gonorrhea from 132 per 100,000 population (1999) to 19 new cases per 100,000 population by 2010.

Gonorrhea is transmitted by intercourse and by oral-genital and anal-genital contact. Because the bacteria need the warmth and moisture provided by the mucous membranes of the vagina, mouth, or anus, it is unlikely (though not impossible) that a person could acquire gonorrhea from using someone else's towel or from sitting on a public toilet seat unless the bacteria has just been deposited there and the area is warm and moist. A male exposed to the bacteria through sexual intercourse has about a 20% chance of developing gonorrhea, whereas a female likewise exposed has about an 80% chance of contracting gonorrhea. The difference is due to the vaginal environment, which is conducive to the growth of the bacteria.

Effects of Gonorrhea

Gonorrhea affects the urogenital tract in both sexes: the urethra in males and the urethra, vagina, and cervix in females. The symptoms, however, are somewhat different in men and women. The early symptoms in men are a milky, bad-smelling discharge from the penis, feelings of urgently having to urinate, and a burning sensation when doing so. If untreated, the infection can cause swelling of the testicles and damage the prostate gland, ultimately resulting in sterility. Additional complications may include kidney and bladder damage.

Whereas infected men are usually aware something is wrong with them, women may not notice the early signs of gonorrhea. One reason for this is that the symptoms are similar to those in common vaginal infections: a slight burning sensation in the genital areas and a mild discharge from the vagina. An estimated 80% of women who have gonorrhea are unaware of it until the disease has become more severe. If left untreated, gonorrhea invades the uterus, fallopian tubes, and ovaries. Pelvic infection may result, causing sterility or requiring surgical removal of infected pelvic organs. An additional concern in women is that gonorrhea can be passed from an infected mother to her infant as it passes through the vaginal canal during delivery, often resulting in blindness. To prevent this from occurring, the eyes of newborns are routinely treated with drops of silver nitrate.

Treatment of Gonorrhea

Diagnosis of gonorrhea is not as simple as it is for some of the other STIs. Diagnosis requires laboratory examination of a sample taken from the infected area with a cotton swab or growing the bacteria under laboratory conditions. The disease usually responds to penicillin treatment. If the patient is allergic to penicillin, tetracycline drugs are used. Concern about penicillin-resistant strains of gonorrhea is growing, and researchers are attempting to develop other drugs that will effectively eradicate the disease.

Those treated for gonorrhea should return for a follow-up examination in about 10 days to be certain that the medication has been effective and that the infection has not reoccurred. During treatment, patients should abstain from sexual intercourse and other sexual activities that may transmit the bacteria.

Syphilis

Known in the past as the "great pox" or the "great impostor" because people thought it resembled smallpox, **syphilis** is now often referred to as just "the syph." Syphilis is caused by the Treponema pallidum, a corkscrewlike organism that resembles bacteria and that is part of a group of such organisms called spirochetes.

Because Treponema pallidum can survive only in the warmth and moisture provided by the mucous membranes of the human body, it quickly dies outside the body. For this reason, syphilis usually cannot be contracted from a toilet seat, unless the spirochete has been deposited there just before someone else with an open sore sits on the seat, the chances of which are extremely remote. Syphilis is transmitted during sexual intercourse, oral-genital or anal-genital contact, or by kissing a person who has a syphilitic sore in the mouth. These activities provide the spirochete with a route of entrance to the body.

In 1999 there were 6,657 cases of syphilis reported, a rate of 2.5 per 100,000 persons. This figure is the lowest number of cases reported since 1959. The 2010 national health objectives establish a target of 1 case per 100,000 by 2010.

Effects of Syphilis

The disease progresses through four stages. In stage 1 (primary stage) a painless sore, called a **chancre** (pronounced shanker), appears 3 to 4 weeks after the spirochete enters the body. The chancre looks like a pimple or wart and appears where the spirochete entered the body, often on the lips or the vaginal wall. Women may not notice the chancre, and men may ignore it because it is painless and disappears in a few weeks without treatment.

sexually transmitted infections (STIs)— Bacterial, viral, and parasitic diseases that are transmitted through sexual contact, which usually affect the genital area and may cause serious disease complications throughout the body.

gonorrhea—An STI caused by a bacterium. Although the disease can be treated with antibiotics, if left untreated it can lead to serious complications, including bladder and kidney disease and diseases of the pelvic and genital areas.

syphilis—A serious STI caused by a spirochete; untreated syphilis has serious complications and is eventually fatal. Treatment includes the use of antibiotics, but some strains of syphilis are resistant to treatment.

chancre—A painless sore on the penis, mouth, or anus or in the vagina where the spirochete that causes syphilis has entered the body.

Stage 2 (secondary stage) occurs about 6 weeks after contact. Symptoms may include a rash over the entire body, welts around the genitals, low-grade fever, headache, hair loss, and sore throat. These symptoms also disappear without treatment. If the symptoms are noticeable, however, most victims see a doctor at this time. Thus, it is uncommon for cases of syphilis in the United States to progress to the third stage.

Stage 3 (latency stage) begins about 2 years after contact (up to 5 years in some people). After a year, the victim cannot transmit the disease to anyone else. The only exception is that a pregnant woman can transmit the disease to her fetus through the placental wall. Latency may last 40 or more years. During this time, the organism infects and irreparably damages the heart, brain, and other organs. By stage 4 (tertiary stage), the disease may lead to heart failure, blindness, other organ damage, and finally death.

Treatment of Syphilis

A simple blood test can detect syphilis. Because it is such a potentially dangerous disease and can be transmitted to unborn babies, most states require a blood test for syphilis before marriage and, in pregnant women, during the prenatal period. Syphilis generally responds well to penicillin or, in some cases, to other antibiotics. Because no immunity develops to the disease, prompt diagnosis and treatment after any possible exposure are essential.

Syphilis passed from the mother to the fetus before birth is known as congenital syphilis. Until the 16th week of pregnancy, a membrane called Langhan's layer protects the fetus from spirochetes. After the 16th week, however, spirochetes can pass through the placental barrier and enter the fetus's bloodstream, causing birth defects, physical abnormalities, and mental retardation.

People who contract syphilis should refrain from all sexual activity that can transmit the spirochete. Treatment should also consist of follow-up examinations to determine whether antibiotics have been effective in eliminating the spirochete. As with gonorrhea and the other STIs, the disease-causing organism needs a route of entry into the body, so use of a condom can help prevent the spread of syphilis.

Genital Herpes

Herpes simplex viruses are of two types. Type 1 causes cold sores in the mouth, and type 2 causes **genital herpes.** Evidence is growing, however, that they are more related than previously thought. Genital herpes now rivals gonorrhea as one of the most prevalent STIs in the United States.

Genital herpes has been diagnosed in 45 million Americans. The 2010 national health objectives seek to reduce genital herpes from 17% of the population to 14% by 2010.

Effects of Herpes

Approximately 2 to 10 days after the virus enters the body, symptoms such as sores and swollen glands (around the groin), flulike symptoms (fever, muscle aches), and pain in the genital area during urination or intercourse may occur. Other symptoms may include fatigue, swelling of the legs, and watery eyes. The disease progresses through four stages:

1. Prodrome stage. An itching or tingling sensation **(prodrome)** develops near the site where the virus invaded the body, with the skin turning red and becoming sensitive. Prodrome is also an early symptom of a recurrent infection or outbreak.

2. Blister stage. A sore or cluster of sores appears; fever, swollen glands, and other symptoms may occur; and after 2 to 10 days, the sores break open (on future outbreaks, fever and swollen glands usually do not occur).

3. Healing stage. Sores shrink; scabs form; and pain, swollen glands, and fever subside (scabs fall off by the end of the 2nd week).

4. Inactive stage. The virus retreats to nearby nerve cells; stress and poor health may cause the virus to reemerge.

Because the virus remains dormant in the nerve cells, people can experience reoccurrences. These reoccurrences, however, are not as frequent as most people believe. Although some people may experience future outbreaks several times monthly, others may encounter them only rarely. Approximately one-third of those with the disease never have a reoccurrence, and another third have outbreaks only rarely. Furthermore, reoccurrences of herpes are usually shorter and less painful than the initial outbreak.

Herpes has potentially more harmful effects on women than it does on men. Women who have herpes genitalis are eight times more likely to develop cervical cancer than noninfected women are. In addition, a herpes-infected pregnant woman has a one in four chance of transmitting the infection to her infant during delivery, and the risks to the infant include death. Consequently, the recommended course of action for pregnant women with herpes is to obtain delivery by cesarean section (incision through the abdomen and uterus to remove the fetus rather than delivery through the vaginal canal).

Treatment of Herpes

Herpes is treated with the drug Acyclovir, which can relieve some symptoms and suppress reoccurrence of the disease. To prevent passing the virus to others, individuals with herpes should refrain from sex from the onset of the prodrome until sores have completely healed and should use a condom at other times.

Chlamydia

Caused by a viruslike bacterium called Chlamydia trachomatis, **chlamydia** is the most prevalent STI. Some estimate that 4 million new cases occur each year, with as many as 500,000 progressing to pelvic inflammatory disease. Others estimate that chlamydia is up to 10 times more prevalent than gonorrhea and may be present in as many as 4% of all pregnant women. Up to 10% of college students may be infected with chlamydia.

Officially, 659,441 new cases of chlamydia were reported in 1999. The 2010 national health objectives seek to reduce the rate of chlamydia from 254 cases per 100,000 population to 3 per 100,000 population by the year 2010.

Effects of Chlamydia

In women, chlamydia can cause infections in the vagina and pelvic inflammatory disease, which can lead to infertility. Symptoms include vaginal discharge, itching and burning of the vulva, and some discomfort when urinating. As many as 70% of female chlamydia infections go undetected, however, until more serious problems develop. As with other STIs, chlamydia can create problems during birth deliveries if the pregnant woman is infected. The newborn can contract conjunctivitis, an inflammation of the eye, during delivery, and blindness can result. Ointments containing tetracycline or erythromycin applied to the newborn's eyes can prevent these conditions.

In men, chlamydia can cause inflammation of the urinary and reproductive tracts and, in extreme circumstances, sterility. Symptoms include a mild burning sensation when urinating, followed by a thin, watery, clear discharge. Left untreated, it can lead to swelling of the testicles.

Treatment of Chlamydia

College health services can easily detect chlamydia with a simple culture test. Once detected, a weeklong administration of the antibiotic drug tetracycline provides effective treatment. As with other treatments consisting of antibiotics, finishing the entire dosage of the tetracycline is important; otherwise, the infection may reoccur and be more resistant to the drug than it was before.

Genital Warts

The result of a viral infection (human papillomavirus, or HPV), **genital warts** occur on most areas of the genitals and anus. In females, the warts typically appear in the lower area of the vagina. In males, they appear on the glans, foreskin (if not circumcised), and shaft of the penis and may appear in the anal area in some homosexual men. The incubation period for HPV is approximately 3 months after contact with an infected person. University health centers report that genital warts are quite prevalent among college students.

Estimates are that more than 20 million women in the United States have genital warts, with three-fourths of their sexual partners infected. Year 2010 national health objectives do not establish a target to reach by the end of the decade, but they specify the intention of reducing the proportion of persons with HPV.

genital herpes—An STI caused by the herpes simplex, type 2 virus. The disease is incurable. Carefully treated, it is not a serious disease, but its spread to the rest of the body can result in serious complications. Genital herpes has been linked to the onset of cervical cancer.

prodrome—An itching or tingling sensation that develops near the site where the herpes simplex, type 2 virus enters the body.

chlamydia—A common STI caused by a viruslike bacterium, it can lead to sterility, inflammation in the reproductive and urinary tracts, and pelvic inflammatory disease. Chlamydia is treated with antibiotics.

genital warts—An STI of the genital and perineal areas of both men and women caused by a virus; linked to increased incidence of cancer.

Effects of Genital Warts

Researchers have found that several strains of HPV are associated with the development of cervical cancer. This revelation has led to a more urgent need for prevention of what was previously thought to be a relatively benign STI.

Some lesions are moist, and some are dry. The moist lesions are the ones that respond well to treatment. Large warts should be biopsied for cancerous cell growth.

Diagnosis is made by the appearance of the warts. In the moist areas of the body, they tend to be white, pink, or white to gray. In the dry areas, they are usually yellow and yellow-gray.

Treatment of Genital Warts

The usual treatment is administration of the drug podophyllin, an irritant that causes the outer skin in the area containing the virus to slough off. Thus, the drug does not kill the virus but merely removes the infected tissue. The health practitioner applies podophyllin to each lesion and allows it to dry, and the patient then washes it off 4 hours later. Sometimes, an antibiotic ointment is prescribed as well to treat infection at the site and help keep the wart moist. The podophyllin is usually applied once a week for 5 or 6 weeks or for the time it takes to control the infection. Genital warts often reoccur after the first bout, however, even if treated. These reoccurrences can be experienced for several months or years until immunity develops. In some cases, warts are removed by laser surgery, electrosurgery, freezing with liquid hydrogen, or surgical incision.

Pelvic Inflammatory Disease

With the exception of AIDS, **pelvic inflammatory disease (PID)** is the most dangerous and the most difficult to diagnose of all the STIs affecting women because its symptoms may not be obvious until damage has occurred. Left untreated, PID can result in infertility and even death.

Eight percent of American women between the ages of 15 and 44 have required treatment for pelvic inflammatory disease. The national health objectives seek to reduce that to 5% by the year 2010.

Effects of Pelvic Inflammatory Disease

Symptoms of PID include abdominal pain or tenderness, pain during intercourse, increased menstrual cramps, profuse bleeding during menstruation, irregular menstrual cycles, vaginal bleeding at times other than when menstruating, lower-back pain, nausea, loss of appetite, vomiting, vaginal discharge, burning sensation during urination, chills, and fever. Unless PID is promptly diagnosed and treated, scar tissue forms inside the fallopian tubes. This scar tissue can result in infertility by blocking the tubes partially or totally, thereby preventing the egg from entering the uterus or the sperm from fertilizing the egg. Scar tissue also increases the risk of a tubal pregnancy (in which the fertilized egg becomes implanted inside the fallopian tube rather than the uterus).

Treatment of Pelvic Inflammatory Disease

Diagnosis of PID is based on medical and sexual history, a pelvic examination, and laboratory tests. Treatment is by administration of an antibiotic and is usually effective. Any structural damage done to pelvic organs, however, may be irreversible or, at the least, require extensive medical treatment.

HIV Infection and AIDS

Acquired immunodeficiency syndrome (AIDS) is a condition caused by infection with the **human immunodeficiency virus (HIV)**. AIDS is called a syndrome because it consists of a number of conditions resulting from a decrease in the ability of the body's immunological system to ward off infections and other threats to health. Among the manifestations of the syndrome are pneumonia, cancer, and other opportunistic infections (infections resulting from lowered resistance of a weakened immune system). HIV is transmitted through bodily fluids, predominantly blood, semen, and vaginal secretions. An infected pregnant woman can transmit HIV to her fetus. To infect someone, HIV must have a route of entry into the body. The most common ways HIV is transmitted are

pelvic inflammatory disease (PID)—An extremely serious STI for women. PID can lead to infertility, tubal pregnancy, and structural damage to pelvic organs.

acquired immunodeficiency syndrome (AIDS)—An STI that weakens the human immune system, leading to serious opportunistic diseases; fatal in the long run.

human immunodeficiency virus (HIV)—Virus transmitted primarily through sexual contact and intravenous drug use that weakens the immune system and often develops into full-blown AIDS.

through sex and use of intravenous drugs. Sexual intercourse, oral-genital sex, or anal intercourse in which bodily fluids are exchanged are particularly risky activities. Intravenous drug use with a shared needle may result in the direct deposit of HIV into the bloodstream.

Prevalence of HIV Infection and AIDS

The number of people infected with HIV and the number of people with AIDS keep increasing, so any figures we give you will soon be outdated. As of the beginning of 1996, the World Health Organization estimated that there were approximately 4.5 million cases of AIDS worldwide and an additional 18.5 million adults and 1.5 million children infected with HIV. In the United States, over three-quarters of a million AIDS cases have been reported to the Centers for Disease Control and Prevention (CDC). That total is larger than the population of the state of Wyoming or the city of Cleveland. As noted in figures 14.4 and 14.5, 46,208 adolescent and adult males and 17,228 females reported having AIDS or HIV in the year 2000. Of course, many more of

our fellow citizens are infected with HIV but have not yet developed AIDS.

Effects of HIV Infection

Once in the body, HIV invades the cells of the immune system, resulting in its becoming less effective over time. Increasing incapacity results, with death being inevitable. Symptoms include loss of appetite, weight loss, fever, night sweats, skin rash, diarrhea, tiredness, lack of resistance to infection, and swollen lymph glands. Among the common conditions of full-blown AIDS, which usually develops some 8 to 10 years after HIV infection, are Kaposi's sarcoma (a form of cancer of the blood vessels that can be evidenced by purple skin lesions), other cancers, pneumonia, and brain dementia.

Treatment of HIV Infection

Rather than testing for the presence of the virus itself, HIV infection is diagnosed with a blood test (called ELISA—enzyme-linked immunosorbent assay) that identifies the presence of antibodies

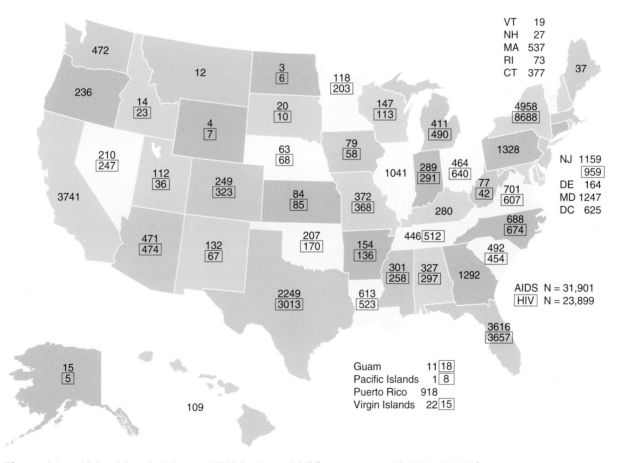

Figure 14.4 Male adult and adolescent HIV infection and AIDS cases reported in 2000, United States.

From Centers for Disease Control and Prevention, 2001, *HIV/AIDS Surveillance Report* 13(2).

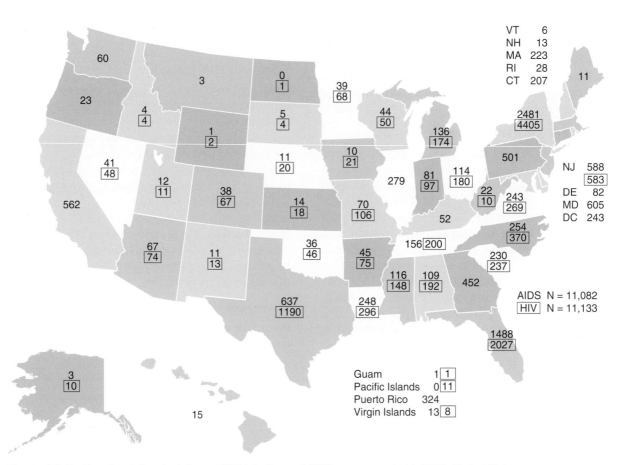

Figure 14.5 Female adult and adolescent HIV infection and AIDS cases reported in 2000, United States.

From Centers for Disease Control and Prevention, 2001, *HIV/AIDS Surveillance Report* 13(2).

that develop in response to HIV. If the test is positive for these antibodies, a more sophisticated test (Western blot) is administered to confirm this result. Anywhere from 3 to 8 months may be required, however, for enough of these antibodies to develop to be identifiable through the AIDS test. Consequently, someone may test negative even though he or she is infected. Furthermore, this person may still transmit the virus to other people.

Although HIV infection is incurable and usually results in death, some medications appear to be effective in prolonging the onset of debilitating symptoms. The most well-known of these drugs is AZT (azidothymidine). Recent studies have found that a combination of AZT with other drugs is most effective in prolonging symptom-free living among people infected with HIV.

A new generation of drugs has produced the most dramatic advancement in the fight against

AIDS to date. The three classes of antiretrovirus therapies are the following:

1. Mucleoside reverse transcriptase (such as zidovudine) that prevents HIV RNA from reproducing
2. Protease inhibitors (such as indinavir) that prevent HIV from replicating and invading T cells
3. Nonnecleoside transcriptase inhibitors (such as delavirdine) that prevent HIV from replicating by blocking reverse transcriptase directly

The result has been that many people with HIV infection have lived relatively long lives with what has come to be viewed as a chronic manageable condition. Yet the length of time that these medications remain effective is now part of the social experimentation phase in which we now find ourselves.

Ways of preventing HIV infection include abstaining from high-risk sexual activities, using a condom if sexually active, limiting the number of sexual partners, maintaining a monogamous relationship with someone who is HIV-free, and refraining from the use of intravenous drugs. For pregnant women who are HIV infected, the administration of AZT can dramatically decrease the risk of their babies being born infected. Therefore, if they have participated in high-risk behaviors (or even if they have not), they might want to have an AIDS test to determine whether AZT is warranted.

The resources in figure 14.6 can provide you with more information on AIDS and other STIs.

Other Diseases and Conditions

Prevention of several other diseases and conditions has also been associated with exercise, including diabetes, kidney disease, obesity, and hypertension.

Diabetes

Diabetes is a disease of the pancreas in which an insufficient amount of insulin is produced to make use of sugars and other carbohydrates in a normal way. The result is increased blood-glucose levels, which can lead to a number of other states of ill health. The sixth-leading cause of death in the United States, diabetes contributes to the development of heart disease, stroke, kidney failure, and blindness. Diabetes is the leading cause of new cases of blindness in adults ages 20 to 74. Each year 12,000 to 24,000 people lose their sight because of this disease. The risk of stroke and heart disease is two to four times higher in people with diabetes. About 60 to 70% of people with diabetes have mild to severe forms of dia-

betic nerve damage (which often includes reduced sensation or pain in the feet or hands and slowed digestion of food in the stomach). Severe forms of diabetic nerve damage can lead to amputation of the lower extremities. More than 86,000 amputations are performed annually among Americans with diabetes. The total annual cost for those amputations is over $1.1 billion (National Center for Health Statistics, 2001).

Diabetes affects African American men at a rate nearly 50% greater than that for Caucasian men. For African American women, the rate of diabetes is nearly 100% greater than that of their White counterparts. Collectively, African Americans experience higher rates of amputation than do Hispanics or Caucasians with diabetes. They are also 1.5 to 2.5 times more likely to have lower-limb amputations.

Diabetes affects Hispanics almost twice as frequently as it does non-Hispanic Whites. Yet the highest rate of diabetes occurs among Native Americans, who have a rate 2.8 times that of non-Hispanic Whites (Norris and Agodoa, 2002). Over the past few decades, the major disease burden faced by Native Americans arises from chronic illnesses, particularly diabetes and its complications. In some tribes, 30 to 50% of the population have diabetes. Of dire concern to public health officials, the highest rate of increase among Native Americans occurred in the 15- to 19-year-old age group, with an increased prevalence of 32% between 1991 and 1997 (Narva, 2002).

Foot disease is the most common complication leading to hospitalization among adults with diabetes. According to the National Diabetes Education Program (NDEP), a partnership among over 200 organizations including the National Institutes of Health and the Centers for Disease Control and Prevention, as many as half of the lower-extremity amputations might be prevented

- CDC National HIV/AIDS and Sexually Transmitted Disease Hotline: 800-342-AIDS
- CDC National STD and AIDS Hotline: 800-227-8922
- CDC National STD and AIDS Hotline (in Spanish): 800-344-7432
- CDC National Prevention Information Network: 800-458-5231
- CDC Hearing Impaired Hotline: 800-243-7889
- National Herpes Hotline: 919-361-8488

Figure 14.6 Contact information for AIDS and STIs.

through simple but effective foot-care practices. With physician approval, people with diabetes are encouraged to engage in regular physical activity. They are advised, however, to examine their feet regularly to identify any emergent foot problems. Exercisers with diabetes should also learn about care of the feet. Finally, they should follow established guidelines for selecting appropriate exercise footwear.

Symptoms of diabetes include frequent urination and thirst, extreme hunger, rapid weight loss, blurred vision or sudden change in visual acuity, overtiredness, and drowsiness. Some of the more than 10 million people with diabetes in the United States need to take insulin into their bodies to help regulate the amount of glucose in their blood. Others, however, can control insulin insufficiency (sometimes called glucose intolerance) by diet and exercise. Exercise uses up the excess blood glucose, and diet can limit the amount of sugar and carbohydrates ingested in the first place.

Kidney Disease

More than 6.2 million Americans may have chronic kidney disease (CKD), the prevalence of which appears to fall disproportionately on African Americans. The incidence of CKD, an insidious illness that causes high mortality, is increasing at an alarming rate in our nation because of its association with hypertension, diabetes, and cardiovascular disease and the fact that it typically results in end-stage renal disease (ESRD). Like diabetes, ESRD occurs at a disproportionately higher rate in ethnic minorities than in white Americans, with a rate per million in the American population of 953 for African Americans, 652 for Native Americans, 386 for Asian Americans, and 237 for Caucasian Americans (U.S. Renal Data System, 2001). In 1999 the incidence of African Americans starting dialysis remained 311% higher than the incidence in Caucasians (U.S. Renal Data System, 1999).

Although many risk factors predispose one to CKD, the higher prevalence of both hypertension and diabetes among racial and ethnic minorities accounts, in part, for the greater incidence of chronic kidney disease in those populations. Diabetes mellitus has become the leading cause of end-stage renal disease (ESRD) in America and accounts for 44% of new cases each year. Native Americans have the highest rate of diabetes-related ESRD, and African Americans have the second highest rate.

Obesity

The relationship between leanness and colon and other cancers, and between body fat, production of estrogen, and subsequent breast cancer, was mentioned earlier in this chapter. Exercise helps reduce body fat, tone muscles, and decrease body weight. When that occurs, the heart does not need to pump as forcefully because blood vessels are not occluded, the blood has less distance to travel, and blood glucose is lower because muscular contractions are using it during physical activity. For those reasons, diet control in conjunction with an exercise program is the best treatment for obesity.

Although the effect of obesity as an independent risk factor for developing heart disease has been documented at length, the economic implications of the effect have not been well examined until recently. Based on data from the 1995 National Health Interview Survey and the 1996 Medical Expenditure Panel Survey (Wang et al., 2002), more than half (54.6%) of the adults in the American population were either overweight or obese. The total medical cost directly associated with overweight and obesity-associated heart disease was conservatively estimated at $22 billion ($31 billion in 2001 dollars). Nearly $12 billion of the cost was attributed to men and $10 billion to women. With the inclusion of indirect costs, such as loss of productivity, the economic effect would be substantially greater. These data demonstrate a critical need to address the excessive prevalence of obesity in the American population today.

Data from these national surveys also support other findings that health risks increase according to the severity of obesity. Although more individuals were overweight than were obese, obesity accounted for more than twice the medical costs imposed by overweight individuals. Obesity, defined as being 20% or more above recommended weight, is related to CHD, stroke, hypertension, diabetes, and other conditions. Furthermore, when the BMI is 30 or greater, mortality rates from all causes, especially CVD, increase by 50 to 100% (Poirier and Despres, 2001). Persons with class 3 obesity (BMI of 40 or more) are at even greater risk (Freedman et al., 2002).

Waist circumference is also emerging as an important measure of obesity-associated risks in adult women. NHANES III reported that waist circumference was more closely linked to cardiovascular disease risk factors than was BMI among the 9,019 Caucasian women participating in the study (Zhu et al., 2002). Some recent evidence also shows that high waist circumference is a strong predictor for stroke in older men but is not as consistent in predicting stroke in older women (Dey et al., 2002). Waist circumference has also been linked to hypertension and functional disability more accurately than has body-mass index in African American women (Rheeder et al., 2002) and elderly Hispanic adults (Chen et al., 2002).

Hypertension

When blood vessels are partially blocked, the heart has to work harder to pump blood through them. This increased tension of the blood against the walls of the blood vessels is called hypertension, or high blood pressure. Blood pressure is measured as diastolic and systolic blood pressure. The recommended blood pressure reading is 120 systolic/80 diastolic. Usually, readings above 140 systolic or 90 diastolic are considered high.

The stress that high blood pressure creates on the walls of the arteries can result in the rupture of those blood vessels. When that happens in the brain, a stroke occurs. In addition, high blood pressure can create small tears on the walls of the coronary arteries, making it easier for plaque to attach and accumulate and CHD to develop.

In many cases, hypertensives need medication for the remainder of their lives. In other cases, however, exercise and diet can help control hypertension. Exercise uses blood fats that otherwise might accumulate on the walls of blood vessels. Exercise also helps the heart become stronger so that it can pump blood as required. In addition, physical activity contracts muscles around blood vessels so that blood moves more efficiently through the circulatory system.

Approximately 50 to 60 million Americans have hypertension, and the prevalence of high blood pressure in adults older than 65 exceeds 50% (Bosworth and Oddone, 2002). At a rate of 71%, the prevalence of hypertension in African Americans is among the highest in the world today (Lea and Nicholas, 2002). The rate of hypertension among Hispanics is similar to that of Caucasians (61% versus 60%, respectively). NHANES III reported that although 68% of individuals are aware of being hypertensive, only 27% of hypertensive patients had their disease under effective control (Burt et al., 1995).

Poor dietary choices, obesity, and sedentary lifestyles may be directly related to the higher prevalence of hypertension among ethnic and racial minorities. Hypertension prevalence and levels of leisure-time physical activity were also studied in 16,246 adult Caucasians, African Americans, and Mexican Americans who participated in NHANES III. Both race and physical activity were independent contributors to hypertension prevalence. Again, Caucasians had a lower prevalence of hypertension than did those in either ethnic minority group, and overall hypertension prevalence was significantly lower in the most active group, compared with sedentary individuals (Bassett et al., 2002).

Summary

Heart Disease   Heart disease is the leading cause of death in the United States. It involves blockage of blood to the heart, thereby depriving it of necessary oxygen and nutrients, without which a heart attack can occur and part of the heart muscle can die. Death can even be the result.

An accumulation of blood fats and other substances on the walls of coronary arteries can occlude, or block, them. This clogging material is known as plaque, and the resulting condition is called atherosclerosis. The fatty particles that can collect on the walls of the arteries are called lipoproteins. Lipoproteins consist of triglycerides, a blood protein, and cholesterol.

HDLs and LDLs are produced in the liver and released into the bloodstream, where they carry cholesterol needed by the body. Excess cholesterol carried by LDLs can accumulate on the artery walls, eventually clogging coronary arteries and causing heart disease. HDLs carry excess cholesterol back to the liver and possibly provide a protective layer of grease to help prevent a buildup of substances on the walls of the arteries. When LDL is elevated and HDL is too sparse, there is a likelihood that arteries will be clogged and CVD will be promoted.

Risk factors for CVD include diets high in fats, hypertension, obesity and overweight, stress, sedentary lifestyle, the use of tobacco, and a family history of heart disease.

Physical activity is an excellent means of preventing CVD because it relates to several risk factors. It exercises the heart muscle, encourages the production of HDL, aids in the control of mild hypertension, develops cardiorespiratory endurance, reduces catecholamines produced in response to stress, helps maintain desirable weight, and discourages cigarette smoking.

Behavioral Change and Motivational Strategies

Many things might interfere with your behaving in ways to prevent CHD and cancer. Here are some barriers (roadblocks) and strategies for overcoming them.

Roadblock

Friends or relatives may smoke cigarettes, which may tempt you to do so yourself. Although we like to think we act independently, the behavior of other people influences us, particularly if we like and respect them. Furthermore, you do not even have to smoke to be subjected to the harmful effects of tobacco products. Just by breathing in secondhand, or sidestream, smoke can affect your susceptibility to CHD and cancer.

Behavioral Change Strategy

Two behavioral change strategies appropriate here are contracting and social support. Find a friend or relative who would like to give up smoking. This will not be difficult. Smokers often try to quit; the problem is that they are usually unsuccessful. Draw up a contract for each of you to reduce the number of cigarettes you smoke gradually over a period of weeks (gradual programming). Use the contract format described in chapter 4. If you do not presently smoke, have your contract address your not starting to smoke and the other person's contract specific to achieving a gradual reduction in the number of cigarettes smoked per week. Each of you then signs the other's contract as a witness. The support that you provide each other and the pressure of a contract that you will periodically evaluate can be just the motivation you need to counteract the influence of smoking friends and relatives.

You may find exercise uncomfortable. Your muscles may ache, your clothes and body may become sweaty, and you may not enjoy the activity itself. With that attitude, you cannot expect to maintain an exercise program even if you are motivated to begin one. After all, most people do not want to feel uncomfortable and will choose to avoid doing so.

Use goal-setting strategies to establish realistic and achievable fitness goals. If you are experiencing aches and pains, you are overtraining or exercising inappropriately. Fitness experts long ago discarded the maxim "no pain, no gain." You should feel good after a workout.

You can also use selective awareness. Focus on the benefits of the exercise: how it will burn up calories, make you look and feel better, help you be healthier, make the clothes you bought when you weighed less fit again, and so forth. If you focus on the benefits rather than on the temporary discomfort caused by perspiration, you will be more likely to maintain your exercise program.

You may enjoy eating foods high in saturated fats. Many of us grew up on french fries, hot dogs, and hamburgers. They taste good, are easy to prepare, and are relatively inexpensive. Unfortunately, they also put us at risk for both CHD and certain cancers.

Use reminder systems to encourage the buying and eating of healthier foods. Put notes on your refrigerator and pantry to remind you to refrain from eating certain foods when you are looking for a snack. Place a picture of a clogged artery at the top of your shopping list to remind you not to buy unhealthy foods.

You can also use covert modeling. Find a friend who eats well, looks good, and whose behavior you would like to follow. Then observe what this friend eats. After obtaining a good picture of how this friend selects and prepares foods, model your behavior on him or her. Eat and prepare similar foods—at least those that you enjoy eating and that are also low in fat and other unhealthy food ingredients.

List roadblocks interfering with your working at preventing CHD and cancer.

1. _____

2. _____

3. _____

Now cite behavioral change strategies that can help you overcome the roadblocks you just listed. If you need to, refer back to chapter 4 for behavioral change and motivational strategies.

1. _____

2. _____

3. _____

Cancer Cancer is a disease involving abnormal cell growth. These cells can spread to other parts of the body by metastasis. Cancer is the second-leading cause of death in the United States. As many as 80% of cancer cases, however, could be prevented with a change in lifestyle.

Chemicals, environmental pollutants, radiation from the sun, or viruses can cause cancer. The greatest cause of cancer, however, is the use of tobacco. Cigarette smoking causes an estimated 75% of all lung cancer cases, and the use of tobacco is associated with cancer of the larynx, pharynx, esophagus, pancreas, and bladder.

The number of cancer cases could be dramatically reduced if people ate diets low in fats and high in fruits and vegetables (in particular, cruciferous vegetables), refrained from smoking cigarettes, eliminated or reduced their consumption of alcohol, and decreased their exposure to the sun.

Moderate physical activity seems to protect people from developing cancer, particularly cancer of the colon, prostate, endometrium, and breast. Theories about why this relationship exists point to the role of exercise in lowering body fat, producing less estrogen, and increasing the rate of transit of food through the digestive tract.

The earlier cancer is detected, the more effective is the treatment. To identify the presence of cancer early, obtain regular medical screenings and perform regular self-examinations (such as breast and testicular self-examinations).

Sexually Transmitted Infections Sexually transmitted infections are diseases primarily contracted through sexual activity. Among STIs are gonorrhea, syphilis, genital herpes, chlamydia, genital warts, pelvic inflammatory disease, and HIV infection and AIDS.

Gonorrhea is caused by the Neisseria gonorrhoeae bacterium and is treated with penicillin. Early symptoms may include painful urination; a milky, smelly discharge; and an urgent need to urinate. Women are often asymptomatic but may experience a slight burning sensation in the genital area and a mild vaginal discharge.

Syphilis is caused by a corkscrew organism called Treponema pallidum and is treated with penicillin. In stage 1 a painless sore (chancre) appears in the infected area.

The herpes simplex virus causes genital herpes. The infection is treated with the drug Acyclovir (although this treatment only diminishes the severity and frequency of outbreaks, because genital herpes is presently incurable). Early symptoms may include sore and swollen glands, flulike symptoms, and pain in the genital area during urination or sexual intercourse. The virus remains dormant in the nerve cells with periodic reoccurrences possible.

Chlamydia, the most prevalent STI, is caused by the Chlamydia trachomatis bacterium and is treated with the antibiotic tetracycline. Symptoms include vaginal discharge, itching and burning of the vulva, and some discomfort when urinating.

Genital warts are caused by the human papillomavirus (HPV) and are treated with the drug podophyllin (sometimes an antibiotic ointment is prescribed as well). Warts tend to reoccur. Laser surgery, electrosurgery, freezing with liquid hydrogen, or surgical incision can sometimes remove them.

Pelvic inflammatory disease (PID), which can cause infertility and even death if left untreated, is treated by administration of an antibiotic. Symptoms include abdominal pain or tenderness, pain during intercourse, increased menstrual cramps, profuse bleeding during menstruation, irregular menstrual cycles, vaginal bleeding at times other than when menstruating, lower-back pain, nausea, loss of appetite, vomiting, vaginal discharge, burning sensation during urination, chills, and fever.

The human immunodeficiency virus (HIV) causes acquired immunodeficiency syndrome (AIDS), which is presently incurable. HIV is transmitted through bodily fluids (blood, semen, vaginal secretions), most commonly encountered through sex or use of intravenous drugs. HIV infection is treated with the drug azidothymidine (AZT) and a combination of other drugs that seem to prolong symptom-free living. Methods of prevention include abstaining from sex, using a latex condom, limiting the number of sexual partners, maintaining a monogamous relationship with an HIV-free partner, and refraining from use of intravenous drugs.

Other Diseases and Conditions Exercise can be effective in preventing or responding to other diseases, including diabetes, kidney disease, obesity, and hypertension. Exercise uses up blood glucose and other blood fats, expends calories, and makes the heart and circulatory system operate more efficiently. As a result, exercise and diet are mainstays in the treatment and prevention of these conditions.

Discovery Activity 14.1

Your Healthy Heart IQ

Name _____ **Date** _____

Answer true or false to the following questions to determine your healthy heart IQ. This activity comprises three sections. At the conclusion of each section, the correct answers appear with an explanation.

Section I: Heart Health IQ

T ___ **F** ___ 1. The risk factors for heart disease that you can do something about are high blood pressure, high blood cholesterol, smoking, obesity, and physical inactivity.

T ___ **F** ___ 2. A stroke is often the first symptom of high blood pressure, and a heart attack is often the first symptom of high blood cholesterol.

T ___ **F** ___ 3. A blood pressure greater than or equal to 140/90 millimeters Hg is generally considered high.

T ___ **F** ___ 4. High blood pressure affects the same proportion of Blacks as it does Whites.

T ___ **F** ___ 5. The best ways to treat and control high blood pressure are to control your weight, exercise, eat less salt (sodium), restrict your intake of alcohol, and take your high blood pressure medicine, if prescribed by your doctor.

T ___ **F** ___ 6. A blood cholesterol of 240 milligrams per deciliter is desirable for adults.

T ___ **F** ___ 7. The most effective dietary way to lower the level of your blood cholesterol is to eat foods low in cholesterol.

T ___ **F** ___ 8. Lowering blood-cholesterol levels can help people who have already had a heart attack.

T ___ **F** ___ 9. Only children from families at high risk of heart disease need to have their blood-cholesterol levels checked.

T ___ **F** ___ 10. Smoking is a major risk factor for four of the five leading causes of death, including heart attack, stroke, cancer, and lung diseases such as emphysema and bronchitis.

T ___ **F** ___ 11. If you have had a heart attack, quitting smoking can reduce your chances of having a second attack.

T ___ **F** ___ 12. Someone who has smoked for 30 to 40 years probably will not be able to quit smoking.

T ___ **F** ___ 13. The best way to lose weight is to increase activity and eat fewer calories.

T ___ **F** ___ 14. Heart disease is the leading killer of men and women in the United States.

Source: National Heart, Lung, and Blood Institute. www.nhlbi.nih.gov/health/public/heart/other/hh_iq.htm

Discovery Activity 14.1 *(continued)*

Answers for Section I

1. **True.** High blood pressure, smoking, and high blood cholesterol are the three most important risk factors for heart disease. On average, each one doubles your chance of developing heart disease. A person who has all three risk factors is therefore eight times more likely to develop heart disease than someone who has none. Obesity increases the likelihood of developing high blood cholesterol and high blood pressure, which increase your risk of heart disease. Physical inactivity increases your risk of heart attack. Regular exercise and good nutrition are essential to reducing high blood pressure, high blood cholesterol, and overweight. People who exercise are also more likely to cut down on or stop smoking.

2. **True.** A person with high blood pressure or high blood cholesterol may feel and look great, but a stroke or heart attack can occur without warning. To find out if you have high blood pressure or high blood cholesterol, you should have a doctor, nurse, or other health professional test you.

3. **True.** A blood pressure of 140/90 mm Hg or greater is generally classified as high blood pressure. Blood pressure that falls below 140/90 mm Hg, however, can sometimes be a problem. If the diastolic pressure, the second or lower number, is between 85 and 89, a person is at increased risk for heart disease or stroke and should have his or her blood pressure checked at least once a year by a health professional. The higher your blood pressure, the greater your risk of developing heart disease or stroke. Controlling high blood pressure reduces your risk.

4. **False.** High blood pressure is more common in Blacks than it is in Whites. It affects 29 out of every 100 Black adults compared with 26 out of every 100 White adults. In addition, with aging, high blood pressure is generally more severe among Blacks than it is among Whites, and it therefore causes more strokes, heart disease, and kidney failure.

5. **True.** Recent studies show that lifestyle changes can help keep blood pressure levels normal even into advanced age and are important in treating and preventing high blood pressure. Limit high-salt foods, including snack foods such as potato chips, salted pretzels, and salted crackers; processed foods such as canned soups; and condiments such as ketchup and soy sauce. If prescribed by your doctor, taking blood pressure medication is extremely important in making sure that your blood pressure stays under control.

6. **False.** A total blood cholesterol of less than 200 milligrams per deciliter is desirable and usually puts you at lower risk for heart disease. A blood-cholesterol level of 240 milligrams per deciliter or above is high and increases your risk of heart disease. If your cholesterol level is high, your doctor will want to check your levels of LDL cholesterol (bad cholesterol) and HDL cholesterol (good cholesterol). A high level of LDL cholesterol increases your risk for heart disease, as does a low level of HDL cholesterol. A cholesterol level of 200 to 239 milligrams per deciliter is considered borderline high and usually increases your risk for heart disease. If your cholesterol is borderline high, you should speak to your doctor to see if you need additional cholesterol tests. All adults 20 years of age or older should have their blood-cholesterol level checked at least once every 5 years.

7. **False.** Reducing the amount of cholesterol in your diet is important, but eating foods low in saturated fat is the most effective dietary way to lower blood-cholesterol levels, along with eating less total fat and cholesterol. Choose low-saturated fat foods such as grains, fruits, and vegetables; low-fat or skim milk and milk products; and lean cuts of meat, fish, and chicken. Trim fat from meat before cooking, bake or broil meat rather than fry, use less fat and oil, and take the skin off chicken and turkey. Reducing overweight will also help lower your level of LDL cholesterol as well as increase your level of HDL cholesterol.

8. **True.** People who have had a heart attack are at much higher risk for a second attack. Reducing blood-cholesterol levels can greatly slow down (and, in some people, even reverse) the buildup of cholesterol and fat in the walls of the arteries and significantly reduce the chances of a second heart attack.

9. **True.** Children from high-risk families, those in which a parent has high blood cholesterol (240 milligrams per deciliter or above) or in which a parent or grandparent has had heart disease at an early age (at 55 years of age or younger), should have their cholesterol levels tested. If a child from such a family has high blood cholesterol, it should be lowered under medical supervision, primarily with diet, to reduce the risk of developing heart disease as an adult. For children who are not from high-risk families, the best way to reduce the risk of adult heart disease is to follow an eating pattern that is low in saturated fat and cholesterol. All children over the age of 2 years and all adults should adopt a heart-healthy eating pattern as a principal way of reducing coronary heart disease.

(continued)

Discovery Activity 14.1 *(continued)*

10. **True.** Heavy smokers are two to four times more likely to have a heart attack than nonsmokers are, and the heart attack death rate among all smokers is 70% greater than that of nonsmokers. Older male smokers are nearly twice as likely to die from stroke than are older men who do not smoke, and the odds are nearly as high for older female smokers. Further, the risk of dying from lung cancer is 22 times higher for male smokers than for male nonsmokers and 12 times higher for female smokers than for female nonsmokers. Finally, 80% of all deaths from emphysema and bronchitis are directly due to smoking.

11. **True.** One year after quitting, ex-smokers cut their extra risk for heart attack by about half or more, and eventually the risk will return to normal in healthy ex-smokers. Even if you have already had a heart attack, you can reduce your chances of a second attack if you quit smoking. Ex-smokers can also reduce their risk of stroke and cancer, improve blood flow and lung function, and help stop diseases like emphysema and bronchitis from becoming worse.

12. **False.** Older smokers are more likely to succeed at quitting smoking than younger smokers are. Quitting helps relieve smoking-related symptoms like shortness of breath, coughing, and chest pain. Many quit to avoid further health problems and take control of their lives.

13. **True.** Weight control is a question of balance. You obtain calories from the foods you eat. You burn off calories by exercising. Cutting down on calories, especially calories from fat, is key to losing weight. Combining calorie reduction with regular physical activity like walking, cycling, jogging, or swimming can help in both losing weight and maintaining weight loss. A steady weight loss of 1/2 to 1 pound a week is safe for most adults, and the weight is more likely to stay off over the long run. Losing weight, if you are overweight, may also reduce your blood pressure, lower your LDL cholesterol, and raise your HDL cholesterol. Being physically active and eating fewer calories will also help you control your weight if you quit smoking.

14. **True.** Coronary heart disease is the number one killer in the United States. Approximately 489,000 Americans died of coronary heart disease in 1990, and approximately half of the deaths were women.

Section II: Cholesterol and Heart Disease IQ

T ___ F ___   1. High blood cholesterol is one of the risk factors for heart disease that you can do something about.

T ___ F ___   2. To lower your blood-cholesterol level you must stop eating meat altogether.

T ___ F ___   3. Any blood-cholesterol level below 240 milligrams per deciliter is desirable for adults.

T ___ F ___   4. Fish-oil supplements will help you lower your blood cholesterol.

T ___ F ___   5. To lower your blood-cholesterol level, you should eat less saturated fat, total fat, and cholesterol, and lose weight if you are overweight.

T ___ F ___   6. Saturated fats raise your blood-cholesterol level more than anything else in your diet does.

T ___ F ___   7. All vegetable oils help lower blood-cholesterol levels.

T ___ F ___   8. Lowering blood-cholesterol levels can help people who have already had a heart attack.

T ___ F ___   9. All children need to have their blood-cholesterol levels checked.

T ___ F ___ 10. Women do not need to worry about high blood cholesterol and heart disease.

T ___ F ___ 11. Reading food labels can help you eat the heart-healthy way.

Discovery Activity 14.1 *(continued)*

Answers for Section II

1. **True.** High blood cholesterol is one of the risk factors for heart disease that a person can do something about. High blood pressure, cigarette smoking, diabetes, overweight, and physical inactivity are the others.

2. **False.** Although some red meat is high in saturated fat and cholesterol and eating it can raise your blood cholesterol, you do not need to stop eating red meat or any other single food. Red meat is an important source of protein, iron, and other vitamins and minerals. But you should cut back on the amount of saturated fat and cholesterol that you eat. One way to do this is by choosing lean cuts of meat with the fat trimmed. Another way is to watch your portion sizes and eat no more than 6 ounces of meat, about the size of two decks of playing cards, each day.

3. **False.** A total blood-cholesterol level of under 200 milligrams per deciliter is desirable and usually puts you at lower risk for heart disease. A blood-cholesterol level of 240 milligrams per deciliter is high and increases your risk of heart disease. If your cholesterol level is high, your doctor will want to check your level of LDL cholesterol (bad cholesterol). A high level of LDL cholesterol increases your risk of heart disease, as does a low level of HDL cholesterol (good cholesterol). An HDL cholesterol level below 35 milligrams per deciliter is considered a risk factor for heart disease. A total cholesterol level of 200 to 239 milligrams per deciliter is considered borderline high and usually increases your risk for heart disease. All adults 20 years of age or older should have their blood-cholesterol level checked at least once every 5 years.

4. **False.** Fish oils are a source of omega-3 fatty acids, which are a type of polyunsaturated fat. Fish-oil supplements generally do not reduce blood-cholesterol levels. In addition, the effect of the long-term use of fish-oil supplements is not known. But fish is a good food choice because it is low in saturated fat.

5. **True.** Eating less fat, especially saturated fat, and less cholesterol can lower your blood-cholesterol level. Generally, your blood-cholesterol level should begin to drop a few weeks after you start on a cholesterol-lowering diet. How much your level drops depends on the amount of saturated fat and cholesterol you used to eat, how high your blood cholesterol is, how much weight you lose if you are overweight, and how your body responds to the changes you make. Over time, you may reduce your blood-cholesterol level by 10 to 50 milligrams per deciliter or even more.

6. **True.** Saturated fats raise your blood-cholesterol level more than anything else does, so the best way to reduce your cholesterol level is to cut back on the amount of saturated fats you eat. Animal products such as butter, cheese, whole milk, ice cream, cream, and fatty meats contain the largest amounts of these fats. Some vegetable oils—coconut, palm, and palm kernel oils—also contain saturated fats.

7. **False.** Most vegetable oils—canola, corn, olive, safflower, soybean, and sunflower oils—contain mostly monounsaturated and polyunsaturated fats, which help lower blood cholesterol when used in place of saturated fats. But a few vegetable oils—coconut, palm, and palm kernel oils—contain more saturated fat than unsaturated fat. A special kind of fat, called trans-fat, forms when vegetable oil is hardened to become margarine or shortening through a process called hydrogenation. The harder the margarine or shortening, the more likely it is to contain trans-fat. Choose margarine containing liquid vegetable oil as the first ingredient. Just be sure to limit the total amount of fats or oils, because even those that are unsaturated are rich sources of calories.

8. **True.** People who have had one heart attack are at much higher risk for a second attack. Reducing blood-cholesterol levels can greatly slow down (and, in some people, even reverse) the buildup of cholesterol and fat in the wall of the coronary arteries and significantly reduce the chances of a second heart attack. If you have had a heart attack or have coronary heart disease, your LDL level should be around 100 milligrams per deciliter, which is even lower than the recommended level of less than 130 milligrams per deciliter for the general population.

9. **False.** Children from high-risk families, those in which a parent has high blood cholesterol (240 milligrams per deciliter or above) or in which a parent or grandparent has had heart disease at an early age (at age 55 or younger), should have their cholesterol levels tested. If a child from such a family has high blood cholesterol, it should be lowered under medical supervision, primarily with diet, to reduce the risk of developing heart disease as an adult. For most children, the best way to reduce the risk of adult heart disease is to follow an eating pattern that is low in saturated fat and cholesterol. All children over the age of 2 years and all adults should adopt a heart-healthy eating pattern as a principal way of reducing coronary heart disease.

(continued)

Discovery Activity 14.1 *(continued)*

10. **False.** Blood-cholesterol levels in both men and women begin to go up around age 20. Women before menopause have levels that are lower than those of men of the same age. After menopause, a women's LDL cholesterol level goes up—and so does her risk for heart disease. For both men and women, heart disease is the number one cause of death.

11. **True.** Food labels have changed. Look on the nutrition label for the amount of saturated fat, total fat, cholesterol, and total calories in a serving of the product. Use this information to compare similar products. Look also for the list of ingredients. The ingredient in the greatest amount is listed first, and the ingredient in the least amount is given last. To choose foods low in saturated fat or total fat, go easy on products that list fats or oil first, or products that list many fat and oil ingredients.

Section III: Physical Activity and Heart Disease IQ

T ___ **F** ___   1. Regular physical activity can reduce your chances of getting heart disease.

T ___ **F** ___   2. Most people get enough physical activity from their normal daily routines.

T ___ **F** ___   3. You don't have to train like a marathon runner to become more physically fit.

T ___ **F** ___   4. Exercise programs do not require a lot of time to be effective.

T ___ **F** ___   5. People who need to lose some weight are the only ones who will benefit from regular physical activity.

T ___ **F** ___   6. All exercises give you the same benefits.

T ___ **F** ___   7. The older you are, the less active you need to be.

T ___ **F** ___   8. You don't need to spend a lot of money or buy expensive equipment to become physically fit.

T ___ **F** ___   9. Many risks and injuries can occur with exercise.

T ___ **F** ___ 10. You should consult a doctor before starting a physical activity program.

T ___ **F** ___ 11. People who have had a heart attack should not start any program of physical activity.

T ___ **F** ___ 12. To help stay physically active, include a variety of activities.

Answers for Section III

1. **True.** Heart disease is almost twice as likely to develop in inactive people. Being physically inactive is a risk factor for heart disease, along with cigarette smoking, high blood pressure, high blood cholesterol, and being overweight. The more risk factors you have, the greater your chance for heart disease. Regular physical activity (even mild to moderate exercise) can reduce this risk.

2. **False.** Most Americans are busy but not active. Every American adult should make a habit of engaging in 30 minutes of low to moderate levels of physical activity daily. Such activities include walking, gardening, and walking up stairs. If you are inactive now, begin by doing a few minutes of activity each day. If you are active only occasionally, try to work something into your everyday routine.

3. **True.** Low- to moderate-intensity activities, such as pleasure walking, stair climbing, yard work, housework, dancing, and home exercises have both short- and long-term benefits. If you are inactive, the key is

Discovery Activity 14.1 *(continued)*

getting started. One excellent way is to take a walk for 10 to 15 minutes during your lunch break. Dog owners can take their pets for a walk every day. At least 30 minutes of physical activity every day can improve your heart health.

4. **True.** You need to spend only a few minutes a day to become more physically active. If you don't have 30 minutes in your schedule for an exercise break, try to find two 15-minute periods or three 10-minute periods. These exercise breaks will soon become a habit you can't live without.

5. **False.** People who are physically active experience many positive benefits. Regular physical activity gives you more energy, reduces stress, and helps you sleep better. Exercise helps lower high blood pressure and improves blood-cholesterol levels. Physical activity helps tone your muscles, burns off calories to help you lose extra pounds or stay at your desirable weight, and helps control your appetite. Activity can increase muscle strength, help your heart and lungs work more efficiently, and let you enjoy your life more fully.

6. **False.** Low-intensity activities—if performed daily—can have some long-term health benefits and lower your risk of heart disease. Regular, brisk, and sustained exercise for at least 30 minutes three to four times a week, such as brisk walking, jogging, or swimming, is necessary to improve the efficiency of your heart and lungs and burn off extra calories. These activities are called aerobic—meaning that the body uses oxygen to produce the energy it needs for the activity. Other activities may give you benefits such as increased flexibility or muscle strength.

7. **False.** Although we tend to become less active with age, physical activity is still important. Older persons who engage in regular physical activity have greater capacity to perform everyday activities. In general, middle-aged and older people benefit from regular physical activity just as young people do. What is important, at any age, is tailoring the activity program to your fitness level.

8. **True.** Many activities require little or no equipment. For example, brisk walking requires only a comfortable pair of walking shoes. Many communities offer free or inexpensive recreation facilities and physical activity classes. Check your shopping malls; many are open early and late for people who do not wish to walk alone, in the dark, or in bad weather.

9. **False.** The most common risk in exercising is injury to the muscles and joints. Such injuries usually result from exercising too hard for too long, particularly if a person has been inactive. To avoid injuries, try to build up your level of activity gradually, listen to your body for warning pains, be aware of possible signs of heart problems (such as pain or pressure in the left or midchest area, left neck, shoulder, or arm during or just after exercising, or sudden lightheadedness, cold sweat, pallor, or fainting), and be prepared for adverse weather.

10. **True.** You should ask your doctor before you start (or greatly increase) your physical activity if you have a medical condition such as high blood pressure, have pains or pressure in the chest and shoulder, feel dizzy or faint, become breathless after mild exertion, are middle-aged or older and have not been physically active, or plan a vigorous activity program. If none of these apply, start slowly and get moving.

11. **False.** Regular physical activity can help reduce your risk of having another heart attack. People who include regular physical activity in their lives after a heart attack improve their chances of survival and can improve how they feel and look. If you have had a heart attack, consult your doctor to be sure that you are following a safe and effective exercise program that will help prevent heart pain and further damage from overexertion.

12. **True.** By picking several different activities that you enjoy doing, you will be more likely to stay with an exercise program. Plan short-term and long-term goals. Keep a record of your progress and check it regularly to see the progress you have made. Persuade your family and friends to join in. They can help keep you going.

From *Physical fitness and wellness, third edition*, by Jerrold S. Greenberg, George B. Dintiman, and Barbee Myers Oakes, 2004, Champaign, IL: Human Kinetics.

Discovery Activity 14.2

Blood Composition Assessment

Name _____ **Date** _____

The composition of your blood is extremely important when it comes to preventing CHD. You can easily have your physician check your blood-fat levels. Sometimes this is done with a simple finger prick, but for greater accuracy blood should be drawn from a vein after you have fasted for about 12 hours. Record the results of that assessment below by checking the appropriate rating.

_____ Total cholesterol below 200: No further evaluation is necessary; recheck in 5 years.

_____ Total cholesterol 200 to 239 (borderline high cholesterol): Evaluate risk factors to see what lifestyle changes you can make (diet, exercise, and so forth). If your physician says that you are not in the high-risk category for CHD, active treatment is not necessary, but you should recheck in 1 to 8 weeks.

_____ Total cholesterol above 240 (high cholesterol): Analyze and measure HDL, LDL, and triglycerides.

After completing the previous assessment, answer the following questions:

Yes   No

___   ___   1. Is your total cholesterol no more than 3.5 times greater than your HDL cholesterol?

___   ___   2. Is your cholesterol-to-HDL ratio at least 5 to 1?

___   ___   3. Is your HDL reading above 35?

___   ___   4. Is your LDL cholesterol less than 160?

If the answers to these questions are yes, your lipid profile is good. Regardless of how your lipid profile turned out, list the changes you can make to lower your total cholesterol and increase your HDL cholesterol over the next 12 months.

1. _____

2. _____

3. _____

4. _____

5. _____

Discovery Activity 14.3

Service-Learning for Preventing Premature Heart Disease and Cancer

In today's busy society, people too often eat the quickest meal rather than the healthiest one. Consequently, fast-food restaurants saturate our neighborhoods to satisfy this desire. If people ate a healthier diet, they would be able to postpone the development of premature chronic conditions such as coronary heart disease and cancer. You can help your neighbors eat a more healthy diet through this service-learning assignment.

Begin by researching the relationship between certain foods and heart disease and cancer. For example, analyze the association between diets high in saturated fats and the occurrence of heart disease and cancer, or study the relationship between fiber and cruciferous vegetables and the incidence of heart disease and cancer. Your research will result in lists of both healthy and unhealthy foods. Next, contact local restaurants and encourage them to identify food choices on their menus that are heart healthy or cancer preventing. You might develop a flyer that identifies healthy and unhealthy foods and ask restaurateurs to distribute them to customers. In this way you will be contributing to the health of your community while learning more about the material discussed in this chapter.

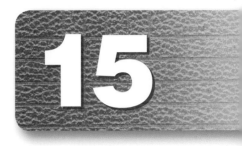

Designing a Program of Lifetime Fitness

Chapter Objectives

By the end of this chapter, you should be able to

1. identify your fitness goals,
2. select physical activities to meet your fitness goals,
3. design an exercise program that is appropriate for you now and that you can continue or adapt for many years to come,
4. list criteria for evaluating an exercise club and selecting exercise equipment to buy, and
5. describe how you can keep fit as you age.

When Mandy was an infant, she crawled around her playpen and on the carpet endlessly. A full day of that type of exercise tired her out, and she had no problem sleeping through the night. When she started school, Mandy participated in physical education and soon learned sport skills she used to become physically fit and healthy. She became enamored with soccer in particular and joined a recreational soccer league that played on the weekends. By the time she enrolled in college, Mandy was interested in weight training and aerobic dance classes. She used the college exercise room to lift weights and signed up for an aerobic dance class to meet the physical education course requirement for graduation. Mandy is now in her 60s and no longer interested in aerobic dance, is not in condition to play soccer, and cannot lift the amount of weight she could when she was younger. Yet Mandy still exercises regularly. She walks daily and joins her contemporaries in the pool for aqua aerobics 4 days a week. She found that the local YMCA has a weight room with a staff person qualified to advise her on the best type of weight training for someone of her age and in her condition, so she weight trains 3 days a week. In a real sense, Mandy is still enrolled in physical education, only this time with a different type of instructor.

Some physical education instructors today understand the nature of physical fitness and how it relates to health and wellness. Unfortunately, many instructors still force individuals to run long distances when they are not in shape to do so or only teach people how to play softball, basketball, or football. These instructors teach individuals to hate running because the long runs tire them out for the rest of the day and create needless aches and pains. Team sports, on the other hand, may be great fun, but once the class is over, getting enough people together to play football, softball, or basketball is difficult. Of course, communities and other organizations offer coed softball leagues, people play pickup basketball games at the local YMCA or community center, and some people still meet on the weekends to play touch football. But most of us would prefer physical activities that require less organization. That may be why we join health clubs and weight train, or why we take up jogging and swimming, or why we play tennis or golf. We can do these lifetime sports activities alone or with only one other person. And our bodies can withstand the activity even into our later years.

Today, more physical education courses of study include instruction on tennis, golf, weight training, and badminton while not neglecting more aerobically intense physical activities such as basketball, soccer, football, and jogging. What is more, they sometimes even add a health and wellness perspective to the courses.

In this chapter, we provide you with the information you need to continue your fitness program for the rest of your life. We do this by helping you determine your fitness goals and showing you how to achieve them. We even help you evaluate fitness and health clubs and identify what you should look for when buying exercise equipment.

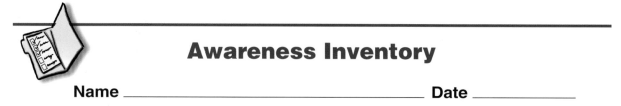

Awareness Inventory

Name _____ **Date** _____

Check the space by the letter T for the statements that you think are true and the space by the letter F for the statements that you think are false. The answers appear following the list of statements. This chapter will present information to clarify these statements for you. As you read the chapter, look for explanations for the reasons why the statements are true or false.

T ___ **F** ___ 1. Although walking is classified as a fitness activity, it does not affect serum cholesterol levels or cardiorespiratory endurance.

T ___ **F** ___ 2. When running or jogging you should avoid excessive forward lean.

T ___ **F** ___ 3. When determining the best length for a jump rope, stand on its center and make sure that the handles are at waist level.

T ___ **F** ___ 4. A singles match of tennis burns approximately 60 more calories than a doubles match does.

T ___ **F** ___ 5. Aerobics instructors know enough about the activity that they can avoid injury.

T ___ **F** ___ 6. When riding a stationary bike, adjust the seat so that your legs extend fully when the pedal is in the low position.

T ___ **F** ___ 7. Most exercise clubs are pretty much the same, so it does not really matter which one you join (except for the cost).

T ___ **F** ___ 8. Treadmills should have a large, heavy-duty roller that keeps the belt centered.

T ___ **F** ___ 9. Exercise equipment that stimulates the muscle electrically is an effective way to develop muscle tone.

T ___ **F** ___ 10. If you adopt a sedentary lifestyle, you cannot do much about it when you get older.

Answers: 1-F, 2-T, 3-F, 4-T, 5-F, 6-F, 7-F, 8-T, 9-F, 10-F

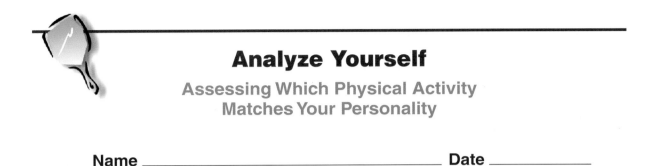

Analyze Yourself

Assessing Which Physical Activity Matches Your Personality

Name _____ **Date** _____

Fitness experts tell us that if you match your personality with your choice of exercise, you will increase your chances of staying with your program. Here is a way to do that. Read the description of each psychosocial personality variable and then rate yourself on the scorecard that follows.

- **Sociability:** Do you prefer doing things on your own or with other people? Do you make friends easily? Do you enjoy parties?
- **Spontaneity:** Do you make spontaneous decisions, or do you plan in detail? Can you change direction easily, or do you become locked in once you make up your mind?
- **Discipline:** Do you have trouble sticking with things you find unpleasant or trying, or do you persist regardless of the obstacles? Do you need a lot of support, or do you just push on alone?
- **Aggressiveness:** Do you try to control situations by being forceful? Do you like pitting yourself against obstacles, or do you shy away when you must assert yourself physically or emotionally?
- **Competitiveness:** Do situations that produce winners and losers bother you? Does your adrenaline flow when you're challenged, or do you back off?
- **Mental focus:** Do you find it easy to concentrate, or do you have a short attention span? Can you be single minded? How good are you at clearing your mind of distractions?
- **Risk taking:** Are you generally adventurous, physically and emotionally, or do you prefer to stick to what you know?

Scorecard
Fill in the appropriate circles and
connect them with a line.

	Very high ⟵⟶ Very Low				
Sociability	O	O	O	O	O
Spontaneity	O	O	O	O	O
Discipline	O	O	O	O	O
Aggressiveness	O	O	O	O	O
Competitiveness	O	O	O	O	O
Mental focus	O	O	O	O	O
Risk-taking	O	O	O	O	O

(continued)

Analyze Yourself *(continued)*

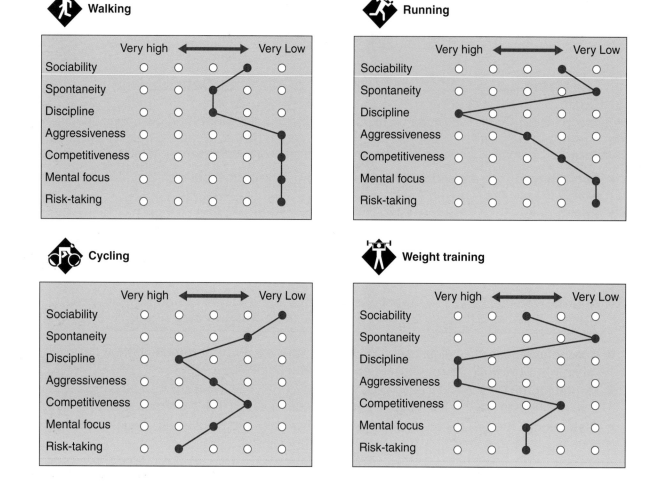

Understanding Your Score

To see how well your profile matches your sport or exercise activity, look at the four sample profiles in this activity. If you have the typical personality of a runner, walker, cyclist, or bodybuilder, your profile should look similar to one of these profiles. If your athletic preference lies elsewhere, turn to the "Your Personality/Your Sport" chart to see where your activities rank on each characteristic. Then compare these rankings with how you scored yourself.

Compared with running, for example, walking is more spontaneous and less aggressive. (Walking is also safe, in terms of physical stress.) Racket sports are high in sociability, spontaneity, competitiveness, and focus but low in discipline. Swimming is fairly high in discipline and low in sociability, spontaneity, and aggressiveness.

If you've been having trouble sticking to a fitness program, these charts may explain why. If you're still looking for a sport, use your findings as a guide.

Analyze Yourself *(continued)*

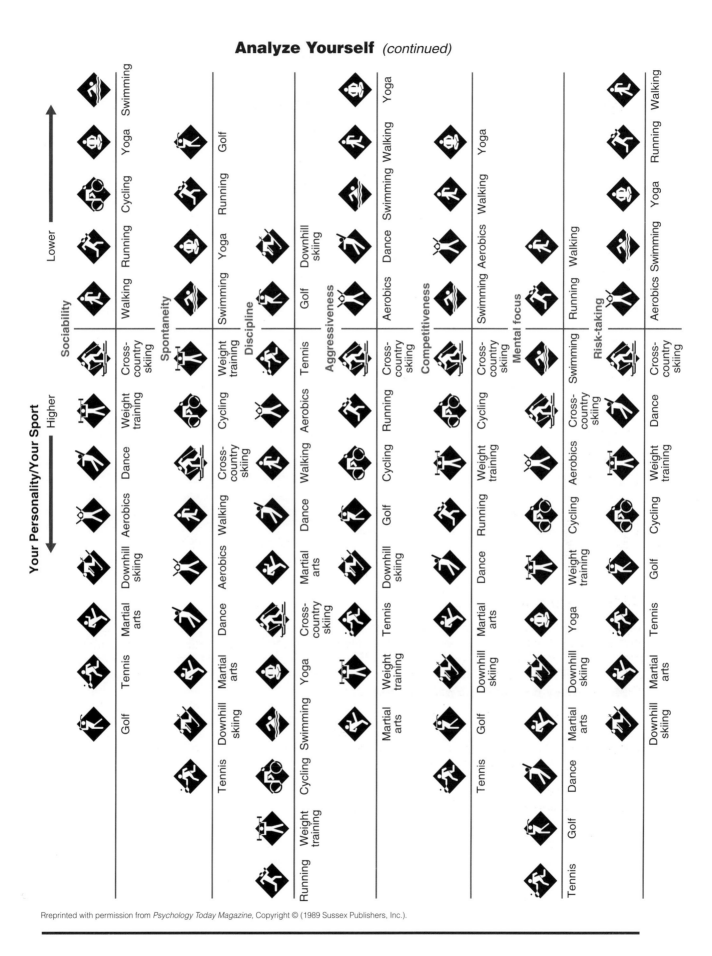

Identifying Your Fitness Goals

Why do you want to engage in physical activity? Some people simply want to be healthy. Others want to look good, to have energy, to develop strength, or to compete for the sake of competing. It stands to reason that if you do not know why you participate in physical fitness activities, you cannot select activities that will help you meet your goals.

Health Promotion and Disease Prevention

One of your fitness goals is probably to maintain good health. We have already discussed the fact that this requires more than simply exercise. For example, you know that to remain healthy, you need to eat nutritionally, use stress-management techniques to prevent illness and disease, and refrain from using chemical substances that can harm you (such as tobacco and illicit drugs). When you do all this, you can prevent, or at least postpone, the onset of cardiovascular diseases (such as coronary heart disease and stroke) as well as precursors of these diseases (such as high blood pressure). You can also decrease your risk of contracting cancer or other life-threatening diseases. But beyond merely preventing illness and disease, you can also enhance your well-being by engaging in a variety of lifestyle behaviors. Although we will now focus on exercise behaviors, do not neglect to consider other lifestyle behaviors when designing a total fitness program for yourself. We will return to this topic at the conclusion of this chapter.

Fitness Activities to Help You Achieve Your Goals

You can participate in a seemingly endless array of physical activities. We will describe several of the more popular and effective exercise options in this section. If we skip your favorite activity, we apologize, but be comforted by knowing that a trip to the library will probably disclose all you ever wanted to know about it.

Walking

Walking is an excellent way to keep fit without putting undue stress on your connective tissue and bones. Studies have shown that adults who

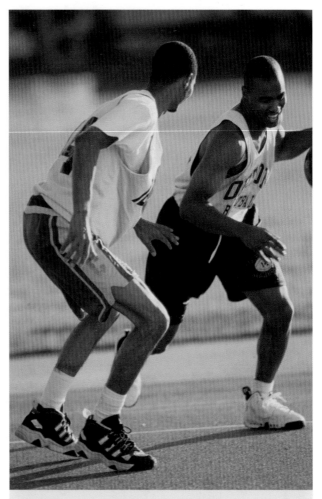

Exercise is important for people of all ages who wish to stay healthy and prevent disease.
PhotoDisc

walk for exercise 2 1/2 to 4 hours a week tend to have less than half the prevalence of elevated serum cholesterol as those who do not walk or exercise regularly. Walking can develop cardiorespiratory endurance (especially if the speed of walking is brisk) and burn a lot of calories. What is more, people of all ages can participate in walking. Finally, walking can have psychological benefits as well, helping to reduce anxiety and depression.

The President's Council on Physical Fitness and Sports offers some tips to help you develop an efficient walking style:

1. Hold your head erect and keep your back straight and your abdomen flat. Your toes should point straight ahead, and your arms should swing loosely at your sides.

2. Land on the heel of your foot and roll forward to drive off the ball of your foot. Walking only on the balls of your feet or flat-footed may cause fatigue and soreness.

3. Take long, easy strides but do not strain for distance. When walking up or down hills or at a rapid pace, lean forward slightly.

4. Breathe deeply (with your mouth open if that is more comfortable).

To help you to begin a walking program, follow the regimen in table 15.1.

Jogging and Running

If walking is too slow for you, try **jogging** or **running.** With either, you can get a comparable workout in a shorter time. Unfortunately, jogging puts stress on your body, subjecting you to a greater chance of injury than walking does. Foot, ankle, knee, and back problems can develop. Yet with the proper precautions (good shoes and not doing more than you are in condition to do), you can minimize jogging injuries.

Having the right running shoes is important if you choose to jog. Many shoes are available from which to choose. We will discuss how to buy shoes in which to run or jog later in this chapter. Personnel in stores selling running shoes can help you select a shoe right for you, but you need to be the final judge. If the shoe feels comfortable and provides enough support, it is probably the right shoe for you.

> **jogging**—Running at pace of 9 minutes per mile or slower.
>
> **running**—Running at a pace faster than 9 minutes per mile.

TABLE 15.1—Sample Walking Program

Week	Warm-up	Target zone exercising	Cool-down	Total time
WEEK 1				
Session A	Walk 5 min	Then walk briskly 5 min	Then walk more slowly 5 min	15 min
Session B	Repeat previous pattern			
Session C	Repeat previous pattern			
CONTINUE WITH AT LEAST THREE EXERCISE SESSIONS DURING EACH WEEK OF THE PROGRAM.				
Week 2	Walk 5 min	Walk briskly 7 min	Walk 5 min	17 min
Week 3	Walk 5 min	Walk briskly 9 min	Walk 5 min	19 min
Week 4	Walk 5 min	Walk briskly 11 min	Walk 5 min	21 min
Week 5	Walk 5 min	Walk briskly 13 min	Walk 5 min	23 min
Week 6	Walk 5 min	Walk briskly 15 min	Walk 5 min	25 min
Week 7	Walk 5 min	Walk briskly 18 min	Walk 5 min	28 min
Week 8	Walk 5 min	Walk briskly 20 min	Walk 5 min	30 min
Week 9	Walk 5 min	Walk briskly 23 min	Walk 5 min	33 min
Week 10	Walk 5 min	Walk briskly 26 min	Walk 5 min	36 min
Week 11	Walk 5 min	Walk briskly 28 min	Walk 5 min	38 min
Week 12	Walk 5 min	Walk briskly 30 min	Walk 5 min	40 min
Week 13 and on	Check your pulse periodically to see whether you are exercising within your target zone. As you become more fit, try exercising within the upper range of your target zone. Gradually increase your brisk walking time to 30 to 60 min, three or four times a week. Remember that your goal is to gain the benefits you are seeking and enjoy your activity.			

From President's Council on Physical Fitness and Sports. 2003, *A guide to physical activity.* http://www.pueblo.gsa.gov/cic_text/health/exercise-heart/index.htm.

The President's Council on Physical Fitness and Sports points out that running for fitness is different from running for speed and power. When you run for fitness, you should maintain a comfortable, economical running style:

- Run in an upright position, avoiding excessive forward lean. Keep your back as straight as you comfortably can and keep your head up. Do not look down at your feet.

- Carry your arms slightly away from your body, with your elbows bent so that your forearms are roughly parallel to the ground. Occasionally shake and relax your arms to prevent tightness in your shoulders.

- Land on the heel of your foot and rock forward to drive off the ball of your foot. If this proves difficult, try a more flat-footed style. Running only on the balls of your feet will tire you quickly and make your legs sore.

- Keep your stride relatively short. Do not force your pace by reaching for extra distance.

- Breathe deeply with your mouth open.

One concern about either walking or running is safety. Recognizing the need to advise runners how to exercise to limit vulnerability, the Road Runners Club of America offers these tips in their booklet titled *Women Running: Run Smart. Run Safe.*

- Stay alert.
  a. Do not wear headphones. If you wear them, you will not hear an approaching car or an approaching attacker.
  b. Run against traffic so that you can observe approaching vehicles.
  c. Practice identifying characteristics of strangers and memorizing license tags.
  d. Tune into your environment, not out of it.
- Avoid isolation.
  a. Run in familiar areas.
  b. Run with a partner or dog.
  c. Write down or leave word about the direction of your run. Tell friends and family of your favorite running routes.
  d. Befriend neighbors and local businesses.
- Use your intuition.
  a. Trust your intuition about an area or a person, avoiding any place or person you are unsure of.
  b. Use discretion in acknowledging verbal harassment by strangers. Look directly at

others and be observant, but keep your distance and keep moving.
  c. Call police immediately if something happens to you or someone else or if you notice anyone out of the ordinary.
- Be prepared.
  a. Carry identification or write your name, phone number, and blood type on the inside of your running shoe.
  b. Do not wear jewelry.
  c. Carry a noisemaker.
  d. Be prepared to scream and break the silence.
  e. Wear reflective material.
  f. Know the location of telephones.
  g. Vary your route.

Jogging or running costs relatively little (good running shoes are the only major expense), can be done almost anywhere (indoors or out of doors), and is an excellent aerobic exercise. To help you begin a jogging and running program, follow the regimen in table 15.2.

Rope Jumping

When one of the authors was 13, he fell in love with 12-year-old, blonde-haired, adorable, vivacious Jill—heart-poundlingly, palm-perspiringly, any-spare-time-spent-with-her in love. The problem was that Steven was also in love with Jill. In the competition to win Jill's heart, the two boys learned how to jump rope that summer. While their friends played basketball and softball, they jumped rope with Jill. They were frantic to avoid being seen by their friends in this sissy activity. If their other friends had seen them, they would have died.

Well, no longer crippled by that thought, we learned that the sex you were born with need not stop you from participating in any enjoyable activity. Rope jumping is an excellent way of developing cardiorespiratory endurance, strength, agility, coordination, and a sense of wellness. Here are some pointers for rope jumping:

- Determine the best length for your rope by standing on the center of the rope. The handles should reach from armpit to armpit.

- When you are jumping, keep your arms close to your body with your elbows almost touching your sides. Have your forearms out at right angles and turn the rope by making small circles with your hands and wrists. Keep your feet, ankles, and knees together.

TABLE 15.2—Sample Jogging Program

Week	Warm-up	Target zone exercising	Cool-down	Total time
WEEK 1				
Session A	Walk 5 min, then stretch and limber up	Then walk 10 min, trying not to stop	Then walk more slowly 3 min and stretch 2 min	20 min
Session B	Repeat previous pattern			
Session C	Repeat previous pattern			
CONTINUE WITH AT LEAST THREE EXERCISE SESSIONS DURING EACH WEEK OF THE PROGRAM.				
Week 2	Walk 5 min, then stretch and limber up	Walk 5 min, jog 1 min, walk 5 min, jog 1 min	Walk 3 min, stretch 2 min	22 min
Week 3	Walk 5 min, then stretch and limber up	Walk 5 min, jog 3 min, walk 5 min, jog 3 min	Walk 3 min, stretch 2 min	26 min
Week 4	Walk 5 min, then stretch and limber up	Walk 4 min, jog 5 min, walk 4 min, jog 5 min	Walk 3 min, stretch 2 min	28 min
Week 5	Walk 5 min, then stretch and limber up	Walk 4 min, jog 5 min, walk 4 min, jog 5 min	Walk 3 min, stretch 2 min	28 min
Week 6	Walk 5 min, then stretch and limber up	Walk 4 min, jog 6 min, walk 4 min, jog 6 min	Walk 3 min, stretch 2 min	30 min
Week 7	Walk 5 min, then stretch and limber up	Walk 4 min, jog 7 min, walk 4 min, jog 7 min	Walk 3 min, stretch 2 min	32 min
Week 8	Walk 5 min, then stretch and limber up	Walk 4 min, jog 8 min, walk 4 min, jog 8 min	Walk 3 min, stretch 2 min	34 min
Week 9	Walk 5 min, then stretch and limber up	Walk 4 min, jog 9 min, walk 4 min, jog 9 min	Walk 3 min, stretch 2 min	36 min
Week 10	Walk 5 min, then stretch and limber up	Walk 4 min, jog 13 min	Walk 3 min, stretch 2 min	27 min
Week 11	Walk 5 min, then stretch and limber up	Walk 4 min, jog 15 min	Walk 3 min, stretch 2 min	29 min
Week 12	Walk 5 min, then stretch and limber up	Walk 4 min, jog 17 min	Walk 3 min, stretch 2 min	31 min
Week 13	Walk 5 min, then stretch and limber up	Walk 2 min, jog slowly 2 min, jog 17 min	Walk 3 min, stretch 2 min	31 min
Week 14	Walk 5 min, then stretch and limber up	Walk 1 min, jog slowly 3 min, jog 17 min	Walk 3 min, stretch 2 min	31 min
Week 15	Walk 5 min, then stretch and limber up	Jog slowly 3 min, jog 17 min	Walk 3 min, stretch 2 min	30 min

From President's Council on Physical Fitness and Sports. 2003, *A guide to physical activity.* http://www.pueblo.gsa.gov/cic_text/health/exercise-heart/index.htm.

- Relax. Do not tense up. Enjoy yourself.
- Keep your body erect, with your head and eyes up.
- Start slowly.
- Land on the balls of your feet, bending your knees slightly.
- Maintain a steady rhythm.
- Jump just 1 or 2 inches off the floor.
- Try jumping to music and maintaining the rhythm of the music.
- When you get good, improvise. Create new stunts. Have fun.

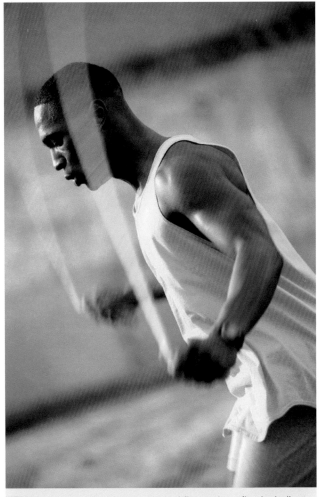

Rope jumping offers many physical fitness benefits, including the development of cardiorespiratory endurance, strength, agility, and coordination.

Getty Images

Swimming

Swimming is both a popular and an excellent physical fitness activity. What's more, it enhances physical fitness while diminishing the chances of injury because it limits the amount of weight your body must bear. When you are submerged up to the neck in water, you experience an apparent loss of 90% of your weight. If you weigh 130 pounds and are in water up to your neck, your feet and legs have to support only 13 pounds. Therefore, you are less apt to injure your legs and feet.

Many people who use swimming for conditioning do lap swimming—that is, they swim back and forth. When you are lap swimming, you should periodically check your heart rate to determine if you are at your target. But lap swimming is not appropriate for everyone. Backyard pools are usually not large enough. Most residential pools are no bigger than 36 feet by 17 feet, with approximately 600 square feet of water surface and depths of 3 to 8 feet. In a swimming pool of this size, you must adjust your workout considerably from that usually practiced in the typical school, college, or athletic club pool. Otherwise, swimming in the backyard pool becomes largely a matter of diving in, gliding across, and climbing out. For most people, it means only inactive bathing. But swimming pools, regardless of size, have high potential as exercise facilities. People can realize that potential by learning how to exercise in limited water areas.

The President's Council on Physical Fitness and Sports recommends an exercise program for limited water areas in its booklet *Aqua Dynamics*. The program involves standing water drills (for example, alternate toe touching, side-straddle hopping, toe bounding, and jogging in place), poolside standing drills (such as stretching the arms out, pressing the back flat against the wall, and raising the knees to the chest), gutter-holding drills (such as knees to chest, hop twisting, front and back flutter kicking, and side flutter kicking), bobbing, and treading water. If you have your own pool and feel it is too small for lap swimming, you might write to the President's Council on Physical Fitness and Sports, 200 Independence Avenue SW, Washington, DC 20201, for the *Aqua Dynamics* booklet. Another good source is Jane Katz's article "The W.E.T. Workout," which was published in the June 1986 issue of *Shape* magazine. Or you can contact your nearest health club, YMCA, or Jewish Community Center to see if they have water aerobics classes.

To help you begin a swimming program, follow the regimen in table 15.3.

Tennis

As with all fitness activities, duration and intensity will determine how much your tennis game contributes to your physical fitness and wellness. A doubles match generally results in a less demanding workout than a singles match does. A doubles match will use up to 330 calories per hour, whereas a singles match will use up to 390 calories per hour.

The contribution of tennis to wellness, however, is another matter. As we have often stated in this book, if your physical health improves while other components of your health suffer, you have not improved your health. Playing tennis or other competitive sports may improve the efficiency of your heart, but if your attitude and behavior on the court compromise your friendships, result in

TABLE 15.3—Swimming

Week	Aerobic training program	Comments
I. VERY BEGINNING		
1st week	Begin by using any stroke and swim for 12-20 min per session at least three times per week.	Swim until out of breath. Continue until you can swim nonstop for the allotted time.
3rd week	Swim three to five times per week. Try to use the freestyle stroke as much as possible.	Swim continuously for 20 min.
6th week	Test yourself in the 1.5 mi test. If your category has changed, move on to the program for rating II. If no change has occurred, remain at this point for 2 more weeks and then retest.	—
II. BEGINNING		
1st week	Begin by using any stroke and swim for 15-22 min per session at least three times per week.	Swim until out of breath. Continue until you can swim nonstop for the allotted time.
3rd week	Swim daily. Use the freestyle stroke as much as possible.	Swim continuously for 22 min.
6th week	Swim daily for 30 min. Test yourself in the 1.5 mi test. If your category has changed, move on to the program for rating III. If no change has occurred, remain at this point for 2 more weeks.	—
III. INTERMEDIATE		
1st week	Swim freestyle for 500 yd per workout, three times per week.	Begin to time your workouts. Aim for a time of 12 min. If you reach 12 min, then aim for 10 1/2 min.
3rd week	Continue swimming 500 yd per workout. Add one additional workout each week.	Try to reach the above target times.
6th week	Test yourself in 1.5 mi test. If your category has changed, move on to the program for rating IV. If no change has occurred, remain at this point for 2 more weeks and then retest.	—
IV. ADVANCED		
1st week	Swim freestyle for 650 yd per workout, four times each week.	Aim for a time of 15 1/2 min.
3rd week	Add one workout in each of the next 2 weeks so that you do six workouts per week.	—
6th week	Test yourself in 1.5 mi test. If your category has changed, move on to the program for rating V. If no change has occurred, remain at this point for 2 more weeks, add 50 yd per workout, and then retest.	—
V. SUPERIOR		
—	Aim to swim freestyle for 1,000 yd per workout. Begin with 700 yd per workout and add 50 yd every two workouts.	Aim for a 1,000 yd time of under 16 1/2 min.
—	Take the 1.5 mi test once monthly to judge the success of your maintenance program.	If you want to improve rather than maintain present level, add 50 yd every three workouts until you reach 2,000 yd. Aim for a time of 34 min.

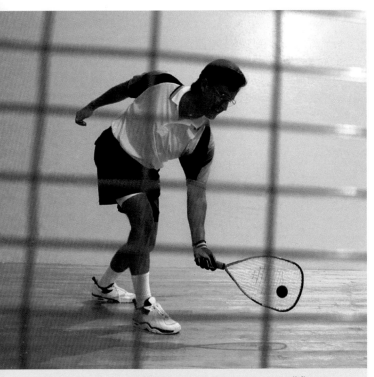

Racquetball is an excellent way to improve your overall fitness, muscular strength, and flexibility.

PhotoDisc

cardiorespiratory endurance, muscular strength and endurance of the legs, flexibility, agility, balance and coordination, and weight control. They are also usually fun. Yet danger is involved in these sports. Every year, over 3,000 eye injuries result from indoor racket sports. That need not be the case if players wear appropriate eye protectors. Eye protectors should offer a complete shield (do not use the kind with narrow bands with openings between them) and be made of polycarbonate.

Another risk of these sports involves the environment in which they are played. Exercising in a hot room can be hazardous unless you take certain precautions. You should drink plenty of water before starting to play and intermittently take breaks to replenish the water you lose through perspiration. You should not play longer than you are in condition to play; to overdo it in a hot room can be risky. Know when to stop.

Finally, you must be in good physical condition before engaging in these sports. They are highly competitive, usually played in a hot environment, and involve dynamic (stop-and-go) and stretching movements. If you are not in good physical condition, you may injure yourself. If you are in good condition, these sports are excellent activities to help you remain fit.

Aerobic Dance

One of the best fitness activities is dance, especially if you're serious about your training. Look at the bodies of dancers. They are remarkably muscular, incredibly supple, and highly prepared to meet the demands that strenuous exercise places on their cardiorespiratory systems. Dance is a good way to develop and maintain physical fitness.

The traditional dance programs are tap, ballet, and modern dance. In recent years, a different form of dance has swept the country and become a significant part of the fitness movement. Aerobic dance, a term coined by Jacki Sorenson in 1979, combines calisthenics and a variety of dance movements, all done to music. It involves, hopping, bouncing, kicking, and various arm movements designed to develop cardiorespiratory endurance, flexibility, and muscular strength and endurance. Dancing to music is an enjoyable activity for many people who would not otherwise seek to exercise. Because aerobic dance is often done in groups, the social contact makes it even more enjoyable.

your not enjoying yourself, or frustrate you, you would be better off not playing at all. In spite of exercising, you are making yourself less well. Two solutions make the most sense to us: Either approach competitive sports with a different attitude or select a less competitive exercise to engage in regularly.

When stroking the ball, if you roll over the shot too much (use too much topspin), you can contribute to tennis elbow. Using too much wrist in the shot will lead you to roll over; instead, you should stroke through the ball with your wrist locked. If tennis elbow does develop, you can switch to a lighter racket to reduce aggravation of the elbow. Applying ice after playing will also help.

A warm-up that includes stretching is a must. Tennis involves dynamic, quick movements with a great deal of stretching to reach the ball. Therefore, if you are not flexible enough, you may be prone to muscle and connective-tissue injuries, such as muscle pulls or sprained ligaments.

Racquetball, Handball, and Squash

The indoor racket sports can be excellent ways to develop and maintain fitness. They contribute to

To maximize the fitness benefits of aerobic dance, you should maintain the dancing for approximately 35 to 45 minutes and work out three or four times a week. In addition, you should check periodically to see if you are maintaining your target heart rate (THR). Because many communities offer aerobic dance classes (some may be called dancercise or jazzercise) through YMCAs, Jewish Community Centers, colleges, local schools, and even morning television programs, maintaining a regular dance regimen should not be difficult. The only equipment you need is a good pair of aerobic dance shoes with good shock absorbency, stability, and outer-sole flexibility and clothes to work out in. One caution: Do not dance on a concrete floor because the constant pounding could result in shin splints. A wooden floor is ideal.

Low-Impact Aerobics

Several factors associated with aerobic dance have led some experts to question the manner in which it is usually conducted. An early study by the American Aerobics Association found that 80% of instructors and students were sustaining injuries during workouts, and another questionnaire administered to instructors revealed that 55% reported significant injuries (Garrick and Requa, 1988). Among the causes of these injuries were bad floors (too hard), bad shoes (too little shock absorbency and stability), and bad routines offered by poorly trained instructors. With the popularity of aerobics, it is not surprising what people do in its name. An aerobics routine has even been developed for the pudgy dog or cat. We should not be surprised that some aerobics instructors are poorly trained and teach routines that are inappropriate and injury producing, using surfaces that cause high-impact injuries.

In response to these concerns, several things have happened. One is the certification of aerobics instructors. Organizations such as the American College of Sports Medicine (ACSM), the Aerobics and Fitness Association of America, National Dance-Exercise Instructor's Training Association, Ken Cooper's Aerobics Way, and the Aerobic Center have all instituted certification programs for aerobics instructors. Unfortunately, the requirements for certification by these organizations vary greatly. Some form of certification, however, is probably better than none.

The development of low-impact aerobics routines is another response to the high injury rate of aerobics. Low-impact aerobics features keeping one foot on the ground at all times and using light weights. The idea is to cut down on the stress to the body caused by jumping and bouncing while at the same time deriving the muscle-toning and cardiorespiratory benefits of high-impact aerobics. These routines have become increasingly popular as the risk of injury from high-impact aerobics has become better known. Something called chair aerobics has even been developed. In this activity, participants do routines while seated in a chair.

Low-impact aerobics is not completely risk free. Injuries to the upper body caused by the circling and swinging movements with weights are not infrequent. Many of these injuries can be treated at home, however, and are not serious. Any form of physical activity includes the chance of injury. The benefits to the cardiorespiratory system and the rest of the body—benefits that we have described throughout this book—are often worth the slight chance of injury.

A recent aerobic dance development is step aerobics, which involves stepping up and down on a small platform (step) to the rhythm of music and the directions of an instructor. The workout can vary from mild to extremely intense depending on the speed, movements, and duration of the exercise. Another variation is double-step aerobics, which involves the use of two platforms. Step aerobics classes are usually offered at the same places where aerobic dance classes are conducted. If you are interested in double-step aerobics, you can read an article about it in the May 1993 issue of *American Health* magazine (Winters, 1993).

Bicycling

To begin a bicycle exercise program, you obviously need a bicycle. A good 10-speed bicycle will cost approximately $400. You can get an adequate 10-speed bike or a mountain bike (a sturdier bike) for less if you shop around or buy one secondhand. You will also need a helmet to protect your head from injury should you fall. Gloves with padded palms can make your ride more comfortable. In addition, think about adding pant clips or clothes designed specifically for bicycling.

Of course, you can exercise with any bike—it need not have 10 speeds or be a mountain bike—if you choose. A good bike, however, will allow you to take trips that add to the enjoyment of cycling in addition to enhancing overall health and wellness.

When you are bicycling, follow this advice:

- Keep your elbows slightly bent.
- Lower your upper body for a streamlined position.
- Do not grip the handlebars too tightly.
- Wear bright clothing so that motorists can easily see you.
- Obey all traffic laws.
- Always lean into the turn.
- Learn and use hand signals that indicate which way you are turning.
- Leave the radio at home so that you can focus on the road and hear vehicles and other potential hazards.
- Keep your bicycle in good working order, well oiled with grease and dirt removed from around the chain and gears.

Some people bicycle for terrific exercise yet go nowhere. They use stationary bikes. Many health clubs have computerized stationary bikes that riders can set for various kinds of riding (for example, hilly or high speed) and for various distances. Other people remove a wheel from a bicycle, raise the frame, and cycle indoors during the winter months. You can buy equipment called a wind trainer that does this for you.

When you ride a stationary bike, you need to adjust the seat and handlebars to the proper height and angle. To work your leg muscles properly, your knee should be slightly bent when the pedal is in the fully down position (see figure 15.1). Too great or too little a bend will result in inefficient use of the leg muscles. You should adjust the handlebars so that you are relaxed and leaning slightly forward (see figure 15.2).

In addition, you should pay attention to the bicycle seat. Urologists disagree about the possibility that males will develop erectile dysfunction (previously referred to as impotence) by riding a bicycle for long periods. Some riders report a numbing sensation in the groin area resulting from pressure on the nerves and blood vessels. But no definitive studies have linked erectile dysfunction with bicycle riding. Still, caution may be warranted. Consequently, you might consider a bicycle seat with holes where this pressure usually occurs, gel-filled seats, or seats with rubber shock absorbers. For some riders, just tilting the front of the seat slightly downward works.

To help you begin a bicycling program, follow the regimen in table 15.4.

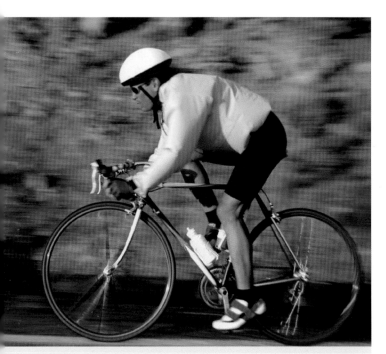

Anyone who rides a bicycle, even for short distances, should wear a helmet at all times.

PhotoDisc

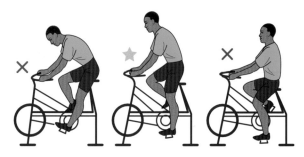

Figure 15.1 Seat adjustment when riding a stationary bike. The middle drawing depicts correct seat height. The seat on the left is too high, and the one on the right is too low. Maintain a slight bend in the lower leg when vertical.

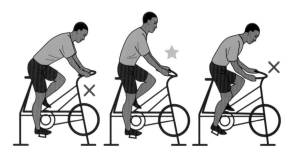

Figure 15.2 Handlebar adjustment when riding a stationary bike. The middle drawing depicts correct handlebar adjustment.

TABLE 15.4—Cycling

Week	Aerobic training program	Comments
I. VERY BEGINNING		
1st week	Ride for 2 mi, three times per week.	Do not be concerned with time during first weeks of your program. Cycle at a pace that allows you to finish 2 mi without undue fatigue.
3rd week	Ride for 2 mi, three times per week. Try to finish the distance in 12 min or less.	Time your ride and attempt to reach the target time.
6th week	Test yourself in the 1.5 mi test. If your category has changed, move on to the program for rating II. If no change has occurred, add one workout and cycle four times each week.	—
II. BEGINNING		
1st week	Ride for 3 mi, three times per week.	Time your ride and aim for a time of 17 min or less.
3rd week	Continue riding for 3 mi but work out four times per week.	Try to lower the time for your ride to 14 min or less.
6th week	Test yourself in the 1.5 mi test. If your category has changed, move on to the program for rating III. If no change has occurred, add one workout and cycle five times each week.	—
III. INTERMEDIATE		
1st week	Ride for 5 mi, three times per week.	Time your ride and aim for a time of 25 min or less.
3rd week	Continue riding for 5 mi but work out four times per week.	—
6th week	Test yourself in the 1.5 mi test. If your category has changed, move on to the program for rating IV. If no change has occurred, add one workout and cycle five times each week.	—
IV. ADVANCED		
1st week	Ride for 8 mi, four times per week.	Aim for a time of 35 min or less.
3rd week	Add one workout and cycle five times per week.	—
V. SUPERIOR		
—	Continue with this workout and try to lower your time to 24 min or less. Take the 1.5 mi test once a month to judge the success of your program.	

Other Fitness Activities

A range of new exercise activities and equipment can challenge fitness aficionados. The stability or exercise ball is a large, soft ball (usually between 42 and 65 centimeters) inflated with air. The exerciser can lie on it in a prone or supine position and do a number of different exercises or hold it against a wall with his or her back while performing a progression of movements.

A variation of the exercise ball is the bosu ball. The bosu ball is like half of an exercise ball. That is, it is an inflated hemisphere. The word *bosu* means "both sides." The ball can be placed with either the flat or the inflated side down. Its proponents say it enhances balance. The bosu ball can even be used for other exercises (for example, abdominal crunches).

More health clubs are offering Pilates classes. Pilates exercises were developed by Joseph Pilates to encourage correct posture and technique—control over core muscles—rather than excessive repetitions or lifting heavy weights. Muscles are worked in more than one direction to prevent muscle imbalance that can lead to injuries.

A variation on Pilates is Gyrokinesis or Gyrotonic, called Gyro for short. Gyro can be performed while seated in a chair, lying down, or standing up. It involves being attached to a special machine and performing circular motions with various parts of the body. Its proponents believe that Gyro enhances flexibility and balance as well as muscular strength.

For those preferring to exercise on stationary bikes, an activity called spinning offers an appealing variation. Spinning is a group activity led by an instructor who encourages the spinners to rise from their bikes at times and to change the pace periodically. Spinning requires a special bike, and spinners often buy special shoes that attach to the pedals and make cycling easier. The music the group listens to while spinning serves as motivation to get a hearty workout, especially if the instructor carefully selects the music.

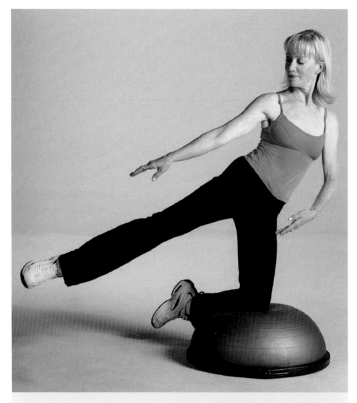

Bosu ball, Gyro, and spinning are fitness activities that provide variety and flexibility to workouts.

Courtesy of FitnessQuest

Being a Fitness Consumer

To remain fit your whole life, you need to be an effective fitness consumer. You need to know how to select a fitness club and buy the right equipment.

Selecting an Exercise Club

Joining a health or fitness club is an excellent strategy for beginning or maintaining your exercise program. The club will encourage your participation in several ways. First, once you shell out the membership fee, you will want to get your money's worth. Second, after working out a few times, you will probably meet other people at the club whom you would like to get to know better. That social contact is reinforcing, and the subtle peer pressure to be there—"Hey, Betty, where were you last Wednesday?"—may be just enough to get you to the club when you do not feel like working out.

Because a health or fitness club can be expensive, inconvenient to get to, or both, you should select one carefully. The club should meet your needs, be safe, and support your exercise goals. Figure 15.3 provides you with a way to evaluate a club and decide whether it is right for you.

Buying Exercise Equipment

Some fitness activities require little if any equipment. A pair of running shoes, shorts, a top, and socks are usually enough for jogging. On the other hand, you cannot play tennis without a tennis racket or bike without a bicycle. In this section, we make brief comments to help you make sensible decisions when you buy exercise equipment.

Athletic Shoes

The major criteria to use when selecting athletic shoes are comfort and support. Here are a few suggestions that will help you buy the right shoe (and the left one, too, for that matter):

- Recognize whether you pronate or supinate. Buy a shoe made specifically for either pronators or supinators.
- Shop for shoes late in the day. Your feet tend to swell as the day goes on. No sense buying a shoe that fits snugly in the morning when you usually, or even occasionally, exercise in the afternoon.
- Try shoes on with the kind of socks you usually wear when you are exercising.

The Fitness Industry Association (FIA) of the United Kingdom recommends that a health club provide the following:

- Two types of basic equipment—resistance and cardiovascular machines
- Possibly a swimming pool and sauna
- Clean changing areas and a number of showers
- Qualified fitness instructors who will be available to give advice on exercise, weight control, and nutrition
- A variety of fitness classes covering a wide timetable
- A basic physical assessment before you exercise
- A nursery or child-care facility for children

Every health club will allow you to take a tour of the facility. Usually someone will accompany you. During this tour you should ask the questions on your mind. Questions you might consider asking include these:

- What are the club's opening times?
- What is the membership fee?
- Is the membership a yearly contract?
- Can membership be canceled or frozen?
- Can I downgrade or upgrade a membership?
- Are off-peak prices available?
- Are showers and changing facilities available?
- Are qualified instructors on hand?
- Is fitness instruction offered?
- Will I be given an exercise program to follow?
- Will I need a doctor's approval?
- Are fitness classes offered?
- Are classes included in the membership price?
- What specific facilities are available?
- How busy does the gym get? At what times?
- Is parking available?
- Are accommodations made for children?
- Is a nursery or child-care facility on site?

Figure 15.3   Is this the club for me?

Data courtesy of: (Thefitmap LTD)—www.thefitmap.com. For more health club ideas visit www.The fitmap.com. Reprinted by permission of THEFITMAP Limited.

- Buy shoes with uppers made of leather or nylon that breathes.
- Look for brands of shoes that come in different widths if you have exceptionally narrow or wide feet.
- Buy a shoe with a last (the form on which the shoe is made) made for your size foot. That means most women ought to buy shoes made for women, and men should buy shoes made for men, because women's and men's lasts differ.
- Shop at a store with experienced salespeople. Discuss your particular concerns with them. For example, if you want a shoe with shock

absorption, one that is extra wide, or one that will hold up, the salesperson should be able to recommend the appropriate shoe. If you want a shoe for tennis or basketball or some other sport, an experienced salesperson should be able to help with that as well.

- When trying the shoes on, perform some of the moves you will use when exercising in them. Jump or twist or bend or stretch. Make sure that the shoe is comfortable during these movements.

- Once you decide which shoe you want to buy, check the price at different stores or from several athletic shoe distributors. You can do this easily by telephone. Also, check the back of sports magazines for distributors who discount the price of shoes.

Replace athletic shoes regularly, before they wear out. Fifty percent of a shoe's shock-absorbing capacity is gone after 300 miles of running or walking or 300 hours of aerobics classes, and 80% is gone at 500 miles and 500 hours. Exercising with shoes whose shock-absorbing capacity is diminished is a recipe for injury.

Orthotics

Some people have problems with their feet that need some form of correction when they are exercising. They may have leg imbalances (one leg longer than the other), or they may **pronate** or **supinate.** Orthotic devices placed in athletic shoes correct these problems and allow people to exercise in comfort. Orthotics also diminish the risk of injury. The devices come in rigid or soft forms. Ready-made inserts are available in drugstores and sporting goods shops and may be all that is needed in some cases. Because each foot is different from every other foot, however, if you have a problem, it is wise to consult an expert.

Bicycles

Many different kinds of bicycles are available: city bikes, all-terrain mountain bikes, touring bikes, racing bikes, and so forth. An experienced salesperson can guide you to the type of bicycle that will best suit the use you wish to make of it. When you buy a bike (usually somewhere between $400

> **pronate**—Rolling the foot inward when it is pushing off.
>
> **supinate**—Rocking the foot to the outside when it is pushing off.

and $1,200), factor in the cost of a helmet, a water bottle, a repair kit for flat tires, shorts, shoes, and gloves. Those items might add another $300. Buy the bike at a store that offers good service and is staffed by professionals who really know bikes. When you think you are interested in a particular bike, test ride it. In addition, test ride others for comparison. Try all the gears. Can you shift the gears easily? Do the brakes work well? How does it corner? Buying the right bicycle will enhance the enjoyment you get out of bicycling and consequently will help you maintain your exercise program.

Home Exercise Equipment

Some people prefer to exercise alone. If you can afford to purchase home exercise equipment, you might consider buying a stationary bike (maybe one with a built-in computer), a recumbent bicycle (a stationary bike that is low to the floor so that your legs are straight out instead of hanging down), a climber (which imitates stair climbing), a rower, a cross-country ski machine, a treadmill, or weights. Because this equipment can be expensive, you should be careful to buy exercise equipment that will help you meet your fitness goals safely.

Because exercise equipment undergoes continuous improvement and prices change frequently, we have decided not to be too specific about particular home exercise equipment in this section. Once you decide you would like to exercise at home, you should consult with an expert in fitness at a local health club, YMCA, or Jewish Community Center (be sure to speak with someone credentialed in exercise physiology or physical fitness), read articles about selecting home exercise equipment in health and fitness journals and magazines at your local library, or speak with a fitness expert at a local college or university.

You should consider the following when you are deciding what equipment to buy:

- What are your fitness goals? If you are trying to develop cardiorespiratory endurance, you should probably buy a treadmill or stationary bike rather than weights.

- Who is going to use the equipment? If more than one person will exercise with the equipment, it should be easily adjustable.

- How much space do you have? You might have room for a stationary bike but not enough space to add a rower as well. In that case, you will need to decide which piece of equipment you want most.

- How much can you spend? In a perfect world, cost would be no object. But you probably do not live in a perfect world, so you will need to decide the best way to spend your limited resources.

Try the equipment before buying it. Is the seat comfortable? Is the climbing motion smooth? Is the machine sturdy? Is the activity fun to do? Do you get the type of workout you want?

Stationary Bikes

Your first decision is whether to buy a standard upright or a recumbent bike. With a recumbent bike, you sit in a reclined position with your legs outstretched. The recumbent bike works your gluteal muscles more than a stationary bike does, but it requires a little more room to store and operate. Make sure any bike you buy has a comfortable seat that is adjustable and can lock in place. The bike should have straps to hold your feet on the pedals. For fast, smooth pedaling, look for a bike with a heavy flywheel (at least 25 pounds) and a high gear ratio (at least 4 to 1, and optimally 7 to 1). If you own a road bike, you might think about buying a bike trainer or rollers that convert it into a stationary bike for indoor workouts. When using rollers, however, the front and rear wheels ride on aluminum drums, so quite a bit of balance is required. Therefore, you might first try a bike trainer that clamps to the rear axle of the bike, providing resistance with a wind mechanism or magnetic flywheel.

Treadmills

A treadmill that costs less than $1,000 is usually noisy, wobbly, and difficult to use. In addition, it will not last very long, especially if you use it often. A treadmill should have at least a 1-horsepower motor, an adjustable incline to simulate hills, and a wide, long running surface with good traction. Make sure that the treadmill has a large, heavy-duty roller that keeps the belt centered. Consider buying a treadmill with a two-ply belt because it will last longer. Treadmills come with many other options. Some offer different programs for your workout, others have low-impact suspension systems, and still others have a safety feature that shuts the machine off if you lose your balance. Of course, in general, the greater the number of features, the higher the cost.

Steppers

Most people who buy a stepper for their home buy one with hydraulic shock absorbers rather than an electronic, computer-controlled stepper like those found in health clubs. These hydraulic steppers are more moderately priced. Some steppers are dual action—that is, they can work the arms as well as the legs. An example is the vertical-ascent machine that simulates ladder climbing. Make sure you buy a stepper that does not wobble (is sturdy) or squeak, that has comfortable foot pedals that are wide enough for your feet, and that provides smooth and relatively quiet motion. Consider a stepper with a glare-free screen that provides feedback such as elapsed time, step rate, total steps, and estimated calories used.

Cross-Country Ski Machines

Some cross-country ski machines have a belt and flywheel for resistance, an abdominal pad for balance, and a friction pulley system threaded with a nylon cord with grips that the skier holds in the hands and pumps during exercise. These machines have independent ski action, with each ski moving independently of the other. Another type of cross-country ski machine has footpads mounted on ski-type tracks and arm poles that pivot on each side of the machine's base. These machines have dependent ski action—as one ski moves forward, the other moves backward. Dependent ski action makes the machine easier to use; independent ski action is sometimes difficult to get used to. Regardless of which type of ski machine you decide to buy, make sure that it is solid and stable, that it has separate resistance adjustments for upper- and lower-body movements, and that the display that provides feedback on elapsed time, estimated calories expended, and the like is easy to read.

Abdominal Exercise Equipment

What do actor Jean-Claude Van Damme and basketball player Michael Jordan have in common? When NordicTrack, a leading exercise equipment manufacturer, asked people in the United States who had the best abs, 39% chose Van Damme and 21% chose Jordan. In the female category, Olympian Jackie Joyner-Kersee was the choice of 44%, far ahead of singer Janet Jackson (19%) and Madonna (8%). Those judged to need the most work on their abdominal muscles were comedienne Roseanne (48%), politician Newt Gingrich (19%), cartoon character Homer Simpson (14%), and President Bill Clinton (12%).

If you are up late at night flipping through the television channels, you are likely to see someone selling abdominal exercise equipment. If it isn't the Ab Blaster®, it's the Ab Flex®, the Total Ab Isolator®, or the Ab Trainer®. The washboard abdomen has, unfortunately, become the ultimate symbol of fitness for many people, or at least the most visible. People are willing to pay anywhere from $30 to $200 for the promise of a rippled belly. Approximately 2.75 million abdominal exercise machines were sold in the United States in 1995. Sales increased in 1996 to between $200 million and $400 million.

If you are thinking about buying one of these machines, think again. The way to acquire a washboard abdomen is through diet and abdominal exercises for which you do not need any equipment. If you have too much fat around the abdominal area, you can do abdominal exercises until the cows come home with little noticeable effect. Only losing fat and then tightening the abs will work. You would be better advised to take the money you were thinking of spending on abdominal exercise equipment and hiring a trainer or taking a class to learn which abdominal exercises to do and how to do them correctly.

The same goes for those electrical muscle stimulators (EMS). These machines purport to develop muscles without work by applying electrical current through the skin that stimulates muscle contraction. The only problem is that they don't work, and they can cost upward of $500. Some users complain of pain similar to a muscle cramp. Now, is all of that worth $500?

Promoting Lifetime Physical Fitness for Disabled Individuals

For the past few decades, myriad organizations have been developed that are designed to facilitate physically active lifestyles for mentally and physically challenged persons of all ages, not just the elite performers who qualify for the Paralympics or the Special Olympics. Physical activity, up to and including high-performance sports, has become important in the rehabilitation process for physically disabled individuals because many research studies find that reduced physical activity and a reduction in muscle mass often occur as a consequence of a variety of progressive neuromuscular diseases (McDonald, 2002; Rejeski and Focht, 2002; Gignac et al., 2002; Specht et al., 2002). This decline negatively affects quality of life, as determined by self-care, productivity, and leisure-time behavior of physically challenged persons.

People with disabilities continue to increase their participation in sports activities because they typically experience the same mental and physical health benefits, enjoyment, opportunity to increase self-esteem, enhanced self-concept, and opportunities to build and engage in social relationships as do nondisabled individuals. Furthermore, research on disabled athletes suggests that with persistent aerobic fitness conditioning or sports participation, many individuals confined to wheelchairs improve both their cardiorespiratory fitness and muscle function. A recent study of wheelchair athletes (Wu and Williams, 2001) found that friends and peers with disabilities were much more influential as continuing socialization agents than were rehabilitation therapists. The researchers also found that disabled athletes participated in sports activities primarily for fitness, fun, health, socialization, and competition.

In the American educational system, physical educators are increasingly encouraged to design a curriculum that includes activities and creates a supportive environment for physically and mentally challenged students. Recently, Shriner's Hospital for Children in Portland, Oregon, developed a 7-minute video titled *Kids Just Want To Have Fun!* about kids with disabilities from age 8 to the early teens and an 8-minute video primarily for middle and high school students titled *What's the Difference*. These videos, designed to promote acceptance and inclusion, show children with disabilities participating in all kinds of sports. The children share their philosophies about remaining active despite their disabilities. From them we learn that disability is as much an attitude as it is a condition.

The Amputee Coalition of America's (ACA's) Youth Activities Program has a new youth fitness program designed for children, parents, and caregivers. Their Bio-Fit Program occurs several times annually around the nation to allow maximal participation by youths, their families, and their caregivers. A monthly electronic newsletter provided by the National Center on Physical Activity and Disability (NCPAD) publicizes organizations and events such as these because they underscore the belief that healthy disabled individuals should remain physically active all their lives. The Web site address for NCPAD is www.ncpad.org.

For decades, we have witnessed the growth of wheelchair athletes at both grassroots and national levels. In fact, wheelchair basketball is the oldest Paralympic sport, dating back to the 1940s. Additionally, wheelchair racing is one of the most popular sporting activities of individuals with spinal cord injuries (Bhambhani, 2002). The first organized disabled sports games were held in 1948 in England. In March 2002 the U.S. Paralympics was formed as a separate division of the U.S. Olympic Committee (USOC). The primary focus of this new division is to enhance programs for Paralympic athletes. U.S. Paralympics and BlazeSports Clubs of America are the two leading sports programs targeting the needs and interests of the 52 million disabled Americans.

The Paralympic Games are held in the same city and during the same year as the Olympic Games. Like the Olympics, the Paralympics have both winter and summer games. The Paralympic Games include 3 winter sports and 18 summer sports. The Paralympics use a classification system so that athletes from six different disability classes can compete together, either individually or as teams. Paralympic sporting events follow the rules and procedures of the Olympic sports as much as possible. National and international competitions such as these send a message that disabled individuals, like nondisabled individuals, are capable of becoming lifelong elite performers.

Keeping Fit As You Age

The Andean village of Vilcabamba in Ecuador and the community of Abkhagia in Georgia share an unusual reputation. They are places where people supposedly live longer and remain more vigorous in old age than do people who live in other places. What factors contribute to the unusual longevity of people in these communities, where men and women who are well beyond 100 years of age are common? In the United States, the average life expectancy is in the 70s (depending on such factors as gender, ethnicity, education, and socioeconomic status), and there are only slightly more than 3 centenarians per 100,000 persons.

Clearly, genetic factors play a major role in the communities just cited. Many of the elderly had parents who also lived to be quite old. Yet when researchers studied these communities, they found other factors related to longevity. Elders are held in high esteem. They receive encouragement to work and be productive community members. Their efforts are appreciated and valued. These 100-year-olds eat low-calorie diets, about 1,800 calories a day, compared with the 3,300-calorie diet of the average American. These communities are located in remote mountainous regions and tend to be agricultural. Daily living in that environment requires significant climbing and descending of steep slopes and vigorous physical activity.

Exercise for the Elderly

We are generally less physically active than the centenarians just described. Only 30% of U.S. residents over 65 years of age exercise regularly. Therefore, we need to plan regular exercise. If we do, we will not only live longer but also live better. We will be less ill, less dependent on other people, more pain-free, and more psychologically healthy.

Planning exercise for elderly people requires attention to some special considerations:

- Skeletal structures are more prone to fracture (especially in older women).
- Connective tissue is more dense, and ligaments and tendons are less elastic. Range of motion may be significantly limited.
- Muscle mass is somewhat diminished, and reaction and reflex times are slower.

For these reasons, careful assessment should be made before prescribing exercise for an elderly individual. Older people must avoid wrenching and twisting movements, as well as sudden starting and stopping or changing direction. Slow, rhythmic stretching activities are best. And frequent rests should be built into the program.

Walking is an excellent activity for older people, especially in groups where they can socialize. Supervised swimming or exercises in the water are other good activities because they decrease weight bearing and tend to be fun. Also, do not forget dancing, which can enhance fitness goals when done rigorously. See table 15.5 for one possible program for elders.

Benefits of Exercise for Elders

Exercising will increase longevity and provide older people with a more fulfilling life. Elders can enhance their wellness when they exercise with other people (social health), when they exercise out of doors and appreciate the surroundings (spiritual health), when they exercise with family members and learn to control emotions that interfere with performing the activity (emotional health), and when they read and learn about the particular exercise and its benefits (mental health). In addition, exercise can postpone the inevitable changes associated with aging. Table 15.6 shows which physical activities relate to the changes brought on by aging.

The U.S. Public Health Service (1996) recognizes that inactivity increases with age. By age 75, about one in three men and one in two women engage in no physical activity. When elders do exercise, walking and gardening or yard work—excellent means of acquiring the benefits

of physical activity—tend to be most popular. The surgeon general goes on to offer the following "key messages":

- Older adults, both male and female, can benefit from regular physical activity.
- Physical activity need not be strenuous to achieve health benefits.
- Older adults can obtain significant health benefits with a moderate amount of physical activity, preferably daily. Longer sessions of moderately intense activities (such as walking) or shorter sessions of more vigorous activities

TABLE 15.5—Good Physical Activities for the Elderly

Activity	Frequency	Duration
Walking	3 times per week	3/4 hour
Swimming	3 times per week	1/2 hour
Dancing	2 times per week	Sets of 20 min with intervals of rest
Stretching and calisthenics	Every day	10-15 min
Golf	2 or 3 times per week	As long as necessary to complete 9 or 18 holes
Horseshoe pitching	According to desire	1/2 hour
Shuffleboard	According to desire	1 hour
Bocce	According to desire	1 hour
Croquet	According to desire	1 hour

TABLE 15.6—Aging Effects and Physical Activities That May Postpone or Reduce Them

Effects	Physical activities
Reduced cardiac output	Aerobic activities, jogging, swimming, cycling
Lowered pulmonary ventilation	Exercises that stretch rib-cage joints, aerobic activities of moderate to high intensity
Elevated blood pressure	Aerobic activities, jogging, swimming, cycling
Decrease in muscular strength	Weight training (resistance training)
Decrease in muscular endurance	Aerobic dance, calisthenics
Decrease in flexibility	Stretching, bending
Increase in percentage of stored body fat	Jogging, running, swimming, cycling
Loss of skin elasticity	Weight training (to maintain muscle tone and fill out skin)
Reduced calcium resorption	Aerobic activities and weight training
Decreased hours of sleep	Aerobic activities

(such as fast walking or stair walking) can provide a moderate amount of activity.

- Older people can gain additional health benefits through performing greater amounts of physical activity by increasing the duration, intensity, or frequency. Because risk of injury increases at high levels of physical activity, elders should take care not to engage in excessive amounts of it.

- Previously sedentary older adults who begin physical activity programs should start with short intervals of moderate physical activity (5 to 10 minutes) and gradually build up to the desired amount.

- Older adults should consult with a physician before beginning a new physical activity program.

- Besides improving their health through cardiorespiratory endurance (aerobic) activity, older adults can benefit from muscle-strengthening activities. Stronger muscles help reduce the risk of falling and improve the ability to perform the routine tasks of daily life.

The surgeon general also makes recommendations for what communities can do to promote physical activity among older people:

- Provide community-based physical activity programs that offer aerobic, strengthening, and flexibility components specifically designed for older adults.

- Encourage malls and other indoor or protected locations to provide safe places for walking in any weather.

- Ensure that facilities for physical activity accommodate and encourage participation by older adults.

- Provide transportation for older adults to parks or facilities that provide physical activity programs.

- Encourage health care providers to talk routinely to their older adult patients about incorporating physical activity into their lives.

- Plan community activities that include opportunities for older adults to be physically active.

Some Last Words on Wellness

You can be fit and achieve a high degree of wellness if you so desire. In choosing a physical fitness program, consider the following:

Myth and Fact Sheet

Myth	Fact
1. Jogging is a better physical fitness activity than walking.	**1.** Walking is as good an activity to develop physical fitness as any other. You simply have to walk for a longer time to gain comparable benefits.
2. Jogging leads to all sorts of injuries.	**2.** You can limit injuries from jogging if you take certain precautions. Wear the appropriate athletic shoes and do not overdo your workout.
3. Rope jumping is for wimps.	**3.** You can get a great workout while having fun if you know several rope-jumping stunts.
4. Most fitness clubs are the same.	**4.** Fitness clubs differ in a number of significant ways. Some clubs do not have enough equipment or enough variety of equipment. Others do not have adequately trained staff, do not offer a safe environment in which to exercise, or cost too much.
5. Elderly people do not need to exercise.	**5.** Everyone can benefit from regular exercise. Exercise can help elderly people enhance not only their physical fitness but also their social, mental, emotional, and spiritual health, thereby helping maintain their overall wellness.

- To be well, pay attention to your body. If you do, you will know when it is doing fine and when it needs special care.

- Pay attention to your mind. When you choose an activity to include in your fitness routine, choose one that is enjoyable, one you look forward to doing. Choosing the right activity will not only improve the chances of your continuing the activity but also increase your wellness by making you feel good.

- Pay attention to your spirit, too. Gain spiritual health from your fitness selections. Feel closer to nature or to a supreme being. Feel connected to your past and your future. To do so is to move toward high-level wellness.

- Be aware of the effects of your fitness choices on your mental and social health. Do your choices add to your knowledge? To your learning? Do they improve your relationships or help you establish new ones?

- Remember that improving one component of your health to the neglect of the others does not achieve wellness. Wellness is coordinating and integrating your physical fitness activities with the mental, social, emotional, and spiritual parts of your life.

We can think of no better image to leave you with than that of the Special Olympics—athletic competition for the mentally and physically challenged. These athletes try their best, train long and hard, and feel good about participating and competing. What better example of wellness is there? The learning (mental health) that must precede the competition, the good feelings that develop between athletes and their coaches and competitors (social health), the satisfaction derived from trying one's best (emotional health), the sense of oneness and closeness developed in competition (spiritual health), and the physical fitness needed to participate in the first place (physical health) provide evidence of the wellness of these competitors. They may not be totally healthy, but they certainly are well.

We wish for all of you the same degree of wellness.

Summary

Identifying Your Fitness Goals   People engage in physical activity for many reasons. Some do so for their health, others to look good or to have energy, and still others to develop strength or because they enjoy the competition. Before you can select activities to meet your fitness goals, you need to identify why you want to become fit.

Fitness Activities to Help You Achieve Your Goals   Many physical activities can contribute to the development of physical fitness, such as walking, jogging, running, rope jumping, swimming, tennis, racquetball, handball, squash, aerobic dance, low-impact aerobics, and bicycling. Some of these help develop cardiorespiratory endurance, others build muscular strength or muscular endurance, and some develop other components of physical fitness. In choosing an activity to engage in regularly, make sure to match it to your personality. You may be sociable, spontaneous, disciplined, aggressive, competitive, able to concentrate well, a risk taker, or a combination of two or more of those traits. Because people have different personalities, their choices of exercise will differ.

Being a Fitness Consumer   When you are deciding whether a fitness club is right for you, determine if the facility and the equipment offered can help you achieve your fitness goals. The staff should be well trained and the equipment abundant enough that you will not have to wait too long to use it. Safety procedures should be in place to minimize your chances of being injured. And the club should be easily accessible to you, have adequate parking, be located not too far from where you live or work, and charge a membership fee within your budget.

You should buy athletic equipment thoughtfully so that you do not waste your money. When buying athletic shoes, choose shoes that are comfortable and consistent with any foot problems you may have (for example, if you pronate or supinate). If you need orthotics because of a foot abnormality, you should consult a podiatrist, although in some cases ready-made shoe inserts are all you may need. Many different kinds of home exercise equipment are available, including stationary bikes, climbers, rowers, cross-country ski machines, treadmills, and weights. In deciding what home exercise equipment to buy, you should determine what your fitness goals are, who is going to use the equipment, how much space you have available to house the equipment, and how much you have to spend.

Promoting Lifetime Physical Fitness for Disabled Individuals   Disabled individuals who engage in physical activity programs typically experience the same mental and physical health benefits, enjoyment, opportunity to increase self-esteem,

Behavioral Change and Motivational Strategies

Many things can interfere with your ability to maintain a lifetime of physical fitness, health, and wellness. Here are some barriers (roadblocks) and strategies for overcoming them.

Roadblock	Behavioral Change Strategy
You will on occasion decide not to work out. You will be too busy, too tired, or too interested in doing something else. Note that the most effective behavioral change programs allow for periodic deviation from the goal. Consider a dieter who diets for 2 months but has an ice cream sundae one weekend. Those who recognize that a deviation need not mean that the diet is ruined are more likely to continue dieting. Those who believe that going off their diets even once means that they have failed are likely to cease dieting after eating the sundae. The situation is similar with exercise. Not exercising when you are supposed to is OK, as long as it does not happen frequently. If it happens often, you need to make an adjustment in your exercise program.	Make a list of the benefits and disadvantages of the exercises that make up your routine. List as many benefits and disadvantages as you can, big ones and little ones. Now go over the list and decide the following: ■ Are the benefits worth the potential disadvantages? ■ Can other physical activities give you similar benefits with fewer or less important disadvantages? ■ Are there ways you can decrease the barriers to engaging in a fitness program? For example, can you exercise closer to home (using chaining to your advantage)? Can you exercise with a friend (using social support)? ■ What changes do you need to make to maintain an exercise regimen?
You have participated in competitive athletics all your life and have maintained a high level of fitness by doing so. Now you are getting older, and the competition is becoming potentially harmful. You are being bumped around too much and are experiencing injuries. In addition, winning is not as important to you as it was when you were younger. Maintaining fitness, health, and wellness is now your exercise goal.	You need to find noncompetitive physical activities that can help you achieve your new fitness goals. Ask friends who are noncompetitive what they do for exercise. Use their help (social support). You can use covert techniques. Imagine yourself participating in noncompetitive activities and reward yourself by thinking of a relaxing image or pleasant thought (covert rehearsal). If that is too much unlike you, imagine someone you know who is not competitive engaging in a noncompetitive physical activity and then substitute yourself for that person (covert modeling).
You dislike exercising but know it is good for you. You need to find ways to continue your fitness program. You are afraid you will give it up before too long.	You can use self-monitoring by keeping a record of the times you engage in exercise activities. Then boast to friends in a considerate way about sticking with your program. You can also make a contract with yourself that if you exercise at least three times a week for at least 20 to 30 minutes each time, you will reward yourself. Think up some really fulfilling rewards. Rewards that are realistic and worth striving for will be most effective. You may also want to question your choice of exercise activity. Unless exercise is enjoyable you are likely to discontinue it before too long. What activities can you substitute for what you have been doing would be more fun but still help you achieve your fitness goals?
List roadblocks interfering with your maintaining a lifetime of physical fitness, health, and wellness. 1. _____ 2. _____ 3. _____	Cite behavioral change strategies that can help you overcome the roadblocks you just listed. If you need to, refer back to chapter 4 for behavioral change and motivational strategies. 1. _____ 2. _____ 3. _____

enhanced self-concept, and opportunities to build and engage in social relationships as do nondisabled individuals. In the school system, physical educators are increasingly encouraged to design a curriculum that includes activities and creates a supportive environment for physically and mentally challenged students. In March 2002 the U.S. Paralympics was formed as a separate division of the U.S. Olympic Committee (USOC) to enhance programs for Paralympic athletes.

Keeping Fit As You Age Exercise can help you live longer and live better. Physical activity also staves off some of the effects of aging. For example, exercise can help with reduced cardiac output, lowered pulmonary ventilation, elevated blood pressure, decreased muscular strength and endurance, diminished flexibility, increased body fat, and loss of skin elasticity. Furthermore, exercise is an excellent way for elders to enhance their overall wellness.

Discovery Activity 15.1

Discover Why You Want to Be Physically Fit

Name _____ **Date** _____

People have many reasons for engaging in physical activity in their efforts to become physically fit. If you know why you exercise, you will be able to choose activities that help you achieve your goals. To determine the reason or reasons why you exercise, place the following statements in rank order.

I exercise because

____ I want to lose or maintain my weight.

____ I want to look good.

____ I want to have a healthy heart and lungs.

____ I want to be strong.

____ I want to make new friends or socialize with my present friends.

____ I want to channel my aggression positively.

____ I like competition.

____ I like to be out in natural surroundings.

____ I want to develop enough energy not to be tired during the day.

____ I want to be flexible.

____ I want to have fun.

Interpretation of Results

Consult chapter 3 to match the reasons you exercise with the benefits of the various physical activities. For example, if you exercise to lose weight, consider activities such as aerobic dance, basketball, or bicycling. If you exercise to make friends, play softball or volleyball. If you exercise to look good, weight train. Matching your fitness goals with activities that can help you achieve those goals is the best way of ensuring that you will maintain your exercise program. Conversely, if you exercise regularly but do not achieve your goals because you have chosen the wrong physical activities, you will probably not continue with your program.

    Mix and match activities so that you achieve more than one of your goals. That way you will further increase the probability that you will become a lifetime participant in physical fitness activities.

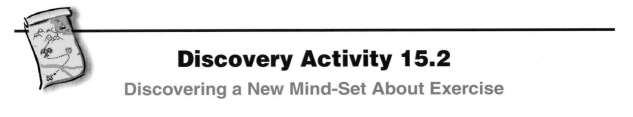

Discovery Activity 15.2

Discovering a New Mind-Set About Exercise

Name _____ **Date** _____

When people try to develop a new habit, thoughts of failure often plague them. During the early stages of your new exercise program, you can become your own worst enemy. Examine the list of excuses. Do any of these look familiar to you? Take a minute to prepare your own list of self-defeating thoughts about exercise. Prepare a list of positive thoughts, too.

Learn to use these lists wisely. When self-defeating thoughts enter your mind, counteract them immediately with positive ones. Write your list of positive thoughts on a card and carry it in your wallet or purse so that you can refer to it when you are about to avoid a scheduled exercise session. List both long-term benefits (such as more energy, weight loss, and prevention of disease) and more immediate benefits (such as using up calories and feeling good).

Negative thoughts about exercise	**Positive thoughts about exercise**
1. I'm too busy to exercise today. I'm working too hard anyway and need a break.	1. I can find time to exercise today. I just have to think about my routine and plan carefully.
2. I'm too tired to exercise today, and if I work out I won't have enough energy to do other things I need to do.	2. I may feel tired today, but I'll do a light exercise routine instead of the heavy one I usually do. If I keep working out on a regular basis, I'll build my stamina so that I won't feel so tired during the day.
3. I missed my workout today. I might as well forget all this fitness stuff. I don't have the self-control to keep at it.	3. Just because I missed one exercise session does not mean that I should give up. I'm not going to let this small setback ruin everything I've accomplished.
4. None of my friends are fit or trim, and they don't worry about it. I'm not going to worry either.	4. What my friends do about exercising has nothing to do with my exercise habits. I'll make additional friends who do exercise.
5. I'm already over the hill. I should just let myself go and enjoy life more.	5. I can get in shape and stay there. All I have to do is stick to my schedule. Knowing I can control my behavior is something I can enjoy every day.

Your own negative thoughts about exercise

1. _____

2. _____

3. _____

4. _____

Your own positive thoughts about exercise

1. _____

2. _____

3. _____

4. _____

Source: Jerrold S. Greenberg and George B. Dintiman, *Exploring Health: Expanding the Boundaries of Wellness* (Englewood Cliffs, NJ: Prentice Hall, 1992), p. 225.

From *Physical fitness and wellness, third edition,* by Jerrold S. Greenberg, George B. Dintiman, and Barbee Myers Oakes, 2004, Champaign, IL: Human Kinetics.

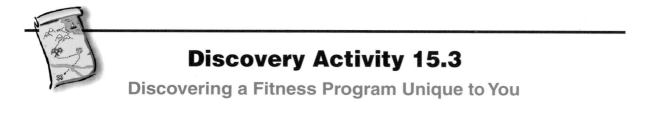

Discovery Activity 15.3

Discovering a Fitness Program Unique to You

Name _____ **Date** _____

By this point in the book you have acquired a great deal of information about physical fitness, about wellness and health, and about your own fitness needs and motivations. You are now ready to use this knowledge to develop a fitness program that is unique to you and, therefore, likely to be successful. To do so, complete each of the following items.

1. My physical fitness needs are the following:

a. _____

_____

b. _____

_____

c. _____

_____

d. _____

_____

e. _____

_____

2. I describe my present level of physical fitness in this way: _____

_____

_____

_____

_____

(continued)

Discovery Activity 15.3 *(continued)*

3. I can use these behavioral change techniques to adopt a program of regular exercise:

a. _____

_____

b. _____

_____

c. _____

_____

d. _____

_____

e. _____

_____

4. I can use these behavioral change techniques to maintain my exercise program:

a. _____

_____

b. _____

_____

c. _____

_____

d. _____

_____

e. _____

_____

Discovery Activity 15.3 *(continued)*

5. I can use behavioral change techniques in the following ways to maintain my program:

a. _____

_____

b. _____

_____

c. _____

_____

d. _____

_____

e. _____

_____

6. The specific components of my exercise program will include the following:

Exercise	Duration	Intensity	Frequency
a. _____	_____	_____	_____
b. _____	_____	_____	_____
c. _____	_____	_____	_____
d. _____	_____	_____	_____
e. _____	_____	_____	_____
f. _____	_____	_____	_____
g. _____	_____	_____	_____
h. _____	_____	_____	_____
i. _____	_____	_____	_____
j. _____	_____	_____	_____

(continued)

Discovery Activity 15.3 *(continued)*

7. I will evaluate the effectiveness of my exercise program based on these criteria (assess not only changes in the specific components of physical fitness but also adherence to your program and psychosocial and spiritual benefits):

a. _____

_____

b. _____

_____

c. _____

_____

d. _____

_____

e. _____

_____

From *Physical fitness and wellness, third edition,* by Jerrold S. Greenberg, George B. Dintiman, and Barbee Myers Oakes, 2004, Champaign, IL: Human Kinetics.

Discovery Activity 15.4

Service-Learning for Running Safely

We periodically read about runners—usually women—who have been assaulted, and sometimes even killed, while out jogging. You can provide a service for people in your community, as well as learn more about keeping yourself safe, if you develop a program to educate runners about how to run safely. You can start with the information provided in this chapter, but you should do additional research. For example, you might read articles, interview police, and inspect jogging trails. After you complete your research, you could develop posters for display in areas where people run. You might place a poster on a tree at the start of a jogging trail that goes through the woods or on a lamppost on a running route in an urban area. You could offer to conduct an educational session on running safely at the start of local races. In addition, you could print up a flyer on running safely for distribution to runners and joggers at various locations: in sports stores that sell running shorts and shoes, at the end of races, in physical education classes, and in recreational areas (for example, parks and community centers).

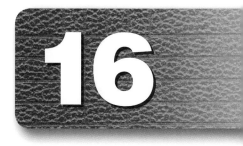

Beyond Fitness: Becoming an Elite Performer

Chapter Objectives

By the end of this chapter, you should be able to

1. distinguish between physical fitness and sports performance training factors;

2. identify the principles you should follow to reach a high level of fitness;

3. develop a weekly workout schedule to meet your training objectives;

4. design a program to increase your strength, speed, power, aerobic fitness, and anaerobic fitness to the elite level;

5. describe a training program that will prepare you to compete in a 5K, 10K, marathon, or triathlon; and

6. understand and use special training programs such as plyometrics, sport loading, and sprint-assisted training.

Carol Ann has always been active as a college student, attending an aerobics class three times weekly, jogging on weekends, and completing two to three 15- to 20-minute weight-training sessions per week. Although her health-related fitness is excellent, Carol Ann has noticed that she is still not in good enough condition to stay up with some of the female runners on the cross-country team or fit enough to participate on the university soccer team. After reaching the excellent level, many people want to test their limits as human beings and often compare themselves with others. Although she would like to elevate her fitness level even higher and move on to more advanced training, Carol Ann just doesn't know how to reach her goal.

This chapter focuses on both of Carol Ann's concerns and presents training programs to move her to the elite fitness category and to prepare her for competitive sports at the recreational, intramural, and varsity levels.

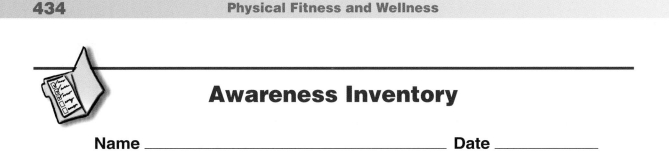

Awareness Inventory

Name _____ **Date** _____

Check the space by the letter T for the statements that you think are true and the space by the letter F for the statements that you think are false. The answers appear following the list of statements. This chapter will present information to clarify these statements for you. As you read the chapter, look for explanations for the reasons why the statements are true or false.

T ___ **F** ___ 1. Towing an individual at superhigh speeds with surgical tubing is referred to as sprint-resisted training.

T ___ **F** ___ 2. The Ironman triathlon in Hawaii requires a 2.4-mile swim, 112-mile cycle, and a 26.2-mile run.

T ___ **F** ___ 3. A triathlon involves three events: swimming, running, and horseback riding.

T ___ **F** ___ 4. To complete a 5K or 10K race in respectable time, it will be necessary to engage in training that involves running about 40 to 60 miles per week.

T ___ **F** ___ 5. Sprinting uphill with a weighted vest or against the resistance of surgical tubing is referred to as sprint-assisted training.

T ___ **F** ___ 6. Pickup sprints that may involve sets of a 25-yard walk, a 25-yard jog, a 25-yard three-quarter stride, and a 25-yard sprint are an example of anaerobic or speed endurance training.

T ___ **F** ___ 7. Jumping, hopping, and bounding movements are a form of plyometric training designed to increase explosive power.

T ___ **F** ___ 8. The squat, deadlift, and bench press are three exercises referred to as power lifts.

T ___ **F** ___ 9. Speed in short distances such as a 40-meter or 100-meter dash is an inherited ability that training cannot improve.

T ___ **F** ___ 10. Long, slow distance training that elevates heart rate to the target level will develop cardiovascular fitness.

Answers: 1-F, 2-T, 3-F, 4-T, 5-F, 6-T, 7-T, 8-T, 9-F, 10-T

Analyze Yourself

Determining Your Involvement in High-Level Fitness Activities

Name _____ **Date** _____

Instructions: Indicate how often each of the following occurs in your daily activities and exercise sessions. Respond to each item with a number from 0 to 3, using the following scale:

0 = Never   **1** = Occasionally   **2** = Most of the time   **3** = Always

____ **1.** I test myself every 6 to 8 weeks to evaluate my improvement in areas such as aerobic fitness, anaerobic fitness, strength, power, and speed.

____ **2.** I run a minimum of 40 miles weekly or engage in an advanced conditioning or aerobics class five or six times per week.

____ **3.** I engage in a 60- to 90-minute strength-training program five or six times per week and follow a program devised by an expert to meet my training objectives.

____ **4.** I follow a total training program similar to one that competitive athletes in the same sport use.

____ **5.** To improve speed in short distances, I use sprint-assisted training, plyometric training, sport loading, and strength training each week.

____ **6.** To improve my ability to complete repeated short sprints, I follow an anaerobic (speed endurance) program at least twice weekly.

____ **7.** I use a series of dynamic stretching exercises in each workout immediately after my warm-up and complete each workout with 10 to 15 minutes of static stretching.

____ **8.** I alternate light and heavy workout days and avoid consecutive days of hard workouts.

____ **9.** I keep my percentage of body fat at the lower end of the recommended ranges given in chapter 8.

____ **10.** If an injury occurs, I discontinue exercise and rest until I am pain-free and able to return to light workouts.

Scoring: Excellent = 25-30

Good = 19-24

Poor = Below 19

From *Physical fitness and wellness, third edition,* by Jerrold S. Greenberg, George B. Dintiman, and Barbee Myers Oakes, 2004, Champaign, IL: Human Kinetics.

Competitive Aerobics

Although most people who enter fitness programs have no desire to compete, many eventually become interested in comparing themselves with others. Such comparisons are possible in a competitive race situation. By reading this section, you have indicated a desire to make such a comparison. The information presented here is designed to help you train to race the most popular road-racing distances of 5,000 meters (approximately 3.1 miles) and 10,000 meters (approximately 6.2 miles).

Your fitness level can help you select the distance you should run. For those who are in the good to superior category on the 1.5-mile test (chapter 2) and are training 20 to 40 miles per week, either distance is appropriate. Those who score below the good category and train less than 20 miles per week should consider increasing training before racing or limiting their effort to a slow 5K race. No matter which race you select, your training will determine your performance.

5,000-Meter (5K) to 10,000-Meter (10K) Racing

Training for 5K to 10K races requires that you put in sufficient mileage weekly just to finish the race safely. If you want speed, training also requires speed work. The amount of mileage and speed work you should do depends on your goal. Practically anyone who scores good or excellent on the 1.5-mile test can finish a 10K race, and nearly anyone can finish a 5K (even slow walkers). Competition implies constantly striving to improve your performance, and improvement comes with increased mileage and speed work. Minimum mileage for a strong performance is 40 miles per week but need not exceed 60 miles per week. This weekly mileage should include 2 days of speed work and 1 day for racing.

You should not attempt the training schedule described in table 16.1 until you have reached a good rating on the 1.5-mile test and are doing at least 35 miles per week. Timing yourself at the 5K distance would be helpful in determining your training pace.

Intervals

Intervals are a type of speed workout with four parts:

1. The distance to be run before each rest interval
2. The total distance to be run in the workout
3. The speed at which you run
4. The rest interval between runs

Your conditioning level and your desired race distance determine the distance you should run. Because this section deals with the 5K and 10K, you should run at least 220 yards, or 200 meters. The total distance of the workout should be 2 to 3 miles for the 5K and 4 to 6 miles for the 10K. The speed should be about 20 seconds faster than your desired race pace. If you want to run a 6-minute-per-mile pace, for example, you should run your quarter miles at 80 seconds, half miles at 2 minutes and 40 seconds, and miles at 5 minutes and 40 seconds. The rest interval varies accord-

intervals—A training routine that manipulates four elements: the intensity of exercise, the duration or length of each workout, the number of repetitions completed per workout, and the rest interval between each repetition.

TABLE 16.1—Typical Training Week

Day	Workout
Sunday	Long, slow distance of 10 to 12 mi at a pace approximately 1 min per mi slower than your racing pace
Monday	7 to 8 mi at a pace about 30 to 45 sec slower than race pace
Tuesday	Speed work day: 3 to 5 mi of intervals at a pace about 20 sec faster than your desired race pace (be realistic here); total workout mileage including warm-up and cool-down is 6 to 9 mi
Wednesday	6 to 9 easy mi
Thursday	Speed work day: 3 to 6 mi of intervals
Friday	4 to 6 mi of easy running if a race is planned for Saturday; 8 mi if no race is scheduled
Saturday	Race 5K to 10K distance

ing to the distance and conditions. For quarters, a set rest interval of 90 seconds is recommended. Some people, however, run a quarter and jog a quarter for rest. For longer distances, you should

TABLE 16.2—5K and 10K Interval Workouts

5K workouts	10K workouts
8 × 1/4 mi	12 × 1/4 mi
1 × 1/2 mi 4 × 1/4 mi 6 × 220 yd	16 × 1/4 mi
2 × 1/2 mi 4 × 1/4 mi	2 × 1/2 mi 8 × 1/4 mi 6 × 220 yd
8 × 1/4 mi 4 × 220 yd	4 × 1/2 mi 6 × 1/4 mi 6 × 220 yd
12 × 1/4 mi	1 × 1 mi 2 × 1/2 mi 4 × 1/4 mi 6 × 200 yd
2 × 1/2 mi 6 × 1/4 mi 6 × 220 yd	2 × 1 mi 2 × 1/2 mi 4 × 1/4 mi
16 × 1/4 mi	2 × 1 mi 2 × 1/2 mi 4 × 1/4 mi 8 × 220 yd
4 × 1/2 mi 6 × 1/4 mi 6 × 220 yd	6 × 1/2 mi 8 × 1/4 mi 8 × 220 yd
1 × 1 mi 2 × 1/2 mi 3 × 1/4 mi 4 × 220 yd	3 × 1 mi 2 × 1/2 mi 5 × 1/4 mi 6 × 220 yd
2 × 1 mi 2 × 1/2 mi 4 × 1/4 mi	1 × 2 mi 2 × 1 mi 3 × 1/2 mi 4 × 1/4 mi
1 × 2 mi 1 × 1 mi 2 × 1/4 mi	1 × 3 mi 2 × 1 mi 3 × 1/2 mi 4 × 1/4 mi

allow your heart rate to return below 120 beats per minute before running the next bout. Table 16.2 describes sample interval workouts for 5K and 10K races. These workouts will improve your conditioning to the level you need to complete the 5K and 10K race. To improve your speed (pace), follow the interval workout schedule shown in table 16.3.

Marathons and Ultramarathons

"What the mind of man can conceive and believe can be achieved." Men and women continue to put this saying to ultimate physical tests. No longer are people satisfied with the marathon. They compete in 100-mile races, 24-hour races, across-the-country races, races that involve parachuting into Death Valley and running out. The human mind seems to be in an endless race with the body to see which will crack first. These long-distance (endurance) contests are not new; races across the United States were waged for thousands of dollars during the 1920s and 1930s. Participants in those early races, as well as in the modern-day ultraraces, were few.

Although the number of participants has declined in the past decade, the marathon (26.2 miles) is still popular. The mystique of the marathon continues to draw runners of all ages and levels of conditioning. Television coverage of the Boston and New York Marathons has generated much national attention. Marathon participants come in all sizes and shapes; some are prepared and some, many of them first-time participants, are not.

Marla Runyan is legally blind from a degenerative eye condition that limits her vision to approximately 15 feet. Nonetheless, she finished first among U.S. female runners and fifth overall in the 2002 New York City Marathon. Throughout the race, Runyan had the assistance of a cyclist who yelled instructions to guide her along the course.

A minimum of 3 months of training is required to run a marathon. Training requires 60 miles per week including at least one long run of 18 miles or more. If you plan to race the marathon, you should be running 40 miles per week before the final 3 training months. You then gradually increase your mileage (approximately 10% per week) to 60 miles a week during the month before the race. A gradual decline occurs during the week just before the race. Table 16.4 provides a suggested training schedule for the marathon.

TABLE 16.3—Sample Interval Workout for Developing Speed for Road Racing

	Conditioned beginner (around 8:00 pace)	Average runner (around 7:00 pace)	Advanced runner (around 6:30 pace)
Repetitions	6	6	10
Distance	220 yd	1/4 mi	1/4 mi
Pace	45 to 50 sec	100 sec	90 sec
Rest interval	90 sec	90 sec	90 sec
Repetitions	4	8	6
Distance	1/4 mi	1/4 mi	1/2 mi
Pace	110 sec	100 sec	3 min
Rest interval	90 sec	90 sec	3 min

All speed workouts begin with a minimum of a 1 mi warm-up of easy running followed by gentle stretching and some short (40 yd) running in which the pace gradually increases to workout pace in the last 15 to 20 yd.

Most distances beyond 1/2 mi are done as repeats in which sufficient rest is taken to allow the heart rate to drop to 120 beats per minute. Distances for repeats can range from 1/2 mi to any distance at which an individual can run faster than desired race pace, that is, 10 mi repeats could be run in preparation for a marathon. Most repeats, however, are in the 1/2 mi to 3 mi range.

Triathlon

Three-event races (swimming, biking, and running), or triathlons, began in Hawaii and are now held throughout the United States, attracting thousands of participants. To be successful, you must train in all three areas and develop what participants call all-around fitness. Keep in mind that the triathlon is not for everyone. The event requires specialized training and a tremendously high level of fitness.

Triathlon distances vary greatly. One is as short as a 400-yard swim, a 4-mile cycle, and a 1-mile run on the beach. The Hawaii event consists of a 2.4-mile swim, a 112-mile cycle, and a 26.2-mile run.

Anaerobic Training (Intense Exercise for a Short Time)

Sports such as tennis, racquetball, handball, squash, football, sprinting, and baseball require all-out efforts in the form of short sprints for several seconds. To make these repetitive short sprints over a period of 30 seconds or more, you must improve your anaerobic conditioning level.

Sprinting forms the foundation of an **anaerobic** training program. Your first step is to apply the principle of specificity (see chapter 3) by designing your sprints over distances similar to those occurring in your sport. Tennis players, for example, rarely must sprint all out for more

than 15 yards. A sound program for tennis, then, is a series of 15- to 50-yard sprints interrupted by short rest intervals, such as the following programs:

- Pickup sprints: This type of anaerobic program involves a gradual increase from a jog to a three-quarter stride to a sprint. In early workouts, jog 10 yards, stride 10, sprint 10, and finish that repetition with a 10-yard walk. As your conditioning level improves, increase the number of repetitions and decrease the rest interval after each. Once weekly, use longer distances of 25, 50, and 75 yards.

- Hollow sprints: This program involves two sprints interrupted by a hollow period of recovery such as walking or jogging. A sample repetition includes a 15-yard sprint, 15-yard jog, 15-yard sprint, and a 15-yard walk for recovery. You can use similar segments of 50, 75, and 100 yards.

Sample workouts using pickup and hollow sprints are shown in table 16.5.

> **anaerobic training**—Anaerobic means "without oxygen" and describes short, all-out exercise effort such as the 100-, 200-, or 400-meter dash and activity in sports such as football and baseball. Participants perform activity at such high intensity that they have insufficient time to use atmospheric oxygen at the tissue level and oxygen debt occurs.

TABLE 16.4—Training for the Marathon

Day	Week 1 (mi)	Week 2 (mi)	Week 3 (mi)	Week 4 (mi)	Week 5 (mi)	Week 6 (mi)
1	10	11	12	13	14	15
2	0	0	0	0	0	3
3	6	6	6	6	7	7
4	7	7	8	8	8	8
5	6	6	6	6	7	7
6	7	7	8	10	10	10
7	4	4	4	4	4	5
Total	40	41	44	47	50	55
Day	Week 7 (mi)	Week 8 (mi)	Week 9 (mi)	Week 10 (mi)	Week 11 (mi)	Race week (mi)
1	15	15	20	15	15	15
2	4	4	0	5	5	5
3	7	7	6	6	6	6
4	9	10	10	10	10	5
5	7	7	7	7	7	4
6	10	10	10	10	10	3
7	6	7	7	7	7	Race day
Total	58	60	60	60	60	

Basic assumptions:

1. You are a serious runner and have been running between 25 and 40 mi a week for at least a year.

2. You have had some race experience at distances of 10K or above.

3. You have at least 3 months to train before the marathon you wish to run.

4. If you plan to race the marathon, you will do one speed workout a week (middle of the week) and will race (no longer than 13.1 mi) every other week.

5. If you miss a workout, you will not double up the next day to make up for it. You will do one long run (15 mi) a week beginning in the 2nd month and will try to have two double-digit runs (10 or more mi) per week.

TABLE 16.5—Sample Pickup and Hollow Sprints

Season	Sprints
Early season (initial 3 to 5 workouts)	Walk or jog 2 mi; jog 15 yd, stride 15, walk 15—repeat 5 times; end workout with a 1 mi jog or walk.
2nd and 3rd weeks	Jog 1 mi nonstop; jog 15 yd, stride 15, sprint 15, walk 15—repeat the 15-yd jog/stride/sprint/walk cycle 6 to 12 times; repeat previous set with 10 yd sprints 6 to 12 times; end workout with a 1 mi jog or walk.
4th to 8th weeks	Jog 1 mi; jog 15 yd, stride 15, sprint 15, walk 15—repeat the 15-yd jog/stride/sprint/walk cycle 6 to 12 times; sprint 50 yd; jog for 10 to 12 sec—repeat 4 times to complete a 440 yd run on the track in less than 90 sec—repeat the 50-yd sprint/jog cycle 6 to 8 times (in later workouts try to reduce the total 440 yd time to 75-80 sec using the sprint-jog cycle); cool down with a 1 to 2 mi slow jog.
In-season workout	Jog 1 mi; jog 15 yd, stride 15, sprint 15, walk 15—repeat 3 to 5 times; jog 25, sprint 15, jog 25, sprint 15, jog 25, sprint 15, jog 25, sprint 15—repeat 6 times; 300 yd all-out run—repeat 2 to 6 times; cool down with a 1 mi slow jog.

Flexibility

The degree of flexibility you need depends on the activity for which you are training. Chapter 6 provides all the information you need to increase your range of motion for basic health, for carrying out everyday chores at home and work, and for successful participation in any activity or sport. The key is to warm up properly for each workout with large-muscle activity such as jogging or the movements of your specific sport or activity until you are perspiring freely. Only then do you engage in 10 to 12 minutes of dynamic stretching. At the very end of each workout, after completing the other training programs, a 15- to 20-minute static stretching session that focuses on all major joints will effectively increase your range of motion to the desired levels. Only a few activities such as ballet, gymnastics, and diving require extremely high levels of flexibility. For others, it is not necessary and can even be dangerous to strive for extreme flexibility that could damage joints.

Strength

Strength is another key component for health-related fitness and for those seeking the elite fitness category. Men and women who hope to become highly fit must engage in a regular strength-training program almost daily, completing upper-body exercises one day and lower-body exercises the next.

Special Strength-Training Programs

Exercises and exact routines can be designed to meet your specific training objectives. Elite fitness participants and athletes in various sports have used a number of unique strength-training programs. Most of these approaches are demanding and involve handling heavy weights. For that reason, we recommend that you do lifting sessions with a partner (spotter). A brief description of some of these programs follows.

Rest-Pause

You perform a single repetition at near-maximal weight (1RM) before resting for 1 to 2 minutes. You then complete a second repetition, rest again, and continue with that pattern until the muscle becomes fatigued and cannot perform even one repetition.

Set System

The use of multiple sets is one of the most popular advanced training methods. You perform several repetitions, rest, repeat the exercise, rest, and repeat it again. Three to four sets of approximately five to six repetitions are generally used for each exercise.

Burnout

For each exercise, you use 75% of your maximum weight to complete as many consecutive repetitions as possible. Without any rest interval, you remove 10 pounds from the starting weight and perform another infinite set. Again, without any rest period you remove another 10 pounds and do a third set. You repeat this procedure until the muscle burns out (cannot respond). Each designated muscle group goes through the same demanding process. A partner should be nearby to help remove weights and assist should premature fatigue occur.

Wipeout

For each exercise, you use 50% of your maximum weight to complete as many consecutive repetitions as possible. This method does not require you to remove weight nor does it include a rest interval. The number of repetitions is infinite until the designated muscle group fails. An assistant should be nearby in the event that premature fatigue occurs. As a variation, you can take a 1-minute rest before attempting a second or third set. Your ultimate goal is to exhaust the muscle group completely.

Supersets

In this approach, you perform a set of exercises for one group of muscles and follow it immediately by a set for their antagonists. A variation of this method is known as super multiple sets and consists of performing three sets of an exercise for one group of muscles followed by the same number of sets for their antagonists. A short rest is taken between sets. For example, you perform one set of arm curls (biceps muscle, agonist) and then perform a set of bench presses (triceps, antagonist).

Groves's Superoverload Method

This procedure has the potential for superior strength gains and is highly applicable to the bench press, leg press, and ankle exercises. Follow these steps:

1. Establish your 1RM.
2. Add 25% more weight to that amount.
3. Have an assistant help you get into the up position (the bench press begins with arms extended overhead, elbows locked; the leg press begins with legs extended and knees locked).
4. Bend the joint slightly (only 2 to 3 inches) on the first repetition.
5. Continue taking the weight downward farther each time until on the seventh repetition you are unable to return the weight to the up position without assistance.
6. Complete three sets of seven repetitions every other day.

At the end of each week, redetermine your 1RM and repeat these steps using the new weight.

Circuit Weight Training (CWT)

This system involves a series of weight-training exercises of approximately 12 to 15 repetitions each using a moderate amount of weight (about 40 to 60% of 1RM). You move quickly from one station to another with minimal rest (15 to 30 seconds) between stations. Generally, the two or three circuits of 10 exercises are designed so that the total workout time is between 25 and 30 minutes. CWT increases aerobic capacity by approximately 5%, compared with 15 to 25% for other aerobic exercise programs. Lean-body mass also increases from 2 to 7 pounds (1 to 3 kilograms), and fat decreases 0.8 to 2.9%. Strength improves 7 to 32%. The energy costs of CWT are similar to jogging at 5 miles per hour. Improvement in strength and maximum oxygen uptake ($\dot{V}O_2$max) depends on work performed, not on the equipment used. CWT will not develop high levels of aerobic fitness, but it can help maintain fitness.

Competitive Weightlifting

Weightlifting comprises two distinct categories. The first is the Olympic Games competition consisting of three specific overhead lifts: the military press, the snatch, and the clean and jerk. The other category is referred to as powerlifting, which involves the squat, deadlift, and bench press. In either category, the primary objective is to lift as much weight as possible in each of the competitive events. Male lifters are divided into 11 body-weight divisions ranging from flyweight (114 1/2 pounds) to super heavyweight (over 242 1/2 pounds). Women have 9 weight divisions, from flyweight (96 1/2 pounds) to heavyweight (over 181 pounds).

Bodybuilding

Bodybuilders are generally more concerned with flex appeal (size, shape, definition, proportion) than muscle strength. They use dumbbells, barbells, and resistance-designed machines to carve out and define individual muscles. Beauty of physique is much more important than feats of strength. Competitors perform posing routines. Judges evaluate them on symmetry (body parts having been equally developed top and bottom, left and right), muscle definition, and poise. Females finish up their competition by engaging in a brief freestyle routine to music, a kind of cross between sport and cabaret.

Power

Power, also referred to as speed strength, is vital to performance in sports and other activities requiring a high level of fitness. Although power output is highly related to strength, it should be treated as a separate fitness component. Explosive actions such as executing a vertical jump, accelerating from a stationary position to full speed, lunging forward or sideways, stopping and starting, and other explosive movements require special training programs such as those described in the following sections. You can also improve power by altering some strength-training workouts to involve rapid, explosive movements against resistance. With free weights, these movements can often simulate the movements of the activity or sport for which you are training, thus applying the principle of specificity to the workout.

Plyometrics

Plyometric training is designed to increase the strength and power of the muscles involved in an activity through a series of jumping, hopping, and bounding movements for the lower body and swinging, quick-action push-offs, catching and throwing of weighted objects (medicine balls,

> **plyometrics**—A series of hopping, jumping, and bounding movements for the lower body and swinging, push-offs, catching, throwing, and arm swings for the upper body designed to increase muscular strength and power.

Myth and Fact Sheet

Myth	Fact
1. You can change the shape of your body and reach the elite fitness level by training three or four times per week for 60 minutes in each session.	**1.** Moving into the elite fitness category in both performance and appearance will take a minimum of 1 to 2 years of training, 6 days weekly with 1 day of rest, and close adherence to the principles of exercise described in chapter 3. To add muscle and acquire definition, daily strength-training and bodybuilding sessions alone will exceed 1 hour (alternating between upper-body movements one day and lower-body movements the next). Other training programs will take an additional 60 to 90 minutes. Be patient and plan your program over a 1- to 2-year period.
2. You can add 1 to 2 pounds of muscle per week with proper training.	**2.** Adding muscle mass through proper nutrition and strength training is a slow process. Plan to pursue a safe, steroid-free program and strive for a maximum of 1/4 pound of added muscle per week, or 1 pound monthly. Such an approach requires about 100 extra calories daily and only a slight increase in protein intake. Consult your physical education instructor about designing a strength-training program to meet this objective.
3. You cannot improve speed in short sprints because this trait is purely genetic.	**3.** Although the amount of fast-twitch fiber in the muscles involved in sprinting is genetically determined, research clearly shows that everyone can improve sprinting speed with proper training that involves programs designed to increase stride rate and stride length, and improve acceleration, anaerobic endurance, and form and technique. These training programs can also convert much of your fast-twitch type IIa fibers to the faster type IIb that is vital to explosive power and speed. Keep in mind that you cannot reach your genetic speed capacity and be as fast as you can be without following a solid speed improvement program.
4. You can perform different training programs in any order you choose in a single workout, as long as you complete the programs.	**4.** The order of use has a significant effect on the benefits you receive. One acceptable order of use for training programs is this: (1) general warm-up—8 to 12 minutes of jogging, running, or performing the skills of your sport that brings about sweating, (2) stretching—10 to 15 minutes of dynamic stretching exercises such as those described in chapter 6, (3) form training—techniques of sprinting, road racing, or sports activities, (4) sprint-assisted training—high-speed towing should occur when you are fatigue free, (5) aerobic or anaerobic training, (6) sport loading, (7) plyometrics, (8) weight training, (9) cool-down and static stretching (see exercises in chapter 6). Speed activities occur early in a workout after warm-up and stretching, and the heavy conditioning activities come near the end of the workout.
5. Running long distances at a slow pace is not an effective training routine for 5K and 10K road races.	**5.** A number of different training methods are used to improve speed in road races (5K and 10K). **Long slow distance (LSD),** fartlek (alternating fast and slow running over varied terrain), and intervals are a few techniques purported to improve speed. Some apply only to running, whereas others such as LSD and intervals can apply to walking, swimming, cycling, and running. As a beginning exerciser, you will experience greater speed with nearly every workout as long as you do not overdo it in any one session. This increased speed is due primarily to increased muscle strength; a direct relationship between speed and strength operates

in early training. Later, cardiovascular efficiency comes into play, and improvement takes place more slowly.

Most people are satisfied with the fitness and speed developed through the LSD approach. For fitness purposes, long slow distance is the only exercise routine required. This method is both safe and effective in improving cardiovascular conditioning. Continued LSD training, however, may fail to develop speed and prepare you only for running long distances at a slow pace.

For racing purposes, experts argue that you must train at a speed faster than you desire to race. For middle- and long-distance cyclists, swimmers, and runners, this means training at short, fast distances at or faster than the eventual race pace. Milers in track, for example, will run fast quarter miles and half miles in training (overspeed training). For running, this chapter includes speed work that uses intervals. Other techniques, such as towing, downhill running, and fartlek, are also valuable for developing speed.

To select the best speed-training techniques for any activity, you should identify activities that closely simulate the actual event. Although calisthenic activities such as rope jumping, push-ups, and jumping jacks are good fitness activities, they do little for developing speed in sports.

---

6. Champion athletes are born, not made.

6. Champions are products of hard work, not heredity. You do not have to be 7 feet tall and weigh 250 pounds to become a champion athlete, nor do you need to be born with superior skill. Keep in mind that heredity deals the cards but environment plays the hand. Some athletes born with superior coordination and physical qualities never reach stardom, while others with only average qualities become champions. The difference is strong dedication to two broad areas: skill development for every aspect of the particular sport and physical development through numerous training programs to allow the body to perform those perfected skills with maximum power, strength, agility, endurance, and speed. Modern-day champions are hardworking, dedicated individuals. They do not develop superior skill or physical qualities in a year. For many, it means one to two workouts daily and countless additional hours of practice time spent on skills over a period of 5 to 12 years. Those who eventually make it are the most persistent, dedicated, and hardworking, not necessarily the most genetically blessed.

---

long slow distance (LSD)—A training program for 5K races, 10K races, and marathons based on high volume (miles completed) rather than intensity.

shot put, sandbags), arm swings, and pulley throws for the upper body. The objective is to improve the ability to generate maximum force in the shortest possible time.

The main concept of plyometrics (loading and unloading) is easy to understand, and you will immediately see that you already apply it in many activities. When you cock your wrist or ankle just before throwing a baseball, hitting a baseball, shooting a basketball, kicking a soccer ball or football, swinging a golf club, or executing any tennis stroke, you are loading or rapidly stretching the muscles to activate the stretch reflex. When you explosively complete the action and throw the ball (or kick it or hit it), you are unloading (the stretch reflex sends a powerful message to the muscles causing them to contract faster and with more power). The same thing occurs when you jump or sprint. The object is to shorten your ground contact time by immediately going into the next repetition of the jump.

Follow these tips to get the maximum benefit from your plyometric workout:

- Avoid plyometrics unless you meet minimum strength standards. For the lower body, you should be able to leg-press 1 1/2 to 2 times your body weight. For the upper body, you should be able to bench-press your body weight.

- Use footwear with good ankle and arch support and a nonslip sole (basketball or aerobic shoe).

- Complete each workout on soft areas, such as grass, padded artificial turf, or wrestling mats. Never perform plyometrics on asphalt or gymnasium floors.

- Avoid depth jumping from boxes higher than 30 inches (0.75 meter).

- Too many workouts per week and too many jumps per workout may result in injury. Do plyometric exercises no more than two times weekly with 2 days of rest between the workouts. The number of jumps per workout should not exceed 80 to 100 for beginners, 100 to 120 for intermediates, and 120 to 140 for elite fitness participants.

- You must train fast to be fast. The quickness of the stretch, not the length of the stretch, is what is important. That means hitting and getting off the ground as quickly as possible.

- Concentrate on an all-out effort on each jump, hop, or bound. You will not automatically sprint at maximum speed, serve at 100 miles per hour in tennis, kick a ball 60 yards, or jump 25 feet without being psyched before performing the movement. You must concentrate on completing this task with your maximum effort.

- The most helpful plyometric exercises are those that closely resemble specific movements of the sport or activity for which you are training.

Low-Intensity Jumps (Beginning Program)

Individuals who have been inactive or are using plyometrics for the first time should complete this beginning program before moving to the medium-intensity jumps. The total number of jumps, leaps, and bounds should not exceed 80 to 100 per workout.

Squat Jump

From an upright position, with hands behind the neck, drop downward to a one-half squat position before exploding upward as high as possible. Land and immediately explode upward again.

Split Squat Jump

This jump is the same as the previous one except that you land with one leg extended forward and the other behind the center of your body in a lunge position (see figure 16.1, a-b).

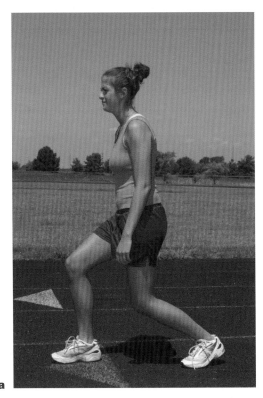 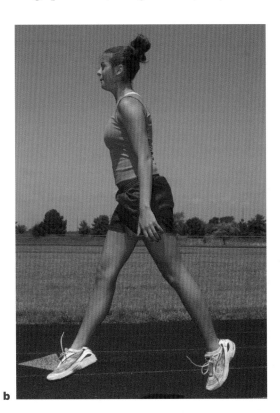

a   b

Figure 16.1a-b Split squat jump.

Double-Leg Ankle Bounce

With arms extended to the sides, jump upward and forward using the ankles. Execute the next jump upon landing.

Lateral Cone or Bench Jump

Stand to one side of a cone or bench, jump laterally to the other side, and jump back to the starting position immediately upon landing.

Medium-Intensity Jumps

Individuals who have used plyometrics in the past and currently exercise a minimum of five times weekly may begin with the medium-intensity jumps. The total number of jumps, leaps, and bounds should not exceed 100 to 120 per workout.

Pike Jump

Begin in an upright position with both arms to the side and feet shoulder-width apart. Compete a vertical jump as you bring both fully extended legs in front of the body and reach out with both hands to touch your toes in a pike position (see figure 16.2). Go into the next jump immediately upon landing.

Double-Leg Tuck Jump

From the starting position described for the pike jump, complete a vertical jump and grasp the knees while in the air, release the grasp before landing, and immediately go into the next jump.

Standing Triple Jump

From the standing broad jump position, use a two-foot takeoff to jump forward as far as possible. Land on the right foot, then immediately jump forward and land on the left foot. Finish with one last jump off the left foot, landing on both feet (figure 16.3, a-b). This jump is identical to the triple jump in track except that you use a two-foot takeoff.

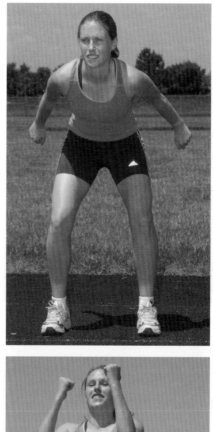

a

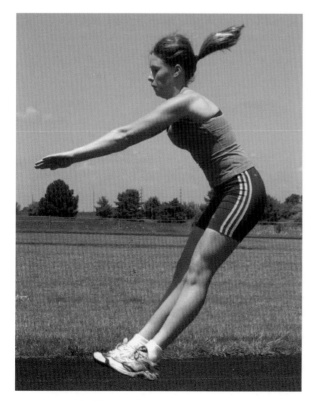

Figure 16.2 Pike jump.

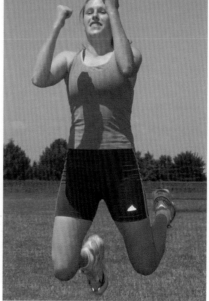

b

Figure 16.3a-b Standing triple jump.

Standing Long Jump

Perform the initial jump described for the standing triple jump, using maximum arm swing and exploding into the next repetition upon landing.

Single-Leg Hop

From a standing broad jump position with one leg slightly forward, rock to the front foot and jump as far and high as possible, driving the lead knee up and out. Land in the starting position on the same foot and continue jumping until you complete the specified number of repetitions.

Double-Leg Bound

From the standing broad jump position, thrust both arms forward as the knees and body straighten and the arms reach for the sky.

Alternate-Leg Bound

Stand upright with one foot slightly ahead of the other. Push off with the back leg as you drive the lead knee up to the chest and try to attain as much height and distance as possible. Continue immediately by repeating this action with the other leg (see figure 16.4, a-c).

Running Bound

Run forward and jump as high as possible on each step, emphasizing height and high knee lift. Land with the center of gravity under you.

High-Intensity Jumps or Short-Response Hops and Bounds

High-intensity jumps are designed for the highly conditioned athlete who has used plyometric training on a regular basis. The total number of jumps, leaps, and bounds should not exceed 120 to 140 per workout.

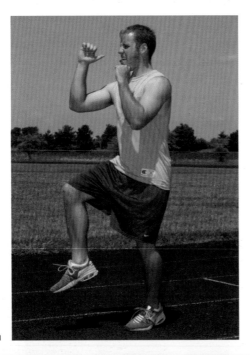

a

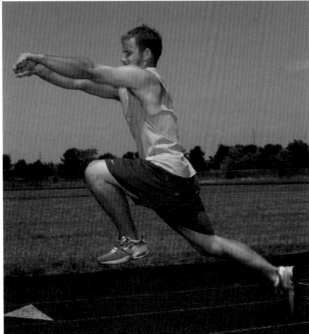

b

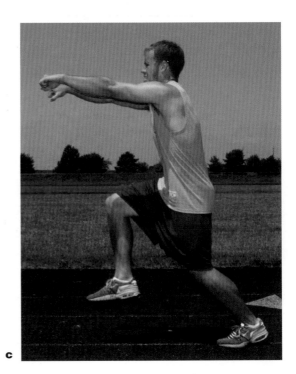

c

Figure 16.4a-c Alternate leg bound.

Double-Leg Vertical Power Jumps

From the standing vertical jump position, thrust both arms upward and jump as high as possible. Immediately jump again upon landing with as little ground contact as possible.

Single-Leg Vertical Jump

Repeat the previous action using a one-leg take-off.

Side Jump and Sprint

Stand to one side of a bench or cone with your feet together. Jump back and forth over the bench 4 to 10 times. On the last jump, sprint forward for 25 yards.

Double-Leg Speed Hop

Assume an upright position with the back straight, shoulders forward, and head up. Jump as high as possible, bringing the feet under the buttocks in a cycling motion at the height of the jump. Jump again immediately upon contacting the ground.

Single-Leg Speed Hop

Repeat the previous exercise taking off on one leg only.

Decline Hop

From a quarter-squat position at the top of a grassy hill with a 3- or 4-degree slope, hop down the hill for speed using the double-leg hop.

Single-Leg Stride Jump

Assume a position to the side and at one end of a bench with only the inside foot on top of the bench. Your arms are at your sides. Drive both arms upward as the inside leg on the bench pushes off to propel the jump as high as possible. Continue jumping until you reach the other end of the bench.

Box Jumps

Step off a box of the correct height and immediately jump upward and outward upon hitting the ground (see figure 16.5, a-b).

A sample 5-week program of plyometrics is presented in table 16.6, showing two workout sessions per week.

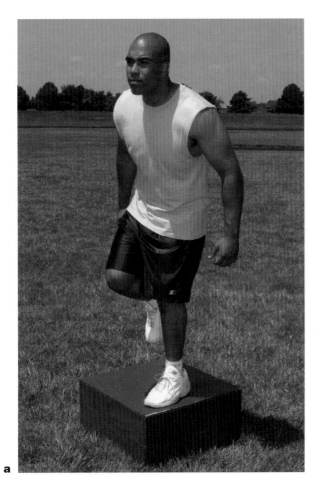
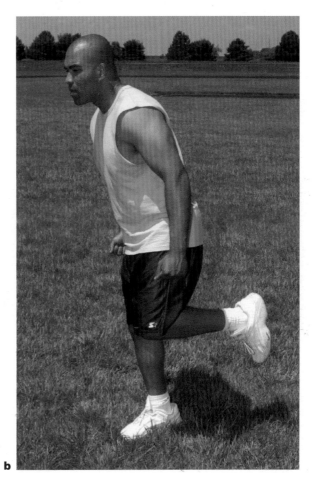

a   b

Figure 16.5a-b Box jumps.

TABLE 16.6—Plyometrics

Week	Routine or distance	Repetitions	Sets	Rest interval
1	Low-intensity program: Master the correct form for each exercise.			
	Squat jump	4	2	2 min between sets
	Double-leg ankle bounce	4	2	2 min
	Lateral cone jump	4	2	2 min
	Split squat jump	4	2	2 min
1	Same as previous workout	4	2	2 min
2	Same as previous workout	5	2	2 min
2	Same as previous workout	6	2	2 min
3	Medium-intensity program:			
	Standing long jump	6	2	2 min
	Alternate-leg bound	6	2	2 min
	Double-leg bound	6	2	2 min
	Pike jump	6	2	2 min
	Double-leg tuck jump	6	2	2 min
	Single-leg hop	6	2	2 min
	Running bound	6	2	2 min
3	Same as previous workout	7	2	2 min
4	Same as previous workout	8	2	2 min
4	High-intensity program:			
	Single-leg vertical jump	6	2	90 sec
	Single-leg speed hop	6	2	90 sec
	Double-leg speed hop	6	2	90 sec
	Multiple box jumps	6	2	90 sec
	Double-leg vertical jump	6	2	90 sec
	Single-leg stride jump	6	2	90 sec
	Box jump	6	2	90 sec
5	Same as previous workout	7	2	90 sec
5	Same as previous workout	8	8	90 sec
6	Maintenance workout: high-intensity exercises	5	2	90 sec

Plyometric workouts should not exceed 80-100 jumps, leaps, and bounds per session for beginners and athletes in early workouts, 100-120 per session for intermediates, and 120-140 for athletes who have had 4-6 weeks of plyometric training. The emphasis is on quality jumps and form, rather than volume.

Sport Loading

Sport loading is a program that trains the muscles involved in starting, running, and sprinting using the resistance of a sled, a slight incline, or stadium stairs. These exercises require more effort than normal sprinting on a flat surface does. Too much resistance, such as a 15- or 20-pound weight, reduces speed and is not effective. Eight to 10 pounds of weight or no more than a 1% incline (hill) will force the biceps femoris and rectus femoris muscles to work harder than they do in all-out sprinting on a flat surface. This kind of activity will effectively train those muscles to improve both speed and anaerobic endurance. This is one example of how more weight is not better. The goal is to apply a light load to the key muscles involved in sprinting and avoid drastic reductions in stride rate, stride length, and speed.

You can use one of the methods described in the succeeding sections and follow the program in table 16.7 (also shows two workout sessions per week), depending on the equipment available.

> **sport loading**—A training technique that involves adding resistance to the body while running and sprinting in the form of weighted vests, a sled, a slight incline, or stadium stairs.

Uphill Sprinting

Locate a 10- to 30-yard incline of 3 to 7 degrees.

Weighted Sleds, Weighted Vests, and Parachutes

You can buy one of numerous inexpensive sleds that are available or make a similar device with a spare tire, rope, and belt for little cost. Metal and plastic models are available that allow quick and easy weight changes. You can buy weighted vests loaded in half-pound increments. For acceleration sprints, small parachutes provide enough resistance without interfering with proper form. Younger athletes tend to enjoy parachutes more than they do other sport-loading methods.

TABLE 16.7—Sport-Loading Program: Hill Sprinting, Stadium Stairs, Weighted Vests, or Sled

Week	Routine or distance	Repetitions	Sets	Rest interval
1	Half-speed power starts in uphill sprinting or sled with no weight for 15 yd.*	3	1	Walk back to the starting position.
1	Repeat previous workout at three-quarter speed.	3	1	Same
2	Repeat previous workout.	3	2	Same
2	Repeat previous workout.	4	2	Same
3	Repeat previous workout. Add weight to sled or vests, accelerate to maximum speed, and hold for 15 yd.	5	2	Same
3	Repeat previous workout, accelerating for 25 yd.	5	2	Same
4	Same as previous workout. Add weight to sled or vest.	5	2	Same
4	Repeat previous workout, accelerating for 30 yd.	4	2	Same
5	Remove weight from sled or vest and return to a slightly reduced incline. Accelerate at maximum speed and sprint for 40 yd.	4	3	Same
5	Repeat previous workout. Finish with one all-out 100 yd acceleration sprint.	5	3	Same
6	Repeat previous workout.	5	3	Same
6	Maintenance load. Remove weight from sled or vest or use no more than a 3% incline. Accelerate to maximum speed and sprint for 40 yd.	4	3	Same

*Distance you pull the sled, sprint with weighted vests, sprint uphill, or sprint up stadium steps

Two-Person Harness

Two athletes of similar weight use the same harness. One provides the resistance, and the other provides the power.

Surgical Tubing

Partners can alternate sprinting against resistance.

Stadium Stairs

You can use stadium stairs or other stairs in the same way that you use uphill sprinting. Staircase acceleration training can be dangerous. Young athletes should avoid that type of training because all-out sprints can cause a fall that produces serious injury.

Sport loading trains the muscles involved in starting, running, and sprinting.

Speed

All of us can improve our sprinting speed. Although heredity is important, keep in mind that heredity only deals the cards; environment and training play the hand. What this means is that regardless of your genetic makeup, you can become faster with proper training. On the other hand, even genetically gifted athletes will not reach their potential unless they follow a complete speed improvement program.

You can improve your speed in only five ways:

1. Increase the number of steps you take per second. You can improve stride rate (steps per second) by using sprint-assisted training, plyometrics, and weight training.

2. Increase the length of each stride. You can increase the length of your stride through weight training, plyometric training, and sport loading.

3. Improve your acceleration and start. Plyometrics, weight training, and sport loading can improve acceleration.

4. Improve your sprinting form. Although no two athletes sprint the same way, basic mechanics are similar for everyone. By mastering proper sprinting technique with

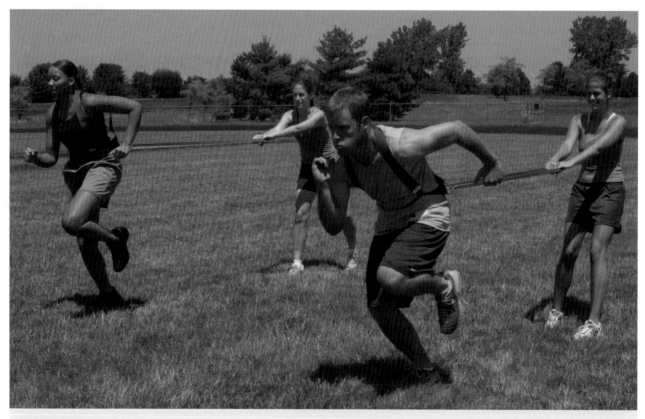

Sport loading can help you to improve speed and anaerobic endurance.

your coach, you can eliminate errors in arm action, body lean, foot contact, overstriding, understriding, and tension.

5. Improve your speed endurance. If your sport requires you to complete many all-out sprints during competition, you must develop your anaerobic conditioning to a level that allows you to maintain your speed for long sprints and prevents you from slowing down as the game progresses because of fatigue. Interval sprint-training programs (pickup sprints and hollow sprints) will improve your speed endurance. With proper training, you will be able to complete each sprint at the same high speed throughout the game or match.

This simple approach works for everyone. We previously discussed anaerobic training, strength training, plyometrics, and sport loading. The next section covers sprint-assisted training.

Sprint-Assisted Training

Sprint-assisted training is designed to improve speed in short sprints by increasing the stride rate. The training forces you to take faster steps than you can take without assistance. These exercises expose both the nervous and muscular systems to higher muscle contraction rates. Research shows that the number of steps an individual takes per second and the length of the stride will improve after 4 to 6 weeks of sprint-assisted training.

You can perform sprint-assisted training using three basic methods. Some require special equipment, and others do not.

Towing

Towing or pulling people so that they sprint faster is not a new approach. Before the use of surgical tubing and two-person pulley arrangements became popular, motor scooters, motorcycles, and even automobiles were used. You can buy a 20-foot piece of surgical tubing with two belts for little cost. To use the tubing, fasten yourself to one end and fasten the opposite end to another person or, to train alone, to a tree or goal post.

> **sprint-assisted training**—A program that forces people to sprint faster and take longer and faster steps than they can without assistance through the use of towing (surgical tubing), downhill sprinting, or high-speed stationary cycling.

You simply back up and stretch the tubing 20 or 30 yards and then use the rubber-band effect to sprint with the pull.

To prevent injury, a coach should provide supervision. Although tubing rarely breaks, improperly tied belts can work loose and cause injury. Tears can occur if the tubing is stretched too far (more than six times the original length). Follow these safety guidelines at all times:

- Make certain that the tubing is tied securely to the belt. After tubing is used a few times, the knots will tighten. Tighten and inspect newly tied belts before each run.
- After putting on the belt, an extra length of belt will remain (the tail). Wrap the tail around the abdomen, thread it again through the loop, and pull securely to form a knot. Repeat this process until you use most of the leftover belt. In other words, attach the belt properly and then tie several additional knots with the tail.
- Inspect the tubing on the first run by letting it slide through your hand as you back up to locate any nicks or rough marks. If you find a nick, discard and replace the tubing.
- Avoid stretching the tubing more than six times its length.
- Avoid standing with the tubing fully stretched for more than 1 or 2 seconds. Knots can come loose during this stretched phase.
- Avoid assuming a three-point stance with tubing fully stretched. If the opposite end comes loose, it could recoil into your face and eyes.
- To avoid soft-tissue injury, warm up properly before using surgical tubing. Jog at least a half mile, stretch thoroughly, and use a sequence of 20- or 25-yard walk-jog-stride-sprint segments for one-fourth to one-half mile.

Towing and other sprint-assisted training programs should occur early in the workout, immediately after your general warm-up and stretching exercises and before you are fatigued from drills, scrimmage, calisthenics, plyometrics, sport loading, weight training, or other conditioning routines. Almost full recovery should occur between repetitions.

At the end of each tow, you should attempt to sprint another 10 yards without the pull at the high speeds attained with its assistance. Some devices allow you to uncouple after receiving the full benefits of the pull.

Examples of specific workout drills follow:

- Attach tubing to a goalpost. For the first five trials, back up an extra 5 yards on each trial to increase the pull as you adjust to running at half speed for the first three trials and at three-quarter speed, but no faster, for the remaining two.

- Allow the tubing to pull you at approximately 4/10 of a second faster than your best 40-yard dash time. A slight pull will produce this effect. Place two marks 40 yards apart and have a partner use a stopwatch to get your time for a 40-yard tow.

- For a two-person drill up and down the field, tubing is attached to two runners. One runner, with the belt turned around so that the tubing is attached to the belt at his or her back, sprints about 30 yards ahead against resistance and stops. The runner who provided resistance (with the tubing attached to the belt in the front) now sprints toward the stopped runner in an overspeed run. Runners continue for 75 to 100 yards before reversing roles.

- Runners repeat the drill sprinting backward.

- One runner in tow can race another who is not assisted by tubing. Reverse the situation and compare the results. A fast runner without a tow can race against a slow one who is being towed.

Downhill Sprinting

If you can locate a hillside 50 yards long with a slope of no more than 3 to 7 degrees (only a slight decline), you can vary your program with downhill sprinting. Too much slope will increase the risk of falling and cause overstriding, landing on the heels of the feet, and ground contact beyond the center of gravity, which produces a "braking effect" that will slow your sprinting speed. The ideal area should allow a 20-yard sprint on a perfectly flat surface so that you can accelerate to near-maximum speed, a 15-yard high-speed sprint downhill on a slope of 2 to 7 degrees to force higher than normal stride rate and speed, and a 15-yard sprint on a flat area to allow you to hold the higher speed without the assistance of gravity. Ask your coach to help you find the right area.

High-Speed Stationary Cycling

Because it eliminates wind resistance, gravity, and body weight, high-speed stationary cycling allows you to complete more revolutions (similar to steps in sprinting) per second than the sprinting action does. This excellent sprint-assisted technique should be used with one other method, such as towing or downhill sprinting. Table 16.8 presents a sample 5-week program, showing two workout sessions per week.

Summary

Competitive Aerobics Competing in 5K and 10K road races, marathons, ultramarathons, and triathlons requires a high level of cardiovascular endurance or aerobic fitness. Training is demanding and must be specific to the activity. Those who were accustomed to exercising for 30 to 60 minutes several times weekly must now train 6 days weekly for several hours in a much more intense fashion that involves sustained effort at 90% of maximum heart rate or greater. With higher training volume, injuries and illnesses are more likely to occur unless exercisers plan workouts carefully, progress slowly, and eat properly.

Anaerobics Executing repeated short sprints at the same high speed with minimum rest after each or having enough reserve to complete a successful kick at the end of a 5K, 10K, or marathon requires a high level of anaerobic fitness. Without proper training, people will slow down because of fatigue after only a few short bursts and be unable to accelerate for a substantial distance at the end of a road race. To improve your anaerobic fitness, you can adapt intervals (for 5K and 10K races) and pickup sprints and hollow sprints (for sports and other activities requiring repeated short sprints) to the specific distances used in the activity for which you are training.

Flexibility After a general warm-up period, you should use dynamic stretching exercises to prepare for each workout. To increase your range of motion, perform static stretching exercises at the end of each exercise session. Most people do not need an extremely high level of flexibility.

Strength Obtaining a high level of strength requires almost daily workouts in the weight room using a variety of different approaches such as the rest-pause method, set system, burnout, wipeout, and techniques designed for competitive weightlifting and bodybuilding. Programs are demanding and require use of a partner who acts as a spotter.

TABLE 16.8—Sprint-Assisted Training—Towing With Surgical Tubing and Downhill Sprinting

Week	Overspeed distance	Repetitions	Rest
1	Half-speed runs toward the pull for 15 yd.	5	1 min
	Half-speed backward runs toward the pull for 15 yd.	3	1 min
1	Three-quarter-speed runs for 20 yd.	5	2 min
	Three-quarter-speed backward runs toward the pull for 20 yd.	3	2 min
2	Three-quarter-speed runs for 25 yd.	5	2 min
	Three-quarter-speed backward runs toward the pull for 25 yd.	3	2 min
	Three-quarter-speed turn-and-runs at a 45-degree angle for 25 yd (right and left).	3	2 min
2	Three-quarter-speed runs toward the pull for 15 yd.	5	2 min
	Maximum-speed sprints toward the pull for 15 yd.	5	2 min
3	Three-quarter-speed runs for 20 yd.	3	2 min
	Maximum-speed sprints for 20 yd.	6	2 1/2 min
3	Three-quarter-speed runs for 25 yd.	3	2 min
	Maximum-speed sprints for 25 yd.	6	3 min
4	Three-quarter-speed sprints for 30 yd.	3	2 min
	Maximum-speed sprints for 30 yd.	6	3 min
4	Three-quarter-speed runs toward the pull for 15 yd.	3	1 min
	Quick feet, short step, low knee lift sprint for 15 yd with rapid arm-pumping action.	3	2 min
	Quick feet, short step, fast high knee lift sprint for 15 yd with rapid arm-pumping action.	3	2 min
	Maximum-speed pulls for 30 yd.	4	3 min
5	High-speed stationary cycling. With the resistance on low to average, warm up for 5-7 min until you perspire freely. Pedal at three-quarter speed for 30 sec.	3	1 min
	Pedal at maximum speed for 2 sec as you say "one thousand and one, one thousand and two."	7	2 min
	Repeat previous for 3 sec.	3	2 min
	Maximum speed for 20 yd.	6	2 1/2 min
5	Repeat the preceding stationary cycling workout.		
	Add two-man pull-and-resist drill for 100 yd.	2	4 min
	Maximum speed sprints for 25 yd.	6	3 min
6	Repeat the preceding stationary cycling workout.		
6	Maintenance program:		
	Three-quarter speed runs toward the pull for 15 yd.	2	2 min
	Quick feet, short step, high knee lift sprint for 15 yd with rapid arm-pumping action.	2	2 min
	Maximum-speed forward pull for 20 yd, plant right foot, and sprint diagonally left for 20 yd. Repeat, planting the left foot and sprinting diagonally right for 20 yd.	3	2 min

Behavioral Change and Motivational Strategies

Many things can prevent you from becoming an elite performer. Here are some of these barriers (roadblocks) and strategies for overcoming them.

Roadblock	Behavioral Change Strategy
You know that training will take time away from family and friends. You are not willing to give up time with them.	Here is the perfect time for you to employ social support. Involve family and friends in your training. Have someone time you. Have another person be in charge of water. Have still another family member or friend keep a log of your progress. In this way, you can train and not have to sacrifice time with loved ones.
You were never a fast runner nor very strong. You believe that having those traits is necessary to be an elite performer.	Some people are born to run fast. Others have a great capacity for endurance. Recognizing these differences will help you determine at which activities you might excel. Using self-talk will allow you to make a more realistic evaluation of your chances of excelling. Statements such as, "With some hard work, there is no reason I cannot increase my strength or endurance," are helpful. You might say, "Others have learned to excel and there is no reason why I should think I cannot." Or you could say, "I have people who can train me and who are knowledgeable, so I certainly should be able to improve significantly."
You think that your body is so stiff that you'll never be able to do the movements required to be an elite performer.	You can improve your flexibility significantly if you work at it. This is a good time to use the behavioral change technique of reminders. Placing a copy of your flexibility training program on the refrigerator will remind you to stretch daily. Keeping a log of the days and times you stretch and your body's reactions can serve as another reminder. Finally, leaving messages on your telephone answering machine regarding your intention to attend a yoga class will remind you of when it is scheduled and keep you from missing that class.
List other roadblocks you are experiencing that interfere with your becoming an elite performer.	Now list the behavioral change strategies that can help you overcome these roadblocks. If you need to, refer back to chapter 4 for behavioral change and motivational strategies.

1. _____

2. _____

3. _____

1. _____

2. _____

3. _____

Power   Power, or speed strength, is a separate fitness component that you can improve through use of plyometrics, sport loading, and specially designed weight-training programs that involve explosive movements through the entire range of motion. Using free weights can improve specificity of training and develop power in the exact movements of a sport or activity.

Speed   Everyone can improve sprinting speed by increasing the number of steps taken per second, increasing the length of each stride, and improv-ing acceleration, form, and speed endurance. Sprint-assisted training (using a slight decline or surgical tubing to force faster steps than you are capable of taking without assistance), sport loading (training with additional resistance in the form of weighted vests, staircase sprinting, or hill sprinting), plyometrics (hopping, jumping, and bounding exercises performed at superhigh speeds), weight training, and speed endurance training are some of the programs you can use to improve sprinting speed for a specific sport or activity.

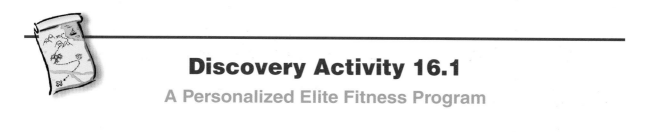

Discovery Activity 16.1

A Personalized Elite Fitness Program

Name _____ **Date** _____

Instructions: Design a total personalized fitness program.

Procedure

1. Establish a goal for each of the fitness areas you wish to develop, as in these examples:

- Be able to run a 10K in under 40 minutes.
- Be able to finish in the top 10% of my age group in a triathlon.
- Improve my strength by 15%.
- Reduce my percentage of body fat to 15%.
- Achieve a combination of all the preceding goals.

_____

_____

_____

_____

_____

2. Establish some specifically stated objectives, such as the following:

- Over a 10-week period, I will do a track workout once a week using the interval schedule from this chapter.
- Using the set system and Groves's superoverload, I will lift three times a week until I reach my goal.
- Using my personal fitness program and information from the nutrition chapter, I will modify my diet to lose ___ pounds in 6 months.

_____

_____

_____

_____

_____

(continued)

Discovery Activty 16.1 *(continued)*

3. Establish some rewards for accomplishing your goals and objectives.

_____

_____

4. Using the goals, objectives, and information from this entire book, establish a total fitness program.

_____

_____

_____

_____

_____

5. Write down your daily workouts, including an objective for each day.

- Be sure to follow the concepts established in chapter 3.
- The workouts should cover a period of at least 3 months.

_____

_____

_____

_____

_____

From *Physical fitness and wellness, third edition,* by Jerrold S. Greenberg, George B. Dintiman, and Barbee Myers Oakes, 2004, Champaign, IL: Human Kinetics.

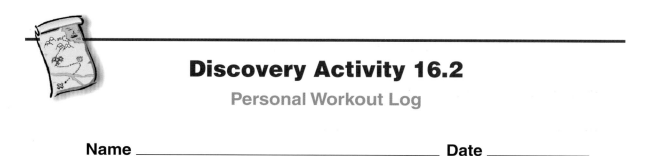

Discovery Activity 16.2

Personal Workout Log

Name _____ **Date** _____

Instructions: Design a personal daily log.

Procedure

1. Do this activity after completing Discovery Activity 16.1.

2. Using the information from Discovery Activity 16.1, design a personal log to record your progress (a 5-inch-by-7-inch spiral notebook is a good size for recording information).

3. Record the following information:

   a. Date and time
   b. Weather, if appropriate
   c. Time or distance covered
   d. For intervals, the length of each repetition, the total number of repetitions, the time, and the rest interval
   e. General impressions and special considerations, such as any unusual pains
   f. Nutritional information, including everything eaten each day

From *Physical fitness and wellness, third edition,* by Jerrold S. Greenberg, George B. Dintiman, and Barbee Myers Oakes, 2004, Champaign, IL: Human Kinetics.

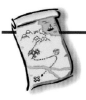

Discovery Activity 16.3

Service-Learning for Elite Fitness Champions

Whether they like it or not, elite athletes are often perceived as role models. That is one reason why it is important for college athletes to behave responsibly. To help elite athletes on your campus serve as positive role models, you could play the role of an agent. That is, you can make contact with the teams' coaches and suggest that team members volunteer to speak with children, youth, and others in the local community about various factors required to be a champion—be that an athletic champion, an educational champion, a champion friend or family member, or a champion citizen. After coaches agree to participate, you can make contacts with community schools, youth organizations, senior citizen centers, after-school centers, and other community organizations and arrange for the athletes to speak before these groups. The elite athletes might discuss the importance of responsible alcohol drinking and the dangers of drinking and driving, the importance of nutrition in staying healthy so that one can participate effectively in the life of the community, the dangers of eating disorders such as anorexia nervosa and bulimia nervosa, the necessity to manage anger and how to use anger-management techniques, or the importance of doing well in school. Community groups may also recommend topics in which they are interested.

From *Physical fitness and wellness, third edition,* by Jerrold S. Greenberg, George B. Dintiman, and Barbee Myers Oakes, 2004, Champaign, IL: Human Kinetics.

Appendix A

Nutritional Content of Common Foods

For this food composition table, foods are listed within the following groups:

1. Breads, cereals, rice, and pasta
2. Vegetables
3. Fruit
4. Milk, yogurt, and cheese
5. Meat, poultry, fish, dry beans, eggs, and nuts
6. Fats, oils, sweets, and alcoholic beverages

Name	Amount	Weight (g)	Energy (calories)	Protein (g)	Carbohydrate (g)	Fiber (g)	Total fat (g)	Saturated fat (g)	Cholesterol (mg)	Sodium (mg)	Vitamin A (RE)	Vitamin C (mg)	Calcium (mg)	Iron (mg)
BREADS, CEREALS, RICE, AND PASTA														
Bagel, plain	1 bagel, 4'' diameter	89	245	9.3	47.5	2.0	1.4	0.2	0	475	0	0	16	3.2
Barley, pearled, cooked	1/2 cup	79	97	1.8	22.2	3.0	0.3	0.1	0	2	1	0	9	1.0
Biscuit	1 biscuit, 2 1/2'' diameter	27	93	1.8	12.8	0.4	4.0	1.0	0	325	0	0	5	0.7
Bread, corn	1 piece	60	188	4.3	28.9	1.4	6.0	1.6	37	467	26	0	44	1.1
Bread, French	1 slice	64	175	5.6	33.2	1.9	1.9	0.4	0	390	0	0	48	1.6
Bread, oatmeal	1 slice	27	73	2.3	13.1	1.1	1.2	0.2	0	162	1	0	18	0.7
Bread, pita, white	1 pita, 6 1/2'' diameter	60	165	5.5	33.4	1.3	0.7	0.1	0	322	0	0	52	1.6
Bread, pita, whole wheat	1 pita, 6 1/2'' diameter	64	170	6.3	35.2	4.7	1.7	0.3	0	340	0	0	10	2.0
Bread, pumpernickel	1 slice	26	65	2.3	12.3	1.7	0.8	0.1	0	174	0	0	18	0.7
Bread, raisin	1 slice	32	88	2.5	16.7	1.4	1.4	0.3	0	125	0	0	21	0.9
Bread, rye	1 slice	32	83	2.7	15.5	1.9	1.1	0.2	0	211	0	0.1	23	0.9
Bread sticks	2 sticks, 7 5/8" × 5/8"	20	82	2.4	13.6	0.6	1.9	0.3	0	131	0	0	4	0.8
Bread stuffing	1/2 cup	100	178	3.2	21.7	2.9	8.6	1.7	0	543	81	0	32	1.1

(continued)

Name	Amount	Weight (g)	Energy (calories)	Protein (g)	Carbohydrate (g)	Fiber (g)	Total fat (g)	Saturated fat (g)	Cholesterol (mg)	Sodium (mg)	Vitamin A (RE)	Vitamin C (mg)	Calcium (mg)	Iron (mg)
BREADS, CEREALS, RICE, AND PASTA *(continued)*														
Bread, white	1 slice	30	80	2.5	14.9	0.7	1.1	0.2	0	161	0	0	32	0.9
Bread, whole grain	1 slice	32	80	3.2	14.8	2.0	1.2	0.3	0	156	0	0.1	29	1.1
Bread, whole wheat	1 slice	28	69	2.7	12.9	1.9	1.2	0.3	0	148	0	0	20	0.9
Buckwheat groats, cooked	1/2 cup	84	77	2.8	16.8	2.3	0.5	0.1	0	3	0	0	6	0.7
Bulgar, cooked	1/2 cup	83	110	3.0	23.5	4.5	0.1	0	0	4	0	0	11	0.5
Bun, hamburger or hot dog	1 roll	43	123	3.7	21.6	1.2	2.2	0.5	0	241	0	0	60	1.4
Cake, angelfood	1/12 of 10'' cake	50	129	3.1	29.4	0.1	0.2	0	0	255	0	0	42	0.1
Cake, chocolate w/frosting	1/8 of 18 oz cake	64	235	2.6	34.9	1.8	10.5	3.1	27	214	16	0.1	28	1.4
Cake, yellow w/icing	1/8 of 18 oz cake	64	243	2.4	35.5	1.2	11.1	3.0	35	216	21	0	23	1.3
Cereal, All-Bran	1/2 cup	30	53	3.7	22.7	15.3	0.9	0.2	0	127	260	17.3	116	5.2
Cereal, Bran Chex	3/5 cup	28	90	2.9	22.6	4.6	0.8	0.1	0	200	6	15.0	17	8.1
Cereal, Cheerios	1 cup	30	110	3.1	22.9	2.6	1.8	0.4	0	284	375	15.0	55	8.1
Cereal, cornflakes	1 cup	28	102	1.8	24.2	0.8	0.2	0.1	0	298	210	14.0	1	8.7
Cereal, Cream of Wheat	1/2 cup	126	67	1.9	13.8	0.9	0.3	0	0	168	0	0	25	5.1
Cereal, Frosted Flakes	3/4 cup	31	119	1.2	28.3	0.6	0.2	0.1	0	200	225	15.0	1	4.5
Cereal, granola	1/2 cup	31	135	3.0	22.4	1.9	4.2	0.6	0	8	0	0.1	24	1.3
Cereal, raisin bran	1 cup	61	186	5.6	47.1	8.2	1.5	0	0	354	250	0	35	5.0
Cereal, Total	3/4 cup	30	105	3.0	23.9	2.6	0.7	0.2	0	199	375	60.0	258	18.0
Cereal, Wheaties	1 cup	30	110	3.2	0.9	2.1	0.9	0.2	0	222	225	15.0	55	8.1
Coffee cake w/topping	1 piece	63	263	4.3	29.4	1.3	14.7	3.7	20	221	21	0.2	34	1.2
Cookie, chocolate chip	1 medium cookie	16	78	0.9	9.3	0.4	4.5	1.3	5	58	26	0	6	0.4
Cookie, fig bar	1 cookie	16	56	0.6	11.3	0.7	1.2	0.2	0	56	1	0	10	0.5
Cookie, fortune	1 cookie	8	30	0.3	6.7	0.1	0.2	0.1	0	22	0	0	1	0.1
Cookie, oatmeal	1 large cookie	18	81	1.1	12.4	0.5	3.3	0.8	0	69	0	0.1	7	0.5
Cookie, sandwich	1 cookie	10	47	0.5	7.0	0.3	0.3	0.4	0	60	0	0	3	0.4
Corn grits, cooked	1/2 cup	121	73	1.7	15.7	0.2	0.2	0	0	0	7	0	0	0.8
Cornmeal, dry	1/4 cup	35	126	2.9	26.8	2.6	0.6	0.1	0	1	14	0	2	1.4
Couscous, cooked	1/2 cup	79	88	3.0	18.2	1.1	0.1	0	0	4	0	0	6	0.3

Name	Amount	Weight (g)	Energy (calories)	Protein (g)	Carbohydrate (g)	Fiber (g)	Total fat (g)	Saturated fat (g)	Cholesterol (mg)	Sodium (mg)	Vitamin A (RE)	Vitamin C (mg)	Calcium (mg)	Iron (mg)
BREADS, CEREALS, RICE, AND PASTA *(continued)*														
Cracker, Crispbread, rye	3 crispbreads	30	110	2.4	24.7	5.0	0.4	0	0	79	0	0	9	0.7
Cracker, Goldfish	24 goldfish	12	70	1.0	8.0	1.0	4.0	0	0	100	0	0	8	0.4
Cracker, graham	3 squares	28	119	2.0	21.3	1.0	2.8	0.4	0	185	0	0	22	1.2
Cracker, matzo	1 matzo	28	112	2.8	23.7	0.9	0.4	0.1	0	1	0	0	4	0.9
Cracker, melba toast	6 pieces	30	117	3.6	23.0	1.9	1.0	0.1	0	249	0	0	28	1.1
Cracker, Ritz	5 crackers	16	79	1.2	10.3	0.3	3.7	0.6	0	124	0	0	24	0.6
Cracker, saltine	10 squares	30	130	2.8	21.5	0.9	3.5	0.9	0	390	0	0	36	1.6
Cracker, whole wheat	6 crackers	24	106	2.1	16.5	2.5	4.1	0.8	0	158	0	0	24	0.7
Croissant, butter	1 medium	57	231	4.7	26.1	1.5	12.0	6.6	38	424	106	0.1	21	1.2
Danish pastry, cheese	1 pastry	71	266	5.7	26.4	0.7	15.5	4.8	11	320	32	0	25	1.1
Doughnut, glazed	1 medium	45	192	2.3	22.9	0.7	10.3	2.7	14	181	1	01	27	0.5
English muffin, plain	1/2 muffin	29	67	2.2	13.1	0.8	0.5	0.1	0	132	0	0	50	0.7
French toast	1 slice	65	149	5.0	16.3	0	7.0	1.8	75	311	86	0.2	65	1.1
Macaroni, cooked	1/2 cup	70	99	3.3	19.8	0.9	0.5	0.1	0	1	0	0	5	1.0
Muffin, blueberry	2'' × 2 3/4''	57	158	3.1	27.4	1.5	3.7	0.8	17	255	5	0.6	32	0.9
Muffin, oat bran	2 1/4'' × 2 1/2''	57	154	4.0	27.5	2.6	4.2	0.6	0	224	0	0	36	2.4
Noodles, chow mein	1/2 cup	23	119	1.9	12.9	0.9	6.9	1.0	0	99	2	0	5	1.1
Noodles, egg, cooked	1/2 cup	80	106	3.8	19.6	0.9	1.2	0.2	653	6	5	0	10	1.3
Noodles, Japanese soba	1/2 cup	57	56	2.9	12.2	0	0.1	0	0	34	0	0	2	0.3
Oatmeal, instant	1 packet	155	153	4.1	31.4	2.6	1.8	0.4	0	234	302	0	105	3.9
Oats, uncooked	1/4 cup	20	78	3.2	27.1	2.1	1.3	0.2	0	1	2	0	11	0.9
Pancake	4'' pancake	38	74	2.0	13.9	0.5	1.0	0.2	5	239	12	0.1	48	0.6
Pasta, cooked	1/2 cup	57	75	2.9	14.2	0	0.6	0.1	19	3	3	0	3	0.7
Popcorn, air-popped	2 cups	16	61	1.9	12.5	2.4	0.7	0.1	0	1	3	0	2	0.4
Popcorn, oil-popped	2 cups	22	110	1.9	12.6	2.2	6.2	1.0	0	194	3	0	2	0.6
Pretzels	10 twists	60	229	5.5	47.5	1.9	2.1	0.5	0	1,029	0	0	22	02.6
Quinoa, uncooked	1/4 cup	43	159	5.6	29.3	2.5	2.5	0.3	0	9	0	0	26	3.9
Rice, brown, cooked	1/2 cup	71	109	2.3	22.9	1.8	0.8	0.3	0	1	0	0	10	0.5
Rice cake	1 cake	9	35	0.7	7.3	0.4	0.3	0	0	29	0	0	1	0.1
Rice, white, cooked	1/2 cup	93	121	2.2	26.6	0.3	0.2	0.1	0	0	0	0	3	1.4
Rice, wild, cooked	1/2 cup	82	83	3.3	17.5	1.5	0.3	0	0	3	0	0	2	0.5

(continued)

Name	Amount	Weight (g)	Energy (calories)	Protein (g)	Carbohydrate (g)	Fiber (g)	Total fat (g)	Saturated fat (g)	Cholesterol (mg)	Sodium (mg)	Vitamin A (RE)	Vitamin C (mg)	Calcium (mg)	Iron (mg)
BREADS, CEREALS, RICE, AND PASTA *(continued)*														
Roll, dinner	1 roll, 2" square	28	84	2.4	14.1	0.8	2.0	0.5	0	146	0	0	33	0.9
Spaghetti, cooked	1/2 cup	70	99	3.3	19.8	1.2	0.5	0.1	0	70	0	0	5	1.0
Taco shell	1 medium	13	62	1.0	8.3	1.0	3.0	0.4	0	49	0	0	21	0.3
Tortilla chips	1 oz	28	142	2.0	17.8	1.8	7.4	1.4	0	150	6	0	44	0.4
Tortilla, corn	1 medium	26	58	1.5	12.1	1.4	0.17	0.1	0	42	0	0	46	0.4
Tortilla, flour	1 medium	49	159	4.3	27.2	1.6	3.5	0.9	0	234	0	0	61	1.6
Wheat germ, toasted	1/4 cup	28	108	8.3	14.1	3.7	3.0	0.5	0	1	0	1.7	13	2.6
VEGETABLES														
Artichoke, cooked	1 medium	120	60	4.2	13.4	6.5	0.2	0	0	114	22	12.0	54	1.5
Arugula, raw	1 cup	20	5	0.5	0.7	0.3	0.1	0	0	3	24	3.0	16	0.1
Asparagus, cooked	6 spears	90	22	2.3	3.8	1.4	0.3	0	0	10	49	9.7	18	0.7
Bamboo shoots, canned	1/2 cup	66	13	1.1	2.1	0.9	0.3	0.1	0	5	1	0.7	5	0.2
Bean sprouts, raw	1/2 cup	35	43	4.6	3.3	0.4	2.3	0.3	0	5	0	5.4	23	0.7
*Beans, baked (plain)	1/2 cup	127	118	6.1	26.0	6.4	0.6	0.1	0	504	22	3.9	64	0.4
*Beans, black, cooked	1/2 cup	86	114	7.6	20.4	7.5	0.5	0.1	0	1	1	0	23	1.8
*Beans, fava, cooked	1/2 cup	85	94	6.5	16.7	4.6	0.3	0.1	0	4	2	0.3	31	1.3
Beans, green snap, cooked	1/2 cup	63	22	1.2	4.9	2.0	0.2	0	0	2	42	6.1	29	0.8
*Beans, kidney, cooked	1/2 cup	89	112	7.7	20.2	6.5	0.4	0.1	0	2	0	1.1	25	2.6
*Beans, lentils, cooked	1/2 cup	99	115	8.9	19.9	7.8	0.4	0.1	0	2	1	1.5	19	3.3
*Beans, lima, cooked	1/2 cup	94	108	7.3	19.6	6.6	0.4	0.1	0	2	0	0	16	2.2
*Beans, navy, cooked	1/2 cup	91	129	7.9	23.9	5.8	0.5	0.1	0	1	0	0.8	64	2.3
*Beans, pinto, cooked	1/2 cup	86	117	7.0	21.9	7.4	0.4	0.1	0	2	0	1.8	41	2.2
*Beans, refried	1/2 cup	126	118	6.9	19.6	6.7	1.6	0.6	10	377	0	7.6	44	2.1
Beans, yellow snap, cooked	1/2 cup	63	22	1.2	4.9	2.1	0.2	0	0	2	5	6.1	29	0.8
Beet greens, cooked	1/2 cup	144	39	3.7	7.9	4.2	0.3	0	0	347	734	35.9	164	2.7
Beets, cooked	1/2 cup	74	37	1.4	8.5	1.7	0.2	0	0	65	3	3.1	14	0.7
Broccoli spears, cooked	2 spears	78	22	2.3	3.9	2.3	0.3	0	0	20	108	58.2	36	0.7
Brussels sprouts, cooked	4 sprouts	84	33	2.1	7.3	2.2	0.4	0.1	0	18	60	52.1	30	1.0
Cabbage, cooked	1/2 cup	75	17	0.8	3.3	1.7	0.3	0	0	6	10	15.1	23	0.1

VEGETABLES *(continued)*

Name	Amount	Weight (g)	Energy (calories)	Protein (g)	Carbohydrate (g)	Fiber (g)	Total fat (g)	Saturated fat (g)	Cholesterol (mg)	Sodium (mg)	Vitamin A (RE)	Vitamin C (mg)	Calcium (mg)	Iron (mg)
Cabbage, raw	1/2 cup	45	11	0.6	2.4	1.0	0.1	0	0	8	6	14.3	21	0.3
Carrot juice	1/4 cup	177	71	1.7	16.4	1.4	0.3	0	0	51	1,938	15.0	42	0.8
Carrots, cooked	1/2 cup	78	35	0.9	8.2	2.6	0.1	0	0	51	1,915	1.8	24	0.5
Carrots, raw	1 medium	62	26	0.6	6.2	1.8	0.1	0	0	21	1,716	5.6	16	0.3
Cauliflower, cooked	1/2 cup	62	14	1.1	2.5	1.7	0.3	0	0	9	1	27.4	10	0.2
Celery, raw	8 sticks	32	5	0.2	1.2	0.5	0	0	0	28	4	2.2	13	0.1
Chard, cooked	1/2 cup	88	18	1.6	3.6	1.8	0.1	0	0	156	275	15.8	51	2.0
Coleslaw, homemade	1/2 cup	60	41	0.8	7.4	0.9	1.6	0.2	5	14	49	19.6	27	0.4
Collards, cooked	1/2 cup	95	25	2.0	4.7	2.7	0.3	0	0	9	297	17.3	113	0.4
Corn, yellow, cooked	1/2 cup	82	89	2.7	20.6	2.3	1.1	0.2	0	14	18	5.1	2	0.5
Cucumber, raw	1/2 cup	52	7	0.4	1.4	0.4	0.1	0	0	1	11	2.8	7	0.1
Eggplant, cooked	1/2 cup	50	14	0.4	3.3	1.2	0.1	0	0	1	3	0.6	3	0.2
Endive, raw	1/2 cup	25	4	0.3	0.8	0.8	0.1	0	0	6	51	1.6	13	0.2
Hominy, canned	1/2 cup	84	94	1.2	11.8	2.1	0.7	0.1	0	173	0	0	8	0.5
Kale, cooked	1/2 cup	65	18	1.2	3.6	1.3	0.3	0	0	15	481	26.7	47	0.6
Lettuce, iceberg	1 cup	55	7	0.6	1.1	0.8	0.1	0	0	5	18	2.1	10	0.3
Lettuce, looseleaf	1 cup	56	10	0.7	2.0	1.1	0.2	0	0	5	106	10.1	38	0.8
Lettuce, romaine	1 cup	56	8	0.9	1.3	1.0	0.1	0	0	4	152	13.4	20	0.6
Mushrooms, cooked	1/2 cup	78	21	1.7	4.0	1.7	0.3	0	0	2	0	3.1	5	1.4
Mushrooms, raw	1/2 cup	35	9	1.0	1.4	0.4	0.1	0	0	1	0	0.8	2	0.4
Mustard greens, cooked	1/2 cup	70	11	1.6	1.5	1.4	0.2	0	0	11	212	17.7	52	0.5
Okra, cooked	1/2 cup	92	26	1.9	5.3	2.6	0.3	0.1	0	3	47	11.2	88	0.6
Onion, raw	1/2 cup	80	30	0.9	6.9	1.4	0.1	0	0	2	0	5.1	16	0.2
Parsnip, raw	1/2 cup	67	50	0.8	12.0	3.2	0.2	0	0	7	0	11.3	24	0.4
*Peas, blackeyed, cooked	1/2 cup	86	100	6.6	17.9	5.6	0.5	0.1	0	3	1	0.3	21	2.2
*Peas, chickpeas (garbanzos)	1/2 cup	82	134	7.3	22.5	6.2	2.1	0.2	0	6	2	1.1	40	2.4
Peas, edible podded	10 peapods	34	14	1.0	2.6	0.9	0.1	0	0	1	5	20.4	15	0.7
Peas, green	1/2 cup	80	62	4.1	11.4	4.4	0.2	0	0	70	54	7.9	19	1.2
*Peas, split, cooked	1/2 cup	98	116	8.2	20.6	8.1	0.4	0.1	0	2	1	0.4	14	1.3
Pepper, green chili, canned	1/2 cup	70	15	0.5	3.2	1.2	0.2	0	0	276	9	23.8	25	0.9

(continued)

Name	Amount	Weight (g)	Energy (calories)	Protein (g)	Carbohydrate (g)	Fiber (g)	Total fat (g)	Saturated fat (g)	Cholesterol (mg)	Sodium (mg)	Vitamin A (RE)	Vitamin C (mg)	Calcium (mg)	Iron (mg)
VEGETABLES *(continued)*														
Pepper, sweet green, raw	1 small	74	20	0.7	4.8	1.3	0.1	0	0	1	47	66.1	7	0.3
Pepper, sweet red, raw	1 small	74	20	0.7	4.8	1.5	0.1	0	0	1	422	140.6	7	0.3
Pickle, dill	1 medium	65	12	0.4	2.7	0.8	0.1	0	0	21	833	1.2	6	0.3
Potato, baked w/skin	1 medium	173	188	4.0	43.5	4.1	0.2	0	0	14	0	22.3	17	2.3
Potato, boiled	1 potato, 2 1/2'' diameter	136	118	2.5	27.4	2.4	0.1	0	0	5	0	17.7	7	0.4
Potato, French fries	10 fries	50	109	1.7	17.0	1.6	4.1	1.9	0	141	0	4.8	5	0.7
Potato, mashed w/milk	1/2 cup	105	81	2.0	18.4	2.1	0.6	0.3	2	318	6	7.0	27	0.3
Potato salad	1/2 cup	125	179	3.4	14.0	1.6	10.3	1.8	85	661	41	12.5	24	0.8
Pumpkin, canned	1/2 cup	123	42	1.3	9.9	3.6	0.3	0.2	0	6	2702	5.1	32	1.7
Radish	13 medium	58	12	0.3	2.1	0.9	0.3	0	0	13.9	1	13.2	12	0.2
Rutabaga, mashed	1/2 cup	120	47	1.5	10.5	2.2	0.3	0	0	24	67	22.6	58	0.6
Sauerkraut, drained	1/2 cup	121	13	0.6	3.0	1.8	0.1	0	0	469	1	10.5	21	1.0
Soybeans, green, boiled	1/2 cup	90	127	11.1	9.9	3.8	5.8	0.7	0	13	14	15.3	131	2.3
Spinach, cooked	1/2 cup	95	27	3.0	5.1	2.9	0.2	0	0	82	739	11.7	139	1.4
Spinach, raw	1 cup	30	7	0.9	1.1	0.8	0.1	0	0	24	202	8.4	30	0.8
Squash, summer, cooked	1/2 cup	90	18	0.8	3.9	1.3	0.3	0	0	1	26	5.9	24	0.3
Squash, Summer, raw	1/2 small squash	59	12	0.7	2.6	1.1	0.1	0	0	1	12	8.7	12	0.3
Squash, winter	1/2 cup	100	39	0.9	8.8	2.8	0.6	0.1	0	1	356	9.6	14	0.3
Sweet potato, baked	1/2 cup	100	103	1.7	24.3	3.0	0.1	0	0	10	2,182	24.6	28	0.5
Sweet potato, canned w/syrup	1/2 cup	100	108	1.3	25.4	3.0	0.3	0.1	0	39	716	10.8	17	1.0
Tomato juice	1/4 cup	182	31	1.4	7.7	1.5	1.4	0	0	18	102	33.3	16	1.1
Tomato, raw	1 medium	123	26	1.0	5.7	1.4	0.4	0.1	0	11	76	23.5	6	0.6
Tomato sauce	1/2 cup	123	37	1.6	1.7	1.7	0.2	0	0	741	120	16.0	17	0.9
Turnip, cooked, mashed	1/2 cup	115	24	0.8	5.6	2.3	0.1	0	0	108	0	13.3	25	0.3
Vegetable juice	3/4 cup	182	35	1.1	8.3	1.5	0.2	0	0	491	213	50.4	20	0.8
Vegetables, mixed	1/2 cup	91	54	2.6	11.9	4.0	0.1	0	0	32	389	2.9	23	0.7
Vegetable soup	1 cup	241	72	2.1	12.0	0.5	1.9	0.3	0	822	301	1.4	22	1.1
Water chestnuts	1/2 cup	70	35	0.6	8.7	1.8	0	0	0	6	0	0.9	3	0.6

Name	Amount	Weight (g)	Energy (calories)	Protein (g)	Carbohydrate (g)	Fiber (g)	Total fat (g)	Saturated fat (g)	Cholesterol (mg)	Sodium (mg)	Vitamin A (RE)	Vitamin C (mg)	Calcium (mg)	Iron (mg)
FRUIT														
Apple	1 medium	138	81	0.3	21.0	3.7	0.5	0.1	0	0	7	7.9	10	0.2
Apple juice	1/4 cup	179	84	0.3	20.7	0.2	0.2	0	0	13	0	44.8	11	0.5
Applesauce, unsweetened	1/2 cup	122	52	0.2	13.8	1.5	0.1	0	0	2	4	25.9	4	0.1
Apricots	2 medium	70	34	1.0	7.8	1.7	0.3	0	0	1	183	7.0	10	0.4
Apricots, dried	9 halves	32	75	1.2	19.4	2.8	0.12	0	0	3	228	0.8	14	1.5
Avocado	1 medium	173	306	3.7	12.0	8.5	30.0	4.5	0	21	105	13.7	19	2.0
Banana	1 medium	118	109	1.2	27.6	2.8	0.6	0.2	0	1	9	10.7	7	0.4
Blackberries	1/2 cup	72	37	0.5	9.2	3.8	0.3	0	0	0	12	15.1	23	0.4
Blueberries	1/2 cup	73	41	0.5	10.2	2.0	0.3	0	0	4	7	9.4	4	0.1
Cantaloupe	1/4 melon 5'' diameter	138	48	1.2	12	11.5	1.1	0.4	0.1	0	12	58.2	15	0.3
Carambola (starfruit)	1 small	70	23	0.4	5.5	1.9	0.2	0	0	1	34	14.8	3	0.2
Cherries, canned in syrup	1/2 cup	128	116	0.9	29.8	1.4	0.1	0	0	9	91	2.6	13	1.7
Cherries, sweet, raw	11 cherries	75	54	0.9	2.3	1.7	0.7	0.2	0	0	16	5.2	11	0.3
Cranberries, raw	1/2 cup	48	23	0.2	6.0	2.0	0.1	0	0	1	2	6.4	3	0.1
Cranberry juice cocktail	1/4 cup	190	108	0	27.3	0.2	0.2	0	0	4	0	67.1	6	0.3
Cranberry sauce	1/4 cup	139	105	0.1	26.9	0.7	0.1	0	0	20	1	1.4	3	0.2
Currants, dried	1/4 cup	36	109	1.5	26.7	2.4	0.1	0	0	3	3	1.7	31	1.2
Dates, dried	`1/4 cup	45	122	0.9	32.7	3.3	0.2	0.1	0	1	2	0	14	0.5
Figs, raw	2 medium	100	74	0.8	19.2	3.3	0.3	0.1	0	1	14	2.0	35	0.4
Fruit cocktail, light syrup	1/2 cup	121	69	0.5	18.1	1.2	0.1	0	0	7	25	2.3	7	0.4
Fruit cocktail, heavy syrup	1/2 cup	124	91	0.5	23.4	1.2	0.1	0	0	7	25	2.4	7	0.4
Fruit cocktail, juice	1/2 cup	119	55	0.5	14.1	1.2	0	0	0	5	37	3.2	9	0.3
Grapefruit	1/2 medium	28	41	0.8	10.3	1.4	0.1	0	0	0	15	44.0	15	0.1
Grapefruit juice	1/4 cup	185	70	1.0	16.6	0.2	0.2	0	0	2	2	54.1	13	0.4
Grapes	12 grapes	60	43	0.4	10.7	0.6	0.3	0	0	1	4	6.5	7	0.2
Guava	1 fruit	90	46	0.7	10.7	4.9	0.5	0.2	0	3	71	165.2	18	0.3
Honeydew	1/8 melon, 5 1/4'' diameter	125	44	0.6	11.5	0.8	0.1	0	0	13	5	31.0	8	0.1
Kiwifruit	1 large	91	56	0.9	13.5	3.1	0.4	0	0	5	16	68.3	24	0.4
Kumquats	5 fruits	100	63	0.9	16.4	6.6	0.1	0	0	6	30	37.4	44	0.4

(continued)

Name	Amount	Weight (g)	Energy (calories)	Protein (g)	Carbohydrate (g)	Fiber (g)	Total fat (g)	Saturated fat (g)	Cholesterol (mg)	Sodium (mg)	Vitamin A (RE)	Vitamin C (mg)	Calcium (mg)	Iron (mg)
FRUIT *(continued)*														
Lemon juice	2 tablespoons	31	6	0.1	2.0	0.1	0.1	0	0	6	1	7.6	3	0
Lemon, with peel	1 fruit	108	22	1.3	11.6	5.1	0.3	0	0	3	3	83.2	66	0.8
Mango	1/2 medium	103	65	0.5	17.0	1.8	0.3	0.1	0	2	389	27.7	10	0.1
Nectarine	1 fruit	136	67	1.3	16.0	2.2	0.6	0.1	0	0	101	7.3	7	0.2
Orange	1 medium	131	62	1.2	15.4	3.1	0.2	0	0	0	28	69.7	52	0.1
Orange juice	3/4 cup	187	82	1.5	18.8	0.4	0.5	0.1	0	2	15	61.6	19	0.3
Papaya	1/2 medium	152	59	0.9	14.9	2.7	0.2	0.1	0	5	43	93.9	36	0.2
Passion fruit	1/2 cup	118	114	2.6	27.6	12.3	0.8	0.1	0	33	83	35.4	14	1.9
Peach, canned in juice	1/2 cup	124	55	0.8	14.3	1.6	0	0	0	5	47	4.4	7	0.3
Peach, raw	1 medium	98	42	0.7	10.9	2.0	0.1	0	0	0	53	6.5	5	0.1
Pear, canned	1/2 cup	124	62	0.4	16.0	2.0	0.1	0	0	5	1	2.0	11	0.4
Pear, raw	1 medium	166	98	0.6	25.1	4.0	0.7	0	0	0	3	6.6	18	0.4
Pineapple, canned in juice	1/2 cup	125	75	0.5	19.5	1.0	0.1	0	0	1	5	11.8	17	0.3
Pineapple, raw	1 slice 3 1/2" × 3 1/4"	84	41	0.3	10.4	1.0	0.4	0	0	1	2	12.9	6	0.3
Plantain, raw	1 medium	179	218	2.3	57.1	4.1	0.3	0		7	6	2.3	5	1.1
Plums	1 1/2 medium	99	55	0.8	13.0	1.5	0.6	0	0	0	32	9.5	4	0.1
Prune juice	1/4 cup	192	136	1.2	33.5	1.9	0.1	0	0	8	0	7.9	23	2.3
Prunes, dried	5 prunes	42	80	1.1	26.3	3.0	0.2	0	0	2	84	1.4	21	1.0
Raisins	1/4 cup	43	129	1.4	34.0	1.7	0.2	0.1	0	5	0	1.4	21	0.9
Raspberries	1/2 cup	62	30	0.6	7.1	4.2	0.3	0	0	0	8	15.4	14	0.4
Rhubarb, raw	1 stalk	51	11	0.5	2.3	0.9	0.1	0	0	2	5	4.1	44	0.1
Strawberries	5 large	90	27	0.6	6.3	2.1	0.3	0	0	1	3	51.0	13	0.3
Tangerine	1 medium	84	40	0.5	'9.4	1.9	0.2	0	0	1	77	25.9	12	0.1
Watermelon	1/16 melon	286	92	1.8	20.5	1.4	1.2	0.1	0	6	106	27.5	23	0.5
MILK, YOGURT, AND CHEESE														
Buttermilk, lowfat	1 cup	245	98	8.1	11.7	0	2.2	1.3	10	257	20	2.5	284	0.1
Cheese, American	2 oz	57	186	11.1	4.1	0	13.9	8.8	36	905	124	0	325	0.5
Cheese, blue	1 1/2 oz	43	150	9.1	1.0	0	12.2	7.9	32	593	97	0	225	0.1
Cheese, cheddar	1 1/2 oz	43	171	10.6	0.5	0	14.1	9.0	45	264	118	0	307	0.3
Cheese, cottage, creamed	1 cup	210	216	26.2	5.6	0	9.5	6.0	32	850	101	0	126	0.3
Cheese, cottage, lowfat (1%)	1 cup	226	163	28.0	6.1	0	2.3	1.5	9	918	25	0	138	0.3

Name	Amount	Weight (g)	Energy (calories)	Protein (g)	Carbohydrate (g)	Fiber (g)	Total fat (g)	Saturated fat (g)	Cholesterol (mg)	Sodium (mg)	Vitamin A (RE)	Vitamin C (mg)	Calcium (mg)	Iron (mg)
MILK, YOGURT, AND CHEESE *(continued)*														
Cheese, cottage, fat free	1 cup	145	123	25.0	2.7	0	0.6	0.4	10	19	12	0	46	0.3
Cheese, cream	2 oz	57	198	4.3	1.5	0	19.8	12.5	62	168	216	0	45	0.7
Cheese, cream, fat free	2 oz	57	55	8.2	3.3	0	0.8	0.5	5	311	159	0	105	0.1
Cheese, feta	1 1/2 oz	43	112	6.0	1.7	0	9.0	6.4	38	475	54	0	210	0.3
Cheese, Mexican	1 1/2 oz	43	151	9.6	1.2	0	12.0	7.6	45	279	27	0	281	0.2
Cheese, Monterey	1 1/2 oz	43	159	10.4	0.3	0	12.9	8.1	38	228	108	0	3,187	0.3
Cheese, mozzarella, part skim	1 1/2 oz	43	108	10.3	1.2	0	6.8	4.3	25	198	75	0	275	0.1
Cheese, parmesan, grated	2 tablespoons	10	46	4.2	0.4	0	3.0	1.9	8	186	17	0	138	0.1
Cheese, process spread	2 oz	56	170	9.1	5.5	0	12.3	8.1	45	839	100	0.1	261	0.1
Cheese, provolone	1 1/2 oz	43	149	10.9	0.9	0	11.3	7.3	29	373	112	0	321	0.2
Cheese, ricotta, part skim	1/2 cup	124	171	14.1	6.4	0	9.8	6.1	38	155	140	0	337	0.5
Cheese, Swiss	1 1/2 oz	43	160	12.1	1.4	0	11.7	7.6	39	111	19	0	409	0.1
Ice cream, chocolate	1 cup	132	285	5.0	37.2	1.6	14.2	9.0	45	100	151	0.9	144	1.2
Ice cream, vanilla, light	1 cup	132	183	5.0	30.0	0	5.7	3.5	18	112	62	1.1	183	0.1
Ice cream, vanilla, rich	1 cup	148	357	5.2	33.2	0	24.0	14.8	90	83	272	1.0	173	0.1
Ice cream, vanilla, soft serve	1 cup	172	370	7.1	38.2	0	22.4	12.9	157	105	265	1.4	225	0.4
Milk, chocolate	1 cup	250	208	7.9	25.9	2.0	8.5	5.3	30	150	73	2.3	280	0.6
Milk, fat free (nonfat)	1 cup	245	86	8.4	11.9	0	0.4	0.3	5	127	149	2.5	301	0.1
Milk lowfat (1%)	1 cup	244	102	8.0	11.7	0	2.6	1.6	10	124	144	2.4	300	0.1
Milk, reduced fat (2%)	1 cup	244	122	8.1	11.7	0	4.7	2.9	20	122	139	2.4	298	0.1
Milk, whole	1 cup	244	149	8.0	11.4	0	8.2	5.1	34	120	76	2.2	290	0.1
Pudding, made with milk	1/2 cup	142	158	4.5	25.6	1.4	4.8	3.0	17	146	37	1.0	158	0.5
Yogurt, frozen, vanilla	1 cup	144	229	5.8	34.8	0	8.1	4.9	3	125	82	1.2	206	0.4
Yogurt, lowfat, plain	8 oz container	227	143	11.9	16.0	0	3.5	2.3	14	159	36	1.8	415	0.2
Yogurt, lowfat, with fruit	8 oz container	227	238	11.0	42.2	0	3.2	2.1	14	148	136	1.6	384	0.2
Yogurt, nonfat, plain	8 oz container	227	127	13.0	17.4	0	0.4	0.3	5	175	5	2.0	342	0.2

(continued)

Name	Amount	Weight (g)	Energy (calories)	Protein (g)	Carbohydrate (g)	Fiber (g)	Total fat (g)	Saturated fat (g)	Cholesterol (mg)	Sodium (mg)	Vitamin A (RE)	Vitamin C (mg)	Calcium (mg)	Iron (mg)
MEAT, POULTRY, FISH, DRY BEANS, EGGS, AND NUTS														
Bacon	3 slices	19	109	5.7	0.1	0	9.4	3.3	19	303	0	0	2	0.3
Bacon, Canadian	2 slices	47	86	11.3	0.6	0	3.9	1.3	27	719	0	0	5	0.4
Beef, 1/2" fat	3 oz	85	344	19.9	0	0	28.7	11.9	78	48	0	0	9	2.1
Beef, corned beef	3 oz	85	213	23.0	0	0	12.7	5.3	73	856	0	0	10	1.8
Beef, ground, extra lean, broiled	3 oz	85	218	21.6	9	9	13.9	5.5	71	60	0	0	6	2.0
Beef, ground, lean, broiled	3 oz	85	231	21.0	0	0	15.7	6.2	74	65	0	0	9	1.8
Beef, ground, regular, broiled	3 oz	85	246	20.5	0	0	17.6	6.9	77	71	0	0	9	2.1
Beef, lean, fat trimmed	3 oz	85	179	25.4	0	0	7.9	3.0	73	56	0	0	7	2.5
Beef liver, braised	3 oz	85	137	20.7	2.9	0	4.2	1.6	331	60	9,011	19.6	6	5.8
Beef ribs, broiled	3 oz	85	306	18.7	0	0	25.1	10.2	70	53	0	0	10	1.8
Chicken breast, w/ skin, roasted	1/2 breast	98	193	29.2	0	0	7.6	2.1	82	70	26	0	14	1.0
Chicken, dark meat, w/skin, roasted	3 oz	85	215	22.1	0	0	13.4	3.7	77	74	49	0	13	1.2
Chicken, dark meat, w/o skin, roasted	3 oz	85	168	22.2	0	0	7.9	2.2	76	76	18	0	12	1.1
Chicken, dark meat, w/skin, fried	3 oz	85	253	18.6	8.0	0	15.8	4.2	76	251	26	0	18	1.2
Chicken, drumstick, w/skin, roasted	1 drumstick	52	112	14.1	0	0	5.8	1.6	47	47	16	0	6	0.7
Chicken, light meat, w/skin, roasted	3 oz	85	189	24.7	0	0	9.2	2.6	71	64	27	0	13	1.0
Chicken, light meat, w/o skin, roasted	3 oz	85	147	26.3	0	0	3.8	1.1	72	65	8	0	13	0.9
Chicken, light meat, w/skin, fried	3 oz	85	235	20.0	8.1	0	13.1	3.5	71	243	20	0	17	1.1
Chicken liver, chopped	1/2 cup	70	110	17.1	0.8	0	3.8	1.3	442	36	3,439	11.1	10	5.9
Chicken, thigh, w/skin, roasted	1 thigh	62	153	15.5	0	0	9.6	2.7	58	52	30	0	7	0.8
Chicken, wing, w/skin, roasted	1 wing	34	99	9.1	0	0	6.6	1.9	29	28	16	0	5	0.4
Egg white, large	1 egg white	33	17	3.5	0.3	0	0	0	0	55	0	0	2	0
Egg, whole, large	1 egg	50	75	6.2	0.6	0	5.1	1.6	213	63	97	0	25	0.7
Egg yolk, large	1 yolk	7	59	2.8	0.3	0	5.1	1.6	213	7	97	0	23	0.6
Fish, catfish, baked/ broiled	3 oz	85	129	15.9	0	0	6.8	1.5	54	68	13	0.7	8	0.7

MEAT, POULTRY, FISH, DRY BEANS, EGGS, AND NUTS (continued)

Name	Amount	Weight (g)	Energy (calories)	Protein (g)	Carbohydrate (g)	Fiber (g)	Total fat (g)	Saturated fat (g)	Cholesterol (mg)	Sodium (mg)	Vitamin A (RE)	Vitamin C (mg)	Calcium (mg)	Iron (mg)
Fish, halibut, baked/broiled	3 oz	85	119	22.7	0	0	2.5	0.4	35	59	46	0	51	0.9
Fish, salmon, baked/broiled	3 oz	85	175	18.8	0	0	10.5	2.1	54	52	13	3.1	13	0.3
Fish, salmon, canned	3 oz	85	130	17.4	0	0	6.2	1.4	37	457	45	0	203	0.9
Fish, salmon, smoked	3 oz	85	99	15.5	0	0	3.7	0.8	20	1,700	22	0	9	0.7
Fish, sardine, canned in oil	1 can (3.75 oz)	92	191	22.7	0	0	10.5	1.4	131	465	62	0	351	2.7
Fish, snapper, baked/broiled	3 oz	85	109	22.3	0	0	1.5	0.3	40	48	30	1.4	34	0.2
Fish sticks	3 sticks	84	228	13.1	19.9	0	10.3	2.6	94	489	26	0	17	0.6
Fish, swordfish, baked/broiled	3 oz	85	132	21.6	0	0	4.4	1.2	4.3	98	35	0.9	5	0.9
Fish, trout, baked/broiled	3 oz	85	162	22.6	0	0	7.2	1.3	63	57	16	0.4	47	1.6
Fish, tuna, canned in oil	3 oz	85	158	22.6	0	0	6.9	1.4	26	337	20	0	3	0.6
Fish, tuna, canned in water	3 oz	85	109	20.1	0	0	2.5	0.7	36	320	5	0	12	0.8
Ham, extra lean	3 oz	85	116	18.0	0.4	0	4.1	1.4	26	965	0	0	5	0.8
Ham, regular	3 oz	85	192	17.5	0.4	0	12.9	4.3	53	800	0	11.9	7	1.2
Lamb, trimmed	3 oz	85	218	20.8	0	0	14.3	6.7	74	65	0	0	14	1.6
Lunch meat, beef pastrami	3 oz	85	297	14.7	2.6	0	248	8.9	79	1,043	0	0	8	1.6
Lunch meat, beef, sliced	3 oz	85	151	23.9	4.9	0	3.3	1.4	35	1,224	0	0	9	0.8
Lunch meat, bologna (beef)	3 slices	85	265	10.4	0.7	0	24.2	10.3	49	834	0	0	10	1.4
Lunch meat, bologna (turkey)	3 slices	85	169	11.7	0.8	0	12.9	4.3	84	747	0	0	71	1.3
Lunch meat, chicken breast	3 oz	85	108	14.3	1.9	0	4.7	1.2	50	1,005	0	0	14	1.3
Lunch meat, franks (beef)	1 frank	57	180	6.8	1.0	0	16.2	6.9	35	585	0	0	11	0.8
Lunch meat, franks (chicken)	1 frank	45	116	5.8	3.1	0	8.8	2.5	45	617	17	0	43	0.9
Lunch meat, ham, lean, sliced	3 slices	85	111	16.5	0.8	0	4.2	1.4	40	1,215	0	0	6	0.6
Lunch meat, liverwurst	3 oz	85	277	12.0	1.9	0	24.2	9.0	134	731	7,059	0	22	5.4
Lunch meat, salami, dry	8 slices	80	334	18.3	2.1	0	27.5	9.8	63	1,488	0	0	6	1.2

(continued)

Name	Amount	Weight (g)	Energy (calories)	Protein (g)	Carbohydrate (g)	Fiber (g)	Total fat (g)	Saturated fat (g)	Cholesterol (mg)	Sodium (mg)	Vitamin A (RE)	Vitamin C (mg)	Calcium (mg)	Iron (mg)
MEAT, POULTRY, FISH, DRY BEANS, EGGS, AND NUTS *(continued)*														
Lunch meat, turkey breast	3 oz	85	94	19.1	0	0	1.3	0.4	35	1,216	0	0	6	0.3
Nuts, almonds	1/3 cup	47	274	10.1	9.3	5.6	24.0	1.8	0	0	0	0	117	2.0
Nuts, cashews, dry roasted	1/3 cup	46	262	7.0	14.9	1.4	21.2	4.2	0	7	0	0	21	2.7
Nuts, chestnuts, dry roasted	1/3 cup	48	117	1.5	25.2	2.4	1.0	0.2	0	1	1	12.4	14	0.4
Nuts, macadamia, dry roasted	1/3 cup	45	321	3.5	6.0	3.6	34.0	5.3	0	2	0	0.3	31	0.3
Nuts, pecans	1/3 cup	36	249	3.3	5.0	3.5	25.9	2.2	0	0	3	0.4	25	0.9
Nuts, pine	1/3 cup	45	257	10.9	6.4	2.0	23.0	3.5	0	2	1	0.8	12	4.2
Nuts, pistachios, dry roasted	1/3 cup	43	244	9.1	11.8	4.4	19.6	2.4	0	4	23	1.0	47	1.8
Nuts, walnuts	1/3 cup	40	262	6.1	5.5	2.7	26.1	2.5	0	1	2	0.5	39	1.2
Peanut butter, chunky	2 tablespoons	32	188	7.7	6.9	2.1	16.0	3.1	0	156	0	0	13	0.7
Peanut butter, smooth	2 tablespoons	32	190	8.1	6.2	1.9	16.3	3.3	0	149	0	0	12	0.6
Peanuts, dry roasted	1/3 cup	49	285	11.5	10.5	3.9	24.2	3.4	0	3	0	0	26	1.1
Pork chop, pan fried	3 oz	85	190	23.5	0	0	10.0	3.7	60	44	2	0.3	4	0.7
Pork ribs, braised	3 oz	85	337	24.7	0	0	25.8	9.5	103	79	3	0	40	1.6
Pork roast	3 oz	85	214	22.9	0	0	12.9	4.5	69	41	3	0	5	0.8
Pumpkin seeds, roasted	1/4 cup	57	296	18.7	7.6	2.2	23.9	4.5	0	10	22	1.0	24	8.5
Sausage, beef	1 sausage	43	134	6.1	1.0	0	11.6	4.9	29	486	0	0	3	0.8
Sausage, pork	1 sausage	67	216	13.4	1.0	0	17.2	6.1	52	618	0	1.3	16	1.0
Sausage, smoked links	3 2" links	48	161	6.4	0.7	0	14.6	6.1	34	454	0	0	5	0.7
Shellfish, clams, canned	3 oz	85	126	21.7	4.4	0	1.7	0.2	57	95	145	18.8	78	23.8
Shellfish, clams, steamed	10 clams	95	140	24.3	4.9	0	1.9	0.2	64	106	542	210	87	26.6
Shellfish, crab, steamed	3 oz	85	82	16.4	0	0	1.3	0.1	45	911	8	6.5	50	0.6
Shellfish, oysters, fried	6 medium	88	173	7.7	10.2	0	11.1	2.8	71	367	79	3.3	55	6.1
Shellfish, shrimp, canned	3 oz	85	102	19.6	0.9	0	1.7	0.3	147	144	15	2.0	50	2.3
Shellfish, shrimp, fried	4 large	30	73	6.4	3.4	0.1	3.7	0.6	53	103	17	0.5	20	0.4
Sunflower seeds, dry roasted	1/4 cup	32	86	6.2	7.7	3.6	15.9	1.7	0	1	0	0.4	22	1.2
Tempeh	1/2 cup	83	160	15.4	7.8	0	9.0	1.8	0	7	0	0	92	2.2

Name	Amount	Weight (g)	Energy (calories)	Protein (g)	Carbohydrate (g)	Fiber (g)	Total fat (g)	Saturated fat (g)	Cholesterol (mg)	Sodium (mg)	Vitamin A (RE)	Vitamin C (mg)	Calcium (mg)	Iron (mg)
MEAT, POULTRY, FISH, DRY BEANS, EGGS, AND NUTS *(continued)*														
Tofu, firm	1/2 cup	126	183	19.9	5.4	2.9	11.0	1.6	0	18	21	0.3	861	13.2
Turkey, dark meat, w/o skin, roasted	3 oz	85	138	24.5	0	0	3.7	1.2	95	67	0	0	22	2.0
Turkey, dark meat, w/skin, roasted	3 oz	85	155	23.5	0	0	6.0	1.8	99	65	0	0	23	2.0
Turkey, light meat, w/o skin, roasted	3 oz	85	119	25.7	0	0	1.0	0.3	73	48	0	0	13	1.3
Turkey, light meat, w/skin, roasted	3 oz	85	139	24.5	0	0	3.9	1.1	81	48	0	0	15	1.4
Veal, sirloin, roasted	3 oz	85	172	21.4	0	0	8.9	3.8	87	71	0	0	11	0.8
Vegetarian bacon, cooked	1 oz	16	50	1.7	1.0	0.4	4.7	0.7	0	234	1	0	4	0.4
Vegetarian franks	1 frank	51	118	12.1	1.5	1.5	7.1	0.8	0	224	0	0	10	1.0
Vegetarian patties	1 patty	67	119	11.2	10.2	4.0	3.8	0.5	0	382	76	0	48	1.2
Vegetarian sausage	1 patty	38	97	7.0	3.7	1.1	6.9	1.1	0	337	24	0	24	1.4
FATS, OILS, SWEETS, AND ALCOHOLIC BEVERAGES														
Alcoholic beverage, beer	1 can or bottle	356	146	1.1	13.2	0.7	0	0	0	18	0	0	18	0.1
Alcoholic beverage, liquor	1.5 oz	42	97	0	0	0	0	0	0	0	0	0	0	0
Alcoholic beverage, wine	5 oz	148	103	0	2.1	0	0	0	0	12	0	0	12	0.5
Beverage, cola	1 can	370	152	0	38.5	0	0	0	0	15	0	0	11	0.1
Beverage, fruit punch	1 cup	247	114	0	28.9	0.2	0	0	0	10	2	108.4	10	0.2
Beverage, kiwi strawberry drink	1 cup	236	113	0.2	27.8	0	0	0	0	10	0	0	0	0
Beverage, lemon-lime soda	1 can	368	147	0	38.3	0	0	0	0	40	0	0	7	0.3
Beverage, tea, bottled, sweetened	1 bottle	480	178	0	40.8	0	0	0	0	0	0	0	0	0
Butter	1 tablespoon	14	102	0.1	0	0	11.5	7.1	31	117	107	0	3	0
Candy, caramels	1 piece	10	39	0.5	7.8	0.1	0.8	0.7	1	25	1	0.1	14	0
Candy, fudge	1 piece	17	65	0.3	13.5	0.1	1.4	0.9	2	11	8	0	7	0.1
Candy, jelly beans	10 large	28	104	0	26.4	0	0.1	0	0	7	0	0	1	0.3
Candy, milk chocolate	1 bar	44	226	3.0	26.0	1.5	13.5	8.1	10	36	24	0.2	84	0.6
Chocolate syrup	2 tablespoons	38	105	0.8	24.4	0.7	0.4	0.2	0	27	1	0.1	5	0.8
Cream, half and half	2 tablespoons	30	39	0.9	1.3	0	3.5	2.2	11	12	32	0.3	32	0

(continued)

Name	Amount	Weight (g)	Energy (calories)	Protein (g)	Carbohydrate (g)	Fiber (g)	Total fat (g)	Saturated fat (g)	Cholesterol (mg)	Sodium (mg)	Vitamin A (RE)	Vitamin C (mg)	Calcium (mg)	Iron (mg)
FATS, OILS, SWEETS, AND ALCOHOLIC BEVERAGES *(continued)*														
Cream, heavy, whipped	1/2 cup	60	206	1.2	1.7	0	22.1	13.8	82	23	252	0.4	39	0
Cream sour	1 tablespoon	12	26	0.4	0.5	0	2.5	1.6	5	6	23	0.1	14	0
Frosting, chocolate	1/12 package	28	151	0.4	24.0	0.2	6.7	2.1	0	70	75	0	3	0.5
Honey	1 tablespoon	21	64	0.1	17.3	0	0	0	0	1	0	0.1	1	0.1
Jam/preserves	1 tablespoon	20	56	0.1	13.8	0.2	0	0	0	6	0	1.8	4	0.1
Lard	1 tablespoon	13	115	0	0	0	12.8	5.0	12	0	0	0	0	0
Marmalade	1 tablespoon	20	49	0.1	13.3	0	0	0	0	11	1	1.0	8	0
Margarine, hard	1 tablespoon	14	101	0.1	0.1	0	11.4	2.1	0	133	113	0	4	0
Margarine, liquid	1 tablespoon	14	102	0.3	0	0	11.4	1.9	0	111	113	0.	9	0
Margarine, soft	1 tablespoon	14	101	0.1	0	0	11.3	2.0	0	152	113	0	4	0
Margarine-like spread	1 tablespoon	14	50	0.1	0.1	0	5.6	1.1	0	138	115	0	3	0
Mayonnaise, fat free	1 tablespoon	16	11	0	2.0	0.3	0.4	0.1	2	120	1	0	1	0
Mayonnaise, regular	1 tablespoon	15	57	0.1	3.5	0	4.9	0.7	4	105	12	0	2	0
Oil, canola	1 tablespoon	14	124	0	0	0	14.0	1.0	0	0	0	0	0	0
Oil, corn	1 tablespoon	14	120	0	0	0	13.6	1.7	0	0	0	0	0	0
Oil, olive	1 tablespoon	14	119	0	0	0	13.5	1.8	0	0	0	0	0	0.1
Popsicle	1 single stick	88	63	0	16.6	0	0	0	0	11	0	9.4	0	0
Salad dressing, blue cheese	2 tablespoons	31	154	1.5	2.3	0	16.0	3.0	5	335	20	0.6	25	0.1
Salad dressing, French	2 tablespoons	31	134	0.2	5.5	0	12.8	3.0	0	427	40	0	3	0.1
Salad dressing, Italian	2 tablespoons	29	137	0.2	3.0	0	14.2	2.1	0	231	7	0	3	0
Salad dressing, Italian light	2 tablespoons	30	32	0	1.5	0	2.9	0.4	2	236	0	0	1	0.1
Sherbet	1/3 cup	74	102	0.8	22.5	0	1.5	0.9	0	34	10	2.3	40	0.1
Shortening, vegetable	1 tablespoon	13	113	0	0	0	12.8	3.2	0	0	0	0	0	0
Sugar, brown	1 tablespoon	14	52	0	13.4	0	0	0	0	5	0	0	12	0.3
Sugar, white	1 tablespoon	13	49	0	12.6	0	0	0	0	0	0	0	0	0
Syrup, corn	1 tablespoon	20	56	0	15.3	0	0	0	0	24	0	0	1	0
Syrup, maple	1/4 cup	79	206	0	52.9	0	0.2	0	0	7	0	0	53	0.9

*Dry beans and peas (legumes) can be counted as servings from the meat, poultry, fish, dry beans, eggs, and nuts group or the vegetables group; data on dry beans are listed under vegetables (see items marked with an asterisk).

Source U.S. Department of Agriculture, Agricultural Research Service. 2001. USDA Nutrient Database for Standard Reference, Release 14I (www.nal.usda.gov/fnic/foodcomp).

Appendix B

Nutritive Values of Popular Fast Foods

Food item	Calories	% Calories from fat	Total fat (g)	Saturated fat (g)	Cholesterol (mg)	Protein (g)	Total carbohydrate (g)	Fiber (g)	Sugars (g)	Sodium (mg)	Calcium (% DRI)
ARBY'S											
Regular Roast Beef	350	43%	16	6	85	21	34	2	NA	950	6%
Super Roast Beef	470	44%	23	7	85	22	47	3	NA	1,130	8%
Beef 'N Cheddar	480	46%	24	8	90	23	43	2	NA	1,240	10%
Grilled Chicken Deluxe	450	44%	22	4	110	29	37	2	NA	1,050	6%
Big Montana®	630	46%	32	15	155	47	41	3	NA	2,080	8%
French Dip Sub	440	36%	18	8	100	28	42	2	NA	1,680	8%
Philly Beef 'N Swiss Sub	700	54%	42	15	130	36	46	4	NA	1,940	30%
Turkey Sub	630	52%	37	9	100	26	51	2	NA	2,170	20%
Grilled Chicken Caesar Salad (no dressing)	230	30%	8	3.5	80	33	8	3	NA	920	20%
Broccoli 'N Cheddar Baked Potato	540	39%	24	12	50	12	71	7	NA	680	25%
Deluxe Baked Potato	650	48%	34	20	90	20	67	6	NA	750	10%
Medium Homestyle Fries	370	38%	16	4	0	4	53	4	NA	710	*
Medium Curly Fries	400	45%	20	5	0	5	50	4	NA	990	*
Cheddar Curly Fries	460	48%	24	6	5	6	54	4	NA	1,290	6%
Potato Cakes (2)	250	56%	16	4	0	2	26	3	NA	490	*
Mozzarella Sticks (4)	470	55%	29	14	60	18	34	2	NA	1,330	40%
Tangy Southwest Sauce™	250	96%	26	4.5	30	0	3	0	NA	290	*
French Toastix, no syrup (6)	370	41%	17	4	0	7	48	4	NA	440	7%
Jamocha Shake	470	30%	15	7	45	10	82	0	NA	390	50%

NA = not available; * = contains less than 2% of the daily value.

Additional food items listed at http://arbys.com/arb06.html.

(continued)

Food item	Calories	% Calories from fat	Total fat (g)	Saturated fat (g)	Cholesterol (mg)	Protein (g)	Total carbohydrate (g)	Fiber (g)	Sugars (g)	Sodium (mg)	Calcium (% DRI)
MCDONALD'S											
Hamburger	280	32%	10	4	30	12	35	2	7	560	20%
Cheeseburger	330	39%	14	6	45	15	35	2	7	800	25%
Quarter Pounder®	420	45%	21	8	70	23	36	2	8	780	20%
Quarter Pounder® with Cheese	530	51%	30	13	95	28	38	2	9	1,250	35%
Big Mac	580	52%	33	11	85	24	47	3	7	1,050	35%
Filet-O-Fish®	470	51%	26	5	50	15	45	1	5	730	20%
McChicken®	430	49%	23	4.5	45	14	41	3	6	840	20%
Chicken McNuggets® (6 pieces)	310	58%	20	4	50	15	18	2	0	680	2%
French Fries (large)	540	43%	26	4.5	0	8	68	6	0	350	2%
Side Salad (no dressing)	15	0	0	0	0	1	3	1	1	10	2%
Grilled Chicken Bacon Ranch Salad (no dressing)	270	44%	13	5	75	28	11	3	4	830	15%
Ranch Dressing (1 pkg)	290	93%	30	4.5	20	1	4	0	3	530	4%
Low-Fat Balsamic Vinaigrette (1 pkg)	40	63%	3	0	0	0	4	0	3	730	*
Chocolate Triple Thick™ Shake (small)	430	26%	12	8	50	11	70	1	61	210	35%
Egg McMuffin®	300	37%	12	5	235	18	29	2	3	840	30%
Bacon, Egg, & Cheese Biscuit	480	58%	31	10	250	21	31	1	3	1,360	15%
Ham, Egg, & Cheese Bagel	550	36%	23	8	255	26	58	2	10	1,500	20%
Hot Cakes w/margarine & syrup	600	25%	17	3	20	9	104	0	40	770	10%
Hash Browns	130	54%	8	1.5	0	1	14	1	0	330	*

*Contains less than 2% of the daily value.

Additional food items listed at www.mcdonalds.com/countries/usa/food/nutrition/categories/nutrition/index.html.

Food item	Calories	% Calories from fat	Total fat (g)	Saturated fat (g)	Cholesterol (mg)	Protein (g)	Total carbohydrate (g)	Fiber (g)	Sugars (g)	Sodium (mg)	Calcium (% DRI)
TACO BELL											
Taco	180	53%	10	4	25	8	13	NA	1	350	6%
Taco Supreme®	220	55%	14	7	40	9	14	NA	2	350	6%
Double Decker® Taco Supreme®	380	42%	18	8	40	15	40	NA	4	820	15%
Soft Taco – Chicken	190	32%	6	2.5	30	14	19	NA	2	550	10%
Burrito Supreme® – Beef	440	36%	18	8	40	18	51	NA	6	1,330	20%
Burrito Supreme® – Steak	420	33%	16	7	35	19	50	NA	5	1,260	20%
Chili Cheese Burrito	390	41%	18	9	40	16	40	NA	3	1,080	30%
Gordita Supreme® – Beef	310	45%	16	7	35	14	30	NA	7	590	15%
Gordita Supreme® – Chicken	290	38%	12	5	45	17	28	NA	7	530	10%
Meximelt®	290	48%	16	8	45	15	23	NA	3	880	25%

Food item	Calories	% Calories from fat	Total fat (g)	Saturated fat (g)	Cholesterol (mg)	Protein (g)	Total carbohydrate (g)	Fiber (g)	Sugars (g)	Sodium (mg)	Calcium (% DRI)
TACO BELL *(continued)*											
Taco Salad with Salsa with Shell	790	48%	42	15	65	31	73	NA	10	1,670	40%
Taco Salad with Salsa without Shell	420	45%	21	11	65	24	33	NA	9	1,400	25%
Nachos Supreme	450	51%	26	9	35	13	42	NA	4	800	10%
Nachos Bell Grande®	780	49%	43	13	35	20	80	NA	6	1,300	20%
Pintos 'N Cheese	180	33%	7	3.5	15	10	20	NA	1	700	15%
Chalupa Supreme – chicken	370	49%	20	8	45	17	30	NA	4	530	10%
Chalupa Baja – beef	430	58%	27	8	30	14	32	NA	4	750	15%

NA = not available.

Additional food items listed at www.tacobell.com.

Food item	Calories	% Calories from fat	Total fat (g)	Saturated fat (g)	Cholesterol (mg)	Protein (g)	Total carbohydrate (g)	Fiber (g)	Sugars (g)	Sodium (mg)	Calcium (% DRI)
PIZZA HUT											
Hand-Tossed Pizza, cheese, 1 slice	240	38%	10	5	10	12	28	2	1	650	20%
Personal Pan® Pizza, pepperoni	620	40%	28	11	30	26	70	5	<2	1,430	30%
Meat Lover's® Stuffed Crust, 1 slice	470	49%	25	11	50	22	40	3	2	1,430	25%
Veggie Lover's® The Big New Yorker, 1 slice	480	42%	22	6	10	19	57	10	<10	1,410	25%
Spaghetti w/ meatballs, 1 serving	850	220	24	10	17	37	120	10	12	1,120	15%
Thin 'N Crispy Pizza, cheese, 1 slice	200	80	9	5	10	10	22	2	1	590	20%
Mild Buffalo Wings, 5 pcs.	200	110	12	3.5	150	23	<1	0	0	510	2%
Breadstick	130	35	4	1	0	3	20	1	1	170	NA
Breadstick Dipping Sauce	30	5	0.5	0	0	<1	5	<1	2	170	NA
Supreme Sandwich	640	250	28	10	28	34	62	4	7	2,150	30%

NA = not available.

Additional food items listed at www.pizzahut.com (click on "Nutritional Info").

Physical Activity and Health: A Report of the Surgeon General

Women

Key Messages

- Physical activity need not be strenuous to promote health benefits.

- Women of all ages benefit from a moderate amount of physical activity, preferably daily. They can obtain the same moderate amount of activity from longer sessions of moderately intense activities (such as 30 minutes of brisk walking) as they can from shorter sessions of more strenuous activities (such as 15 to 20 minutes of jogging).

- Women can gain additional health benefits through engaging in greater amounts of physical activity. Those who can maintain a regular routine of physical activity of longer duration or of greater intensity are likely to derive greater benefit. They should avoid excessive amounts of activity, however, because risk of injury increases with greater activity, as does the risk of menstrual abnormalities and bone weakening.

- Previously sedentary women who begin physical activity programs should start with short intervals (5 to 10 minutes) of physical activity and gradually build up to the desired level of activity.

- Women with chronic health problems, such as heart disease, diabetes, or obesity, or who are at high risk for these conditions, should first consult a physician before beginning a new program of physical activity. Women over age 50 who plan to begin a new program of vigorous physical activity should first consult a physician to be sure that they do not have heart disease or other health problems.

- The emphasis on moderate amounts of physical activity makes it possible to vary activities to meet individual needs, preferences, and life circumstances.

Facts

- More than 60% of U.S. women do not engage in the recommended amount of physical activity.

- More than 25% of U.S. women are not active at all.

- Physical inactivity is more common among women than it is among men.

- Social support from family and friends has been consistently and positively related to regular physical activity.

Benefits of Physical Activity

- Reduces the risk of dying from coronary heart disease and of developing high blood pressure, colon cancer, and diabetes

- Helps maintain healthy bones, muscles, and joints

- Helps control weight, build lean muscle, and reduce body fat

- Helps control joint swelling and pain associated with arthritis

- May enhance the effect of estrogen and replacement therapy in decreasing bone loss after menopause

- Reduces symptoms of anxiety and depression and fosters improvements in mood and feelings of well-being

- Can help reduce blood pressure in some women with hypertension

What Communities Can Do

- Provide environmental inducements to physical activity, such as safe, accessible, and attractive trails for walking and bicycling, and sidewalks with curb cuts

- Open schools for community recreation, form neighborhood watch groups to increase safety, and encourage malls and other indoor or protected locations to provide safe places for walking in any weather

- Encourage employers to provide supportive worksite environments and policies that offer opportunities for employees to incorporate moderate physical activity into their daily lives
- Provide community-based programs to meet the needs of older women, women with disabilities, women of racial and ethnic minority groups, and women with low incomes; include child-care arrangements to encourage participation of women with children
- Encourage health care providers to talk routinely to female patients about incorporating physical activity into their lives

Persons With Disabilities

Key Messages

- Physical activity need not be strenuous to promote health benefits.
- People with disabilities can obtain significant health benefits from a moderate amount of physical activity, preferably daily. They can gain the same moderate amount of activity from longer sessions of moderately intense activities (such as 30 to 40 minutes of wheeling themselves in a wheelchair) as they can from shorter sessions of more strenuous activities (such as 20 minutes of wheelchair basketball).
- People with disabilities can gain additional health benefits through engaging in greater amounts of physical activity. People who can maintain a regular routine of physical activity of longer duration or of greater intensity are likely to derive greater benefit.
- Previously sedentary people who begin physical activity programs should start with short intervals of physical activity (5 to 10 minutes) and gradually build up to the desired level of activity.
- People with disabilities should first consult a physician before beginning a program of physical activity to which they are unaccustomed.
- The emphasis on moderate amounts of physical activity makes it possible to vary activities to meet individual needs, preferences, and life circumstances.

Facts

- People with disabilities are less likely to engage in regular moderate physical activity than people without disabilities are, yet they have similar needs to promote their health and prevent unnecessary disease.
- Social support from family and friends has been consistently and positively related to regular physical activity.

Benefits of Physical Activity

- Reduces the risk of dying from coronary heart disease and developing high blood pressure, colon cancer, and diabetes
- Can help people with chronic, disabling conditions improve their stamina and muscle strength
- Reduces symptoms of anxiety and depression, improves mood, and promotes general feelings of well-being
- Helps control joint swelling and pain associated with arthritis
- Can help reduce blood pressure in some people with hypertension

What Communities Can Do

- Provide community-based programs to meet the needs of persons with disabilities
- Ensure that environments and facilities conducive to being physically active are available and accessible to people with disabilities, such as offering safe, accessible, and attractive trails for bicycling, walking, and wheelchair activities
- Ensure that people with disabilities are involved at all stages of planning and implementing community physical activity programs
- Provide quality, preferably daily, K through 12 accessible physical education classes for children and youths with disabilities
- Encourage health care providers to talk routinely to their patients with disabilities about incorporating physical activity into their lives

Older Adults

Key Messages

- Older adults, both male and female, can benefit from regular physical activity.

- Physical activity need not be strenuous to promote health benefits.
- Older adults can obtain significant health benefits with a moderate amount of physical activity, preferably daily. They can obtain a moderate amount of activity in longer sessions of moderately intense activities (such as walking) or in shorter sessions of more vigorous activities (such as fast walking or stair walking).
- They can gain additional health benefits through engaging in greater amounts of physical activity by increasing duration, intensity, or frequency. Because risk of injury increases at high levels of physical activity, they should avoid engaging in excessive amounts of activity.
- Previously sedentary older adults who begin physical activity programs should start with short intervals of moderate physical activity (5 to 10 minutes) and gradually build up to the desired amount.
- Older adults should consult with a physician before beginning a new physical activity program.
- Besides developing cardiorespiratory endurance (aerobic) activity, older adults can benefit from muscle-strengthening activity. Stronger muscles help reduce the risk of falling and improve the ability to perform the routine tasks of daily life.

Facts

- The loss of strength and stamina attributed to aging is caused in part by reduced physical activity.
- Inactivity increases with age. By age 75, about one in three men and one in two women engage in no physical activity.
- Among adults aged 65 years and older, walking, gardening, and yard work are, by far, the most popular physical activities.
- Social support from family and friends has been consistently and positively related to regular physical activity.

Benefits of Physical Activity

- Helps maintain the ability to live independently and reduces the risk of falling and fracturing bones
- Reduces the risk of dying from coronary heart disease and of developing high blood pressure, colon cancer, and diabetes

- Can help reduce blood pressure in some people with hypertension
- Helps people with chronic, disabling conditions improve their stamina and muscle strength
- Reduces symptoms of anxiety and depression and fosters improvements in mood and feelings of well-being
- Helps maintain healthy bones, muscles, and joints
- Helps control joint swelling and pain associated with arthritis

What Communities Can Do

- Provide community-based physical activity programs that offer aerobic, strengthening, and flexibility components specifically designed for older adults
- Encourage malls and other indoor or protected locations to provide safe places for walking in any weather
- Ensure that facilities for physical activity accommodate and encourage participation by older adults
- Provide transportation for older adults to parks or facilities that provide physical activity programs
- Encourage health care providers to talk routinely to their older adult patients about incorporating physical activity into their lives
- Plan community activities that include opportunities for older adults to be physically active

Adults

Key Messages

- Physical activity need not be strenuous to promote health benefits.
- Men and women of all ages benefit from a moderate amount of daily physical activity. They can obtain the same moderate amount of activity in longer sessions of moderately intense activities (such as 30 minutes of brisk walking) as they do in shorter sessions of more strenuous activities (such as 15 to 20 minutes of jogging).
- They can gain additional health benefits through engaging in greater amounts of physical activity. Adults who maintain a regular routine of physical activity of longer duration or of greater intensity are likely to derive greater benefit. Because risk of injury increases with

greater amounts of activity, however, they should avoid engaging in excessive amounts of activity.

- Previously sedentary people who begin physical activity programs should start with short sessions (5 to 10 minutes) of physical activity and gradually build up to the desired level.

- Adults with chronic health problems, such as heart disease, diabetes, or obesity, or who are at high risk for these conditions should first consult a physician before beginning a new program of physical activity. Men over age 40 and women over age 50 who plan to begin a new program of vigorous activity should consult a physician to be sure they do not have heart disease or other health problems.

Facts

- More than 60% of U.S. adults do not engage in the recommended amount of activity (see figure C.1).

- Approximately 25% of U.S. adults are not active at all.

- Physical inactivity is more common among women than it is among men, among African American and Hispanic adults than it is among Whites, among older adults than it is among younger adults, and among less affluent people than it is among more affluent people.

- Social support from family and friends has been consistently and positively related to regular physical activity.

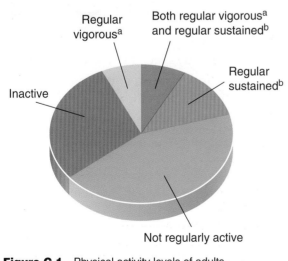

Figure C.1 Physical activity levels of adults.

[a]Regular vigorous—20 minutes three times per week of vigorous intensity
[b]Regular sustained—30 minutes five times per week of any intensity
CDC 1992 Behavioral Risk Factor Study

Benefits of Physical Activity

- Reduces the risk of dying from coronary heart disease and of developing high blood pressure, colon cancer, and diabetes

- Can help reduce blood pressure in some people with hypertension

- Helps maintain healthy bones, muscles, and joints

- Reduces symptoms of anxiety and depression and fosters improvements in mood and feelings of well-being

- Helps control weight, develop lean muscle, and reduce body fat

What Communities Can Do

- Provide environmental inducements to physical activity, such as safe, accessible, and attractive trails for walking and bicycling, and sidewalks with curb cuts

- Open schools for community recreation, form neighborhood watch groups to increase safety, and encourage malls and other indoor or protected locations to provide safe places for walking in any weather

- Provide community-based programs to meet the needs of specific populations, such as racial and ethnic minority groups, women, older adults, persons with disabilities, and low-income groups

- Encourage health care providers to talk routinely to their patients about incorporating physical activity into their lives

- Encourage employers to provide supportive worksite environments and policies that offer opportunities for employees to incorporate moderate physical activity into their daily lives

Adolescents and Young Adults

Key Messages

- Adolescents and young adults, both male and female, benefit from physical activity.

- Physical activity need not be strenuous to promote health benefits.

- People of all ages should engage in moderate amounts of daily physical activity. They can obtain this amount in longer sessions of moderately intense activities, such as brisk walking for 30 minutes, or in shorter sessions of more intense activities, such as jogging or playing basketball for 15 to 20 minutes.

- Greater amounts of physical activity are even more beneficial, up to a point. Excessive amounts of physical activity can lead to injuries, menstrual abnormalities, and bone weakening.

Facts

- Nearly half of American youths aged 12 to 21 are not vigorously active on a regular basis (see figure C.2).

- About 14% of young people report no recent physical activity. Inactivity is more common among females (14%) than it is among males (7%) and among Black females (21%) than it is among White females (12%).

- Participation in all types of physical activity declines strikingly as age or grade in school increases.

- Only 19% of all high school students are physically active for 20 minutes or more, five days a week, in physical education classes.

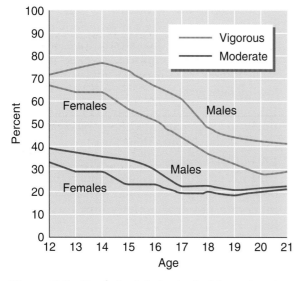

Figure C.2 Physical activity levels of adolescents and young adults, by age and sex.

From CDC National Health Interview Survey Youth Risk Behavior Survey 1992.

- Daily enrollment in physical education classes dropped from 42% to 25% among high school students between 1991 and 1995.

- Well-designed school-based interventions directed at increasing physical activity in physical education classes have been shown to be effective.

- Social support from family and friends has been consistently and positively related to regular physical activity.

Benefits of Physical Activity

- Helps build and maintain healthy bones, muscles, and joints

- Helps control weight, build lean muscle, and reduce fat

- Prevents or delays the development of high blood pressure and helps reduce blood pressure in some adolescents with hypertension

What Communities Can Do

- Provide quality, preferably daily, K through 12 physical education classes and hire physical education specialists to teach them

- Create opportunities for physical activities that are enjoyable, that promote adolescents' and young adults' confidence in their ability to be physically active, and that involve friends, peers, and parents.

- Provide appropriate physically active role models for youths

- Provide a range of extracurricular programs in schools and community recreation centers to meet the needs and interests of specific adolescent and minority groups, females, persons with disabilities, and low-income groups

- Encourage health care providers to talk routinely to adolescents and young adults about the importance of incorporating physical activity into their lives

Source: U.S. Public Health Service, *Physical Activity and Health: A Report of the Surgeon General: Executive Summary* (Washington, DC: U.S. Department of Health and Human Services, 1996), p. 2.

Prevention and Emergency Treatment of Common Exercise Injuries

Injury	General comments	Prevention and treatment	Need for a physician
EXTREMITIES			
Ankle	Most injuries involve inversion sprains (outer edge of foot turns inward). Ankles are not strong enough for most sports, and the muscles and ligaments that poorly support them often stretch and tear from high-speed direction changes, cutting, and contact.	Improved muscle strength offers some protection, along with preventive taping (inversion sprains only). RICE therapy is the preferred treatment. Use crutches for 2 or 3 days if pain is severe.	If swelling or pain remains for 3 days; if ligament or tendon damage is present; if pain prevents walking; if symptoms of fracture exist.
Bruise (charley horse)	A charley horse is nothing more than a thigh contusion from a direct blow to a relaxed thigh muscle (the impact compresses the tissue against the bone). Bruises to other areas occur in similar fashion.	Prevention involves use of proper equipment in contact sports. RICE therapy is the preferred emergency and home treatment. Replace ice with heat on the 3rd or 4th day.	If pain and discoloration do not disappear with rest, treatment, and mild exercise; if numbness, weakness, or tingling occurs, or if there are signs of vascular compromise, immediate referral is necessary.
Elbow (tennis and pitcher's)	The movement causing the condition is a forceful extension of the forearm and a twisting motion (serve in tennis, curve in baseball). The more you play and the older you are, the more likely you are to be afflicted. Pain is present over the outer (lateral epicondyle) or inner (medial epicondyle) elbow and may radiate down the arm. Pain is produced by tears, inflammation, and scar tissue at the attachment of the extensor muscles to the bony prominence of the elbow.	Prevention centers on using a proper warm-up; correcting poor stroke mechanics; avoiding use of wet tennis balls and heavy, inflexible rackets; and reducing the frequency of curve ball pitches (which should be greatly restricted in Little League baseball with growing youngsters).	If condition remains more than 2 or 3 weeks; if pain makes exercise impossible; if severe swelling is present; if night pain occurs.
Fractures	A fracture should be suspected in most injuries where pain and swelling exist over a bone.	Apply ice packs and protect and rest the injured part for 72 hours. In severe cases, splint the bone where the victim lies and transport to emergency room.	If limb is cold, blue, or numb; if pelvis or thigh are involved; if limb is crooked or deformed; if shock symptoms are present; if rapid, severe swelling occurs.
Hamstring strains	Vigorous exercise can strain the large-muscle group in the back of the upper leg. Pain is severe and prohibits further activity. In a few days, discoloration may appear.	Prevention includes proper stretching before exercise, proper diet, improved flexibility, and care in running around wet areas. For treatment use RICE therapy followed by heat application in 3 or 4 days.	If severe discoloration occurs; if pain and discomfort remain after 10 to 15 days of treatment; if numbness, weakness, or tingling occurs; or if there are signs of vascular compromise, immediate referral is necessary.

(continued)

Injury	General comments	Prevention and treatment	Need for a physician
EXTREMITIES *(continued)*			
Knee	The knee is a vulnerable joint that depends on ligaments, cartilage, and muscles for support. Chondromalacia of the patella, or roughing of the undersurface of the kneecap, is the most common injury; kneecap pain and grating symptoms are evident. A tear of the cartilage is the second most common injury. Pain is evident along the inner or outer part of the knee joint along with swelling. Ligament tears are less common but occur from a blow to the leg. Swelling and knee instability result.	Prevention involves flexibility and strength training. Exercise should stretch and strengthen the hamstrings, quadriceps, and Achilles tendon. Chondromalacia is treated through use of arch supports or by bulking up the inner part of the heel of the shoe. Aspirin, ibuprofen, or naproxen sodium and quadriceps exercises also help. Serious knee injury (cartilage and ligament damage) requires examination by an orthopedic surgeon. Use of the arthroscope to examine and insert small tools through puncture wounds offers effective treatment and rapid recovery.	If swelling and pain persist more than 3 to 5 days; if ligament or cartilage damage is suspected; if chondromalacia is suspected.
Shin splints	A shin splint is merely an inflammation of the anterior and posterior tendons of the large bone in the lower leg. This overuse syndrome develops in poorly conditioned individuals in the beginning of their training programs. Hard surfaces add to the problem.	Avoid hard surfaces, too much mileage, doing too much too soon, using improperly fitted shoes, and running on banked tracks or road shoulders. RICE therapy is recommended for 2 to 4 days, followed by taping, heat therapy, and stretching exercises.	If condition remains more than 2 to 3 weeks; if condition reoccurs after reconvening the exercise routine; if signs or symptoms of a stress fracture occur.
Tendinitis	The location of the pain and swelling of tendons varies by sport. Considerable running affects the Achilles tendon. Sports involving repeated movement of the upper arms (swimming, baseball) affect the shoulder tendon. The snapping or rotation of the elbow involved in tennis and handball affects the elbow tendon.	For both prevention and treatment, stretch the involved tendon daily and exercise lightly until pain disappears. RICE therapy is helpful in the early stages for 3 to 4 days (see Elbow, this table). Pain may disappear during a workout only to return and worsen later.	If pain and inflammation continue after 2 to 3 weeks of treatment.
Varicose veins	Varicose veins are nothing more than abnormally lengthened, dilated veins. Surrounding muscles support deep veins, whereas superficial veins have little support. In some individuals, vein valves that prevent blood from backing up become defective, enlarged, and lose their elasticity. The condition is uncommon in young people.	Prevention and treatment for those with symptoms or a family history include bed rest and leg elevation, avoiding long periods of standing, using elastic bandages and support stockings, surgery for severe cases, and removal of intra-abdominal pressure (obesity, tumor, tight girdles).	If pain is severe enough to make walking difficult; if cosmetic problem is bothersome; if swelling in the calf or foot is present.
FEET AND HANDS			
Athlete's foot	Athlete's foot is caused by a fungus and is accompanied by a bacterial infection. Itching, redness, and a rash on the soles, toes, or between the toes is common.	Prevention and treatment are similar; wash between the toes with soap and water, dry thoroughly, use medication containing antifungal preparation twice daily, and place fungistatic foot powder in shoes and sneakers.	If treatment does not relieve symptoms in 2 to 3 weeks.
Blisters	Friction causing the top skin layer to separate from the second layer produces blisters. Blisters can become severely inflamed or infected unless properly treated. You can buy a porous inner sole that almost completely eliminates getting blisters on the feet.	Use clean socks, comfortably fitting shoes, and Vaseline to reduce friction. Avoid breaking open blisters (skin acts as a sterile bandage). If the blister breaks, trim off all loose skin and apply antibiotic salve. Avoid use of tincture of benzoin and powder that increases friction, because doing so is more likely to cause blisters than prevent them.	If inflammation and soreness develop; if redness occurs in the involved limb; if pain or sensitivity occurs under the arms or in the groin area; if a blood blister is present.
Bunions	Bunions are growths on the head of the first or fifth toe that produce inflammation (swelling, redness, pain).	You can prevent bunions by wearing properly fitted shoes.	If symptoms of infection occur.
Corns	Hard corns may result from poorly fitted shoes. Inflammation and thickening of soft tissue (top of toes) occur. Excessive foot perspiration and narrow shoes are often the cause of soft corns. The corn forms between the fourth and fifth toes in most cases.	Prevention and treatment involve use of properly fitted shoes, soaking feet daily in warm water to soften the area, and protecting the area with a small felt or sponge rubber doughnut. Trim and file corns to reduce pressure.	If a change of shoes and treatment do not improve the condition.

Injury	General comments	Prevention and treatment	Need for a physician
FEET AND HANDS *(continued)*			
Heel bruise	The most common cause of heel pain is plantar fascitis—inflammation of the broad band of fibrous tissue that runs from the base of the toes back to the heel and inserts on the inner aspect of the heel. Mild tears and severe bruises are also common.	Prevention involves proper stretching and use of a plastic heel cup. Aspirin can reduce inflammation (two tablets, four times daily); rest is indicated for 5 to 7 days.	If pain persists for more than 5 to 7 days after rest and treatment.
Ingrown toenails	The edge of the toenail grows into the soft tissue, producing inflammation and infection.	Prevention and treatment involve proper nail trimming, soaking the toe in hot water two to three times daily, and inserting a small piece of cotton under the nail edge to lift it from the soft tissue.	If infection occurs.
Stress fracture	A stress fracture is a small crack in a bone's surface, generally a foot, leg, or hand. Unexplained pain may exist over one of the small bones in the hand or foot. X ray will not reveal small cracks until the bone heals and a callus (scar tissue) forms.	Prevention involves not running too many miles, not increasing mileage too fast, running on soft surfaces, and taking care to progress slowly in a fitness program. Treatment requires rest and proper equipment (especially footwear).	If unexplained pain exists in the lower back, hip, ankle, wrist, hand, or foot; if night pain occurs; if pain increases with activity.
HEAD AND NECK			
Cauliflower ear	A deformed outer ear is common in wrestling, rugby, and football from friction, hard blows, and wrenching in a headlock position. With poor circulation to the ear, fluid is absorbed slowly, and the ear remains swollen, sensitive, and discolored.	Use protective ear guards, apply Vaseline to reduce friction, and apply ice as soon as a sore spot develops. Once a deformed ear develops, only a plastic surgeon can return the ear to normal appearance.	If symptoms of infection develop; if cosmetic surgery is desired.
Concussion	Any injury to the head producing dizziness or temporary unconsciousness is serious.	Apply ice to the area. Observe the patient for 72 hours for alertness, unequal pupil size (although about one person in four has unequal pupil size all the time), and vomiting. Pressure inside the skull may develop within the 72-hour observation period.	If unconsciousness occurred; if bleeding occurs from ears, eyes, or mouth; if there is unequal pupil size, lethargy, fever, vomiting, convulsions, speech difficulty, stiff neck, or limb weakness.
Dental injuries	Dental injuries are common in basketball and contact sports from elbow contact.	*Chipped tooth—avoid hot and cold drinks. *Swelling due to abscess—apply ice pack. *Excessive bleeding of socket—place gauze over socket and bite down. *Toothache—aspirin and ice packs.	If tooth is chipped, abscess is present, or bleeding of socket or toothache is present; if tooth is bleeding or knocked out (place in proper solution and see dentist immediately).
Eye (object in eye, contusion from a ball or elbow)	Eye injuries are more common in racket sports and handball from ball contact and in contact sports from elbow contact. In racket sports, the ball may ricochet off the top of the racket into the eye, or ball may hit a victim who turns to see where his or her partner is hitting the ball in doubles play.	You should wear protective eye guards in racquetball and handball. Never turn your head in doubles play. Avoid rubbing—you could scratch the cornea. Close both eyes to allow tears to wash away a foreign body. Grasp the lashes of the upper lid and draw out and down over the lower lid. If it feels like an object is in the eye but none is visible, cornea scrape probably occurred and will heal in 24 to 48 hours. To remove the object, moisten the corner of a handkerchief and touch the object lightly.	If the object is on the eye itself; if the object remains after washing; if the object could have penetrated the globe of the eye; if blood is visible in eye; if vision is impaired; if pain is present after 48 hours; if pain is present after object has been removed.
Nasal fracture	The blow may come from the side or front. The side hit causes more deformity. Hemorrhage is profuse (mucous lining is cut), and swelling is immediate.	Prevention in football involves use of a face guard. Bleeding should be controlled immediately (see Nosebleed).	If bleeding continues; if deformity and considerable swelling are present.

(continued)

Injury	General comments	Prevention and treatment	Need for a physician
HEAD AND NECK (*continued*)			
Neck	Neck injuries are more common in contact sports and require immediate and careful attention. Assume that a vertebra is involved and avoid movement of any kind until a physician or rescue squad arrives.	Neck flexibility exercises should be a part of your warm-up routine. Neck-strengthening exercises are a necessity for contact sport participants.	If any injury to the neck occurs.
Nosebleed	Nosebleed may occur even from mild contact to the nose.	Do not lie down when bleeding starts. Squeeze the nose between the thumb and forefinger just below the hard portion for 5 to 10 minutes while seated with the head tilted forward. Do not lean the head backward. Avoid blowing the nose or placing cold compresses on the bridge of the nose.	If bleeding occurs frequently and is associated with a cold; if victim has a history of high blood pressure; if emergency treatment fails to stop the bleeding.
TORSO			
Back	The first 7 vertebrae control the head, neck, and upper back. The next 12 provide attachments for the ribs. The 5 lumbar vertebrae of the lower back support the weight of the upper half of the body. This area plagues millions of people.	Avoid exercise motions that arch the back. Muscular and ligamentous sprains, mechanical instability, arthritis, and ruptured discs may cause back pain. Most problems will improve with rest, ice, pain medication, and an exercise program.	If pain, weakness, or numbness in legs is present; if pain remains after rest and ice therapy; if aching sensation occurs in buttocks or farther down the leg.
Chest pain	Chest pain provides a heart attack scare to everyone over age 30. Pain could be in the chest wall (muscle, rib, ligament, rib cartilage), the lungs or outside covering, or the pleura, diaphragm, skin, or other organs in the upper part of the diaphragm. Sharp pain that lasts a few seconds, pain at the end of a deep breath or one that worsens with a deep breath, pain on pressing a finger on the spot of discomfort, and painful burning when the stomach is empty are all symptoms that are probably not associated with a heart attack.	Any of the symptoms to the right require immediate hospitalization and physician care.	If any of the following symptoms are present: mild to intense pain with a feeling of pressure or squeezing on the chest; pain beneath the breastbone; accompanying pain in the jaw or down the inner side of either arm; accompanying nausea, sweating, dizziness, or shortness of breath; or pulse irregularity.
Groin strain	Running, jumping, and twisting can easily tear the groin muscles (area between the thigh and abdominal region). Preventing and curing this injury is difficult. Pain, weakness, and internal bleeding may occur.	Prevention involves proper stretching before exercise. RICE therapy is the recommended treatment.	If symptoms remain after several days of rest and mild exercise.
Hernia	A hernia is the protrusion of viscera (body organs) through a portion of the abdominal wall. Hernias associated with exercise and sports generally occur in the groin area.	Prevention involves attention to proper form in weightlifting and weight training and care in lifting heavy objects.	If a protrusion protrudes further with coughing.
Hip pointer	A hard blow to the iliac crest or hip produces what is commonly called a hip pointer. The injury is severely handicapping and produces both pain and spasm.	Prevention involves the use of protective hip pads in contact sports. RICE therapy is the recommended treatment.	If symptoms of a fracture are present.
Jock itch	Jock itch is acquired by contact and is associated with bacteria, fungi, molds, and ringworm.	Prevention and treatment involve practicing proper hygiene (showering in warm water, use of antiseptic soap and powder, proper drying); drinking enough water; regularly changing underwear, supporter, and shorts; disinfecting locker benches, mats, and other equipment; and avoiding long periods of sitting in warm, moist areas.	If condition persists for more than 10 days.

Injury	General comments	Prevention and treatment	Need for a physician
TORSO *(continued)*			
Wind knocked out	A hard blow to the right place, such as a relaxed midsection, can temporarily hamper breathing. Although you will have trouble convincing the victim, breathing will return. The blow has only increased abdominal pressure, produced pain, and interfered with the diaphragmatic cycle reflex because of nerve paralysis or muscle spasm.	The victim should try to breathe slowly through the nose (no easy task for someone who is gasping, dizzy, and convinced that death is only seconds away). Loosen clothing at the neck and waist and apply ice to the abdomen.	If breathing is still not normal in 1 to 2 minutes; if breathing stops (start CPR); if pain persists in the midsection.
SHOULDER			
Tendinitis	Tendinitis is common in tennis and baseball. Soreness results on the front of the shoulder when elevating the arm from the side.	Ice and aspirin are used. Prevention and treatment involve flexibility and weight-training exercises. Flexibility movements concentrate on back stretching, and weight-training choices are lateral lifts and military bench presses.	If soreness remains for 7 to 10 days.
THORAX			
Rib fracture and bruises	Fractures may occur from direct contact or, uncommonly, from muscular contraction. A direct blow may displace the bone and produce jagged edges that cut the tissue of the lungs, causing bleeding or lung collapse.	The type of contact helps reveal rib fracture. Pain when breathing and palpitation are also signs. Initiate RICE therapy immediately.	If pain is present when breathing after a direct blow to the thorax; if fracture is suspected; if shortness of breath or difficulty in breathing persists.
MISCELLANEOUS INJURIES AND ILLNESSES			
Abrasions	Superficial skin layers are scraped off. The injury imposes no serious problem if cleaned properly.	Clean with soap and warm water. Use a bandage if the wound oozes blood. Remove loose skin flaps with sterile scissors if dirty; allow them to remain if clean. Check to see whether victim has been immunized for tetanus within the last 10 years.	If all dirt and foreign matter cannot be removed; if infection develops.
Common cold	Shaking hands with an infected person or breathing in particles after a sneeze are two ways of getting a cold virus. Contributing factors may be low resistance, improper nutrition, tension, bacteria entering the respiratory tract, and remaining indoors in winter months, which increases the likelihood of close contact with a contagious person.	A cold will typically last about 7 days. There is no known protection or cure. Antihistamines, decongestants, and cold tablets are of little value. Taking acetaminophen, combined with rest and plenty of fluids, is sound advice. Exercise only lightly and include 1 or 2 days of rest. Do not exercise if you have a fever or muscle soreness.	If fever or sore throat lasts more than a week; if pain is present in one or both ears.
Fainting and dizziness	Lack of blood flow to the brain commonly occurs with increasing age and may result in temporary loss of vision or light-headedness.	Place the victim in a lying position with the feet elevated. If it is not possible to lie down, an alternative position is a sitting posture with the head lowered between the legs.	If loss of consciousness occurs; if dizziness occurs frequently; if dizziness or fainting occurs with exercise.
Frostbite	Frostbite, a destruction of tissue by freezing, is more likely to occur on outer parts of the nose, cheeks, ears, fingers, and toes.	Thaw rapidly in a warm water bath. Avoid rubbing areas with snow. Water should be comfortable to a normal, unfrozen hand (not over 104°F). When a flush reaches the fingers, remove the frostbitten part from the water immediately. For an ear or nose, use cloths soaked in warm water.	Always see a doctor.
Heat exhaustion and heat-stroke	The body loses heat to the environment and maintains normal temperature in several ways: Evaporation—sweat evaporates into the atmosphere. Radiation—with body temperature higher than air temperature, heat loss occurs. Convection—as body heat loss occurs, air is warmed. This warmed air rises and cooler air moves in to take its place, cooling the body. Conduction—heat moves from deeper body organs to skin through blood vessels. The skin acts as a radiation surface for heat loss to the air.	Symptoms of heat exhaustion include nausea, chills, cramps, and rapid pulse. Treatment requires immediate cooling with ice packs to the head, torso, and joints and maintenance of proper water and electrolyte balance.	If rapid improvement is not evident; if multiple cramps occur; if core temperature does not immediately return to normal; if lethargy or confusion is present; if skin is warm and dry.

(continued)

Injury	General comments	Prevention and treatment	Need for a physician
MISCELLANEOUS INJURIES AND ILLNESSES *(continued)*			
Hypothermia	With extremely cold temperatures and high windchill, core body temperature may drop below normal levels.	Prevention involves following the steps outlined in the section "Dress Properly for the Weather" on page 348. Treatment calls for warming with blankets, heating pads, replacing wet clothing, and administering warm drinks.	If core temperature drops below 94°F; if lethargy or confusion is present.
Infected wounds	Bacterial infection in the bloodstream (septicemia).	Keep the area clean by changing the bandage and soaking and cleaning in warm water twice daily. Up to 10 or 12 days may be needed for normal healing.	If fever is above 100°F; if thick pus and swelling occur the second day.
Minor cuts	Minor cuts can develop into serious problems if mistreated or neglected. Avoid use of antiseptics that may destroy tissue and actually retard healing.	Clean the wound with soap and water or hydrogen peroxide, removing all dirt and foreign matter. Use a butterfly bandage or steri-strip to bring the edges of the wound tightly together without trapping the fat or rolling the skin beneath.	If the cut occurs to the face or trunk; if a deep cut involves tendons, nerves, vessels, or ligaments; if blood is pumping from a wound; if tingling or limb weakness occurs; if the cut cannot be pulled together without trapping the fat; if direct pressure fails to stop the bleeding.
Muscle soreness	You may experience two different types of soreness: general soreness that appears immediately after your exercise session and disappears in 3 or 4 hours, or localized soreness appearing 8 to 24 hours after exercise. The older you are, the longer the period is between exercise and soreness.	You can help prevent soreness by warming up properly, avoiding bouncing-type stretching or flexibility exercises, and progressing slowly in your program. Doing too much too soon is a common cause. You can expect to have some soreness after your first few workouts, especially if you have been inactive. Do not stop exercising; soreness will only reoccur later.	If muscle soreness persists after the second week.
Muscle cramps	Muscular cramps commonly occur in three areas: back of lower leg (calf), back of upper leg (hamstring group), and front of upper leg (quadriceps group). Cramps may be related to fatigue; tightness of the muscles; or fluid, salt, and potassium imbalance.	Stretch before you exercise and drink water freely. If a cramp occurs, stretch the area carefully.	If multiple cramps occur; if symptoms of heat exhaustion are present.

Edited by Gary W. Karkuff, PT, CSCS, president, First Choice Rehabilitation Specialists, Harrisburg, PA.

References and Resources

Chapter 1

Banks-Wallace, J., and V. Conn. 2002. "Interventions to Promote Physical Activity Among African American Women." *Public Health Nurse* 19(5): 321-335.

"Behavior Kills More in U.S. Than Anything." 1994. *Nation's Health* (Jan.): 13.

Blair, S.N., H.W. Kohl, R.S. Paffenbarger, D.G. Clark, K.J. Cooper, and L.W. Gibbons. 1989. "Physical Fitness and All-Cause Mortality: A Prospective Study of Healthy Men and Women." *Journal of the American Medical Association* 262: 2395-2401.

Brandon, J.E., and J.M. Lofton. 1991. "Relationship of Fitness to Depression, State and Trait Anxiety, Internal Health Locus of Control, and Self-Control." *Perceptual and Motor Skills* 73: 563-568.

Brownson, R., A. Eyler, A. King, D. Brown, Y. Shyu, and J. Sallis. 2000. "Patterns and Correlates of Physical Activity Among U.S. Women 40 Years and Older." *American Journal of Public Health* 90: 264.

Brownson, R.C., E.A. Baker, R.A. Housemann, L.K. Brennan, and S.J. Bacak. 2001. "Environmental and Policy Determinants of Physical Activity in the United States." *American Journal of Public Health* 91: 1995-2003.

Bungum, T.J., D.L. Peaslee, A.W. Jackson, and M.A. Perez. 2000. "Exercise During Pregnancy and Type of Delivery in Nulliparae." *Journal of Obstetric, Gynecologic, and Neonatal Nursing* 29: 258-264.

"Can Exercise Reduce Diabetes Risk in Postmenopausal Women?" 2001. *Physical Activity Today* 7: 1.

Carter, J.H. 2002. "Religion/Spirituality in African American Culture: An Essential Aspect of Psychiatric Care." *Journal of the National Medical Association* 94(5): 371-375.

Caspersen, C., and R. Merritt. 1995. "Physical Activity Trends Among 26 States, 1986-1990." *Medicine and Science in Sports and Exercise* 27: 713.

Centers for Disease Control and Prevention. 1999. "Neighborhood Safety and the Prevalence of Physical Inactivity—Selected States, 1998." *Morbidity and Mortality Weekly Report* 48: 143-146.

Crespo, C., B. Ainsworth, S. Keteyian, G. Heath, and E. Smith. 1999. "Prevalence of Physical Inactivity and Its Relation to Social Class in U.S. Adults: Results From the Third National Health and Nutrition Examination Survey, 1988-1994." *Medicine and Science in Sports and Exercise* 31: 1821.

Donahue, R.P., R.D. Abbott, Q.M. Reed, and K. Yano. 1988. "Physical Activity and Coronary Heart Disease in Middle-Aged and Elderly Men: The Honolulu Heart Program." *American Journal of Public Health* 78: 683-685.

Eyler, A., E. Baker, L. Cromer, A. King, R. Brownson, and R. Donatelle. 1998. "Physical Activity and Minority Women: A Qualitative Study." *Health Education Behavior* 25: 640.

Eyler, A.E., S. Wilcox, D. Matson-Koffman, K.R. Evenson, B. Sanderson, J. Thompson, J. Wilbur, and D. Rohm-Young. 2002. "Correlates of Physical Activity Among Women From Diverse Racial/Ethnic Groups." *Journal of Women's Health and Gender-Based Medicine* 11(3): 239-253.

Felton, G., and M. Parsons. 1994. "Factors Influencing Physical Activity in Average Weight and Overweight Young Women." *Journal of Community Health Nursing* 11: 109.

Felton, G.M., M. Dowda, D.S. Ward, R.K. Dishman, S.G. Trost, R. Saunders, and R.R. Pate. 2002. "Differences in Physical Activity Between Black and White Girls Living in Rural and Urban Areas." *Journal of School Health* 17(4): 451-460.

Gordon-Larsen, P., L.S. Adair, and B.M. Popkin. 2002. "Ethnic Differences in Physical Activity and Inactivity Patterns and Overweight Status." *Obesity Research* 10(3): 141-149.

Kimm, S.Y., N.W. Glynn, A.M. Kriska, B.A. Barton, S.S. Kronsberg, S.R. Daniels, P.B. Crawford, Z.I. Sabry, and K. Liu. 2002. "Decline in Physical Activity in Black Girls and White Girls During Adolescence." *New England Journal of Medicine* 347(10): 709-715.

King, A., C. Castro, S. Wilcox, A. Eyler, J. Sallis, and R. Brownson. 2000. "Personal and Environmental Factors Associated With Physical Inactivity Among Different Racial/Ethnic Groups of U.S. Middle- and Older-Aged Women." *Health Psychology* 19: 354.

Krucoff, C. 2000. "Couch Potatoes Don't Make It in the Sack." *Washington Post*, May 5, p. 9.

Krucoff, C. 1992. "Exercise and Cancer: Moderate Activity May Help Reduce Risk of Some Tumors." *Washington Post Health*, January 14, p. 16.

Kujala, U.M., J. Kaprio, S. Sarna, and M. Koskenvuo. 1999. "Future Hospital Care in a Population-Based Series of Twin Pairs Discordant for Physical Activity Behavior." *American Journal of Public Health* 89: 1869-1872.

Kusaka, Y., H. Kondou, and K. Morimoto. 1992. "Healthy Lifestyles Are Associated With Higher Natural Killer Cell Activity." *Preventive Medicine* 21: 602-615.

Leon, A.S., and J. Connett. 1991. "Physical Activity and 10.5 Year Mortality in the Multiple Risk Factor Intervention Trial (MRFIT)." *International Journal of Epidemiology* 20: 690-697.

Maxwell, A.E., R. Bastani, P. Vida, and U.S. Warda. 2002. "Physical Activity Among Older Filipino-American Women." *Women and Health* 36(1): 67-79.

McGuire, M.T., P.J. Hannan, D. Neumark-Sztainer, N.H. Cossrow, and M. Story. 2002. "Parental Correlates of Physical Activity in a Racially/Ethnically Diverse Adolescent Sample." *Journal of Adolescent Health* 30(4): 253-261.

Mosca, L., C. McGillen, and M. Rubenfire. 1998. "Gender Differences in Barriers to Lifestyle Change for Cardiovascular Disease Prevention." *Journal of Women's Health* 7: 711.

Musgrave, C.F.R., C.E. Allen, and G.J. Allen. 2002. "Spirituality and Health for Women of Color." *American Journal of Public Health* 92(4): 557-560.

Mussolino, M.E., A.C. Looker, and E.S. Orwoll. 2001. "Jogging and Bone Mineral Density in Men: Results From NHANES III." *American Journal of Public Health* 91: 1056-1059.

Paffenbarger, R.S., R.T. Hyde, A.L. Wing, and C.-C. Hsieh. 1986. "Physical Activity, All-Cause Mortality, and Longevity of College Alumni." *New England Journal of Medicine* 314: 605-613.

Palaniappan, L., M.N. Anthony, C. Mahesh, M. Elliott, A. Killeen, D. Giacherio, and M. Rubenfire. 2002. "Cardiovascular Risk Factors in Ethnic Minority Women Aged < or = 30 Years." *American Journal of Cardiology* 89(5): 524-529.

"Physical Activity Trends—United States, 1990-1998." 2001. *Morbidity and Mortality Weekly Report* 50: 166-169.

Rakowski, W., and V. Mor. 1992. "The Association of Physical Activity With Mortality Among Older Adults in the Longitudinal Study of Aging." *Journal of Gerontology* 47: M122-M129.

Rojas, D.Z. 1996. "Spiritual Well-being and Its Influence on the Holistic Health of Hispanic Women." In Torres S., ed. *Hispanic Voices: Hispanic Health Educators Speak Out.* New York: NLN Press, 213-229.

Sallis, J.F., L. Greenlee, T.L. McKenzie, S.L. Broyles, M.M. Zive, C.C. Berry, J. Brennan, and P.R. Nader. 2001. "Changes and Tracking of Physical Activity Across Seven Years in Mexican-American and European-American Mothers." *Women's Health* 34(4): 1-14.

Schoenborn, C.A., and P.M. Barnes. 2002. "Leisure-Time Physical Activity Among Adults: United States, 1997-98." *Advanced Data From Vital Health Statistics,* 325 (April 7).

Seefeldt, V., R.M. Malina, and M.A. Clark. 2002. "Factors Affecting Levels of Physical Activity in Adults." *Sports Medicine* 32(3): 143-168.

Shepard, R.J. 1989. "Nutritional Benefits of Exercise." *Journal of Sports Medicine* 29: 83-90.

Spector, R.E. 2000. *Cultural Diversity in Health and Illness.* 5th ed. Stamford, CT: Appleton and Lange.

Steinhardt, M., L. Greenhow, and J. Stewart. 1991. "The Relationship of Physical Activity and Cardiovascular Fitness to Absenteeism and Medical Care Claims Among Law Enforcement Officers." *American Journal of Health Promotion* 5: 455-460.

Tucker, L. A., S.G. Aldana, and G.M. Friedman. 1990. "Cardiovascular Fitness and Absenteeism in 8,301 Employed Adults." *American Journal of Health Promotion* 5: 140-145.

U.S. Department of Health and Human Services. 1996. *Physical Activity and Public Health: A Report of the Surgeon General.* Atlanta, GA: U.S. Department of Health and Human Services, Centers for Disease Control and Prevention, National Center for Chronic Disease Prevention and Health Promotion.

U.S. Public Health Service. 1996. *Physical Activity and Health: A Report of the Surgeon General.* Washington, DC: U.S. Department of Health and Human Services.

Verloop, J., M.A. Rookus, K. van der Kooy, and F.E. van Leeuwen. 2000. "Physical Activity and Breast Cancer Risk in Women Aged 20-54 Years." *Journal of the National Cancer Institute* 92: 128-135.

Welty, T., E. Lee, J. Yeh, et al. 1995. "Cardiovascular Disease Risk Factors Among American Indians." *American Journal of Epidemiology* 142: 269.

Chapter 2

American College of Sports Medicine. 1999. *ACSM Guidelines for Exercise Testing and Prescription.* 6th ed. Baltimore: Williams and Wilkins.

Baechle, Thomas R. (Ed). 1994. *Essentials of Strength Training and Conditioning.* Champaign, IL: Human Kinetics.

Balady, G., B. Chaitman, D. Driscoll, C. Foster, E. Froelicher, N. Gordon, R. Pate, J. Rippe, and T. Bazarre. 1998. "Recommendations for Cardiovascular Screening, Staffing, and Emergency Policies at Health/Fitness Facilities." *Medicine and Science for Sport and Exercise* 30: 1009-1018.

Baumgartner, R., and A. Jackson. 1987. *Measurement for Evaluation and Exercise Science.* Dubuque, IA: Brown.

Buckley, J.G., D. O'Driscoll, and S.J. Bennett. 2002. "Postural Sway and Active Balance Performance in Highly Active Lower-Limb Amputees." *American Journal of Physical Medicine and Rehabilitation* 81: 13-20.

Chin, T., S. Sawamura, H. Fujita, S. Nakajima, H. Oyabu, Y. Nagakura, I. Ojima, H. Otsuka, and A. Nakagawa. 2002. "Physical Fitness of Lower Limb Amputees." *American Journal of Physical Medicine and Rehabilitation* 81: 321-325.

Cooper Institute for Aerobic Research. 1992. *The Prudential FITNESSGRAM Test Administration Manual.* Dallas: Author.

Gaesser, G.A. 1999. "Thinness and Weight Loss: Beneficial or Detrimental to Longevity?" *Medicine and Science in Sports and Exercise* 31: 1118-1128.

Gordon, P., J. Senf, and D. Campos-Outcalt. 1999. "Is the Annual Complete Physical Examination Necessary?" *Archives of Internal Medicine* 159: 909-910.

Kennedy, J. 2001. "Unmet and Undermet Need for Activities of Daily Living and Instrumental Activities of Daily Living Assistance Among Adults With Disabilities: Estimates from the 1994 and 1995 Disability Follow-Back Surveys." *Medical Care* 39(12): 1305-1312.

Morrey, M., and D. Hensrud. 1999. "Risk of Medical Events in a Supervised Health and Fitness Facility." *Medicine and Science in Sports and Exercise* 31: 1233-1236.

NATA News. 1966. *American Heart Association Issues: Nation's First Guidelines for Identifying Athletes at Risk of Sudden Cardiac Death.*

Penninx, B.W., S.P. Messier, W.J. Rejeski, J.D. Williamson, M. DiBAri, C. Cavazzini, W.B. Applegate, and M. Pahor. 2001. "Physical Exercise and the Prevention of Disabilities in Activities of Daily Living in Older Persons With

Osteoarthritis." *Archives of Internal Medicine* 161(19): 2309-2316.

Pollock, M.L., and Wilmore, J.H. 1990. *Exercise in Health and Disease.* 2nd ed. Philadelphia: W.B. Saunders.

President's Council on Physical Fitness and Sports. 1996. *Presidential Sports Award.* Washington, DC: Author.

Reuter, I., and M. Engelhardt. 2002. "Exercise Training and Parkinson's Disease: Placebo or Essential Treatment." *Physician and Sportsmedicine* 30(3): 43-50.

Safrit, J. 1995. *Complete Guide to Youth Fitness Testing.* Champaign, IL: Human Kinetics.

Sharkey, B.K. 2002. *Fitness and Health.* Champaign, IL: Human Kinetics.

Sjostrom, L. 1993. "Impacts of Body Weight, Body Composition, and Adipose Tissue Distribution on Morbidity and Mortality." In *Obesity: Theory and Therapy,* 2nd ed., edited by A.J. Stunkard and T.A Wadden. New York: Raven Press.

Slawta, J.N., J.A. McCubbin, A.R. Wilcox, S.D. Fox, D.J. Nalle, and G. Anderson. 2002. "Coronary Heart Disease Risk Between Active and Inactive Women With Multiple Sclerosis." *Medicine and Science in Sports and Exercise* 34(6): 905-912.

Steadward, R.D., and C. Peterson. 1999. *Paralympics: Where Heroes Come.* Alberta, One Shot Holdings Publishing Division.

Stevens, J., J. Cal, E.R. Pamuk, D.F. Williamson, M.J. Thun, and J.L. Wood. 1998. "The Effect of Age on the Association Between Body-Mass Index and Mortality." *New England Journal of Medicine* 338: 1-7.

Stuifbergen, A.K., and G.J. Roberts. 1997. "Health Promotion Practices of Women With Multiple Sclerosis." *Archives of Physical and Medical Rehabilitation* 78(Suppl 5): S3-S9.

Tesch, P. 1984. "Anaerobic Testing: Practical Applications." *NSCA Journal* 6(5): 44-73.

Van der Woude, L.H.V., C. Bouten, H.E.J. Veeger, and T. Gwinn. 2002. "Aerobic Work Capacity in Elite Wheelchair Athletes." *American Journal of Physical Medicine and Rehabilitation* 81: 261-271.

Walcott-McQuigg, J.A., S.P. Chen, K. Davis, E. Stevenson, A. Choi, and S. Wangsrikhun. 2002. "Weight Loss and Weight Loss Maintenance in African-American Women." *Journal of the National Medical Association* 94(8): 686-694.

Washburn, R.A., W. Zhu, E. McAuley, M. Frogley, and S.F. Figoni. 2002. "The Physical Activity Scale for Individuals With Physical Disabilities: Development and Evaluation." *Archives of Physical Medicine and Rehabilitation* 83(2): 193-200.

Chapter 3

ACOG Committee on Obstetric Practice. 2002. "Exercise During Pregnancy and the Postpartum Period," Committee Opinion No. 267. *International Journal of Gynecology and Obstetrics* 77(1): 79-81.

ACOG Committee on Obstetric Practice. 1994. "Exercise During Pregnancy and the Postpartum Period," Committee Opinion No. 189. *International Journal of Gynecology and Obstetrics* 45(1): 65-70.

American College of Sports Medicine. 1999. *ACSM Guidelines for Exercise Testing and Prescription.* 6th ed. Baltimore: Williams and Wilkins.

Baechle, T.R. (Ed). 1994. *Essentials of Strength Training and Conditioning.* Champaign, IL: Human Kinetics.

Balady, G., B. Chaitman, D. Driscoll, C. Foster, E. Froelicher, N. Gordon, R. Pate, J. Rippe, and T. Bazarre. 1987. "Recommendations for Cardiovascular Screening, Staffing, and Emergency Policies at Health/Fitness Facilities." *Medicine and Science for Sport and Exercise* 30: 1009-1018.

Baumgartner, T., and A. Jackson. 1987. *Measurement for Evaluation and Exercise Science.* Dubuque, IA: Brown.

Carey, G.B., T.J. Quinn, and S.E. Goodwin. 1997. "Breast Milk Composition After Exercise of Different Intensities." *Journal of Human Lactation* 13(2): 115-120.

Cooper Institute for Aerobic Research. 1992. *The Prudential FITNESSGRAM Test Administration Manual.* Dallas: Author.

Ebbehoj, N.E., F.R. Hansen, M.S. Harreby, and C.F. Lassen. 2002. "Low Back Pain in Children and Adolescents. Prevalence, Risk Factors and Prevention." *Ugeskr Laeger* 164(6): 755-758.

Eyler, A.E., S. Wilcox. D. Matson-Koffman, K.R. Evenson, B. Sanderson, J. Thompson, J. Wilbur, and D. Rohm-Young. 2002. "Correlates of Physical Activity Among Women From Diverse Racial/Ethnic Groups." *Journal of Women's Health and Gender-Based Medicine* 11(3): 239-253.

Gordon, P., J. Senf, and D. Campos-Outcalt. 1999. "Is the Annual Complete Physical Examination Necessary?" *Archives of Internal Medicine* 159: 909-910.

Koltyn, K.F. 2001. "The Association Between Physical Activity and Quality of Life in Older Women." *Women's Health Issues* 11(6): 471-480.

Morrey, M., and D. Hensrud. 1999. "Risk of Medical Events in a Supervised Health and Fitness Facility." *Medicine and Science in Sports and Exercise* 31:1233-1236.

NATA News. 1996. *American Heart Association Issues: Nation's First Guidelines for Identifying Athletes at Risk of Sudden Cardiac Death.*

NCPAD News. 2002. "Tips for Evaluating a Potential Exercise Facility for People With Disabilities." *National Center on Physical Activity and Disability Electronic Newsletter* 1(6).

News Brief. 2002. "New ACOG Recommendations Encourage Exercise in Pregnancy." *Physician and Sportsmedicine* 30(3): 9-10.

Noren, L., S. Ostgaard, G. Johansson, and H.C. Ostgaard. 2002. "Lumbar Back and Posterior Pelvic Pain During Pregnancy: A 3-Year Follow-up." *European Spine Journal* 11(3): 267-271.

Penninx, B.W., S.P. Messier, W.J. Rejeski, J.D. Williamson, M. DeBari, C. Cavazzini, W.B. Applegate, and M. Pahor. 2001. "Physical Exercise and the Prevention of Disability in Activities of Daily Living in Older Persons With Osteoarthritis." *Archives of Internal Medicine* 161(19): 2309-2316.

President's Council on Physical Fitness and Sports. 1996. *Presidential Sports Award.* Washington, DC: Author.

Ringdahl, E.N. 2002. "Promoting Postpartum Exercise." *Physician and Sportsmedicine* 30(2): 31-36.

Safrit, J. 1995. *Complete Guide to Youth Fitness Testing.* Champaign, IL: Human Kinetics.

Sharkey, B.J., 2002. *Fitness and Health.* Champaign, IL: Human Kinetics.

Stevens, J., J. Cal, E.R. Pamuk, D.F. Williamson, M.J. Thun, and J.L. Wood. 1998. "The Effect of Age on the Association Between Body-Mass Index and Mortality." *New England Journal of Medicine* 338: 1-7.

Taylor, W.C., T. Baranowski, and D.R. Young. 1998. "Physical Activity Interventions in Low-Income, Ethnic Minority, and Populations With Disability." *American Journal of Preventive Medicine* 15(4): 334-343.

Tesch, P. 1984. "Anaerobic Testing: Practical Applications." *NSCA Journal* 6(5): 44-73.

U.S. Public Health Service. 1996. *Physical Activity and Health: A Report of the Surgeon General.* Washington, DC: U.S. Department of Health and Human Services.

Van der Bij, A.K., M.G. Laurant, and M. Wensing. 2002. "Effectiveness of Physical Activity Interventions for Older Adults: A Review." *American Journal of Preventive Medicine* 22(2): 120-133.

Van Valdhoven, N.H., A. Vermeer, J.M. Bogaard, M.G. Hessels, L. Wijnroks, W.T. Colland, and E.E. van Essen-Zandvliet. 2001. "Children With Asthma and Physical Exercise: Effects of an Exercise Programme." *Clinical Rehabilitation* 15(4): 360-370.

Vincent, R.W., Braith, R.A., et al. 2002. "Resistance Exercise and Physical Performance in Adults Aged 60-83." *American Geriatric Society* 50: 1100-1107.

World Health Organization (WHO). 2002. *2002 Guidelines for the Promotion of Physical Activity for Older Persons.* World Health Day 2002 Report. Geneva, Switzerland.

Chapter 4

Airhihenbuwa, C., S. Kumanyika, T. Agurs, and A. Lowe. 1995. "Perceptions and Beliefs About Exercise, Rest, and Health Among African-Americans." *American Journal of Health Promotion* 9: 426.

Annesi, J.J. 2002. "Relationship Between Changes in Acute Exercise-Induced Feeling States, Self-Motivation, and Adults' Adherence to Moderate Aerobic Exercise." *Perceptual Motivational Skills* 94(2): 425-539.

Banks-Wallace, J., and V. Conn. 2002. "Interventions to Promote Physical Activity Among African American Women." *Public Health Nursing* 19(5): 321-335.

Barnett, T.A., J. O'Loughlin, and G. Paradis. 2002. "One- and Two-Year Predictors of Decline in Physical Activity Among Inner-City Schoolchildren." *American Journal of Preventive Medicine* 23(2): 121-128.

Bent, N., A. Jones, I. Molloy, M.A. Chamberlain, and A. Tennant. 2001. "Factors Determining Participation in Young Adults With a Physical Disability: A Pilot Study." *Clinical Rehabilitation* 15(5): 552-561.

Bull, F.C., A.A. Eyler, A.C. King, and R.C. Brownson. 2001. "Stages of Readiness to Exercise in Ethnically Diverse Women: A U.S. Survey." *Medicine and Science in Sports and Exercise* 33(7): 1147-1156.

Carter-Nolan, P., L. Adams-Campbell, and J. Williams. 1996. "Recruitment Strategies for Black Women at Risk for Non-Insulin-Dependent Diabetes Mellitus Into Exercise Protocols: A Qualitative Assessment." *Journal of the National Medical Association* 88: 558.

Clark, D.O. 1997. "Physical Activity Efficacy and Effectiveness Among Older Adults and Minorities." *Diabetes Care* 20(7): 1176-1182.

Conn, V. 1998. "Older Women's Beliefs About Physical Activity." *Public Health Nursing* 15: 370.

Eyler, A., R. Brownson, R. Donatelle, D. Brown, and J. Sallis. 1999. "Physical Activity Social Support and Middle- and Older-Aged Minority Women: Results From a U.S. Survey." *Social Science Medicine* 49: 781.

Eyler, A., E. Baker, L. Cromer, A. King, R. Brownson, and R. Donatelle. 1998. "Physical Activity and Minority Women: A Qualitative Study." *Health Education Behavior* 25: 640.

Eyler, A.E., S. Wilcox, D. Matson-Koffman, K.R. Evenson, B. Sanderson, J. Thompson, J. Wilbur, and D. Rohm-Young. 2002. "Correlates of Physical Activity Among Women From Diverse Racial/Ethnic Groups." *Journal of Women's Health and Gender-Based Medicine* 11(3): 239-253.

Faulkner, G., and S. Biddle. 2001. "Predicting Physical Activity Promotion in Health Care Settings." *American Journal of Health Promotion* 16(2): 98-106.

Felton, G.M., M. Dowda, D.S. Ward, R.K. Dishman, S.G. Trost, R. Saunders, and R.R. Pate. 2002. "Differences in Physical Activity Between Black and White Girls Living in Rural and Urban Areas." *Journal of School Health* 72(6): 250-255.

Fischer, I., D. Brown, C. Blanton, M. Casper, J. Croft, and R. Brownson. 1999. "Physical Activity Patterns of Chippewa and Menominee Indians: The Intertribal Heart Project." *American Journal of Preventive Medicine* 17: 189.

Glanz, K., and B.K. Rimer. 1997. *Theory at a Glance: A Guide for Health Promotion Practice.* Washington, DC: U.S. Department of Health and Human Services.

Hagger, M.S., N. Chatzisarantis, and S.J. Biddle. 2001. "The Influence of Self-Efficacy and Past Behavior on the Physical Activity Intentions of Young People." *Journal of Sports Science* 19(9): 711-725.

Harnack, L., M. Story, and B. Rock. 1999. "Diet and Physical Activity Patterns of Lakota Indian Adults." *Journal of American Dietetic Association* 99: 829.

Johnson, C., S. Corrigan, P. Dubert, and S. Grambling. 1990. "Perceived Barriers to Exercise and Weight Control Practices in Community Women." *Women's Health* 16: 177.

Johnston-Brooks, C.H., M.A. Lewis, and S. Garg. 2002. "Self-Efficacy Impacts Self-Care and HbA1c in Young Adults With Type I Diabetes." *Psychosomatic Medicine* 64(1): 43-51.

Kaplan, G., N. Lazarus, R. Cohen, and D. Leu. 1991. "Psychosocial Factors in the Natural History of Physical Activity." *American Journal of Preventive Medicine* 7: 12.

Kaplan, M.S., J.T. Newsom, B.H. McFarland, and L. Lu. 2001. "Demographic and Psychosocial Correlates of Physical Activity in Late Life." *American Journal of Preventive Medicine* 21(4): 306-312.

Kimm, S.Y., N.W. Glynn, A.M. Kriska, B.A. Barton, S.S. Kronsberg, S.R. Daniels, P.B. Crawford, Z.I. Sabry, and K. Liu. 2002. "Decline in Physical Activity in Black Girls and White Girls During Adolescence." *New England Journal of Medicine* 347(10): 709-715.

King, A., C. Castro, S. Wilcox, A. Eyler, J. Sallis, and R. Brownson. 2000. "Personal and Environmental Factors Associated With Physical Inactivity Among Different Racial/Ethnic Groups of U.S. Middle- and Older-Aged Women." *Health Psychology* 19: 354.

Lee, R.E., C.R. Nigg, C.C. DiClemente, and K.S. Courneya. 2001. "Validating Motivational Readiness for Exercise Behavior With Adolescents." *Research Quarterly for Exercise and Sport* 72(4): 401-410.

Litt, M.D., A. Kleppinger, and J.O. Judge. 2002. "Initiation and Maintenance of Exercise Behavior in Older Women: Predictors From the Social Learning Model." *Journal of Behavioral Medicine* 25(1): 83-97.

Maxwell, A.E., R. Bastani, P. Vida, and U.S. Warda. 2002. "Physical Activity Among Older Filipino-American Women." *Women and Health* 36(1): 67-79.

Miller, Y.D., S.G. Trost, and W.J. Brown. 2002. "Mediators of Physical Activity Behavior Change Among Women With Young Children." *American Journal of Preventive Medicine* 23(2S): 98-103.

Moore, S. 1996. "Women's Views of Cardiac Rehabilitation Programs." *Journal of Cardiopulmonary Rehabilitation* 16: 123.

Mosca, L., C. McGillen, and M. Rubenfire. 1998. "Gender Differences in Barriers to Lifestyle Change for Cardiovascular Disease Prevention." *Journal of Women's Health* 7: 711.

Mullineaux, D.R., C.A. Barnes, and E.F. Barnes. 2001. "Factors Affecting the Likelihood to Engage in Adequate Physical Activity to Promote Health." *Journal of Sports Science* 19(4): 279-288.

Nies, M., M. Vollman, and T. Cook. 1999. "African American Women's Experiences With Physical Activity in Their Daily Lives." *Public Health Nursing* 16: 23.

Norcross, J.C., M.S. Mrykalo, and M.D. Blagys. 2002. "Auld Lang Syne: Success Predictors, Change Processes, and Self-Reported Outcomes of New Year's Resolvers and Nonresolvers." *Journal of Clinical Psychology* 58(4): 397-405.

Norman, A., R. Bellocco, F. Vaida, and A. Wolk. 2002. "Total Physical Activity in Relation to Age, Body Mass, Health and Other Factors in a Cohort of Swedish Men." *International Journal of Obesity and Related Metabolic Disorders* 26(5): 670-675.

Pender, N.J., O. Bar-Or, B. Wilk, and S. Mitchell. 2002. "Self-Efficacy and Perceived Exertion of Girls During Exercise." *Nursing Research* 51(2): 86-91.

Prochaska, J.O., C.C. DiClemente, and J.C. Norcross. 1992. "In Search of How People Change: Applications to Addictive Behaviors." *American Psychologist* 47: 1102-1114.

Resnick, B. 2002. "Testing the Effect of the WALC Intervention on Exercise Adherence in Older Adults." *Journal of Gerontological Nursing* 28(6): 40-49.

Rhodes, R.E., A.D. Martin, and J.E. Taunton. 2001. "Temporal Relationships of Self-Efficacy and Social Support as Predictors of Adherence in a 6-Month Strength-Training Program for Older Women." *Perceptual Motor Skills* 93(3): 693-703.

Rich, S.C., and M.E. Rogers. 2001. "Stage of Exercise Change Model and Attitudes Toward Exercise in Older Adults." *Perceptual Motor Skills* 93(1): 141-144.

Ronda, G., P. Van Assema, and J. Brug. 2001. "Stages of Change, Psychosocial Factors and Awareness of Physical Activity Levels in The Netherlands." *Health Promotions International* 16(4): 305-314.

Scharff, D., S. Homan, M. Krueter, and L. Brennan. 1999. "Factors Associated With Physical Activity in Women Across the Lifespan: Implications for Program Development." *Women's Health* 29: 115.

Seefeldt, V., R.M. Malina, and M.A. Clark. 2002. "Factors Affecting Levels of Physical Activity in Adults." *Sports Medicine* 32(3): 143-168.

Shin, Y., H. Jang, and N.J. Pender. 2001. "Psychometric Evaluation of the Exercise Self-Efficacy Scale Among Korean Adults With Chronic Diseases." *Research in Nursing Health* 24(1): 68-76.

Skelly, A., J. Marshall, B. Haughey, P. Davis, and R. Dunford. 1995. "Self-Efficacy and Confidence in Outcomes as Determinants of Self-Care Practices in Inner-City, African American Women With Non-Insulin-Dependent Diabetes." *Diabetes Education* 21: 38.

Sternfeld, B., B. Ainsworth, and C. Quesenberry. 1999. "Physical Activity Patterns in a Diverse Population of Women." *Preventive Medicine* 28: 313.

Thompson, J.G., S.M. Davis, J. Gittelson, S. Going, A. Becenti, L. Metcalf, E. Stone, L. Harnack, and K. Ring. 2001. "Patterns of Physical Activity Among American Indian Children: An Assessment of Barriers and Support." *Journal of Community Health* 26(6): 423-445.

Troped, P., and R. Saunders. 1998. "Gender Differences in Social Influence on Physical Activity at Different Stages of Exercise Adoption." *American Journal of Health Promotion* 13: 112.

Walcott-McQuigg, J.A., J.J. Zerwic, A. Dan, and M.A. Kelley. 2001. "An Ecological Approach to Physical Activity in African American Women." *Medscape Womens Health* 6(6): 3.

Wilcox, S., D.L. Richter, K.A. Henserson, M.L. Greaney, and B.E. Ainsworth. 2002. "Perceptions of Physical Activity and Personal Barriers and Enablers in African-American Women." *Ethnic Disease* 12(3): 353-362.

Woods, C., N. Mutrie, and M. Scott. 2002. "Physical Activity Intervention: A Transtheoretical Model-Based Intervention Designed to Help Sedentary Young Adults Become Active." *Health Education Research* 17(4): 451-460.

Wu, T., and N. Pender. 2002. "Determinants of Physical Activity Among Taiwanese Adolescents: An Application of the Health Promotion Model." *Research Nursing Health* 25(1): 25-36.

Young, D.R., J. Gittelson, J. Charleston, K. Felix-Aaron, and L.J. Appel. 2001. "Motivations for Exercise and Weight Loss Among African-American Women: Focus Group Results and Their Contribution Towards Program Development." *Ethnic Health* 6(3-4): 227-245.

Chapter 6

Adler, S.S., D. Beckers, and M. Buck. 1993. *PNF in Practice: An Illustrated Guide.* New York: Springer-Verlag.

Alter, M.J. 1998. *Sport Stretch.* Champaign, IL: Human Kinetics.

Apostolopoulos, N. 2001. "Performance Flexibility." In *High-Performance Sports Conditioning,* ed. Bill Foran. Champaign, IL: Human Kinetics.

Bandy, W.D., and J.M. Irion. 1994. "The Effect of Time on Static Stretch on the Flexibility of the Hamstring Muscles." *Physical Therapy* 74(9): 845-852.

Barbosa, A.R., J.M. Santarem, W.J. Filho, and M.F. Marucci. 2002. "93 Effects of Resistance Training on the Sit-and-Reach Test in Elderly Women." *Journal of Strength Conditioning Research* 16(1): 14-18.

Burbank, P.M., D. Reibe, C.A. Padula, and C. Nigg. 2002. "Exercise and Older Adults: Changing Behavior With the Transtheoretical Model." *Orthopedic Nursing* 21(4): 51-61.

Ebbehoj, N.E., F.R. Hansen, M.S. Harreby, and C.F. Lassen. 2002. "Low Back Pain in Children and Adolescents. Prevalence, Risk Factors and Prevention." *Ugeskr Lfaeger* 164(6): 755-758.

Fatouros, I.G., K. Taxildaris, S.P. Tokmakidis, V. Kalapotharakos, N. Aggelousis, S. Athanasopoulos, I. Zeris, and I. Katrabasas. 2002. "The Effects of Strength Training, Cardiovascular Training and Their Combination on Flexibility on Inactive Older Adults." *International Journal* 23(2): 112-119.

George, S.Z., and A. Delitto. 2002. "Management of the Athlete With Low Back Pain." *Clinical Sports Medicine* 21(1): 105-120.

Grimshaw, P., A. Giles, R. Tong, and K. Grimmer. 2002. "Lower Back and Elbow Injuries in Golf." *Sports Medicine* 32(10): 655-666.

Hardy, L. 1985. "Improving Active Range of Hip Flexion." *Research Quarterly for Exercise and Sport* 56(2): 111-114.

King, M.B., R.H. Whipple, C.A. Gruman, J.O. Judge, J.A. Schmidt, and L.I. Wolfson. 2002. "The Performance Enhancement Project: Improving Physical Performance in Older Adults." *Archives of Physical Medicine and Rehabilitation* 83(8): 1060-1069.

Kurz, T. 1994. *Stretching Scientifically: A Guide to Flexibility Training,* 3rd ed. Island Point, VT: Station.

Lively, M.W. 2002. "Sports Medicine Approach to Low Back Pain." *South Medicine Journal* 95(6): 642-646.

Lubell, A. 1989. "Potentially Dangerous Exercises: Are They Harmful to All?" *Physician and Sportsmedicine* 17(1): 187-192.

Manniche, C., K. Ostergaard, and A. Jordan. 2002. "Training of Back and Neck in the Year of 2002." *Ugeskr Laeger* 164(14): 1910-1913.

Marom-Klibansky, R., and Y. Drory. 2002. "Physical Activity for the Elderly." *Harefuah* 141(7): 646-650.

McAtee, R.E. 1993. *Facilitated Stretching.* Champaign, IL: Human Kinetics.

Pratt, M. 1989 "Strength, Flexibility, and Maturity in Adolescent Adolescents." *American Journal of Diseases of Children* 143(5): 560-563.

Quittan, M. 2002. "Management of Back Pain." *Disability Rehabilitation* 24(8): 423-434.

Stevenson, J.M., C.L. Weber, J.T. Smith, G.A. Dumas, and W.J. Albert. 2001. "A Longitudinal Study of the Development of Low Back Pain in an Industrial Population." *Spine* 26(12): 1370-1377.

Tritilanunt, T., and W. Wajanavisit. 2001. "The Efficacy of an Aerobic Exercise and Health Education Program for the Treatment of Chronic Low Back Pain." *Journal of the Medical Association Thai.* 84(Suppl 2): S528-533.

Van Tulder, M.W. 2001. "Treatment of Low Back Pain: Myths and Facts." *Schmerz* 15(6): 499-503.

Chapter 7

Baechle, T., ed. 1994. *Essentials of Strength Training and Conditioning.* Champaign, IL: Human Kinetics.

Baechle, T., and R.W. Earle. 1989. *Weight Training: A Text Written for the College Student.* Omaha: Creighton University.

Baechle, T.R., and Earle, R.W. 1995. *Fitness Weight Training.* Champaign, IL: Human Kinetics.

Bompa, T., and L. Cornacchia, 1999. *Serious Strength Training: Periodization for Building Muscle Power and Mass.* Champaign, IL: Human Kinetics.

Centers for Disease Control. 2001. *CDC Fact Book: 2000-2001.* Department of Health and Human Services.

Courneya, K.S., J.R. Mackey, and D.C. McKenzie. 2002. "Exercise for Breast Cancer Survivors." *Physician and Sportsmedicine* 30(8): 33-42.

Drechsler, A.J. 1998. *The Weight Lifting Encyclopedia.* Flushing, NY: A Communications.

Dunstan, D.W., R.M. Daly, N. Owen, D. Jolley, M. De Courten, J. Shaw, and P. Zimmet. 2002. "High-Intensity Resistance Training Improves Glycemic Control in Older Patients With Type 2 Diabetes." *Diabetes Care* 25(10): 1729-1736.

Faigenbaum, A., and W. Westcott, 2000. *Strength and Power for Young Athletes.* Champaign, IL: Human Kinetics.

Fleck, S., and W. Kraemer. 1997. *Designing Resistance Training Programs.* Champaign, IL: Human Kinetics.

Grimby, G. 1993. "Clinical Aspects of Strength and Power Training." In *Strength and Power in Sport,* ed. P. Komi, 338-354. London: Blackwell Scientific.

Hakkinen, K., ed. 1998. *International Conference on Weight Lifting and Strength Training Conference Book.* Lahti: Gummerus Printing.

Hass, C., L. Garzarella, D. DeHoyos, and M. Pollock. 2000. "Single Versus Multiple Sets in Long-Term Recreational Weight Lifters." *Medicine and Science in Sport and Exercise* 32: 235-242.

Headley, S., M. Germain, P. Mulhern, B. Ashworth, J. Burris, B. Brewer, B. Nindl, M. Coughlin, R. Welles, and M. Jones. 2002. "Resistance Training Improves Strength and Functional Measures in Patients With End-Stage Renal Disease." *American Journal of Kidney Disease* 40(2): 355-364.

Kraemer, W., and S. Fleck, 1993. *Strength Training for Young Athletes.* Champaign, IL: Human Kinetics.

Lombardi, V.P. 1989. *Beginning Weight Training: The Safe and Effective Way.* Dubuque, IA: Brown.

Morrissey, M., W. Harman, and M. Johnson. 1995. "Resistance Training Modes: Specificity and Effectiveness." *Medicine and Science in Sports and Exercise* 27: 648-660.

Reuter, I., and M. Engelhardt. 2002. "Exercise Training and Parkinson's Disease." *Physician and Sportsmedicine* 30(3): 43-50.

Ritzdorf, W. 1999. "Strength and Power Training in Sport." In *Training in Sport*, ed. B. Elliott. Chichester: Wiley.

Santa-Clara, H., B. Fernhall, M. Mendes, and L.B. Sardinha. 2002. "Effect of a 1 Year Combined Aerobic- and Weight-Training Exercise Programme on Aerobic Capacity and Ventilatory Threshold in Patients Suffering From Coronary Artery Disease." *European Journal of Applied Physiology* 87(6): 568-575.

Tesch, P.A. 1999. *Target Bodybuilding: Precision Lifting for More Mass and Greater Definition.* Champaign, IL: Human Kinetics.

Ward, P.E., and R.D. Ward. 1991. *Encyclopedia of Weight Training.* Laguna Hills, CA: QPT.

Westcott, W.L. 1996. *Building Strength and Stamina.* Champaign, IL: Human Kinetics.

Chapter 8

AHA Science Advisory. 2001. "Lyon Diet Heart Study: Benefits of a Mediterranean-Style, National Cholesterol Education Program/American Heart Association Step I Dietary Pattern on Cardiovascular Disease." #71-4979; 0202. *Circulation* 103: 1823-1825; Editorial: "Can a Mediterranean-Style Diet Reduce Heard Disease?" *Circulation* 103: 1821-1822.

AHA Scientific Statement. 1994. "Guidelines for Weight Management Programs for Healthy Adults." #71-4979; 0053. *Heart Disease and Stroke* 3: 221-228.

Allan, J.D. 1998. "Explanatory Models of Overweight Among African American, Euro-American, and Mexican American Women." *Western Journal of Nursing Research* 29: 45-66.

Anderson, R.E., T.A. Wadden, S.J. Bartlett, B. Zemel, T.J. Verde, and S.C. Franckowiak. 1999. "Effects of Lifestyle vs. Structured Aerobic Exercise in Obese Women: A Randomized Trial." *Journal of the American Medical Association* 281: 335-340.

Applebaum, M.P. Vague, O. Ziegler, C. Hanotin, F. Thomas, and E. Leutenegger. 1999. "Long-term Maintenance of Weight Loss After a Very Low-Calorie Diet: A Randomized Blinded Trail of the Efficiency and Tolerability of Sibutramine." *American Journal of Medicine* 106: 179-184.

Barr, S.L. 1997. "You Really Can Shrink Your Stomach." *Good Housekeeping*, July.

Boutelle, K.N., and D.S. Kirschenbaum. 1998. "Further Support for Consistent Self-Monitoring As a Vital Component of Successful Weight Control." *Obesity Research* 6: 219-224.

Bray, G.A., and B.M. Popkin. 1998. "Dietary Fat Intake Does Affect Obesity." *American Journal of Clinical Nutrition* 68: 1157-1173.

Bray, G.A., and F.L. Greenway. 1999. "Current and Potential Drugs for Treatment of Obesity." *Endocrinology Reviews* 20: 805-875.

Bronner, Y., and E.A. Boyington. 2002. "Developing Weight Loss Maintenance Interventions for African-American Women: Elements of Successful Models." *Journal of the National Medical Association* 94: 224-235.

Chamberlin, L.A., S.N. Sherman, A. Jain, S.W. Powers, and R.C. Whitaker. 2002. "The Challenge of Preventing and Treating Obesity in Low-Income, Preschool Children: Perceptions of WIC Health Care Professionals." *Archives of Pediatric Adolescent Medicine* 156(7): 662-668.

Clark, J.M., L.R. Bone, R. Stallings, A.C. Gelber, A. Barker, S. Zeger, M.N. Hill, and D.M. Levine. 2001. "Obesity and Approaches to Weight in an Urban African-American Community." *Ethnic Disease* 11(4): 676-686.

Crovetti, R., M. Porrini, A. Santangelo, and G. Testolin. 1998. "The Influence of Thermic Effect of Food on Satiety." *European Journal of Clinical Nutrition* 52: 482-488.

Flegal, K.M., D. Carroll, R.J. Kuczmarski, and C.L. Johnson. 1998. "Overweight and Obesity in the United States: Prevalence and Trends. 1960-1994." *International Journal of Obesity* 22: 39-47.

Gutierrez-Fisac, J.L., G.E. Lopez, F. Rodriguez-Artalejo, J.R. Banegas, and P. Guallar-Castillon. 2002. "Self-Perception of Being Overweight in Spanish Adults." *European Journal of Clinical Nutrition* 56(9): 866-872.

Hill, J., and E. Melanson. 1999. "Overview of Determinants of Overweight and Obesity: Current Evidence and Research Issues." *Medicine and Science in Sports and Exercise* 31: 5515-5521.

Ivy, J., T. Zderic, and D. Fogt. 1999. "Prevention and Treatment of Non-Insulin-Dependent Diabetes Mellitus." In *Exercise and Sports Science Reviews*, vol. 27, ed. J. Holloszy, 1-36. Indianapolis: American College of Sports Medicine.

Kempen, K., W. Saris, and K. Westerterp. 1995. "Energy Balance During an 8-Week Restricted Diet With and Without Exercise in Obese Women." *American Journal of Clinical Nutrition* 62: 722-729.

Lee, C.D., A.S. Jackson, and S.N. Blair. 1998. "U.S. Weight Guidelines: Is It Important to Consider Cardiorespiratory Fitness?" *International Journal of Obesity* 22(Suppl. 2): S2-S7.

Jakicic, J.M., K. Clark, E. Coleman, J.E. Donnelly, J. Foreyt, E. Melanson, J. Volek, and S.L. Volpe. 2001. "American College of Sports Medicine Position Stand. Appropriate Strategies for Weight Loss and Prevention of Weight Regain for Adults." *Medicine and Science in Sports and Exercise* 33(12): 2145-2156.

Kottke, T.E., M.M. Clark, L.A. Aase, C.L. Brandel, M.J. Brekke, L.N. Brekke, S.W. DeBoer, S.N. Hayes, R.S. Hoffman, P.A. Menzel, and R.J. Thomas. 2002. "Self-Reported Weight, Weight Goals, and Weight Control Strategies of a Midwestern Population." *Mayo Clinic Proceedings* 77(2): 114-121.

Lowry, R., D.A. Galuska, J.E. Fulton, H. Weschler, and L. Kann. 2002. "Weight Management Goals and Practices Among U.S. High School Students: Associations With Physical Activity, Diet, and Smoking." *Journal of Adolescent Health* 31(2): 133-144.

Mellin, A.E., D. Neumark-Sztainer, M. Story, M. Ireland, and M.D. Resnick. 2002. "Unhealthy Behaviors and Psychosocial Difficulties Among Overweight Adolescents: The Potential Impact of Familial Factors." *Journal of Adolescent Health* 31(2): 145-153.

Miller, W.C., D.M. Koceja, and E.J. Hamilton. 1997. "A Meta-Analysis of the Past 25 Years of Weight Loss Research Using Diet, Exercise, or Diet Plus Exercise Intervention." *International Journal of Obesity* 21: 941-947.

Mokdad, A.H., M.K. Serdula, W.H. Dietz, B.A. Bowman, J.S. Marks, and J.P. Koplan. 1999. "The Spread of the Obesity Epidemic in the United States, 1991-1998." *Journal of the American Medical Association* 282: 1519-1522.

Mokdad, A.H., M. Serdula, W. Dietz, et al. 2000. "The Continuing Obesity Epidemic in the United States." *Journal of the American Medical Association* 284: 1650-1651.

Mokdad, A.H., B.A. Bowman, E.S. Ford, et al. 2001. "The Continuing Epidemics of Obesity and Diabetes in the United States." *Journal of the American Medical Association*: 286(10): 1195-1200.

Mulrine, A. 2003. "Washington Whispers." *U.S. News and World Report*. Aug. 11, p. 5.

Must, A., J. Spadano, E.H. Coakley, A.E. Field, G. Colditz, and W.H. Dietz. 1999. "The Disease Burden Associated With Overweight and Obesity." *Journal of the American Medical Association* 282: 1523-1529.

National Heart, Lung, and Blood Institute. 1998. "Clinical Guidelines on the Identification, Evaluation, and Treatment of Overweight and Obesity in Adults: The Evidence Report." *Obesity Research* 6(Suppl. 2): 51S-209S.

National Institutes of Health. 1998a. *Clinical Guidelines on the Identification, Evaluation, and Treatment of Overweight and Obesity in Adults*. Bethesda, MD: Department of Health and Human Services; National Institutes of Health; National Heart, Lung, and Blood Institute.

National Institutes of Health. 1998b. *First Federal Obesity Clinical Guidelines Released*. NIH News Release, June 17.

Paeratakul, S., M.A. White, D.A. Williamson, D.H. Ryan, and G.A. Bray. 2002. "Sex, Race/Ethnicity, Socioeconomic Status, and BMI in Relation to Self-Perception of Overweight." *Obesity Research* 10(5): 345-350.

St. Jeor, S.T., R.L. Brunner, M.E. Harrington, et al. 1997. "A Classification System to Evaluate Weight Maintainers, Gainers, and Losers." *Journal of the American Dietary Association* 967: 481-488.

Stunkard, A.J., and T.A. Wadden (Editors). 1993. *Obesity: Theory and Therapy*, Second Edition. New York: Raven Press.

Tufts University Diet and Nutrition Letter. 1988. Vol. 5, no. 12, February.

U.S. News and World Report. 2001. "Breast-Fed Babies Make Leaner Kids." May 28.

Wadden, T.A., R.A. Vogt, R.E. Anderson, et al. 1997. "Exercise in the Treatment of Obesity: Effects of Four Interventions on Body Composition, Resting Energy Expenditure, Appetite, and Mood." *Journal of Consulting Clinical Psychology* 65: 269-277.

Walcott-McQuigg, J.A., S. Schen, D. Davis, E. Stevenson, A. Choi, and S. Wangsrikhun. 2002. "Weight Loss and Weight Loss Maintenance in African-American Women." *Journal of the National Medical Association* 94(8): 686-694.

Weinsier, R.L., G.R. Hunter, Y. Schutz, P.A. Zuckerman, and B.E. Darnell. 2002. "Physical Activity in Free-Living, Overweight White and Black Women: Divergent Responses by Race to Diet-Induced Weight Loss." *American Journal of Clinical Nutrition* 76(4): 736-742.

Chapter 9

Barnette, M. 1993. "The Perfect Body." *Allure*, August, 97-110, 146.

Barry, D.T., and C.M. Grilo. 2002. "Eating and Body Image Disturbances in Adolescent Psychiatric Inpatients: Gender and Ethnicity Patterns." *International Journal of Eating Disorders* 32(3): 335-343.

Begley, S., and M. Brant. 1999. "The Real Scandal." *Newsweek*, February 15, 48-54.

Crago, M., C.M. Shisslak, and L.S. Estes. 1996. "Eating Disturbances Among American Minority Groups: A Review." *International Journal of Eating Disorders* 19(3): 239-248.

"Dying to Win." 1994. *Sports Illustrated* 80: 52-60.

Field, A.E., L. Cheung, A.M. Wolf, D.B. Herzog, S.L. Gortmaker, and G.A. Colditz. 1999. "Exposure to the Mass Media and Weight Concerns Among Girls." *Pediatrics* 103: 36.

Garner, D.M. 1997. "The 1997 Body Image Survey Result." *Psychology Today* 30: 30-44.

Goodale, Kimberly R., P.L. Watkins, and B.J. Cardinal. 2001. "Muscle Dysmorphia: A New Form of Eating Disorder." *American Journal of Health Education* 32: 260-266.

Gordon, K.H., M. Perez, and T.E. Joiner Jr. 2002. "The Impact of Racial Stereotypes on Eating Disorder Recognition." *International Journal of Eating Disorders* 32(2): 219-224.

National Center for Health Statistics. 1999. *The National Health and Nutrition and Examination Study*. Hyattsville, MD: National Center for Health Statistics.

National Institute on Drug Abuse. 1999. *Anabolic Steroids*. Research Report Series. DHHS Publication No. (ADM), 91-1810.

Nobakht, M., and M. Dezhkam. 2000. "An Epidemiological Study of Eating Disorders in Iran." *International Journal of Eating Disorders* 28(3): 265-271.

Perez, M., Z.R. Voelz, J.W. Pettit, and T.E. Joiner Jr. 2002. "The Role of Acculturative Stress and Body Dissatisfaction in Predicting Bulimic Symptomatology Across Ethnic Groups." *International Journal of Eating Disorders* 31(4): 442-454.

Rubinstein, S., and B. Caballero. 2000. "Is Miss America an Undernourished Role Model?" *Journal of the American Medical Association* 238: 1569.

Wardlow, G. *Contemporary Nutrition Issues and Insights*. 1997. Madison, WI: Brown and Benchmark.

Williams, M.H. 1996. *Lifetime Fitness and Wellness*. Madison, WI: Brown and Benchmark.

Chapter 10

AHA Conference Proceedings. 2001. "Summary of the Scientific Conference on Dietary Fatty Acids and Cardiovascular Health." #71-4979;0200. *Circulation* 103: 1034-1039.

AHA Science Advisory. 2001. "Wine and Your Heart." #71-4979;0199. *Circulation* 103: 472-475.

AHA Science Advisory. 1996. "Fish Consumption, Fish Oil, Lipids, and Coronary Heart Disease." #71-4979;0096. *Circulation* 94: 2337-2340.

AHA Scientific Statement. 2000. "AHA Dietary Guidelines: Revision 2000." #71-4979;0193. *Circulation* 102: 2284-2299; *Stroke* 31: 2751-2766.

AHA Scientific Statement. 1997. "Trans Fatty Acids, Lipids, and Risk of Developing Cardiovascular Disease." #71-4979;0116. *Circulation* 95: 2588-2590.

AHA Scientific Statement. 1990. "The Cholesterol Facts: A Summary of Evidence Relating Dietary Fats, Serum Cholesterol, and Coronary Heart Disease." #71-4979;1019. *Circulation* 181: 1821-1733.

American College of Sports Medicine. 1996. "Position Stand: Exercise and Fluid Replacement." 28(1), January.

American College of Sports Medicine, American Dietetic Association, and the Dietitians of Canada. 2000. "Joint Position Statement on Nutrition and Athletic Performance." *Medicine and Science in Sports and Exercise.* 32(12): 2130-2145, October.

American Heart Association. 2000. *An Eating Plan for Healthy Americans.*

Brecher, L.S., S.C. Pomerantz, B.A. Snyder, D.M. Janora, K.M. Klotzbach-Shimomura, and T.A. Cavalieri. 2002. "Osteoporosis Prevention Project: A Model Multidisciplinary Educational Intervention." *Journal of the American Osteopathic Association* 102(6): 327-335.

Calle, E.E., C. Rodriguez, K. Walker-Thurmond, and M.J. Thun. "Overweight, Obesity, and Mortality from Cancer in a Prospectively Studied Cohort of U.S. Adults." *New England Journal of Medicine* 248 (17).

Centers for Disease Control. 2000. *CDC Fact Book: 2000-2001.* Department of Health and Human Services.

Duncan, C.S., C.J.R. Blimkie, C.T. Cowell, S.T. Burke, J.N. Briody, and R. Howman-Giles. 2002. "Bone Mineral Density in Adolescent Female Athletes: Relationship to Exercise Type and Muscle Strength." *Medicine and Science in Sports and Exercise* 34(2): 286-294.

Food and Nutrition Board. 1992. *Recommended Daily Allowances,* 8th ed. Washington, DC: National Academy of Sciences.

Foster-Powell, K., and J. Miller. 1995. "International Tables of Glycemic Index." *American Journal of Clinical Nutrition* 62: S871-890.

Kanter, M. 1995. "Free Radicals and Exercise: Effects of Nutritional Antioxidant Supplements." In *Exercise and Sports Science Reviews.* Ed. J. Holloszy. Baltimore: Williams and Wilkins.

Krauss, R.M., R.H. Eckel, B. Howard, et al. 2000. "AHA Dietary Guidelines Revision 2000: A Statement for Health Care Professionals From the Nutrition Committee of the American Heart Association." *Circulation* 102: 2284-2299.

Journal of NIH Research. 1995. 7: 42.

Piaseu, N., K. Schepp, and B. Belza. 2002. "Causal Analysis of Exercise and Calcium Intake Behaviors for Osteoporosis Prevention Among Young Women in Thailand." *Health Care Women International* 23(4): 364-376.

Scientific Committee of the Norwegian Food Control Authority. 2002. *Risk Assessment of Acrylamide Intake From Foods With Special Emphasis on Cancer Risks.* Report From the Scientific Committee of the Norwegian Food Control Authority, 6 June.

U.S. Department of Agriculture, Agricultural Research Service, Dietary Guidelines Advisory Committee. 1995. *Report of the Dietary Guidelines Advisory Committee on the Dietary Guidelines for Americans.* Washington, DC: Secretary of Health and Human Services and Secretary of Agriculture.

U.S. Department of Health and Human Services. 1995. Home and Garden Bulletin No. 232, December.

U.S. News and World Report. 1996. May 13, p. 93.

Vegetarian Resource Group (VRG). *A 2000 National Zogby Poll.* Baltimore.

Wallace, L.S. 2002, "Osteoporosis Prevention in College Women: Application of the Expanded Health Belief Model." *American Journal of Health Behavior* 26(3): 163-172.

Watson, R., and S. Mufti, eds. 1996. *Nutrition and Cancer Prevention.* Boca Raton, FL: CRC Press.

Williams, Melvin H. 1999. *Nutrition for Health, Fitness, and Sport.* Champaign, IL: Human Kinetics.

Chapter 11

AHA Science Advisory. 2001. "Wine and Your Heart." #71-0199. *Circulation* 103:472-475.

AHA Science Advisory. 1996. "Alcohol and Heart Disease." #71-0097. *Circulation* 94:3023-3025.

King, D.S., R.L. Sharp, M.D. Vukovich, G.A. Brown, T.A. Reifenrath, N.L. Uhl, and K.A. Parsons. 1999. "Effect of Oral Androstenedione on Serum Testosterone and Adaptations to Resistance Training in Young Men: A Randomized Controlled Trial." *Journal of the American Medical Association* 21:2020-2028.

Kuipers, H., J.A. Wijnen, F. Hartgens, and S.M. Willems. 1991. "Influence of Anabolic Steroids on Body Composition, Blood Pressure, Lipid Profile and Liver Functions in Body Builders." *International Journal of Sports Medicine* 4:413-418.

Marks, J. 1999. "Oral Creatine Supplementation: Separating Fact From Hype." *Physician and Sportsmedicine* 27(5).

Myhal, M., and C. Wilson. 1999. "Muscle-Building and Fat-Burning Supplements." 13th Annual Gatorade Sports Science Institute Scientific Conference, June 25-26: Chicago, IL: Gatorade Company.

National Household Survey on Drug Abuse (NHSDA), 2001. Office of Applied Studies, Substance Abuse and Mental Health Services Administration (HAMHSA).

PRIDE. 1996. *Press Release: Student Use of Most Drugs Reaches Highest Level in Nine Years—Most Report Getting "Very*

High, Bombed, or Stoned." Atlanta: PRIDE, September 25.

Rosenbloom, C. 1998. "Androstenedione: Its Potential Safety Concerns." *Scan's Pulse* 18:4-6.

Schnirring, L. 1998. "Androstenedione et al.: Nonprescription Steroids." *Physician and Sportsmedicine* 26:1-6.

Substance Abuse and Mental Health Services Administration. 2001. *National Household Survey on Drug Abuse.* Rockville, MD: Substance Abuse and Mental Health Services Administration.

U.S. Department of Health and Human Services, 2002. "Annual Smoking-Attributable Mortality, Years of Potential Life Lost, and Economic Costs—United States, 1995-1999." *Morbidity and Mortality Weekly Report.*

Yesalis, C. 1999. "Medical, Legal, and Societal Implications of Androstenedione Use." *Journal of the American Medical Association* 281:2043-2044.

Chapter 12

Anderson, M.B., and J.M. Williams. 1988. "A Model of Stress and Athletic Injury: Prediction and Prevention." *Journal of Sport and Exercise Physiology* 10: 294-306.

Bromberger, J., E. Newton, N. Avis, S. Harlow, H. Kravitz, and A. Cordal. 2002. "Depressive Symptoms in Midlife African American and White Women." *Annals of Epidemiology* 12(7): 504.

Chabrol, H., A. Montovany, K. Chouicha, and E. Duconge. 2002. "Study of the CES-D on a Sample of 1,953 High-School Students." *Encephale* 28(5): 429-432.

Faith, M., P. Matz, and M. Jorge. 2002. "Obesity-Depression Associations in the Population." *Journal of Psychosomatic Research* 53(4): 935.

Fleck, M.P., A.F. Lima, S. Louzada, G. Schestasky, A. Henriques, V.R. Borges, and S. Camey. 2002. "Association of Depression Symptoms and Social Functioning in Primary Care Service, Brazil." *Review Saude Publication* 36(4): 431-438.

Goodman, E., and R.C. Whitaker. 2002. "A Prospective Study of the Role of Depression in the Development and Persistence of Adolescent Obesity." *Pediatrics* 110(3): 497-504.

Greenberg, J.S. *Comprehensive Stress Management,* 7th ed. 2002. New York: McGraw-Hill.

Herrman, H., D.L. Patrick, P. Diehr, M.L. Martin, M. Fleck, G.E. Simon, and D.P. Buesching. 2002. "Longitudinal Investigation of Depression Outcomes in Primary Care in Six Countries: The LIDO Study. Functional Status, Health Service Use and Treatment of People With Depressive Symptoms." *Psychological Medicine* 32(5): 889-902.

Iwata, N., and S. Buka. 2002. "Race/Ethnicity and Depressive Symptoms: A Cross-Cultural/Ethnic Comparison Among University Students in East Asia, North and South America." *Social Science Medicine* 55(12): 2243-2252.

Leppamaki, S., T. Partonen, and J. Lonnqvist. 2002. "Bright-Light Exposure Combined With Physical Exercise Elevates Mood." *Journal of Affective Disorders* 72(2): 139.

Myers, H.F., I. Lesser, N. Rodriguez, C.B. Mira, W.C. Hwang, C. Camp, D. Anderson, L. Erickson, and M. Wohl. 2002.

"Ethnic Differences in Clinical Presentation of Depression in Adult Women." *Cultural Diversity & Ethnic Minority Psychology* 8(2): 138-156.

Penninx, B.W., W.J. Rejeski, J. Pandya, M.E. Miller, M. DiBari, W.B. Applegate, and M. Pahor. 2002. "Exercise and Depressive Symptoms: A Comparison of Aerobic and Resistance Exercise Effects on Emotional and Physical Function in Older Persons With High and Low Depressive Symptomatology." *Journal of Gerontology Behavior & Psychology Science Social Science* 57(2): P124-132.

Rugulies, R. 2002. "Depression As A Predictor for Coronary Heard Disease." *American Journal of Preventive Medicine* 23(1): 51-61.

Rushton, J.L., M. Forcier, and R.M. Schectman. 2002. "Epidemiology of Depressive Symptoms in the National Longitudinal Study of Adolescent Health." *Journal of the American Academy of Child and Adolescent Psychiatry* 41(2): 199-205.

Scarinci, I.C., B.M. Beech, W. Naumann, K.W. Kovach, L. Pugh, and B. Fapohunda. 2002. "Depression, Socioeconomic Status, Age, and Marital Status in Black Women: A National Study." *Ethnic Disease* 12(3): 421-428.

Strawbridge, W.J., S. Deleger, R.E. Roberts, and G.A. Kaplan. 2002. "Physical Activity Reduces the Risk of Subsequent Depression for Older Adults." *American Journal of Epidemiology* 156(4): 349-352.

Chapter 13

Andrews, J.R., G.L. Harrelson, and K.E. Wilk. 1998. *Physical Rehabilitation of the Injured Athletes,* 2nd ed. Philadelphia: Saunders.

Armstrong, L. 2000. *Performance in Extreme Environments.* Champaign, IL: Human Kinetics.

Beers, M.H., and R. Berkow, eds. 1999. *Merck Manual of Diagnosis and Therapy,* 17th ed. Whitehouse Station, NJ: Merck Research Laboratories.

Bloomfield, J., P.A. Fricker, and K.P. Fitch, eds. 1992. *Textbook of Science and Medicine in Sport.* Champaign, IL: Human Kinetics.

Carpenter, D., and B. Nelson. 1999. "Low Back Strengthening for the Prevention and Treatment of Low Back Pain." *Medicine and Science in Sports and Exercise* 31: 18-24.

Dircks, J.H., ed. 1997. *Stedman's Concise Medical Dictionary for the Health Professions.* Baltimore: Williams & Wilkins.

Houglum, P.A. 2001. *Therapeutic Exercises for Athletic Injuries.* Champaign, IL: Human Kinetics.

Liebenson, C., ed. 1996. *Rehabilitation of the Spine: A Practitioner's Manual.* Baltimore: Williams & Wilkins.

Michlovitz, S.C. 1996. *Thermal Agents in Rehabilitation.* Philadelphia: F.A. Davis.

Plunkett, B., and W. Hopkins. 1996. "The Cause and Treatment of Side Pain 'Stitch.'" *Medicine and Science in Sports and Exercise* 27: S23.

Reid, D. 1992. *Sports Injury Assessment and Rehabilitation.* New York: Churchill Livingston.

Young, A. 1988. "Human Adaptation to Cold." In *Human Performance Physiology and Environmental Medicine at*

Terrestrial Extremes, ed. K. Pandolf, M. Sawka, and R. Gonzalez. Indianapolis: Benchmark.

Chapter 14

Adams-Campbell, L.L., L. Rosenberg, R.S. Rao, and J.R. Palmer. 2001. "Strenuous Physical Activity and Breast Cancer Risk in African-American Women." *Journal of the National Medical Association* 93(7-8): 267-275.

Aghassi-Ippen, M., M.S. Green, and T. Shohat. 2002. "Familial Risk Factors for Breast Cancer Among Arab Women in Israel." *European Journal of Cancer Prevention* 11(4): 327-331.

American Cancer Society. 2002. *Cancer Facts and Figures 2002.* Atlanta, GA: American Cancer Society, p. 33.

American Heart Association. 1992. *Statement on Exercise: Benefits and Recommendations for Physical Activity Programs for All Americans.* Dallas, TX: American Heart Association.

Bassett, D.R., E.C. Fitzhugh, C.J. Crespo, G.S. King, and J.E. McLaughlin. 2002. "Physical Activity and Ethnic Differences in Hypertension Prevalence in the United States." *Preventive Medicine* 34(2): 179-186.

Borrayo, E.A., and S.R. Jenkins. 2001. "Feeling Healthy: So Why Should Mexican-Descent Women Screen for Breast Cancer?" *Qualitative Health Research* 11(6): 812-823.

Bosworth, H.B., and E.Z. Oddone. 2002. "A Model of Psychosocial and Cultural Antecedents of Blood Pressure Control." *Journal of the National Medical Association* 94(4): 236-248.

Burt, V., P. Whelton, E.J. Roccella, et al. 1995. "Prevalence of Hypertension in the U.S. Adult Population: Results From the Third National Health and Nutrition Examination Survey, 1988-1991." *Hypertension* 25: 305-313.

Chen, H., O.I. Bermudez, and K.L. Tucker. 2002. "Waist Circumference and Weight Change Are Associated With Disability Among Elderly Hispanics." *Journals of Gerontology Series A: Biological Sciences and Medical Sciences* 57(1): M19-25.

Dey, D.K., E. Rothenberg, V. Sundh, I. Bosaeus, and B. Steen. 2002. "Waist Circumference, Body Mass Index, and Risk for Stroke in Older People." *Journal of the American Geriatrics Society* 50(9): 1510-1518.

Freedman, D.S., L.K. Khan, M.K. Serdula, D.A. Galuska, and W.H. Dietz. 2002. "Trends and Correlates of Class 3 Obesity in the United States From 1990 Through 2000." *Journal of the American Medical Association* 288(14): 1758-1761.

Friedman, M., and R.H. Rosenman. 1974. *Type A Behavior and Your Heart.* Greenwich, CT: Fawcett.

Lea, J.P., and S.B. Nicholas. 2002. "Diabetes Mellitus and Hypertension: Key Risk Factors for Kidney Disease." *Journal of the National Medical Association* 94(8) (Suppl.): 7S-15S.

Narva, A.S. 2002. "Kidney Disease in Native Americans." *Journal of the National Medical Association* 94(8): 738-742.

National Center for Health Statistics. 2001. "Final Data for 1999." *National Vital Statistics Reports* 49(8), Hyattsville, MD.

National Center for Health Statistics. 2000. *Health, United States, 2000.* Washington, DC: National Center for Health Statistics.

Norris, K.C., and L.Y. Agodoa. 2002. "Race and Kidney Disease: The Scope of the Problem." *Journal of the National Medical Association* 94(8) (Suppl.): 1S-6S.

Poirier, P., and J.P. Despres. 2001. "Exercise in Weight Management of Obesity." *Cardiology Clinics* 19(3): 459-470.

Rheeder, P., R.P. Stolk, J.F. Veenhouwer, and D.E. Grobbee. 2002. "The Metabolic Syndrome in Black Hypertensive Women—Waist Circumference More Strongly Related Than Body Mass Index." *South African Medical Journal* 92(8): 637-641.

Sauter, E.R., T. Welch, A. Magklara, G. Klein, and E.P. Diamandis. 2002. "Ethnic Variation in Kallikrein Expression in Nipple Aspirate Fluid." *International Journal of Cancer* 100(6): 678-682.

Sewell, J.L., B.R. Malasky, C.L. Gedney, T.M. Gerber, E.A. Brody, E.A. Pacheco, D. Yost, B.R. Masden, and J.M. Galloway. 2002. "The Increasing Incidence of Coronary Artery Disease and Cardiovascular Risk Factors Among a Southwest Native American Tribe: The White Mountain Apache Heart Study." *Archives of Internal Medicine* 162(12): 1368-1372.

Surveillance, Epidemiology, and End Results Program, 1973-98. 2001. Division of Cancer Control and Population Studies. American Cancer Society: Cancer Facts & Figures 2002. National Cancer Institute, Bethesda, MD.

U.S. Renal Data System. 2001. *USRDS 2001 Annual Data Report: Atlas of End-Stage Renal Disease in the United States.* Bethesda, MD: National Institutes of Health, National Institute of Diabetes and Kidney Diseases.

U.S. Renal Data System. 1999. *USRDS 1999 Annual Data Report.* Bethesda, MD: National Institutes of Health, National Institute of Diabetes and Digestive and Kidney Diseases.

Wang, G., Z. Zheng, G. Heath, C. Macera, M. Pratt, and D. Buchner. 2002. "Economic Burden of Cardiovascular Disease Associated With Excess Body Weight in U.S. Adults." *American Journal of Preventive Medicine* 23(1): 1-6.

Wenten, M., F.D. Gilliland, K. Baumgartner, and J.M. Samet. 2002. "Associations of Weight, Weight Change, and Body Mass With Breast Cancer Risk in Hispanic and Non-Hispanic White Women." *Annals of Epidemiology* 12(6): 435-444.

Zhu, S., Z. Wang, S. Heskha, M. Heo, M.S. Faith, and S.B. Heymsfield. 2002. "Waist Circumference and Obesity-Associated Risk Factors Among Whites in the Third National Health and Nutrition Examination Survey: Clinical Action Thresholds." *American Journal of Clinical Nutrition* 76(4): 699-700.

Chapter 15

Bhambhani, Y. 2002. "Physiology of Wheelchair Racing in Athletes With Spinal Cord Injury." *Sports Medicine* 32(1): 23-51.

Garrick, J., and R.K. Requa. 1988. "Aerobic Dance: A Review." *Sports Medicine* 6(3): 169-179.

Gignac, M.A., C. Cott, and E.M. Badley. 2002. "Adaptation to Disability: Applying Selective Optimization With Compensation to the Behaviors of Older Adults With Osteoarthritis." *Psychology of Aging* 17(3): 520-524.

Katz, J. 1986. "The W.E.T. Workout." *Shape,* June, 82-86.

McDonald, C.M. 2002. "Physical Activity, Health Impairments, and Disability in Neuromuscular Disease." *American Journal of Physical and Medical Rehabilitation* 81(11 Suppl.): S108-120.

National Center on Physical Activity and Disability (NCPAD). 2002. Fact sheet titled *Paralympics*. www.ncpad.org/Factshthtml/paralympics.htm.

President's Council on Physical Fitness and Sports. Undated. *Aqua Dynamics*. Washington, DC: President's Council on Physical Fitness and Sports.

Rejeski, W.J., and B.C. Focht. 2002. "Aging and Physical Disability: On Integrating Group and Individual Counseling With the Promotion of Physical Activity." *Exercise and Sport Science Reviews* 30(4): 166-170.

Road Runner's Club of America. *Women Running: Run Smart. Run Safe.* Used by permission.

Specht, J., G. King, E. Brown, and C. Foris. 2002. "The Importance of Leisure in the Lives of Persons With Congenital Physical Disabilities." *American Journal of Occupational Therapy* 56(4): 436-445.

U.S. Public Health Service. 1996. *Physical Activity and Health: A Report of the Surgeon General: Executive Summary.* Washington, DC: U.S. Department of Health and Human Services.

Winters, C. 1993. "For Step Aerobic Addicts, a Challenging New Workout: Doing the Two-Step." *American Health,* May, 92.

Wu, S.K., and T. Williams. 2001. "Factors Influencing Sport Participation Among Athletes With Spinal Cord Injury." *Medicine and Science in Sports and Exercise* 33(2): 177-182.

Chapter 16

Alter, M.J. 1998. *Sport Stretch.* Champaign, IL: Human Kinetics.

Baechle, T., ed. 1994. *Essentials of Strength Training and Conditioning.* Champaign, IL: Human Kinetics.

Baechle, T., and R.W. Earle. 1989. *Weight Training: A Text Written for the College Students.* Omaha: Creighton University.

Bompa, T., and L. Cornacchia. 1999. *Serious Strength Training: Periodization for Building Muscle Power and Mass.* Champaign, IL: Human Kinetics.

Chu, D. 1999. *Explosive Power and Strength.* Champaign, IL: Human Kinetics.

Chu, D. 1998. *Jumping Into Plyometrics.* Champaign, IL: Human Kinetics.

Dintiman, G.B., and R. Ward. 2003. *Sportspeed III,* 3rd ed. Champaign, IL: Human Kinetics.

Douillard, J. 1995. *Body, Mind, and Sport: The Mind-Body Guide to Lifelong Fitness, and Your Personal Best.* New York: Crown.

Foran, B., ed. 2001. *High Performance Sports Training.* Champaign, IL: Human Kinetics.

Gambetta, V. 1998. *Soccer Speed.* United States: Gambetta Sports Training.

Gambetta, V., and M. Clark. 1999. "Hard Core Training." *Training and Conditioning* 9:34-40.

Inglis, R. 2000. "Training for Acceleration in the 100m Sprint." In *Sprint and Relays: Contemporary Theory, Technique and Training,* 5th ed. Mountain View, CA: Tafnews Press, pp. 35-39.

Morgan, G.T., and G.H. McGlynn. 1997. *Cross-Training for Sports.* United States: Versa Press.

Polquin C., and I. King. 1992. "Theory and Methodology of Strength Training." *Sports Coach,* 6-18.

Index

About the Authors

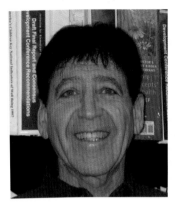

Jerrold S. Greenberg, EdD, is a professor in the department of public and community health at the University of Maryland. Dr. Greenberg was selected as an Alliance Scholar of the American Alliance for Health, Physical Education, Recreation and Dance (AAHPERD) in 1996, and also received the Scholar Award from the American Association for Health Education (AAHE) in 1995.

Dr. Greenberg has authored more than 40 books and 80 articles, and he has made numerous presentations on wellness, fitness, and community health. He has served on numerous committees for AAHPERD and AAHE and for the American School Health Association. The leading scorer and most valuable player of his college basketball team, Dr. Greenberg remains active in basketball, tennis, aerobic activities, and weight training.

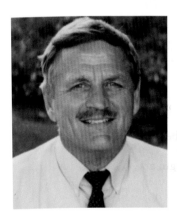

George Blough Dintiman, EdD, is professor emeritus at Virginia Commonwealth University, where he previously served as division chair and professor of health and physical education from 1968 to 1998. He is the author of 40 books and numerous videos on fitness and wellness, nutrition, weight control, general health, and speed improvement. He continues to conduct research on fitness and conditioning and is actively involved in consulting and writing.

Dr. Dintiman is cofounder and president of the National Association of Speed and Explosion, and he is an internationally known expert on the improvement of speed for team sports. He starred in football, basketball, and track in high school and college; was an NFL draft choice; and had his football jersey retired by Lock Haven University, where he still holds many rushing and scoring records. He was inducted into the Capital Area Chapter of the Pennsylvania Sports Hall of Fame in 1993.

Dr. Dintiman has two daughters, one son, and three grandchildren. He and his wife, Carol Ann, live on the Outer Banks of North Carolina where they are avid participants in tennis, running, cycling, kayaking, and weight training.

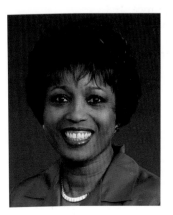

Barbee Myers Oakes, PhD, is the director of multicultural affairs at Wake Forest University. Dr. Oakes is one of the first African American women in the American College of Sports Medicine to receive a doctorate. She has taught and researched in physical fitness and wellness for nearly 20 years, and she has published numerous articles and coauthored five books on related topics as well as presented at national and international conferences.

Dr. Oakes has focused much of her research efforts on minority and women's health issues. She is a member of the Steering Committee for the Maya Angelou Research Center on Minority Health at the Wake Forest University School of Medicine. She has been a member of the board of directors for the Association of Black Cardiologists and was a charter member of the International Society for Hypertension in Blacks. Dr. Oakes stays active by walking, cycling, and gardening.